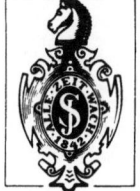

Alan Daneman

Pediatric Body CT

With 317 Figures

Springer-Verlag
London Berlin Heidelberg New York
Paris Tokyo

Alan Daneman, MBBCh, BSc, MRACR, FRCP(C)

Associate Professor of Radiology,
University of Toronto, Ontario, Canada.

Staff Radiologist, Head, Division of Ultrasound and Body CT
Department of Radiology, The Hospital for Sick Children,
555 University Avenue, Toronto, Ontario M5G 1X8, Canada

ISBN-13:978-1-4471-3139-7   e-ISBN-13:978-1-4471-3137-3
DOI: 10.1007/978-1-4471-3137-3

Library of Congress Cataloging-in-Publication Data
Daneman, Alan, 1947–
Pediatric body CT.
Includes bibliographies and index.
1. Tomography. 2. Pediatric radiography. I. Title. [DNLM: 1. Tomography, X-Ray Computed
– in infancy and childhood. WN 240 D179p] RJ51.T65D36 1986 618.92'007'572 86–3795
ISBN-13:978-1-4471-3139-7 (U.S.)

The use of registered names, trademarks etc. in this publication does not imply, even in the absence of a specific statement, that such names are exempt from the relevant laws and regulations and therefore free for general use.

Product Liability: The publisher can give no guarantee for information about drug dosage and application thereof contained in this book. In every individual case the respective user must check its accuracy by consulting other pharmaceutical literature.

Filmset by Computerised Typesetting Services Limited, Finchley, London N12 8LY

2128/3916 543210

*Dedicated to Louise,
Natasha, and Nadine.*

Preface

Pediatric body CT began in earnest in 1976 when for the first time a body CT machine was installed in a pediatric institution, the Hospital for Sick Children in Toronto. The first images were received with great enthusiasm. More recently, newer equipment with faster scan times and better resolution has enabled us to delineate disease processes with even greater accuracy. In the past 9 years we have performed more than 5000 body scans in children. With this experience our examination techniques have changed and the indications for CT in children have been modified. CT has come to occupy an important and specific place in the management of pediatric patients. The performance of body CT studies in children is not always easy. Excellent diagnostic studies can be obtained only with a special understanding of the problems of pediatric patients and pediatric pathology. The information contained herein is a review of our experience with pediatric body CT, how we use body CT in children, and its relationship to other modalities in this department.

This book illustrates the CT appearances of the normal anatomy and the common as well as the rare pathological entities involving the chest, abdomen, pelvis, neck, and musculoskeletal system in children. In the Radiology Department at the Hospital for Sick Children in Toronto, CT studies of the head, face, and spinal cord are supervised by our pediatric neuroradiologists. These areas have thus been excluded from consideration. For a detailed account of the use of CT metrizamide myelography in children, the reader is referred to *CT and Myelography of the Spine and Cord*, authored by Drs. Holger Pettersson and Derek Harwood-Nash, which deals extremely well with our departmental approach to CT of the spine in children. However, the relationship of CT metrizamide myelography to general body CT studies is described in the present book in the sections dealing with paraspinal and vertebral lesions.

Most of the illustrations are from studies performed with the General Electric 9800 (2-s scanner) and 8800 (4.8-, 5.7-, 9.6-s scanner) CT machines and thus reflect imaging with state of the art equipment. A few illustrations are from studies performed with our original Ohio Nuclear Delta 50 scanner (2-min scan time). The reason for including these old images is either that they illustrate rare conditions that we have not had the opportunity to study on our newer scanners at the Hospital for Sick Children, or because at that time CT was used more commonly to delineate certain entities that are now better delineated with other less expensive modalities.

The information contained in this book will be of vital interest not only to all pediatric radiologists, but also to adult radiologists who are involved with performing body CT examinations in children, as well as to pediatricians, pediatric oncologists and radiotherapists, pediatric general surgeons, thoracic surgeons, and orthopedic surgeons. It is hoped that the information provided will be of assistance to these groups of physicians, will help others in making accurate diagnoses, and will aid in the efficient management of pediatric patients.

At the time of writing, the use of nuclear magnetic resonance scanning in children is still in its infancy. The role of nuclear magnetic resonance and its relationship to body CT in the pediatric age group have thus yet to be defined and will require continuing critical reassessment of our use of CT. It is hoped, however, that the information set forth will lay a foundation for the understanding of the cross-sectional images also obtained with nuclear magnetic resonance.

Acknowledgements

I would like to express my gratitude to the following people:

Dr. David Martin (presently at the Ottawa Children's Hospital) and Dr. Gordon Culham (presently at the Vancouver Children's Hospital), who taught me the uses and technique of body CT in children. Their hours of teaching and encouragement laid the foundations for this book.

My radiological colleagues, including Drs. David Martin, Gordon Culham, Bernard Reilly, and David Stringer, who have taken part in body CT studies in the Radiology Department of the Hospital for Sick Children, Toronto, in the past and at present, for their advice and professional contributions.

Dr. Derek Harwood-Nash, Radiologist-in-chief, the Hospital for Sick Children, Toronto, for his constant encouragement, advice, and enthusiasm.

Dr. Charles Fitz, former Head, Division of Special Procedures, for his cooperation and advice.

Dr. Helen Chan, Division of Hematology and Oncology, Department of Pediatrics, for her enthusiasm, advice, and endless hours of work in obtaining clinical information on the patients reported in our previous papers and in this book.

The technical and nursing staff in the Radiology Department, whose valuable expertise plays an important role in the continuing performance of high-quality body CT examinations in this institution.

The secretaries, in particular Lori Fearon, Julete Harris, and Gladys Clarke for their hours toiling over the manuscript so efficiently and also more recently Karen Fennell.

The photographic personnel in the Department of Visual Education, for their expertise and cooperation.

The past and present Fellows of our department who have helped in the performance of body CT studies and who have also taken part in the numerous projects that have been published and presented at radiological meetings, in particular Veronica Donoghue, Chris Farrelly, Peter Liu, Geoff Robey, Piyoosh Kotecha and Alan Sprigg.

Lastly, and most important of all, I would like to thank my wife and daughters for still accepting me as part of the family during the preparation of this book.

Ontario, February 1986   Alan Daneman

Contents

SECTION II: CHEST

SECTION V: MUSCULOSKETAL SYSTEM

Section I:

INTRODUCTION

Section A.

INTRODUCTION

Chapter 1

General Considerations

Introduction

Computed tomography (CT) was initially introduced into our department at the Hospital for Sick Children, Toronto in 1976, and since that time we have come to use CT routinely to evaluate extracranial pathology. Indeed CT has become a vital part of our imaging armamentarium and in many instances has replaced other more invasive modalities. Figures 1.1–1.4 show the overall radiological studies performed in our department, as well as the numbers of special procedures, including those of CT, ultrasound, and nuclear medicine. It is of interest that the numbers of body CT studies are less than the numbers of head CT studies, and it is also significant to compare the way the numbers of body CTs have slowly increased, as opposed to the dramatic rise in the numbers of sonography studies and the somewhat decreasing number of radionuclide studies.

The role of CT in the evaluation of various pathological states in children can only be determined by considering the value of other imaging modalities in the investigation of specific disease entities. Other modalities include conventional radiography, sonography, radionuclide scans, angiography, and, more recently, magnetic resonance imaging.

Conventional radiography is often the investigation of choice in many instances and may indeed be the definitive investigation in skeletal diseases and some abdominal and thoracic diseases. However, the density scale that can be appreciated on plain radiographs is limited, and one may only be able to delineate bone, calcification, soft tissue, fat, and gas. The use of contrast agents to outline the genitourinary and gastrointestinal tracts enhances the ability of more conventional techniques to delineate disease. Radionuclide scans are somewhat organ specific and have certain specific values in many disorders. The value of sonography and CT is that they are not organ specific. Both of these modalities are able to delineate viscera and structures that could only be documented previously with more invasive or multiple techniques.

Sonography has the advantage that the study can be performed at the bedside and that sections can be made in any plane. Children are ideally suited to investigation with sonography because of their relative lack of fat and their small size. Sonography does have certain drawbacks, in that obese and very large children may be difficult to examine as the ultrasound beam will not penetrate fat or long distances. The beam will also not penetrate gas or bone, and these structures may hide vital disease processes. It is difficult to use sonography in the immediate postoperative or posttraumatic period, when there may be significant tenderness, open wounds, bandages, and drains. Sonography is a more difficult technique to perform and interpret. Clinicians in particular find the images more difficult to interpret than those obtained by CT.

RADIOLOGICAL EXAMINATIONS

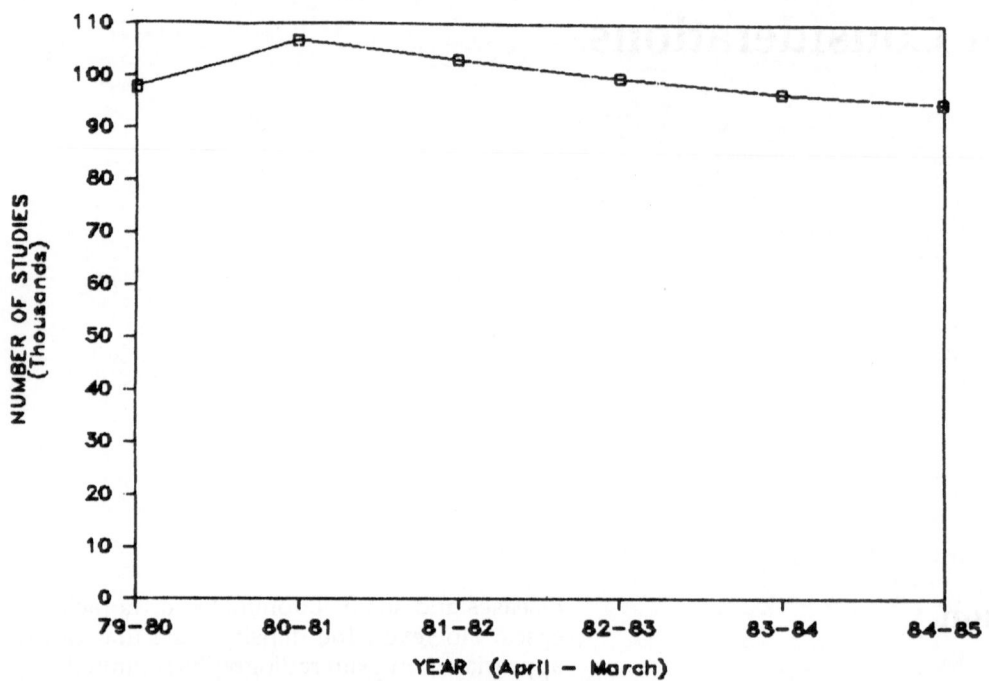

Fig. 1.1. Total number of annual radiological examinations, 1979–1985, Hospital for Sick Children, Toronto.

COMPUTED TOMOGRAPHY EXAMINATIONS

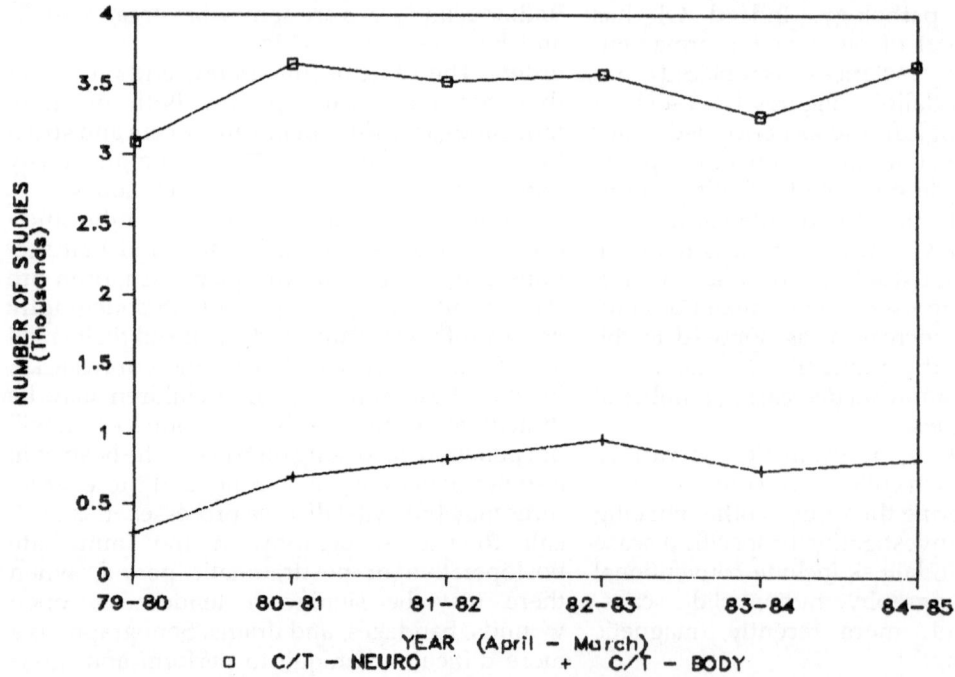

Fig. 1.2. Total number of annual CT examinations of the central nervous system compared with body studies, 1979–1985, Hospital for Sick Children, Toronto.

ULTRASOUND EXAMINATIONS

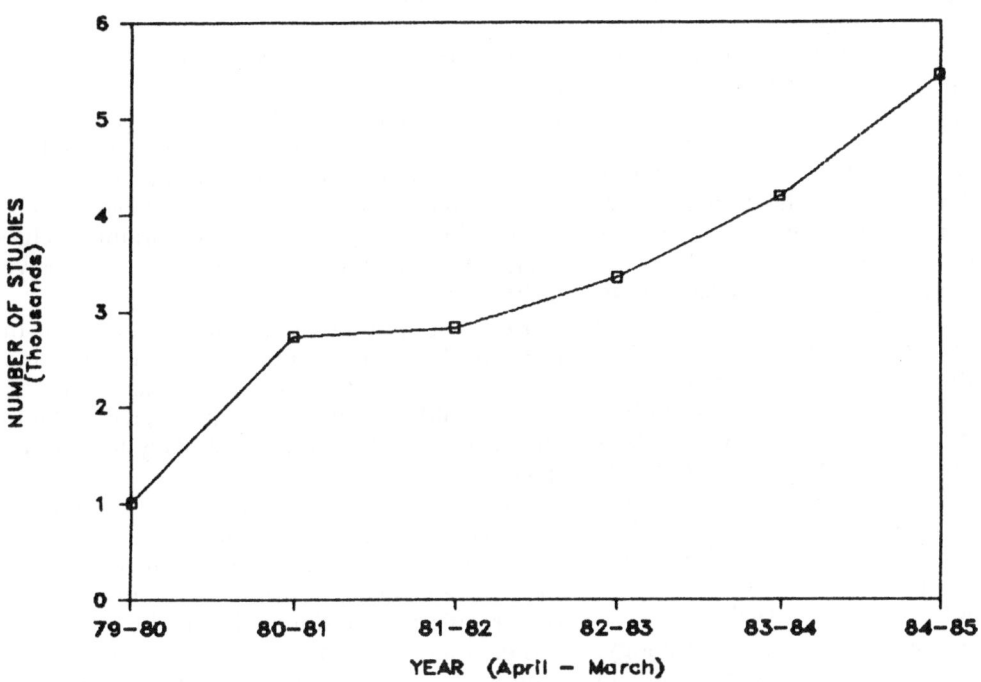

Fig. 1.3. Total number of annual sonographic studies, 1979–1985, Hospital for Sick Children, Toronto.

NUCLEAR MEDICINE EXAMINATIONS

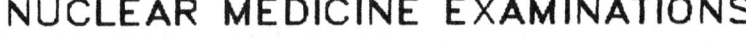
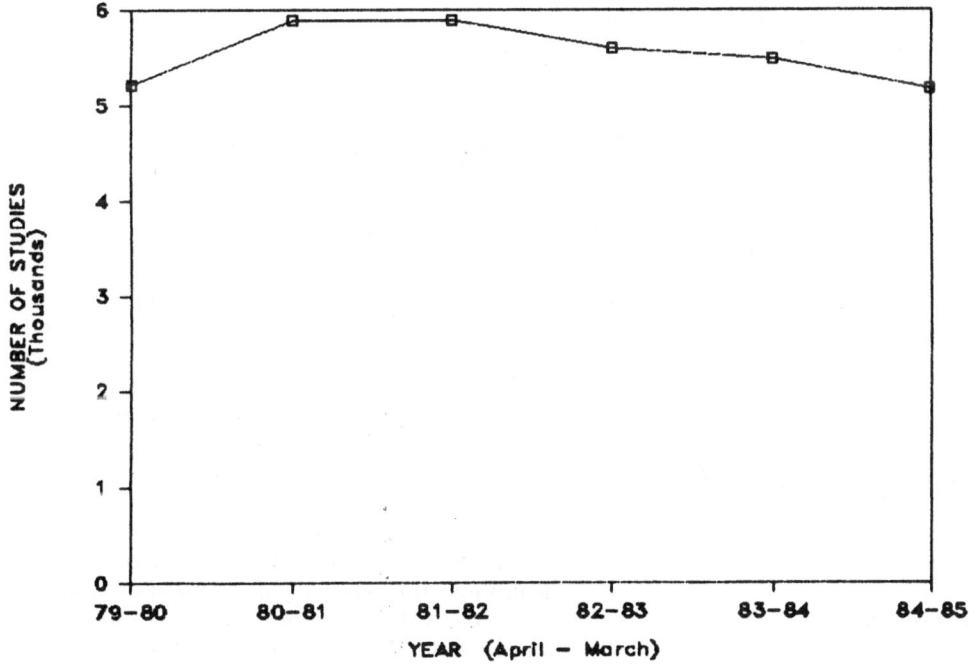

Fig. 1.4. Total number of annual nuclear medicine studies, 1979–1985, Hospital for Sick Children, Toronto.

The advantages of CT are the high density and spatial resolution and the ability to delineate structures in a transverse plane without overlap. CT should not be considered a totally noninvasive procedure. It involves the use of ionizing radiation, and often intravenous and gastrointestinal contrast agents must be given to patients, who may have to be sedated. (These features are outlined in more detail in Chap. 2, see p. 9.) The anatomy of viscera and structures in children may be more difficult to delineate than in adults because of the relative lack of fat; however, when meticulous attention is paid to technique with regard to patient sedation and restraint, and the adequate administration of contrast, CT provides valuable information that may not be obtained with a variety of other modalities. Among the advantages of CT are the fact that bone and gas do not impede the formation of high-quality CT images and that this modality can be easily used in the postoperative period, despite the presence of tenderness, bandages, open wounds, or plaster casts.

In the investigation of extracranial pathology, CT is seldom used as the initial modality of choice. Patients undergoing body CT examinations have usually been studied previously either with conventional radiographic techniques or with sonography, depending on their disease. In certain specific instances (e.g., in suspected metabolically active neoplasms), CT may be used as the initial modality of choice, as information obtained from other modalities may not be helpful. CT has indeed proved extremely valuable in the evaluation of patients with congenital, traumatic, infective, or neoplastic lesions involving extracranial structures. Over recent years the way in which these disorders have been investigated has changed dramatically as a result of the introduction of this modality.

The rapid advance of magnetic resonance imaging technology will force radiologists to reevaluate the role of CT in the future.

Factors Affecting Choice of Modalities

General Considerations

When choosing an initial modality and a sequence of subsequent modalities in the investigation of a child, one should keep the following principles in mind:

1. Keep the radiation exposure to the child to a minimum.
2. Save the child as much trauma as possible by choosing less invasive techniques. In children with malignant lesions, it is difficult to avoid high radiation exposure and invasive techniques, but it is particularly important in children with benign lesions to choose less invasive techniques.
3. Keep the time factor as short as possible. In order to diminish the time stay in hospital and also to enable a diagnosis to be made rapidly, e.g., in children with severe trauma, it is better to choose one study that is most likely to give the diagnosis.
4. Save costs as much as possible. The cost of multiple procedures is tremendous. It is often more cost effective to choose a single more costly procedure if this can supply all the information one requires and diminish the hospital stay rather than to choose many less expensive studies that together may cost even more.

Clinical and Radiological Factors

Clinical Picture

All too often when situations are discussed regarding the choice of modalities, typical clinical situations are used as examples. In such situations the choice of imaging procedures and the order in which they are performed is often very easy and follows logically on from the clinical findings. Indeed, based on these typical clinical situations, protocols can be formulated whereby clinicians and radiologists, in consultation, can easily choose a logical sequence of imaging procedures in order to delineate a particular disease prior to commencing therapy. Unfortunately, many patients do not always present in a typical textbook fashion, and the radiographic changes in any particular patient may not always be typical of the disease that the child has. In these situations the choice of modalities may be extremely difficult. For that reason I do not believe in a rigid set of protocols but believe that the sequence of studies should be tailored to suit the individual child.

The choice of imaging modalities by clinicians should be influenced by their continuing consultation with their radiological colleagues. Occasionally the choice is incorrect. In some of these instances, even when viewed in retrospect, there is very little that the radiologist would have done in consultation prior to the performance of a particular study that would have changed the choice of modality. Although the initial study chosen may be incorrect, adequate clinical and radiological consultation is imperative to ensure the correct sequence of subsequent studies, the first study acting as a guide to further investigation.

An additional problem is that clinicians learn to interpret the images from newer modalities much more slowly than radiologists. Therefore, they may remain reluctant to make important decisions regarding patient management based on these images and may request further studies. It behooves radiologists to teach their clinical colleagues how to interpret these images and to make them aware of the potential uses and pitfalls of these newer modalities, in order that the clinicians become comfortable with these techniques. Such cooperation is certainly in the best interests of the patient.

Availability of State of the Art Modalities

A problem facing radiologists when choosing a modality today is the question of what is available at the particular institution. Not all new modalities are available at all institutions, and adequate images may not be obtained with older equipment.

The rate at which new modalities have been added to the armamentarium and the rate at which technical advances have been made with each modality have made the choice of these modalities extremely difficult; there must be a constant reassessment of the place of each modality as new technical advances are made.

An example of this occurred at The Hospital for Sick Children in Toronto. In 1979, sonography was introduced into our department and made delineation of abdominal mass lesions easier than with our 2-min CT scanner. The introduction at the end of 1979 of a new CT scanner with a 4- and 5-s scan time and, more recently, a 2-s scanner forced us to reevaluate the value of CT, which now gives us far more anatomical detail than sonography.

Radiological Expertise

As new modalities are introduced into a hospital it takes time for radiologists to become familiar with the potential benefits and pitfalls of these modalities and discover how each modality compares with the others. Even when the use of a particular modality is firmly established within an institution, new refinements and technological advances force radiologists continually to reassess the comparative benefits of each modality. The clinician should therefore choose a modality in which the radiologist is experienced. This applies to larger institutions just as much as to smaller ones.

For example, on many occasions a patient is referred to our hospital after preliminary studies have been performed at a referring hospital where the radiologist may not be accustomed to performing sonographic studies on children and where experience with childhood pathology is limited. In this situation, a well-performed excretory urogram is very much more meaningful than a poorly performed and poorly interpreted sonographic study. Furthermore, a pediatric radiologist experienced in a particular modality is obviously far better suited for the use of this modality in children than a radiologist who is an expert in the modality but has no knowledge of pediatric problems and pathology.

Radiological Appearances

All lesions may present with atypical radiological appearances, as noted on all types of imaging modalities. These appearances may occasionally be so atypical that the radiologist will require further studies to delineate the disease process adequately. The more studies that are carried out, the greater should be the certainty of the diagnosis. However, absolute certainty cannot be achieved in every patient.

Radiation Considerations

When comparing the value of different modalities the use of ionizing radiation has always been considered a disadvantage [1,2]. All radiation hazards are important at all ages, but particularly in childhood. In comparison to the radiation hazards of other radiological techniques, the hazards from CT are indeed relatively small. The dose to the skin of the entire circumference of the scanned volume is between 1 and 2 rads. This compares with the skin entrance dose of a lateral lumbosacral spine radiograph. It is certainly much less than the dose from angiography and cardiac catheterization. The skin of the posterior chest may be exposed to between 6 and 10 rads during cardiac catheterization. It should also be compared with the skin entrance dose from exposure for a newborn chest film of 0.005 rads. Natural background radiation for the whole body per year is approximately 0.08 rads.

At our institution, the vast majority of children undergoing body CT examinations have already been examined with conventional radiography, sonography, or nuclear medicine. The decision to perform a body CT examination is determined by the type of information that is required regarding the patient's disease process. If it is felt that CT will provide more information than other less invasive procedures, the CT examination should be performed and not forbidden on radiation grounds alone. Although the use of ionizing radiation is one aspect of the relative invasiveness of CT, there are other aspects that may consitute a greater hazard. These include the hazards of sedation, intravenous contrast enhancement, and the movement of infants out of their incubators.

Despite the low radiation hazard with CT, one should make every attempt to limit the amount of radiation that any child undergoing body CT receives. In our institution all body CT studies are performed only after a close consultation between clinician and radiologist. This consultation includes review of all the patient's previous studies, including plain radiographs, sonograms, and radionuclide studies. In this way it is possible to determine which patients will benefit most from body CT and exclude those in whom CT may contribute less valuable information. The greatest impact of body CT in our institution has been in the field of oncology. The radiation that these children receive from multiple body CT examinations is quite insignificant in comparison to the doses of therapeutic radiation and the risks from chemotherapy that they have already received. Indeed, in these children the benefits of the CT examinations done at the time of diagnosis and at follow-up far outweigh any of the potential hazards either from the study or from their malignancy. However, one should be more critical when examining patients with benign processes.

When performing a body CT study every effort should be made to cut down the amount of radiation that the child receives by performing the least number of slices possible to define the extent of disease adequately without allowing any room for doubt. Other factors that may be considered are the reduction of the mA and the use of the shortest scan times possible.

In summary, the radiation hazards from CT are relatively low. When considering whether to use body CT in a specific child one should weigh up the potential benefits of such a study against the small potential hazards of the study and the hazards from the disease process, which are often much greater.

References

1. Brasch RC, Cann CE (1982) Computed tomographic scan in children: part II, an updated comparison of radiation dose and resolving power of commercial CT scanners. AJR 138:127–133
2. Brasch RC, Boyd DP, Gooding CA (1978) Computed tomographic scanning in children: comparison of radiation dose and resolving power of commercial CT scanners. AJR 131:95–101

Chapter 2

Techniques

Introduction

The purpose of this chapter is to describe in general terms the CT techniques that are used at the Hospital for Sick Children, Toronto. More details of the techniques pertinent to the various body regions are given in the chapters relating to technique in the relevant sections. The exact technique used in any child having a CT examination will depend on the area of the body that is being examined and the reason for the examination. Most CT examinations are performed only after the use of other less expensive noninvasive modalities. These studies may include conventional radiographs, including contrast studies, fluoroscopy, sonography, and radionuclide scans. Before performing a CT examination the attending radiologist should review these previous studies thoroughly. This serves two purposes. Firstly, the radiologist should be familiar with the findings of these studies before deciding whether the CT study is indicated. Secondly, the radiologist will be in the best position to choose the optimum type of technique to be used in a particular patient. Tailoring the technique used to the individual patient will ensure that the maximum information is obtained from each study.

Prescan Preparation

Decisions on how the study is going to be performed should be made well before the child reaches the scan room. This will enable advance preparations to be made and will limit delays when the patient arrives in the radiology department. In our busy department, time on the CT scanner is at a premium; it is therefore important for studies to progress rapidly and efficiently to ensure patient safety and to make good use of the available time.

The major considerations are as follows:

1. *Will the child need sedation and if so what type of sedation?*
If there is any evidence of cardiac, pulmonary, or airway disease a decision to sedate such a child should be made only after thorough consultation with the attending clinician. The relative merits of the study as opposed to the hazards of sedating such a child should be considered. This type of consultation and decision making is best done well before the child is called to the CT room.

2. *Will the child require intravenous contrast material?*
Most of our studies performed to examine the mediastinum and abdomen are performed with

intravenous contrast administration. If the child is to be sedated and/or if the child is young, it is best to have an intravenous line in place before the child is called to the CT room. This can then be used for intravenous contrast administration without disturbing a child who is either sedated or frightened.

3. *Will the child require oral or rectal contrast administration?*

The vast majority of abdominal and pelvic studies are performed only after the administration of oral contrast material, and occasionally rectal contrast material is also required. Patients with full stomachs do not like to drink large quantities of fluid prior to an examination and they may also be induced to vomit following the administration of intravenous contrast material. For this reason we prefer that patients who require intravenous contrast together with oral contrast should fast for at least 4 h prior to the examination. In this way we can be more confident that the child will ingest the required contrast volume and that the possibility of vomiting following intravenous contrast administration will be lessened. Patients who are uncooperative or who are to be sedated should have a feeding tube placed with its tip in the stomach prior to being called to the scan room. This will allow administration of the contrast material directly into the stomach.

Patient Care

Instructions and Monitoring

On arrival in the department, the patient who is old enough to understand should be shown around the CT room and be given an explanation of the basic principles. Explanations to accompanying parents or relatives are also well received and help to allay the fears of both the child and the parents. It is also extremely helpful to allow one or both parents or relatives to stay in the room with the patient while the scan is being performed.

The various phases of the scanning procedure such as the ingestion and the injection of contrast should be explained. While the patient is being examined on the table it is most important to monitor the child's vital signs at regular intervals. In our department we have a closed circuit video camera that relays an image of the patient directly to a television screen above the technician's console and allows the technician to see the patient, lying on the table in the gantry, closely. Patients who are unstable or who are somewhat uncooperative may require a nurse to remain in the room with them. In our department a loud speaker system is provided so that a patient on the table can talk to the technician in the console room.

Sedation

The decision to sedate a patient will depend on the patient's age and ability to cooperate. Neonates are usually called to the department with their previous feed having been withheld. They are then fed in the department and hopefully they fall asleep immediately. Older patients below the age of about 5 years usually require sedation. In our department we use 6 mg/kg Nembutal intramuscularly for all patients requiring body CT. We have found this to be a safe drug, and a further 2 mg/kg can be administered after 1 h if the patient has not fallen asleep. This dose is given to a maximum of 15 kg, above which a dose of 5 mg/kg intramuscularly is used, with a resedation 1 h later of 2.5 mg/kg if the patient has not fallen asleep. We have found that this type of sedation is effective in almost all patients who require body CT. In a very small proportion of patients this drug is not effective, and the patient should then be brought back on another day and sedation attempted with CM_3 (Phenergan, 6.25 mg/ml; Demerol hydrochloride, 25 mg/ml; chlorpromazine, 6.25 mg/ml). This is given in a dose of 0.1 ml/kg intramuscularly, with no resedation if the patient does not fall asleep. If this is ineffective, a general anesthetic has to be used; however, this is extremely rare in our department. In those patients with cardiac, pulmonary, or airway disease, in whom sedation may compromise their stability, it is always best to have an anesthetist on stand-by in the room to care for the child. Our anesthetic department has been extremely helpful in this regard.

Immobilization

Whether the patient is sedated or not, adequate immobilization of the child is imperative in order to obtain high-quality scans which are free of motion artifact. The contraptions that may be used to ensure patient stability include Velcro straps, tape, blankets, pillows, and sponges. Our technicians have learned to use these contraptions expertly in order to achieve patient immobilization as well as patient comfort. A comfortable patient is less likely to fidget and move around during the scans than one who is in pain or uncomfortable. Many children become somewhat bored lying in the scan gantry during a long procedure, and adequate immobilization will help to ensure a first-class study. Scanning through these contraptions does not cause any artifact.

Patients are usually scanned in the supine position, and, because children are smaller, they tend to lie in the scoop of the table quite comfortably. Different positions may have to be used for patients in pain or those who cannot lie in the supine position, and in this regard the technician's ability to improvise and maintain patient comfort as well as immobilization is extremely valuable.

Environment

Neonates must obviously be removed from the warm environment of the incubator before they can be examined in the scanner. These young patients may not be able to control their temperature well and may become very cold during lengthy scans. For this reason it is extremely important to keep these patients warm. In our department we have a heating blanket, through which warm water is pumped, and also have a heating lamp, which can be placed over the patient. The blanket produces no artifact around the patient. The temperature of these devices can be easily controlled but must be closely monitored.

Contrast Administration

Oral contrast should be administered to the patients prior to their entering the scan room in order to allow adequate passage through the gastrointestinal tract. Rectal contrast is administered through a Foley catheter placed in the rectum when the child is lying on the CT scan table. Intravenous contrast is usually injected as a bolus during scans. The value of the intravenous contrast administration is not only to define the vascularity of lesions but also to determine their relationship to the major vessels. This is particularly important in scans through the upper mediastinum and upper abdomen. This

injection can be made into the peripheral venous line that has been inserted before the patient comes to the scan room or, in older children, into a line that is set up in the scan room.

Scan Technique

Computed Radiograph (Scoutview)

After the patient is adequately immobilized on the table computed radiographs can be obtained (Fig. 2.1). These are usually obtained in the anteroposterior direction, but lateral views are particularly helpful when examining regions such as the neck, spine, or sacroiliac joints. From these computed radiographs one can choose the region of the body to be examined and can accurately define the limits of the transverse axial scans. Skin markers may help to define the location of lesions that are palpable clinically (Fig. 2.2).

Axial Scans

Transverse axial scans are usually obtained with a 2-s scan time. The scans are usually 1 cm thick and adjacent to one another. Cuts of 5 mm are extremely helpful in small patients or in areas where more detail is required. Scans which are 1 cm apart from one another may be adequate when examining large patients or large lesions.

If intravenous contrast material is to be administered as a bolus, approximately one-third of the dose is given prior to starting the transverse scan. The scans are then performed while the remaining two-thirds of the dose is injected as a rapid bolus. In this way the major vessels of the chest, abdomen, or neck may be delineated with maximal enhancement. Occasionally delayed scans following contrast injection may also be helpful. Scans without intravenous contrast enhancement are valuable in the search for calcification and in the evaluation of many skeletal problems. All images should be viewed at various window settings so that all structures in the scan field can be optimally displayed. It is important for the radiologist to be present to monitor the examination closely by viewing images in this way. Important decisions can then be made immediately regarding variations of scan technique.

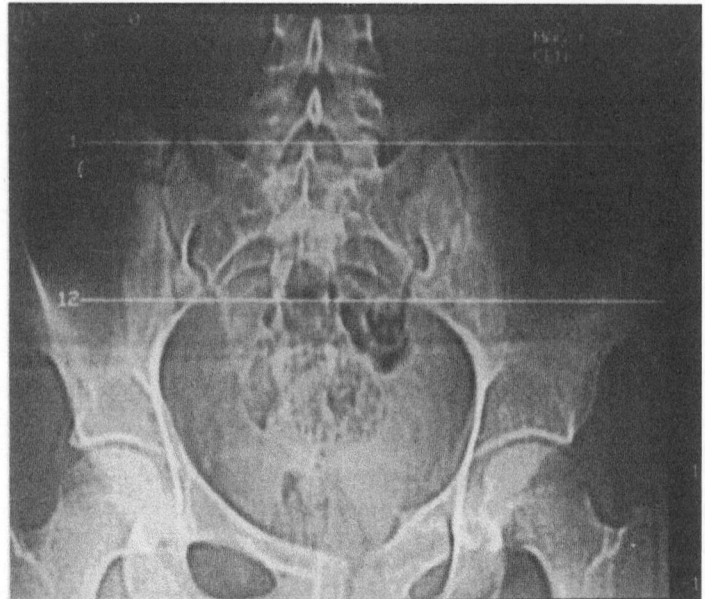

a

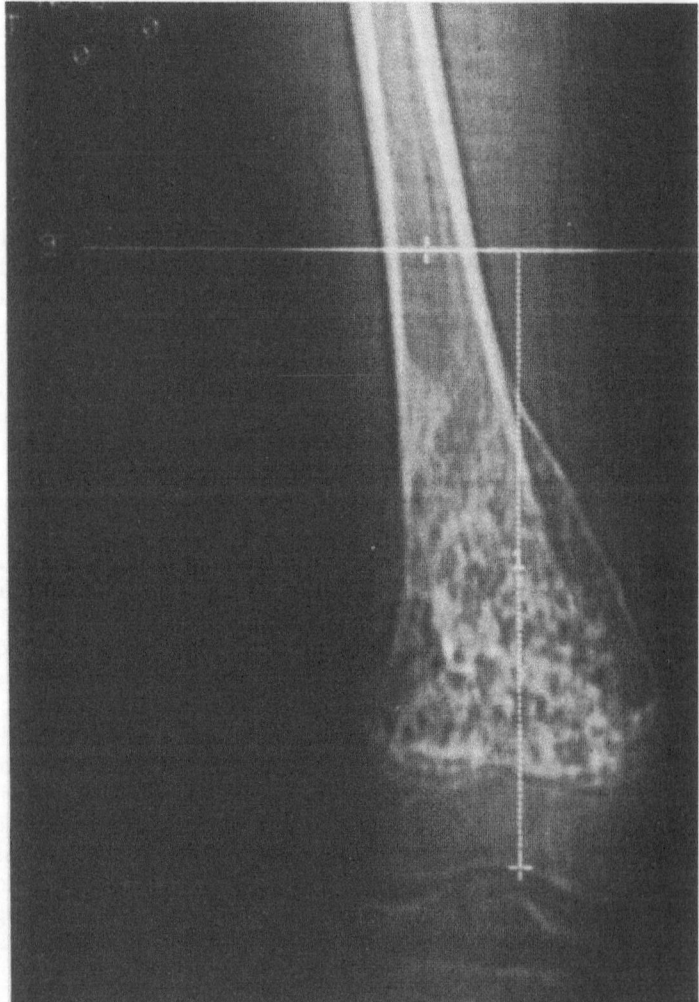

b

Fig. 2.1. a. A scout radiograph of the pelvis shows excellent anatomical detail to allow one to choose an area to be covered by the transverse axial scans. In this instance the sacroiliac joints were being evaluated, and the lines representing the scans at the limits of the joints (scan *1* and scan *12*) can be easily posted on the scout radiograph as shown. This technique is extremely useful, particularly when outlining mass lesions, as illustrated in Chapter 7. **b** A scout radiograph of the right femur shows an osteogenic sarcoma of the metaphyseal region following chemotherapy. Scan line *9* shows the upper limit of the lesion as assessed from features on the transverse axial scan. The distance from this line to the joint line can be easily measured (*vertical line 1*) by the computer.

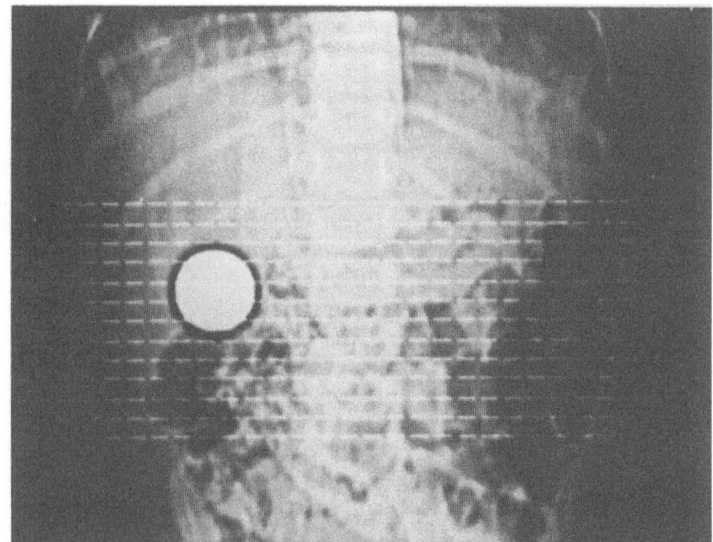

a

Fig. 2.2a,b. When lesions occur on the posterior surfaces of the body it is often useful to scan the patient in the prone rather than the supine position so that there is no distortion to the soft tissues of the posterior surfaces. In the patient illustrated in this figure a small soft tissue mass was present on the back, to the right of the midline. Because it was small a small coin was placed over the mass so that the area could easily be visualized on the initial scout radiograph (**a**). Transverse axial scans can then be chosen to go through this particular area and into the normal tissue above and below to document accurately the extent of the lesion. These lines have been posted on the scout following the study and show their correlation to the main part of the mass. **b** The mass is noted posterior to the right kidney. It is fairly well demarcated and has a somewhat low attenuation value. The lesion represented an angiolipoma of the muscles of the back.

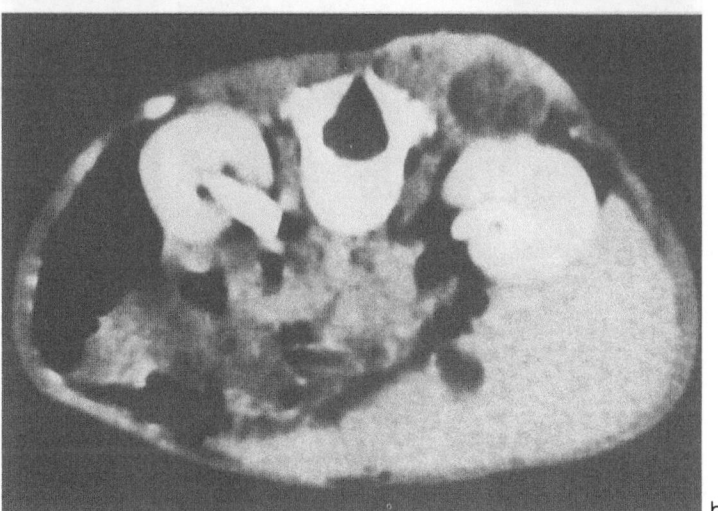

b

Postscan Techniques

Following the completion of the scans, the lines that mark the edges of a lesion can be posted on the computed radiograph (Figs. 2.1, 2.2). This is of particular value to surgeons or radiotherapists. Magnification of parts of the field of view is a valuable method for displaying small details. Sagittal and coronal reconstruction images may be obtained, although we have found that these seldom add much useful information (Fig. 2.3). Direct coronal or sagittal images may occasionally be helpful (see Fig.

4.29, p. 49) particularly in smaller children, who may be able to fit into the gantry in these positions.

A computer program may enhance spatial and contrast discrimination by giving target reconstruction of the raw data obtained during scanning. This program enables back projection of part of the total field of view on very small pixels. We have found it particularly useful for evaluation of bone lesions. With this program the window scale is extended and no additional radiation dose is involved. On newer equipment these images can be obtained immediately during scanning. This saves time as the scans do not have to be reformatted after scanning.

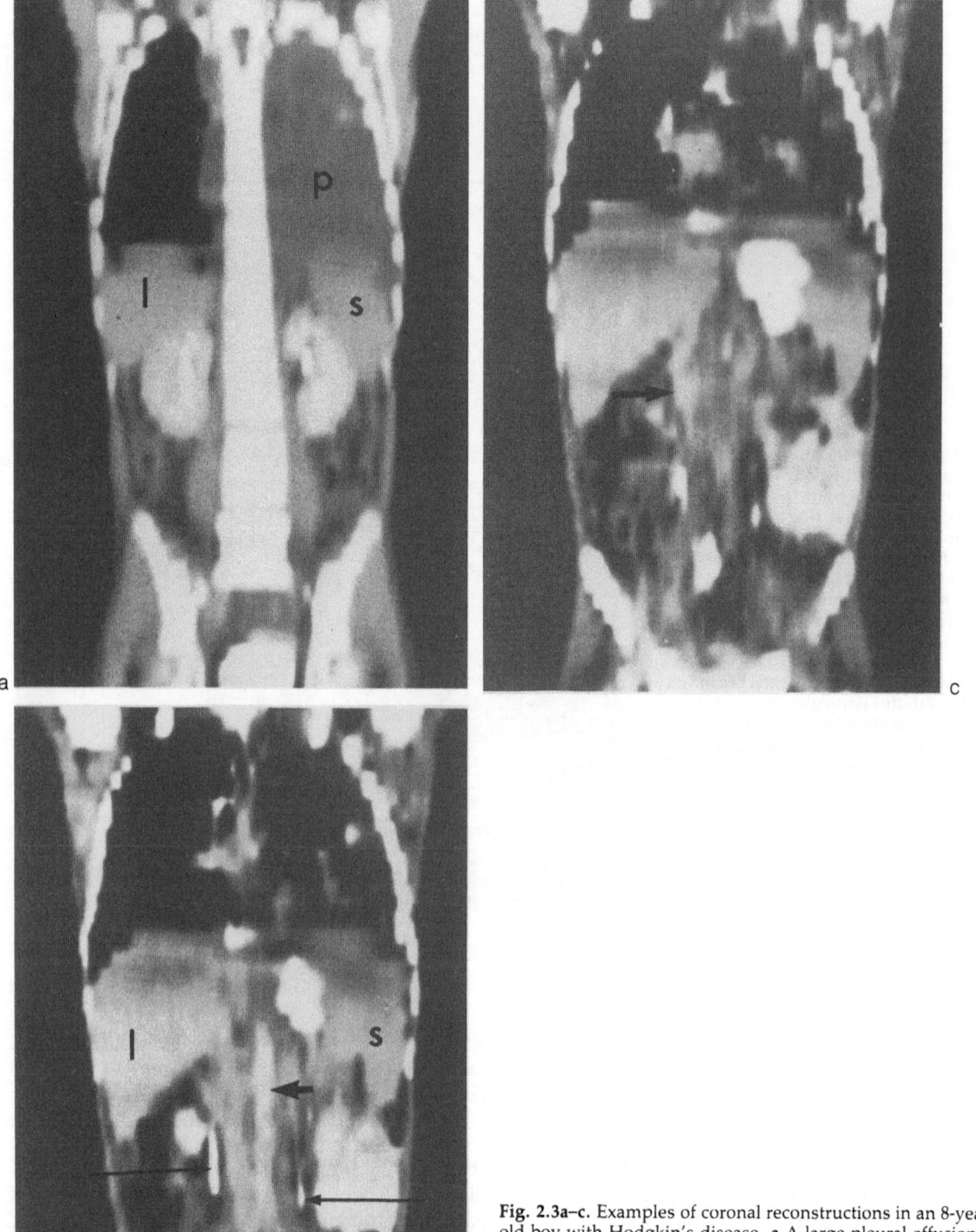

Fig. 2.3a–c. Examples of coronal reconstructions in an 8-year-old boy with Hodgkin's disease. **a** A large pleural effusion is noted on the left (*p*). The liver (*l*) and spleen (*s*) are easily visualized, as well as the kidneys and psoas muscles adjacent to the vertebral column. **b** In more anterior reconstructed images the aorta (*short arrow*) is noted, together with segments of the ureters (*long arrows*). The aortic bifurcation is easily noted. On either side of the aorta the enlarged retroperitoneal nodes are noted. **c** The inferior vena cava (*short arrow*) is noted, displaced to the right by the enlarged retroperitoneal nodes.

Guidance Procedures

CT has been extensively used at other institutions as a guide to drainage of abscesses and fluid collections and also for the biopsy of tumors. At the Hospital for Sick Children, Toronto, we have used sonography extensively for these purposes. In the vast majority of instances sonography has proved valuable, providing the necessary information and therapeutic effects. In none of these patients have we had any complications.

However, CT has been used at our institution in certain instances when ultrasound would be less desirable. CT is particularly useful when the lesions to be biopsied are small and may be less well delineated by sonography. An example of this is shown in Fig. 2.4, where small metastases were present in the liver. These were far more easily delineated with the CT scan performed after contrast injection than could be appreciated on sonography. The use of the grid and cursor measurements helps in the localization of these lesions and facilitates the procedure.

In addition, CT is valuable when lesions are either hidden by bowel gas, bone, or the lungs. An example of this is shown in Fig. 2.5. This patient had a large fluid collection just below the right hemidiaphragm. It was felt that drainage under sonographic guidance might be hazardous. CT was thus chosen as the modality to guide drainage of this fluid collection because of its proximity to the lungs.

Patients undergoing biopsy or drainage procedures under CT guidance should receive appropriate doses of analgesics such as Demerol hydrochloride prior to the procedure. In those patients who are uncooperative or extremely young, a general anesthetic is preferable, as

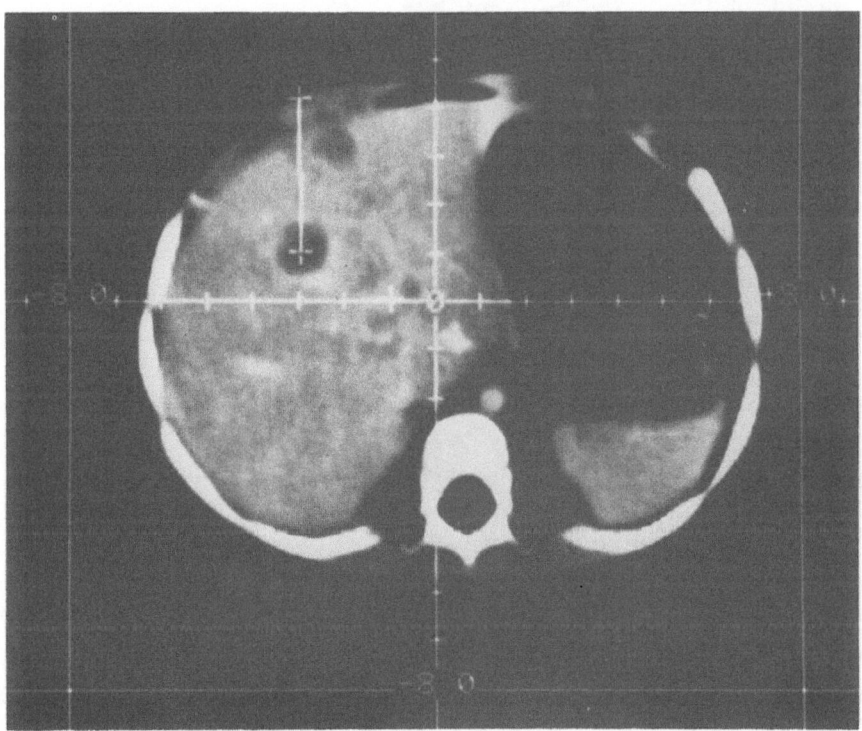

Fig. 2.4. The use of CT in guidance of biopsy. This 6-month-old boy had stage IV S neuroblastoma treated. Residual lesions were noted in the liver on CT but were extremely poorly delineated on sonography. CT was thus chosen as the modality to aid the guidance of biopsy of these lesions. This transverse axial scan shows the lesions during intravenous contrast injection. The grid and cursor measurements aid in the delineation of the lesions and help to provide adequate guidance for the needle into the appropriate position.

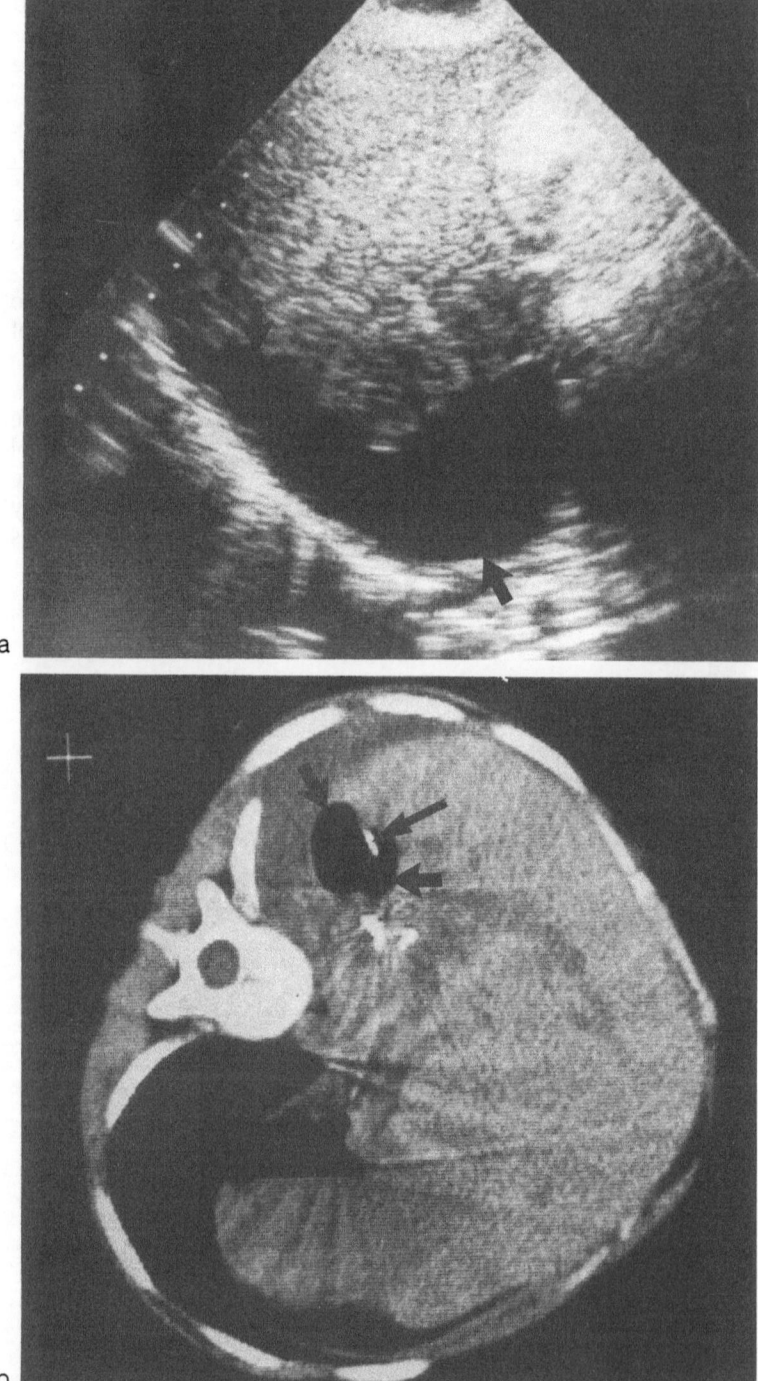

Fig. 2.5a,b. A 10-year-old girl with previously resected fibrolamellar hepatic carcinoma from the right lobe of the liver. **a** Postoperative follow-up ultrasound shows a large fluid collection (*arrows*) below the right hemidiaphragm. Because of the proximity of this collection to the adjacent lung, sonography was not used to guide drainage of this fluid. **b** A transverse axial CT scan with the patient in the left lateral decubitus position shows the fluid collection adjacent to the posterior aspect of the liver. CT was considered to be a more ideally suited modality for the drainage of this cavity and was indeed effective. Note the gas (*short arrows*) which has leaked into the cavity from the drainage tube (*long arrow*). Note the proximity of the cavity to the adjacent surgical clips. The cavity was a biloma related to a local leak from bile ducts damaged during the operation. (This is the same patient illustrated in Fig. 13.10.)

sedation may not be sufficient to stop the patients moving during the procedure.

The procedure should be performed in the following manner. A scout radiograph is obtained. The area in question is chosen from this radiograph, and a number of transverse axial scans are performed through this area, with the patient in the appropriate position for biopsy or drainage. The scan considered most appropriate for guidance of the needle is chosen, and this level is marked on the skin of the patient. The patient is then brought out of the scanner gantry, and the necessary skin sterilization and local anesthetic procedures are performed while the patient remains on the table. It is important that the patient does not move between the transverse axial scan and the time of the placement of the needle. Once the needle has been placed, fluid can be directly aspirated. Alternatively, the table can be pushed back into the gantry and the designated area scanned again to check that the needle is in fact in the appropriate position. The use of the grid and cursor measurements on the transverse axial scan are extremely helpful in determining the site of placement of the needle.

Summary

When attempting to perform a body CT scan on any patient the prescan preparations outlined above are extremely useful in facilitating the efficient performance of the scan as well as ensuring maximal patient safety and comfort. It is important to decide prior to calling the patient to the scan room whether sedation and oral and intravenous contrast will be necessary. Once the patient arrives in the scan room the procedures should be explained to the patient as well as the parents so as to allay fears. Instructions regarding breathing should be adequately explained to the patient. Adequate sedation and immobilization are imperative for the performance of high-quality scans. In young children a warm environment is extremely important, and in children who have been sedated or are unstable constant monitoring by a nurse is mandatory.

Routine scan techniques include the performance of preliminary computed radiographs, from which the transverse axial scans can be chosen. Selected postscan techniques may add to the value of the study for the clinician.

Section II:

CHEST

Chapter 3

Technique

Introduction

The two commonest indications for performing chest CT are in the search for pulmonary metastases and in the investigation of mediastinal masses. The general techniques outlined in Chapter 2 apply to chest CT as they do elsewhere in the body. However, there are certain facets of the examination that should be stressed at this time.

Suspension of respiration during the scans is important to eliminate artifacts caused by respiratory motion. For this reason, patients should be carefully instructed how to stop breathing at the same level of inspiration for each scan so that each scan taken through the chest will be in sequence. If scans are performed at varying levels of respiration, areas of the lung will be out of sequence; indeed, some areas may be missed. Patients who are uncooperative or too young to understand how to suspend respiration should be sedated in the manner described in Chapter 2 (see p. 10). Scans are then performed during quiet respiration. It should be stressed that the decision to sedate a patient with severe cardiac, airway, or pulmonary pathology should be made only after adequate consultation with the attending clinicians. The shortest scan time possible should be used (2 s). Even with this scan time some artifact is noted as a result of the cardiac motion, but this does not usually degrade the image significantly.

CT of the chest during general anesthesia may reveal areas of pulmonary collapse as a result of the anesthetic (see Fig. 10.3d, p. 128). For this reason general anesthesia should be avoided if the CT is performed primarily to assess the lungs.

Ideally patients should be immobilized in the scan gantry with their arms raised above their heads. If necessary, the arms should be securely fastened in this position. Velcro straps can help to immobilize the abdomen.

The transverse axial display of the mediastinal structures on CT is an advantageous depiction of this complex anatomical compartment, showing individual structures which cannot be seen without superimposition on conventional chest radiographs and which cannot even be easily distinguished with conventional tomography. With the newer fast (2-s) high-resolution scanners available many of the mediastinal structures can be differentiated, even in young children and infants. These include the brachiocephalic vessels, thymus, aorta, pulmonary arteries, airways, and esophagus. However, the relative paucity of mediastinal fat in children does not allow as clear a differentiation of these various structures as is seen on CT examinations in adults. Therefore, in order to visualize these structures more easily, intravenous contrast enhancement is used routinely in the evaluation of mediastinal structures in all children. Indeed, the mediastinum and upper abdomen are the two areas of the body that are best interpreted when the scan has been performed with intravenous contrast enhancement. Scans should be performed during intravenous injection of contrast material so that the vasculature may be visualized during the phase of maximal enhancement. In patients with situs solitus it is best to inject the bolus of contrast into a vein in the dorsum of the left hand so that the left brachiocephalic vein can be maximally enhanced and can then easily be differentiated from the thymus anteriorly. Injection into the right hand or feet will not enhance this vein to the same degree and may make it difficult to exclude an anterior mediastinal mass. The anatomy of the mediastinum is shown in Fig. 4.1 (see p. 28). Slight dextroconvexity to the mediastinal contents in the azygo-esophageal recess is a normal variant in children.

Window Settings

In scans of the chest, the densities range widely from the high negative values of the air in the lungs and trachea through the densities of fat and soft tissues all the way up to the high positive values of the bony thorax. All of the structures cannot be optimally visualized at any one particular window setting. For this reason, it is imperative that each scan of the chest be viewed at a number of different window settings so that the examiner satisfies himself that he has visualized all the anatomical structures at each level. The examination is incomplete if this is ignored.

When changing the window level and width, the following principles should be kept in mind:

1. The pulmonary parenchyma (diffuse disease or nodules) is best viewed with the window centered at lung density in the high negative range and with wide window width (poor contrast).
2. Soft tissues of the chest wall and mediastinum should be imaged with the window centered at soft tissue density in the low positive range and with a relatively narrow window width, giving a higher degree of contrast.
3. The skeleton is best visualized with the window set at bone density at high positive values with a wide window width. We have previously viewed the skeleton with reversal of the normal color display so that bone and contrast material

appear black. We have felt that this gave a somewhat clearer display of the bony and contrast detail. However, with the newer equipment we have relied heavily on targetted images to depict bony detail. This has been found to be optimally viewed in the normal color display, showing bone white.

For the inexperienced operator, these guidelines are extremely useful for visualization of the various structures in each scan of the chest. However, the necessary window adjustments are readily learned, and the settings then become automatic adjustments depending on what structures the operator wishes to view. Optimal window settings for any particular structure vary from patient to patient. For this reason, exact numerical values for the window level and width need not necessarily be memorized. The window should be adjusted by each individual operator in such a way as to provide the best visualization of a particular structure in a particular patient.

In order to obtain maximum information from each scan slice, it is important for the consulting radiologist to be present at the doctor's console of the CT scanner during each chest CT examination. At the Hospital for Sick Children, Toronto, all CT scans are closely monitored by a physician (staff radiologist or radiology fellow). In this way, the radiologist can personally adjust the window level and width when viewing each slice and will obtain the maximum amount of information to be recorded on hard copy film. This is a far superior approach than viewing the films that have been taken by the technician after the examination is complete.

Moreover, the consulting radiologist can make further decisions regarding variations of technique while the patient is still on the CT table rather than repeating the procedure at a later date. Immediate decisions can then be made if further views are necessary, which may involve changing the patient's position into a prone or a lateral decubitus position. Further injections of contrast material may be necessary to give better definition of anatomical structures. It may be useful to have direct coronal and sagittal views. Certain technical computer manipulations may be performed, e.g., sagittal and coronal reconstructions and magnification views to enlarge small structures. It is important to be able to make these decisions to suit the needs of each individual patient. For all these reasons, it is imperative that the consulting radiologist monitors the scan closely.

Pseudomasses and Anatomical Variations

Bones

Often normal anatomical structures masquerade as chest wall lesions projecting into the lung field, particularly when scans are viewed with the window set for viewing the lungs. The true nature of these pseudomasses is revealed when the window is reset to view the bones and soft tissues of the chest wall. Scans may average part of the lung and the adjacent bone into one image. These structures are normal, prominent, bony protuberances and anteriorly include the medial ends of the clavicles and anterior ends of the ribs, and posteriorly the heads of the ribs. These bony pseudomasses are most often seen anteriorly in the upper chest because of the natural slope of the chest wall in this region.

An easy method for determining the normal anatomical structure causing the pseudomass is to place the cursor on the suspected mass when viewing the scan with the window set to view the lung. Leaving the cursor in position, change the window setting to view the bones and soft tissues. The tissue under the cursor will now be recognized to have bony density and conform to the shape of the adjacent normal bones (Fig. 3.1).

Vessels

Some vascular structures may also masquerade as pseudomasses when viewing scans with a window set to the view of the lungs. Along the inner aspect of the anterior chest wall, the internal mammary vessels course inferiorly, bilaterally. They should not be mistaken for subpleural or pleural metastases. The fact that these densities are found bilaterally and can be followed superiorly and inferiorly in adjacent scans helps to make this differentiation.

Prominent, normal mediastinal vessels or vascular variations may also masquerade as mass lesions of the mediastinal pleura or adjacent lung. These structures include the superior vena cava on the right and the subclavian artery on the left. Changing the window to view the mediastinal structures with greater contrast will reveal the normal vessels as the cause for the pseudomass. If lack of mediastinal fat makes delineation of these vessels poor with appropriate window settings, further scans can be

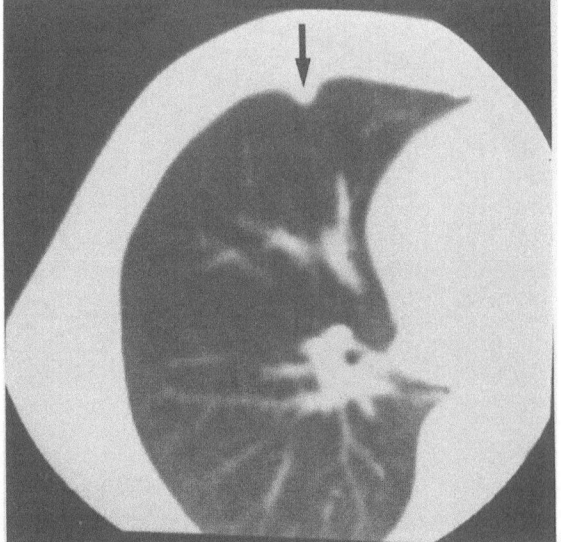

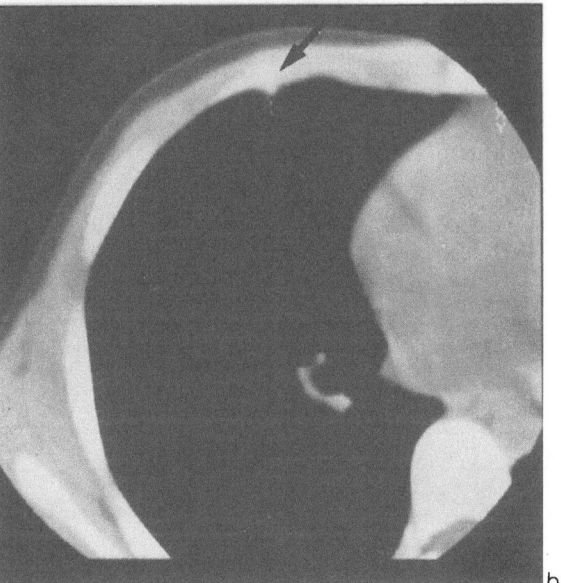

Fig. 3.1a,b. Anterior pseudomass noted in scan **a** (*arrow*). In scan **b** this area is noted to be the bulbous anterior end of a rib (*arrow*). When the study is viewed at the window width set for lung in scan **a** the small cursor is placed over the mass. The window is then changed to view the chest wall and mediastinum as in scan **b**, and at this time the small *cursor* can be seen adjacent to the rib end.

obtained during the rapid intravenous injection of contrast material. In this way these vessels will be well opacified and their true nature confirmed.

Anatomical vascular variations that may cause unusual mass densities include (1) the azygous vein when an azygous lobe is present (Fig. 3.2) and (2) azygous continuation of the inferior vena

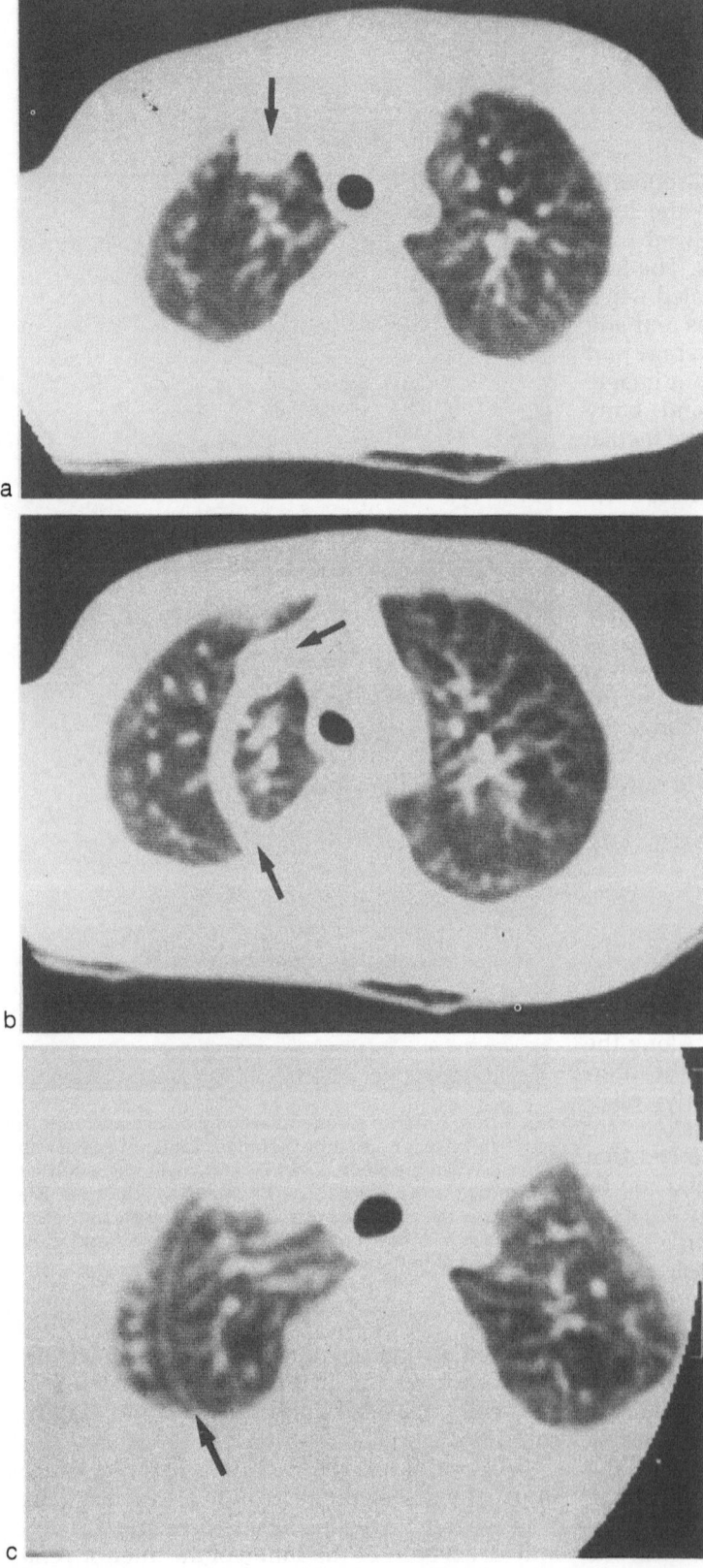

Fig. 3.2a–c. Azygous vein and fissure. The azygous vein is seen in scans **a** and **b** (*arrows*) passsing from the posterior mediastinum anteriorly lateral to the azygous lobe to drain into the superior vena cava. In scan **c** the lower limit of the azygous fissure (*arrow*) is noted as a curvilinear density within the lung. Note that the lung immediately adjacent to either side of the fissure is relatively avascular.

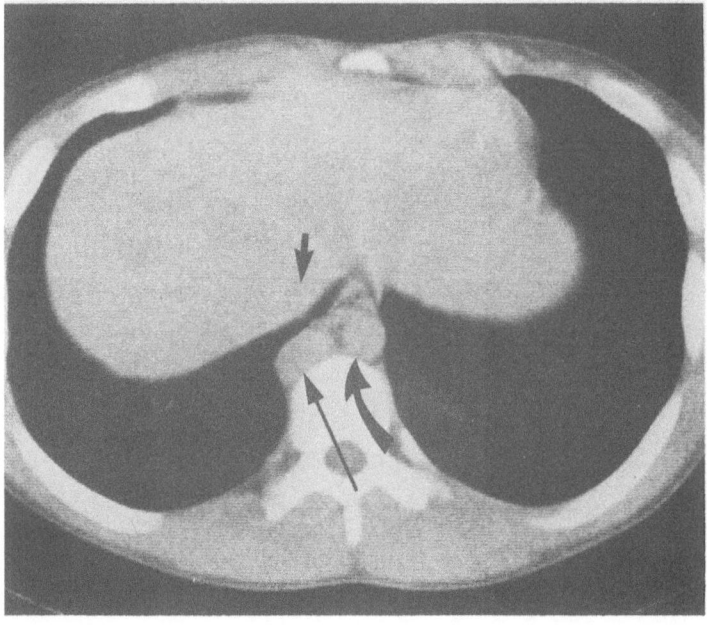

Fig. 3.3. Example of azygous continuation of the inferior vena cava. At this level of scan the normal position of the inferior vena cava is indicated by the *short arrow*. The *long arrow* indicates the large azygous continuation of the inferior vena cava lying to the right of the aorta (*curved arrow*).

cava (Fig. 3.3). When an azygous lobe is present, the azygous vein passes from the posterior mediastinum forward through the azygous fissure in the right upper lobe to drain into the superior vena cava. This causes a curvilinear density to be seen passing through the mid portion of the right upper lobe. A mass in the posterior mediastinum on the right lying anterolateral to the vertebral bodies may represent the azygous continuation of the inferior vena cava as it courses to the superior mediastinum to drain into the superior vena cava. Other anomalies that may be related to visceral heterotaxy or the asplenia/polysplenia syndrome may be further delineated by perform-

ing scans during rapid intravenous injection of contrast. However, cardiac and abdominal ultrasound should be considered first in delineation of the vascular anatomy in such patients. Other vascular anomalies are illustrated in Figs. 4.4 (p. 32), 4.7 (p. 33), and 4.30d (p. 50).

Most of the above-mentioned structures pose at one time or another as pseudomasses to all physicians involved in body CT. The need to use the cursor or intravenous contrast injection to clarify these structures diminishes with increased experience. One learns to accept these normal variations and their appearances at variable window settings on CT.

Chapter 4
Mediastinum

Anatomical Compartments

The mediastinum is the anatomical space in the midline of the thorax, lying between the two lungs and their visceral pleura. It extends from the thoracic inlet superiorly to the central tendon of the diaphragm inferiorly and from the vertebral column posteriorly to the sternum anteriorly. Anatomically the mediastinum can be divided into a superior and an inferior compartment, and the inferior compartment further divided into anterior, middle, and posterior compartments. Hope et al. [24] and Kirks and Korobkin [26] have pointed out that these classic anatomical divisions of the mediastinum are somewhat impractical for the radiological analysis and differential diagnosis of mediastinal abnormalities. These authors have offered modifications of this division which they feel are useful [26]. The division of the mediastinum used here is a simplified approach, merely dividing the entire mediastinum into three components — anterior, middle, and posterior — and thus differing somewhat from previous approaches.

1. The *anterior* mediastinum is situated between the sternum anteriorly and the great vessels, heart, and pericardium posteriorly. It contains the thymus, lymph nodes, and some areolar tissue and fat.
2. The *middle* mediastinum contains the great vessels, major airways, heart and pericardium, hilar regions, lymph nodes, and upper esophagus, together with a small amount of areolar tissue and fat.
3. The *posterior* mediastinum lies behind the above-mentioned structures and includes the paravertebral gutters, together with the sympathetic chains and nerve roots. In the lower thorax the descending thoracic aorta, azygous and hemiazygous veins, thoracic duct, and esophagus, together with some lymph nodes, should be considered part of the posterior mediastinum. In children, the majority of posterior mediastinal masses do in fact arise in the region of the paravertebral gutters.

The anatomical components of the mediastinum are illustrated in Fig. 4.1.

Thymus

The main mass of the thymus lies in the superior part of the anterior mediastinum behind the manubrium and in front of the great vessels. It extends to a variable extent down into the inferior portion of the anterior mediastinum in front of the heart and pericardium.

The thymus varies in size at all ages and is largest in young infants, in whom it is seen on plain radiographs and CT to bulge with a lobulated border bilaterally (Fig. 4.2). Occasionally, its shape may vary considerably. In older children the thymus may be seen easily on CT, even

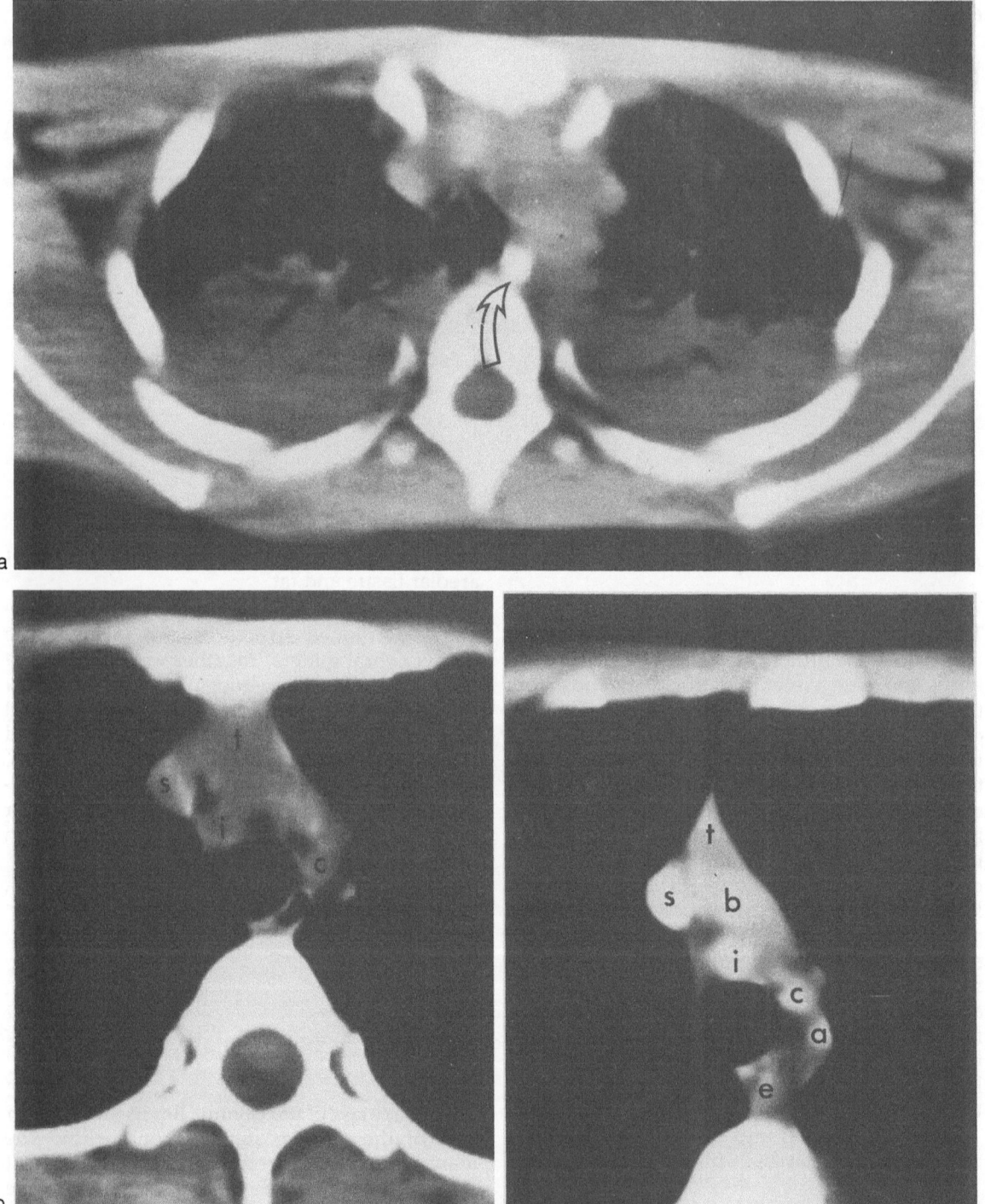

Fig. 4.1. a A 6-year-old boy following chest and abdominal trauma. Note how poorly the mediastinal structures are defined when intravenous contrast is not administered as a rapid bolus. *Curved arrow,* feeding tube in esophagus. Note severe collapse of dependent portions of lung with air bronchograms. **b** Mediastinal structures above the level of the aortic arch in scan without contrast administration. **c** Note how much better these structures are defined in another patient in whom intravenous contrast was given as a rapid bolus injection. *t,* thymus; *s,* superior vena cava; *b,* brachiacephalic vein; *i,* innominate artery; *c,* left common carotid artery; *a,* left subclavian artery; *e,* esophagus. In **b** the esophagus is air filled posterolateral to trachea on left. The left subclavian artery is seen as a small opacity posterolateral to the left common carotid artery in **b**.

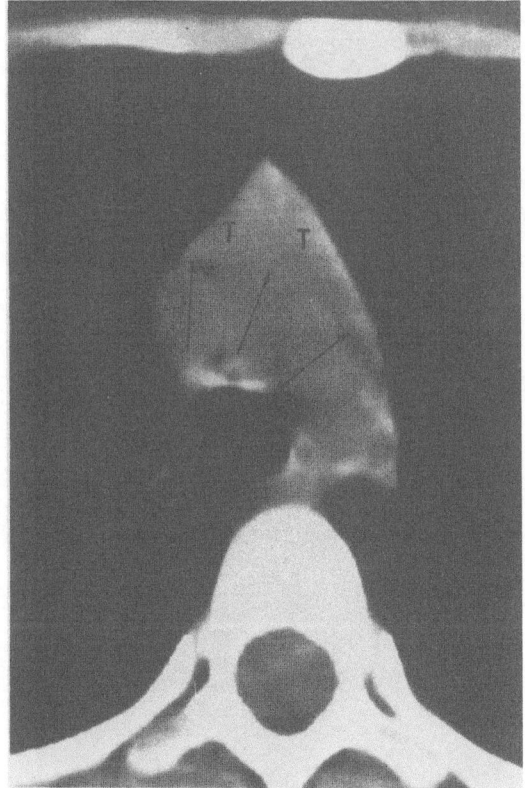

a

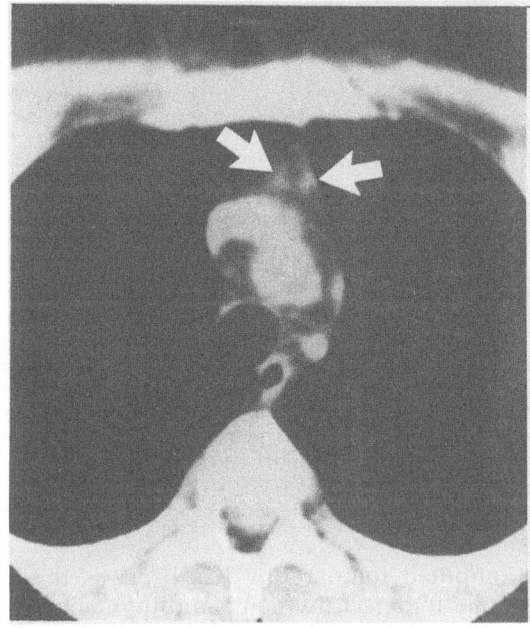

b

Fig. 4.2a,b. Examples of normal thymus. **a** A 10-year-old showing residual thymus (*T*) in the anterior mediastinum. *Arrows* mark the posterior surface of the thymus. Note the tongue of thymus extending posteriorly lateral to the mediastinal vessels. The mediastinal anatomy shows poor contrast in this scan performed without intravenous contrast.
b 12-year-old boy with residual thymus in fat in anterior mediastinum (*arrows*).

when plain chest radiographs fail to reveal its presence (Fig. 4.2). The normal range of thymic sizes on CT at various ages has been estimated by Baron et al. [2]. These authors studied the transverse CT scans in 11 cases between the ages of 6 and 19 years. The mean measurements of the long axis of the lobes of the thymus were found to be: 2.0 cm (SD = 0.55) right; 3.3 cm (SD = 1.1) left. The mean thickness (perpendicular to long axis) of each lobe measured: 1.0 cm (SD = 0.39) right; 1.1 cm (SD = 0.40) left. These values are useful in determining whether there is thymic enlargement on CT or not [1, 2]. The thymus has a homogeneous soft tissue attenuation on CT and enhances homogeneously with intravenous contrast injection [2]. The shape of the gland varies greatly. The two lobes may be easily visualized on CT and may appear triangular, particularly in older children and young adults (Fig. 4.2). Focal or diffuse fatty infiltration gradually occurs in adults [2, 33].

In children it may be extremely difficult to differentiate a normal prominent thymus from a pathologically enlarged thymus on chest radiographs as well as on CT. A widened superior mediastinum resulting from a normal thymus on a chest radiograph of an older child appears less dense than when the thymus is pathologically enlarged. In the past we have found pneumomediastinograms useful to document the outline of the normal thymus in this situation. However, CT is an excellent noninvasive technique to define the outline as well as the attenuation of the various parts of the gland. The thymus should be considered to be pathologically enlarged when its lateral borders have an unusual shape, when there is displacement and compression of the adjacent vessels and airways, and when the attenuation of the gland on CT is inhomogeneous, particularly after intravenous contrast administration [26]. If these changes are not evident on CT, it is impossible to differentiate a normal prominent gland from a pathological one. Occasionally, the thymus has an unusual shape that may simulate disease but represents a normal variation. Rarely, it may be impossible even with CT to differentiate this from a focal thymic lesion (Fig. 4.3).

It should be remembered that although the thymus shrinks in response to stress, it may rebound in size following stress [11]. This has been seen after many different conditions and may also occur in patients who have been treated for malignant disease [11]. Widening of the mediastinum on a chest radiograph in these patients who have completed therapy should

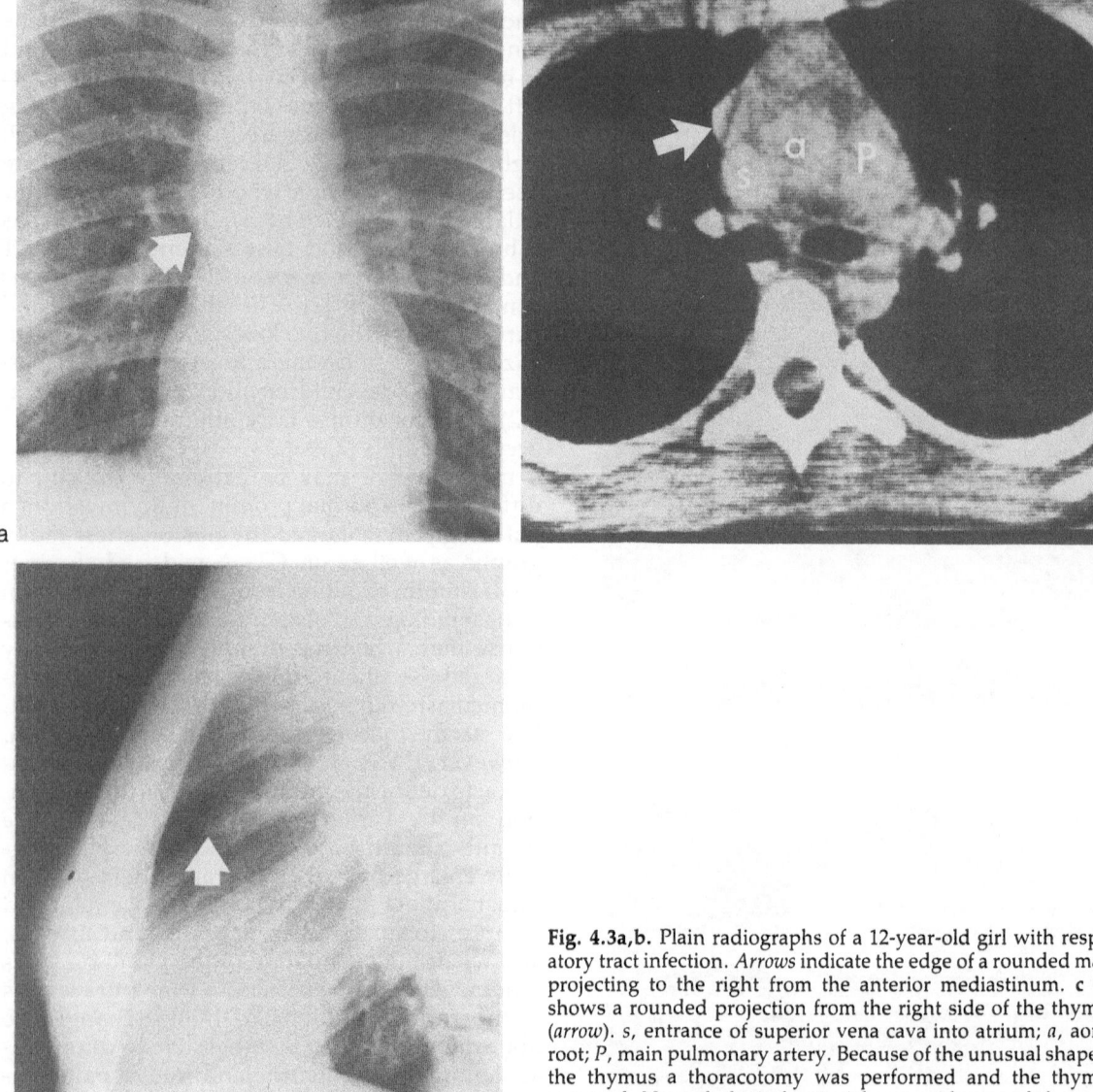

Fig. 4.3a,b. Plain radiographs of a 12-year-old girl with respiratory tract infection. *Arrows* indicate the edge of a rounded mass projecting to the right from the anterior mediastinum. **c** CT shows a rounded projection from the right side of the thymus (*arrow*). *s*, entrance of superior vena cava into atrium; *a*, aortic root; *P*, main pulmonary artery. Because of the unusual shape of the thymus a thoracotomy was performed and the thymus removed. No pathological material was evident, and the mass represents an unusual shape of a normal thymus.

not be considered as necessarily representing malignant disease of the anterior mediastinum. Cohen et al. [11] have suggested following such children with chest radiographs at frequent intervals and have relied on biopsy in five of seven such patients. The use of CT in differentiating normal thymic rebound from a malignant anterior mediastinal mass has not yet been assessed.

Computed tomography has been used successfully to detect thymoma and thymic hyperplasia in adults with myasthenia gravis, even when chest radiographs appeared normal [18]. We agree with others that this type of CT investigation is unrewarding in children [26]. Mass lesions of the thymus are discussed in the section on anterior mediastinal masses (see p. 36).

Trachea

The trachea begins superiorly at the lower level of the cricoid cartilage and extends inferiorly to its bifurcation at the carina, roughly at the level of the sternomanubrial joint [7, 8, 17, 20, 28, 32]. The initial 1–2 cm of trachea are extrathoracic (see Fig. 20.1, p. 294) and the remainder lies in the middle mediastinum within the thorax. With the patient lying supine, CT scans taken through the trachea are at an angle to the longitudinal axis of the trachea; this was measured by Griscom in 1982 [21] as approximately 6°. The transverse axial scans of CT, therefore, do not depict the true transverse cross section of the trachea but rather, oblique sections. The true transverse area and diameter can be estimated by an equation [21]. The trachea may have a horseshoe, elliptical, or circular configuration. The posterior tracheal membrane may protrude slightly into the tracheal air column occasionally. The intrathoracic trachea most commonly has a round or oval shape. Sometimes, however, it may be more horseshoe shaped. Occasionally, different shapes may be noted at different levels in the same subject [21, 22]. Just above the carina the trachea may develop an oval configuration with a longer transverse diameter just prior to bifurcating into the major bronchi. The tracheal wall cannot be discerned, owing to the lack of surrounding fat.

In 1983, Griscom [22] assessed the cross-sectional shape of the trachea on CT in 19 children aged 1–19 years. Scans of the trachea were mostly done during breath-holding at capacities not far from total lung capacity. Griscom found that in this age group, under these circumstances, the trachea is slightly narrow just below the larynx and broadens above the bifurcation. At other levels it was found to be only mildly or moderately off circular (see Fig. 4.13). Mild variations were documented from patient to patient and level to level, but no abrupt changes in size or shape were evident. The severely off-circular shape documented on CT in older adults was not encountered. Our own experience agrees with the above-mentioned findings. However, patients who are scanned during sedation tend to have a more horseshoe-shaped trachea rather than a fully circular trachea.

The value of CT in the estimation of the tracheal caliber in children has been documented by Griscom in 1982 [21] and Effman et al. in 1983 [15]. The usefulness of CT in assessing caliber changes in children with neck or thoracic masses has been stressed [21]. Any mass lesion in any of the compartments of the mediastinum may cause narrowing of the airway. The airway should thus be closely assessed in all scans performed to assess the extent of mediastinal masses [27]. Approximately one-third of the cross-sectional area of the trachea has to be compromised before symptoms of respiratory compromise are evident [27].

The use of CT in the evaluation of intrinsic abnormalities of the trachea in children has not previously been stressed. In 1984, Liu and Daneman [30] reported eight cases of tracheal abnormalities. The patients were six males and two females, whose age at the time of CT examination ranged from 10 days to 4.5 years. This group included three patients with tracheal stenosis, three patients with tracheomalacia, one patient with an acquired tracheoesophageal fistula, and one with a tracheal scar from a previous tracheostomy.

Tracheal stenosis is a rare and potentially fatal condition characterized by the absence of the membranous part of the trachea and the presence of complete circular cartilaginous tracheal rings [5, 16, 25]. The diameter of the trachea is markedly narrowed in these patients. Usually the entire length of the trachea is involved and occasionally the main stem bronchi as well. The diagnosis is usually made by invasive studies such as endoscopy and tracheobronchography. Endoscopy may reveal the proximal end of the narrowing but may not be able to determine its length as the endoscope may not be able to negotiate the airway. CT offers a relatively noninvasive technique in the assessment of the degree and length of tracheal narrowing in these patients. These changes were exquisitely documented in all three of our patients with this type of lesion (Fig. 4.4). The diameter of the entire length of the trachea and main stem bronchi was obviously narrowed for children of their age, and accurate computer measurements were indeed unnecessary. The cross section of the trachea appeared as a perfect circle.

There is an increased incidence of congenital thoracic vascular anomalies in children with tracheal stenosis [29, 30]; in fact this was noted in all three of our patients. It is therefore suggested that scans be performed during rapid bolus injection of intravenous contrast material when examining patients suspected of having tracheal stenosis. These scans will define the relationship of the mediastinal vessels to the tracheal wall. If anomalies are defined, more detailed anatomical

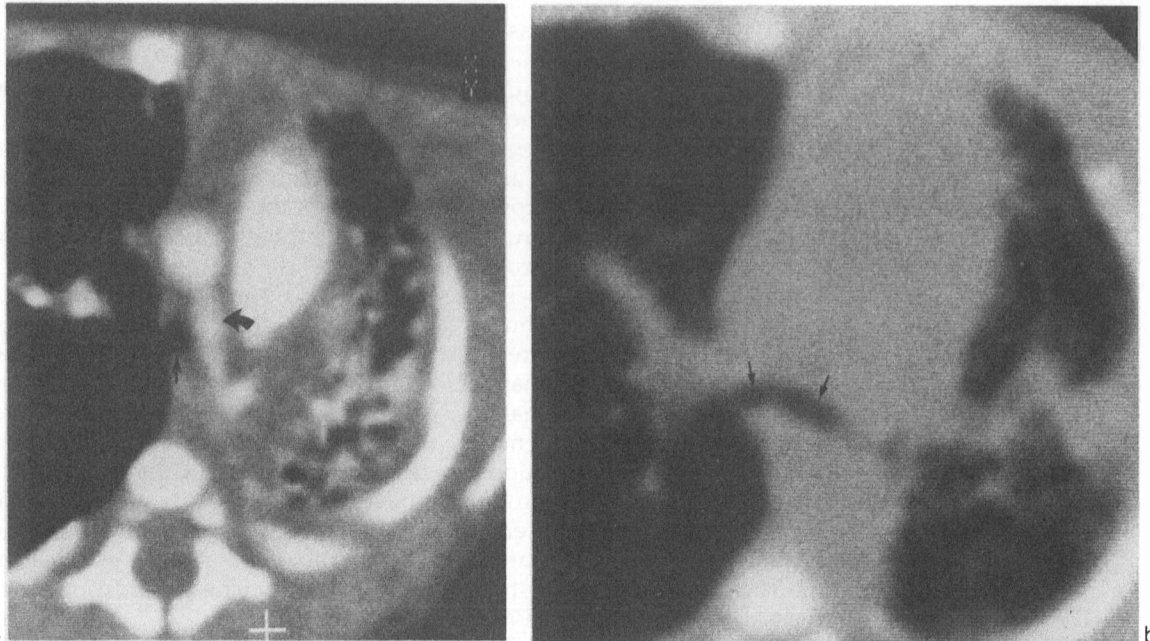

Fig. 4.4a,b. A 23-day-old boy with respiratory distress. CT shows congenital stenosis involving the entire length of the trachea and both main bronchi (*small arrows*). The trachea is round in shape. Note the partial atelectasis of the left lung and the narrow transverse arch of the aorta (*curved arrow*). He had multiple vascular anomalies. In this patient CT was a relatively noninvasive modality for delineating the entire length of the narrowed airway and gave further information regarding vascular anomalies. (Liu and Daneman 1984 [30])

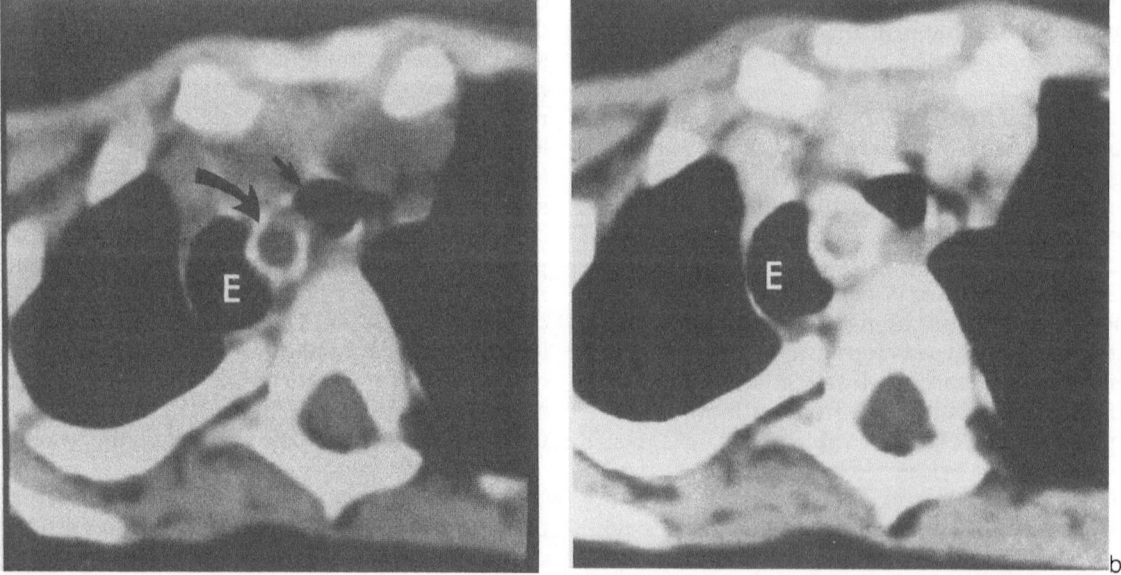

Fig. 4.5a,b. A 4½-year-old boy with respiratory distress. He had been born with a congenital tracheoesophageal fistula, and tracheoplasty had been performed to alleviate respiratory distress caused by tracheomalacia. CT before (**a**) and after (**b**) contrast administration at the time of recurrent respiratory distress showed that the mesh (*curved arrow*) which had been used for the tracheoplasty is lying separate from the trachea (*straight arrow*). Note the compression of the trachea posteriorly on the right by the mesh and the enhancement of tissue around the mesh in **b**, which was found to be vascular granulation tissue at operation. *E,* dilated proximal esophagus. These changes could not be appreciated on plain chest radiographs, and the findings obviated the need for invasive endoscopy with its attendant morbidity. The findings provided essential preoperative information. (Liu and Daneman 1984 [30])

information regarding the vasculature may be required, necessitating cardiac catheterization and angiography after CT.

Tracheomalacia is a condition characterized by weakness of the tracheal cartilages, which may be incompletely developed. This leads to instability of the tracheal wall and marked changes in caliber of the trachea during different phases of respiration. Tracheomalacia most commonly occurs in association with esophageal atresia and tracheoesophageal fistula. The cartilages are incompletely formed and are usually weakened, particularly adjacent to the area of insertion of the fistula into the trachea [3]. Tracheomalacia may also be seen in association with lesions that compress and weaken the tracheal cartilages. This compression may be from an anomalous innominate artery or adjacent mediastinal masses [4, 31].

Fluoroscopy is the most useful modality in assessing the dynamic changes in tracheal caliber that occur in association with tracheomalacia. We have used CT to assess the tracheal caliber in three patients with this condition. In one patient obvious narrowing of the trachea was noted in association with the innominate artery compression syndrome. In the second patient, however, artifact was present owing to the rapid respiratory rate caused by the patient's dyspnea, and scans were consequently of extremely poor quality. In a third patient CT delineated tracheal caliber changes exquisitely, as well as the abnormal position of the previously inserted mesh for tracheoplasty (Fig. 4.5). In this patient none of these changes were evident on the chest radiograph.

In the child thought to have an acquired tracheoesophageal fistula, CT not only defined the position of the fistula accurately but was also useful in excluding the presence of a foreign body (Fig. 4.6). In the child who had a previous tracheostomy, CT was useful in defining the level of the tracheal scar and resultant tracheal narrowing more accurately than plain radiography.

We felt that CT provided valuable information in six of the above-mentioned patients; however, fluoroscopy should still remain the method of choice in the investigation of patients suspected of having tracheomalacia. CT accurately defines the caliber of the airway and documents the site and extent of caliber changes as well as giving detailed information about the tissues and vessels adjacent to the airway (Fig. 4.7). It will easily document the extent of airway involvement in those children in whom endoscopy reveals air-

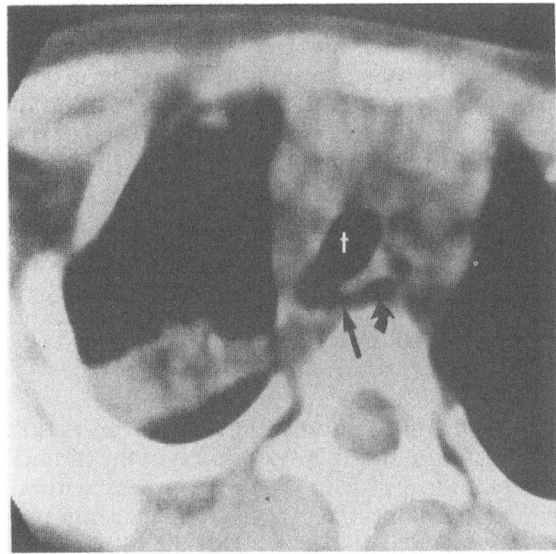

Fig. 4.6. A 4-year-old girl with recurrent acquired tracheoesophageal fistula (*straight arrow*). CT not only defines the site of the fistula between the esophagus posteriorly and the trachea more anteriorly but excludes the presence of an associated foreign body within these structures and in the soft tissues. Note the partial atelectasis of the right lung. *t*, trachea; *curved arrow*, esophagus. (Liu and Daneman 1984 [30])

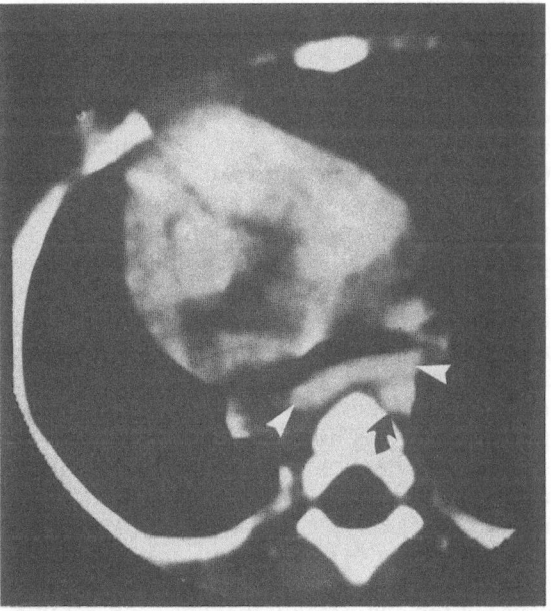

Fig. 4.7. A 2-year-old boy with dextrocardia and respiratory distress. An upper gastrointestinal series showed an indentation in the back of the trachea. CT during the intravenous injection of contrast material shows an aberrant left pulmonary artery (*arrow heads*) lying behind the bifurcation of the trachea. *Curved arrow*, descending aorta.

way narrowing but in whom the endoscope cannot negotiate the involved area to determine its length. On rare occasions CT may be used to define the presence of foreign bodies within the airway [6]. Finally, as has been stressed above, CT is invaluable in the assessment of the airway in association with mediastinal masses [27].

Heart and Pericardium

The heart and pericardium occupy the middle mediastinum in the lower portion of the thoracic cavity and appear in scans performed without contrast enhancement as a somewhat homogeneous soft tissue density. The chambers of the heart are readily visualized when scans are performed during rapid bolus injection of intravenous contrast material. Even with the new fast scanners (2-s scans), minor artifact caused by cardiac motion is still present in scans taken through the level of the heart, but this does not usually cause degradation of the image. Linear artifacts are often seen, particularly close to the cardiac margin anteriorly.

Echocardiography is the method of choice in delineating lesions of the heart and pericardial effusion in children. The main advantages of this technique are the ease of the examination and the absence of ionizing radiation. Furthermore, examinations can be done at the bedside. Nevertheless, echocardiography does have some technical limitations and interpretive pitfalls. Occasionally, abnormalities may be suspected in the pericardium or adjacent to the heart and pericardium on echocardiography. It is in these rare instances that we have used CT to delineate the heart and pericardium specifically and their relationship to the other mediastinal structures in order to confirm or exclude suspicious abnormalities that have been noted on echocardiography. Despite the introduction of gated cine CT studies, the heart and pericardium are still not routinely studied by this technique at most institutions.

In the presence of large pericardial or pleural effusions, CT is often helpful in delineating the cause of the abnormality that has been noted on plain chest radiographs. With the use of intravenous contrast material the transverse axial display of CT shows the pleural, pericardial, cardiac, chest wall, mediastinal, and pulmonary components that contribute to the appearance on the chest radiograph without overlap (see Fig. 6.16, p. 80). This is also particularly helpful in patients who have complications following thoracotomy (see Fig. 4.30).

The pericardium can respond to injury by fibrin production, cellular proliferation, and fluid output [35]. These three mechanisms may occur concomitantly or independently. The normal pericardium is difficult to define in children, and CT examinations are rarely performed in children to define pericardial abnormalities. The pericardium may, however, be easily demonstrated in the presence of pericardial effusions, particularly after the injection of intravenous contrast material. Pericardial effusions can be recognized as a band of fluid density around the heart (see Fig. 6.16, p. 80). Pericardial fluid tends to accumulate initially in the most caudal portions of the pericardial sac, and with increasing volumes the fluid extends dorsally initially and then more ventrally to the heart as well. The heart may ultimately appear to float in very large collections of pericardial fluid.

We have stressed that in all patients undergoing chest CT for pulmonary metastases we routinely view the images with both a wide and a narrow window width (see Chap. 5, p. 63). This technique proved extremely useful in two patients with osteogenic sarcoma in whom ossified cardiac metastases within the heart were evident on the images viewed with the narrow window width but not with the wide window width used to assess the lungs for pulmonary metastases (Fig. 4.8). In only one of these two patients was the ossified lesion very faintly visible on the chest radiograph [13].

During the 64-year period 1919–1982, 45 patients were recorded at the Hospital for Sick Children, Toronto as having metastatic disease involving the heart and pericardium [9]. During this time 5103 patients with malignant disease were seen at this institution. In this series the commonest tumors with metastatic disease involving the heart were non-Hodgkin's lymphoma (42%) and neuroblastoma (29%). The two patients mentioned above represent the only two patients with cardiac metastases from osteogenic sarcoma. Only 13% of all children with cardiac metastases in this series were diagnosed prior to death [9]. Definitive antemortem diagnosis was made by CT, angiocardiography, inferior vena cavography, and two-dimensional echocardiography.

Osteogenic sarcoma is said to be the commonest sarcoma with cardiac metastases [14]. In 1978, Dalal et al. [12] reviewed the literature and

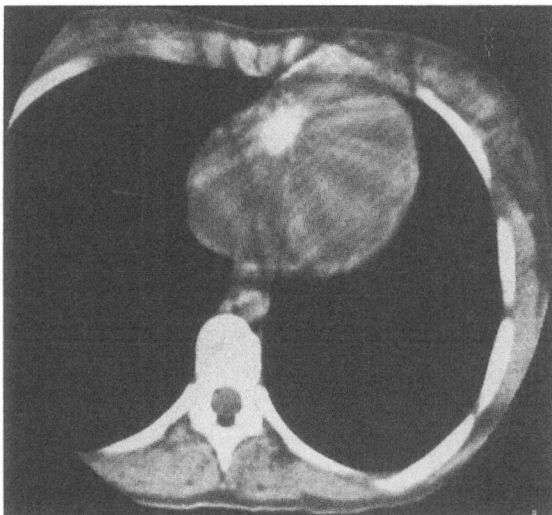

Fig. 4.8. A 16-year-old girl with above-knee amputation 18 months previously for a distal femoral osteogenic sarcoma. Follow-up CT viewed with a narrow window width shows a heavily ossified metastasis from the osteogenic sarcoma in the right ventricle. This study emphasizes the technical point that all patients undergoing chest CT in the search for pulmonary metastases should have the image viewed with both a wide and narrow window width. (Daneman et al. 1983 [13])

found only ten cases reported with cardiac metastases caused by osteogenic sarcoma. In 1981, Dunnick et al. [14] reported another case in which the antemortem diagnosis was confirmed by CT. The CT appearance in this patient was similar to that noted in our two patients. In 1982, Seibert et al. [36] reported three additional cases of cardiac metastases and reviewed the literature

of those cases which had been reported in detail previously. These authors found that the cardiac metastases from osteogenic sarcoma are much more commonly found on the right side of the heart than on the left and that intracavitary lesions are more common than lesions in the wall of the heart. Lesions in the epicardium are unusual. One patient had lesions on both sides of the heart. In 1982, Romeo et al. [34] reported the only other case in whom an ossified cardiac metastasis was faintly visible on a plain chest radiograph.

The symptoms and signs of cardiac metastases are nonspecific [14, 36] and often disproportionately few compared with the large size of many of the lesions. The prognosis is usually poor, but surgical resection has been reported in some patients [14]. Although a solitary cardiac metastasis has been reported [12], widespread metastatic disease is usually present at the time of diagnosis [12, 14]. With the use of more aggressive therapy, antemortem detection of cardiac metastases may become clinically significant [14].

Tumor thrombi may extend up the inferior vena cava and into the heart as well (Fig. 4.9). In children, this may be seen in patients with Wilms' tumor or adrenal carcinoma. Indeed, calcified Wilms' tumor has been documented on CT in the inferior vena cava. We have had the opportunity to perform CT of the chest in a patient with Wilms' tumor in whom cardiac catheterization had been attempted previously. Contrast was injected directly into the tumor thrombus, which extended from the right renal vein up the inferior vena cava and into the right atrium. On CT, the

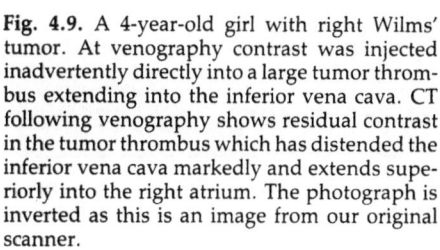

Fig. 4.9. A 4-year-old girl with right Wilms' tumor. At venography contrast was injected inadvertently directly into a large tumor thrombus extending into the inferior vena cava. CT following venography shows residual contrast in the tumor thrombus which has distended the inferior vena cava markedly and extends superiorly into the right atrium. The photograph is inverted as this is an image from our original scanner.

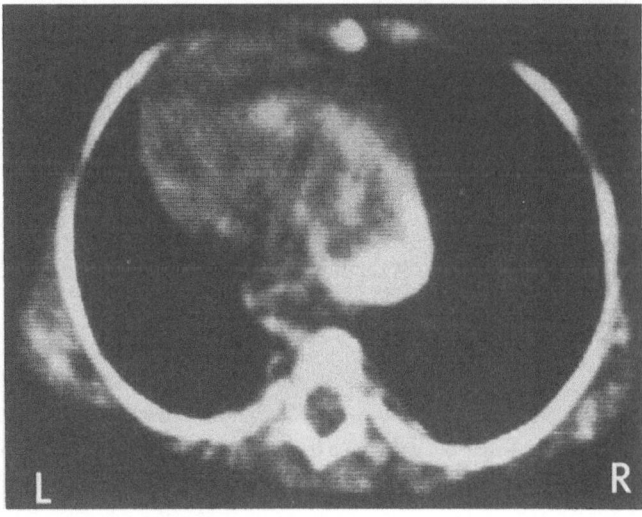

contrast could be seen in the tissue of the tumor thrombus within the inferior vena cava and the right atrium (Fig. 4.9). The high-density resolution of CT is valuable for detection of catheters that break and become lodged in the great vessels but cannot be detected on plain radiographs (Fig. 4.10).

Mediastinal Masses

In children, the mediastinum is the commonest site for thoracic mass lesions. One-third of all mediastinal masses occur in patients under 15 years of age, and three-quarters of children with mediastinal masses have at least mild symptoms [26]. This may be due to the relatively small size of the thorax and the higher frequency of malignant lesions as compared with adults, as well as the large size of many tumors when they present.

Computed tomography plays a major role in delineating the nature and extent of mediastinal mass lesions in children. The lesion is shown free of overlap of surrounding structures. Often a specific diagnosis is possible based on the CT findings, as the site of origin of the lesion is usually easily documented and its attenuation coefficients readily measured. CT is also critical in assessing the response of mediastinal mass lesions to chemotherapy and/or radiotherapy and also in assessing the mediastinum postoperatively in the search for early recurrent lesions. With many malignant mass lesions of the mediastinum the entire thorax should be scanned to assess the lungs for metastatic disease rather than confining the examination to the area of the mass.

The causes of mediastinal masses are summarized in Table 4.1.

Anterior Mediastinum

Of all pediatric mediastinal tumors at the Hospital for Sick Children, Toronto, 35% occur in the anterior mediastinum. Most of these are malignant lesions and arise in the thymus and lymph nodes.

Benign

Inflammatory lesions of the anterior mediastinum are indeed rare. We have had the opportunity to study four cases of anterior mediastinal abscesses. In all cases CT was extremely useful in the delineation of the exact extent of the lesion. Abscesses fail to enhance centrally but may have an enhancing rim, and the presence of gas within the abscess (Fig. 4.11) helps to confirm the diagnosis.

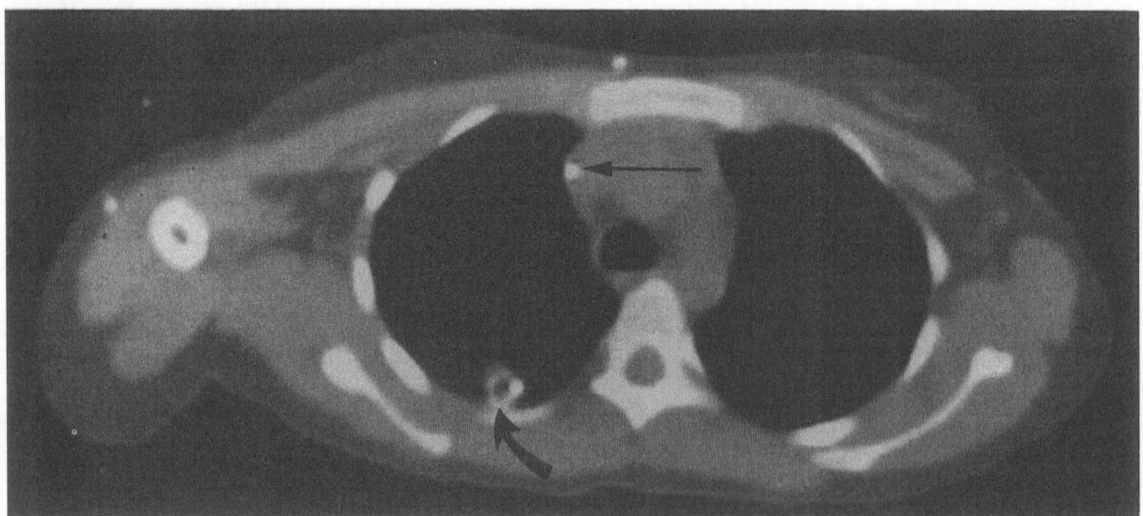

Fig. 4.10. A 12-year-old girl with a broken fragment of catheter from a central venous line (*arrow*) passing from the superior vena cava into the right atrium. This fragment could not be visualized on plain radiographs but is easily noted on CT. *Curved arrow*, intercostal drain.

Table 4.1. Causes of mediastinal masses

Anterior
1. Thymus
   a) normal prominent thymus
   b) cyst
   c) thymoma
   d) lymphoma
   e) leukemia
2. Lymph nodes
   a) non-Hodgkin's and Hodgkin's lymphoma
   b) histiocytosis
   c) leukemia
3. Teratoma and other germ cell tumors
4. Others
   a) lipoma
   b) cystic hygroma
   c) abscesses

Middle
1. Bronchopulmonary foregut malformations
   (cysts, duplications, sequestration)
2. Lymphadenopathy
   a) inflammatory
   b) malignant

Posterior
1. Neurogenic
   a) neuroblastoma
   b) ganglioneuroma
   c) pheochromocytoma
   d) neurofibroma
2. Soft tissue sarcomas
3. Vertebral neoplasms
4. Hemangiomas
5. Inflammatory abscesses
6. Neurenteric cysts

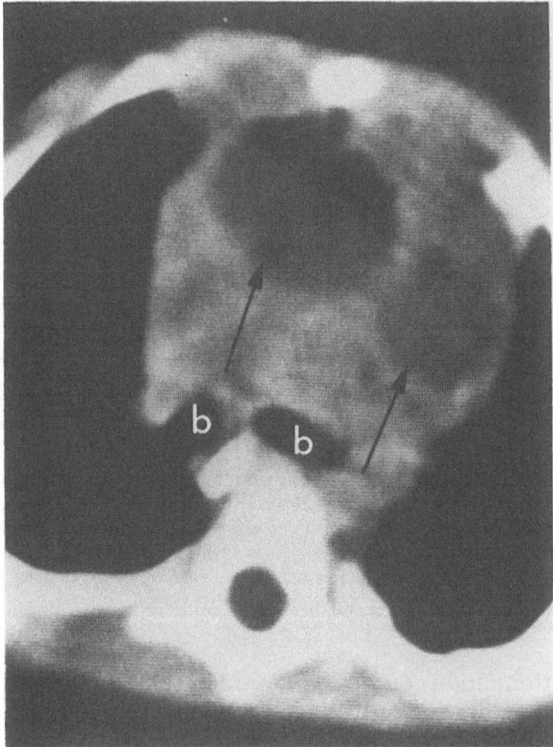

Fig. 4.11. A 6-month-old boy with two large anterior mediastinal abscesses (*arrows*) following a traumatic laryngoscopy for subglottic stenosis. The scan has been performed after the intravenous injection of contrast material. The abscesses have failed to enhance and have extremely irregular outlines. *b*, major bronchi.

Teratomas are a less common cause of anterior mediastinal masses in children than are lymphomas. The presence of calcification, fat, or cystic areas within the mass is highly suggestive of a benign teratoma rather than a lymphoma (Figs. 4.12, 4.13). The more solid portions of the mass may enhance with intravenous contrast administration. Occasionally, the entire mass may just appear as a solid soft tissue lesion without any of the other features described above, and in these instances it is impossible to make a differentiation from lymphoma.

The high-density resolution of CT can also help to characterize other rare masses of the anterior mediastinum. The fatty density of lipomas (Fig. 4,.14) and the fluid characteristics of lymphangiomas may be extremely well delineated on CT, as well as the extent of the masses.

Malignant

The commonest cause of an anterior mediastinal mass is lymphoma; this is usually seen in children early in the second decade of life but may be seen at any time after infancy. Malignant lymphoma may be of Hodgkin or non-Hodgkin type (Figs. 4.15–4.17). The commonest type of Hodgkin's disease in children in the anterior mediastinum is the nodular sclerosing type, but the others (mixed cellularity, lymphocyte predominant, and lymphocyte depleted) are occasionally seen. The non-Hodgkin type of lymphoma includes Burkitt's, histiocytic, T cell, and poorly differentiated types [26]. It has been reported that 60% of children with Hodgkin's disease and almost 40% of those with non-Hodgkin's lymphoma present with enlarged nodes on chest radiographs [26]. The vast majority of these involve the anterior mediastinum; less commonly the middle mediastinum is involved.

On CT these masses appear as lobulated soft tissue lesions in the anterior mediastinum. Extension may occasionally be seen into the middle mediastinum or up into the neck. The soft tissue masses have a fairly homogeneous

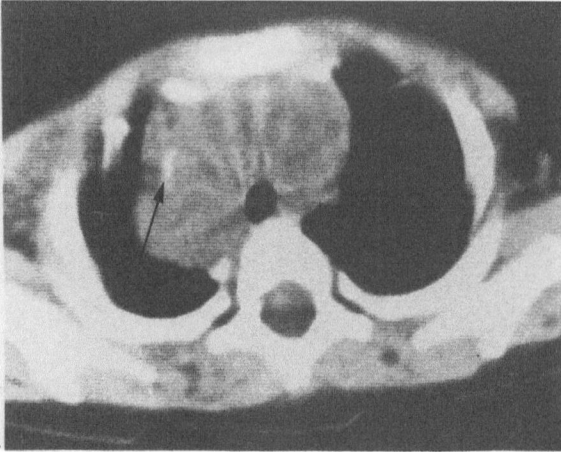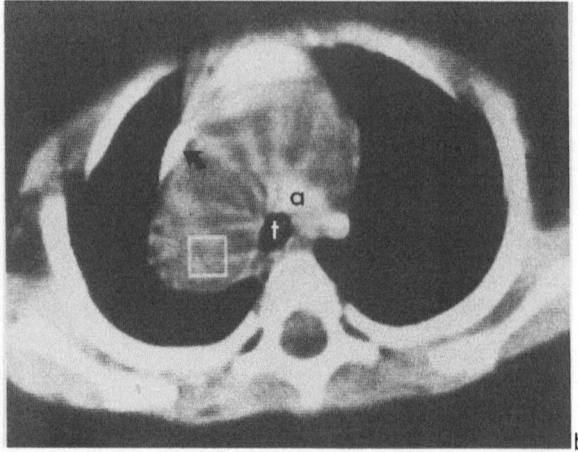

Fig. 4.12a,b. A 1-year-old boy with large anterior mediastinal benign dermoid. Scans before (**a**) and during (**b**) intravenous contrast injection. A large anterior mediastinal mass is present and this extends posteriorly toward the right. **a** A curvilinear area of calcification is noted in the right side of the mass (*arrow*). **b** The relationship of the mass to the adjacent major vessels of the upper mediastinum is clearly visible. The mass extends posteriorly between the superior vena cava (*curved arrow*) and aortic arch (*a*) and trachea (*t*). There were no cystic or fatty elements in this dermoid lesion.

attenuation on CT and enhance, sometimes quite dramatically (Fig. 4.15). Often there are areas of lower attenuation within these masses, and these are better seen after intravenous contrast injection (see Fig. 20.8, p.302). Occasionally, large necrotic areas may be present. Calcification is not a feature of these masses and may be seen occasionally following chemotherapy and/or radiotherapy (Fig. 4.18).

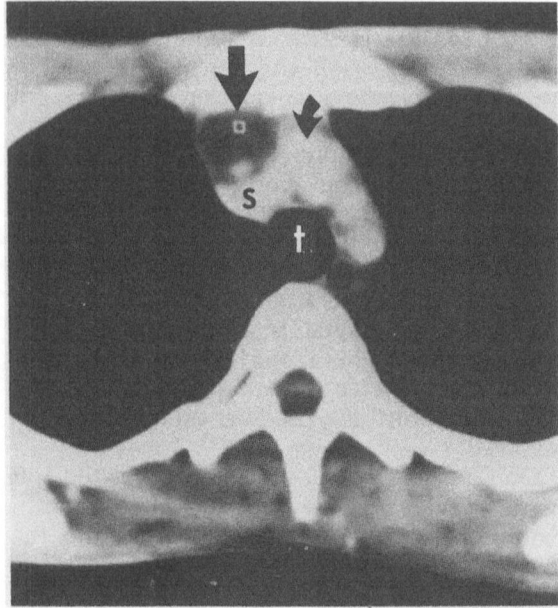

In the investigation of patients with anterior mediastinal masses, CT is valuable, offering information that may not be obtained with more conventional radiographic techniques. The finding of calcification or fat within the mass is more in keeping with a teratoma than with lymphoma. CT delineates the exact extent of the mass well and may give valuable information with regard to the radiotherapy that is necessary. Posterior extension and extension into the chest wall may not be appreciated on plain radiographs but will be easily noted on CT, for example in the patient with histiocytosis X shown in Fig. 4.19. The effects of the mass on the airway, which may not be apparent on more conventional techniques, are readily assessed. Small pleural effusions may also be evident. In patients with Hodgkin's disease the entire chest and abdomen are studied with CT in an attempt to document the presence or absence of associated lung nodules and enlarged nodes in other areas, particularly the retroperitoneum. Follow-up scans in patients with lymphomas are mandatory, as CT is the most accurate means of assessing response to therapy (see Fig. 4.18).

Fig. 4.13. A 12-year-old boy with anterior mediastinal benign dermoid (*large arrow*). The mass is easily visualized lying anterior to the superior vena cava (*s*). *Curved arrow* indicates the three major branches of the aortic arch. *t*, trachea. A small amount of globular calcification is noted in the posterior part of the mass. No fatty elements were present.

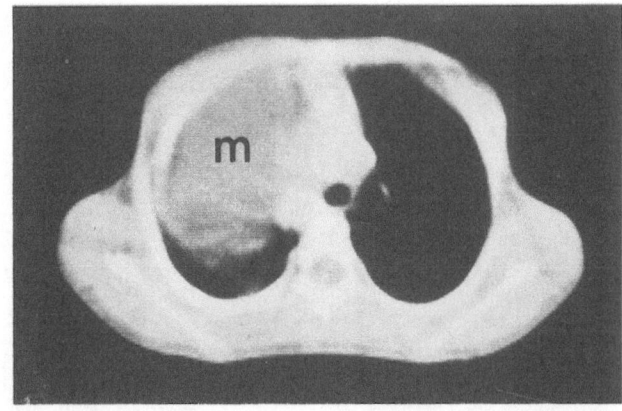

Fig. 4.14. A large lipoma (*m*) is noted extending from the anterior mediastinum far over toward the left. The measurements in this lesion were negative values throughout. The photograph is inverted as this is an image from our original scanner.

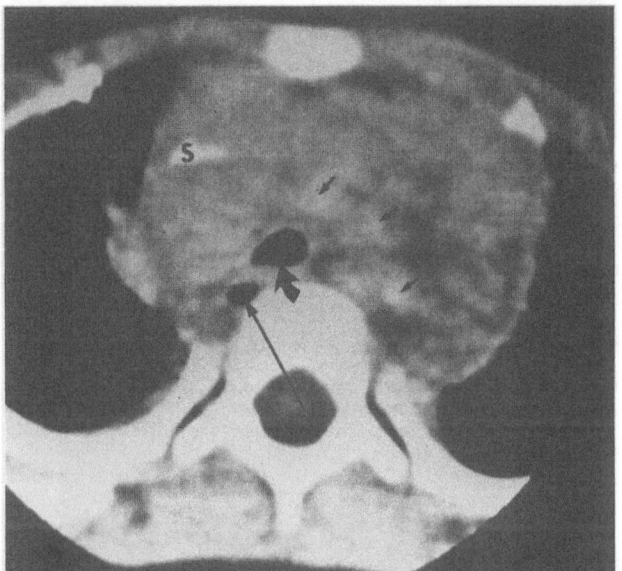

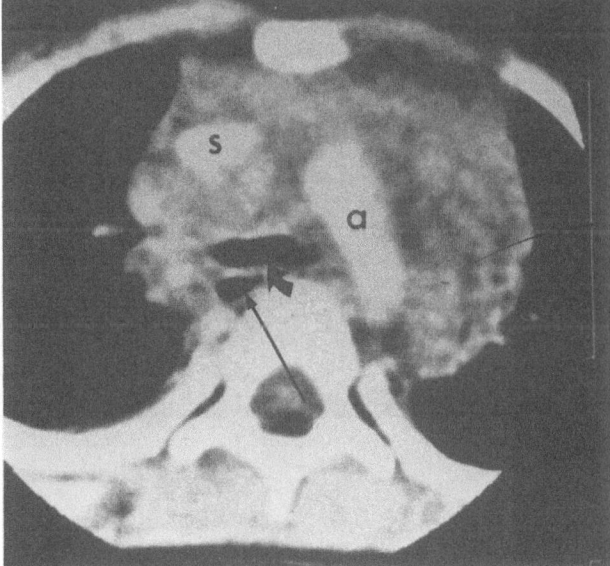

Fig. 4.15a,b. A 15-month-old boy with anterior mediastinal mass caused by non-Hodgkin's lymphoma. Scans performed during intravenous contrast injection. The mass has an inhomogeneous attenuation. **a** The mass infiltrates between the branches of the aortic arch (*small arrows*) and behind the superior vena cava (*s*) and compresses the right side of the trachea (*curved arrow*). **b** The mass extends far over to the left side of the aortic arch (*a*) and infiltrates between the arch and the superior vena cava (*s*) and compresses the region of the carina (*curved arrow*). *Long arrow*, gas-filled esophagus.

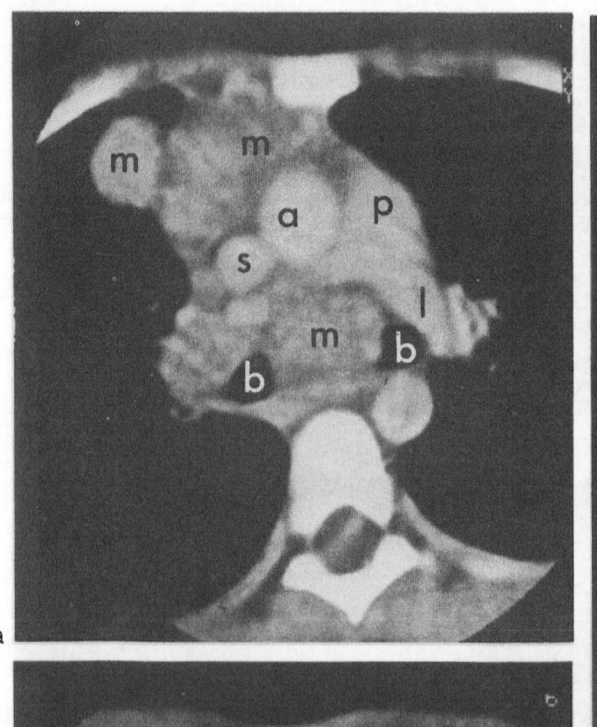

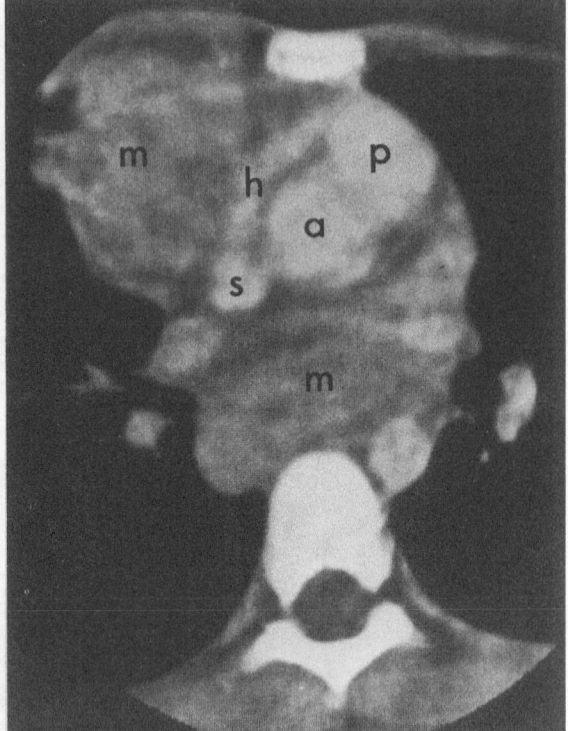

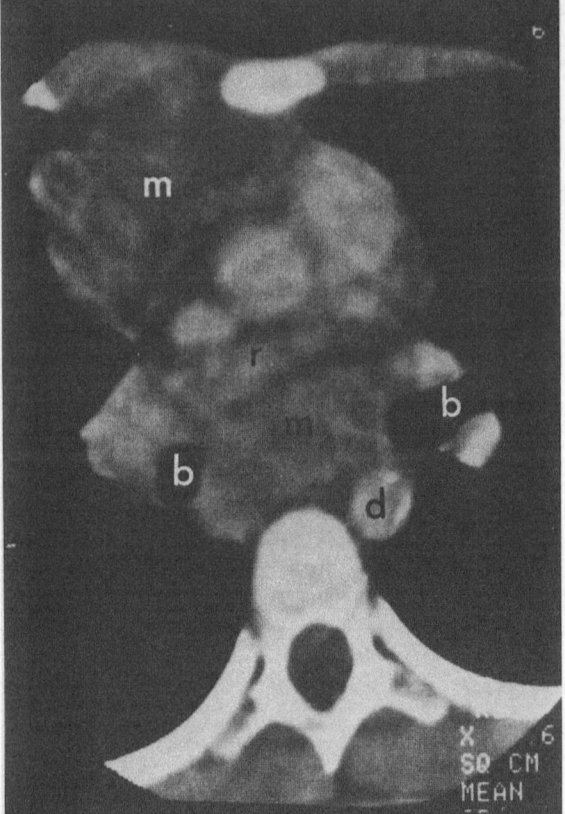

Fig. 4.16a–c. A 14-year-old boy with Hodgkin's disease. Large masses (*m*) are noted in the scans, which were performed during the intravenous injection of contrast. These lesions are noted mainly in the anterior and middle mediastinum. Large subcarinal lymph nodes are noted in **a** between the major bronchi (*b*). The exact extent of the disease is exquisitely shown in these transverse images. *s*, superior vena cava; *a* aortic root; *p*, main pulmonary artery; *l*, left pulmonary artery; *r*, right pulmonary artery; *d*, descending aorta; *h*, right atrium.

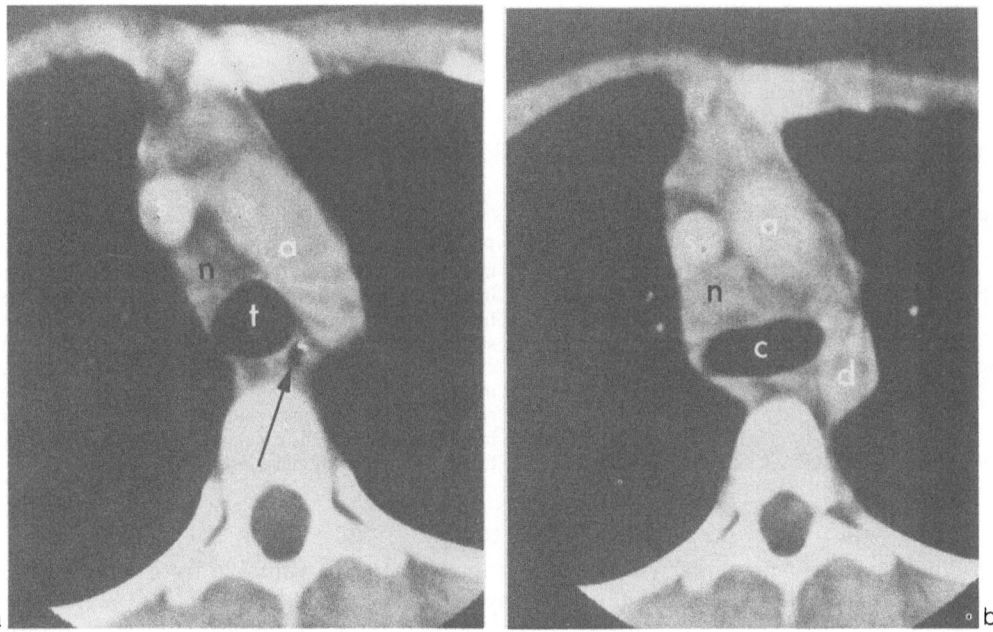

Fig. 4.17a,b. A 12-year-old girl with Hodgkin's disease. The thymus in the anterior mediastinum is nodular and there are also enlarged nodes (*n*) between the superior vena cava (*s*), aortic arch (*a*) and trachea (*t*). Note how these nodes bulge toward the right. *c*, carina; *d*, descending aorta.

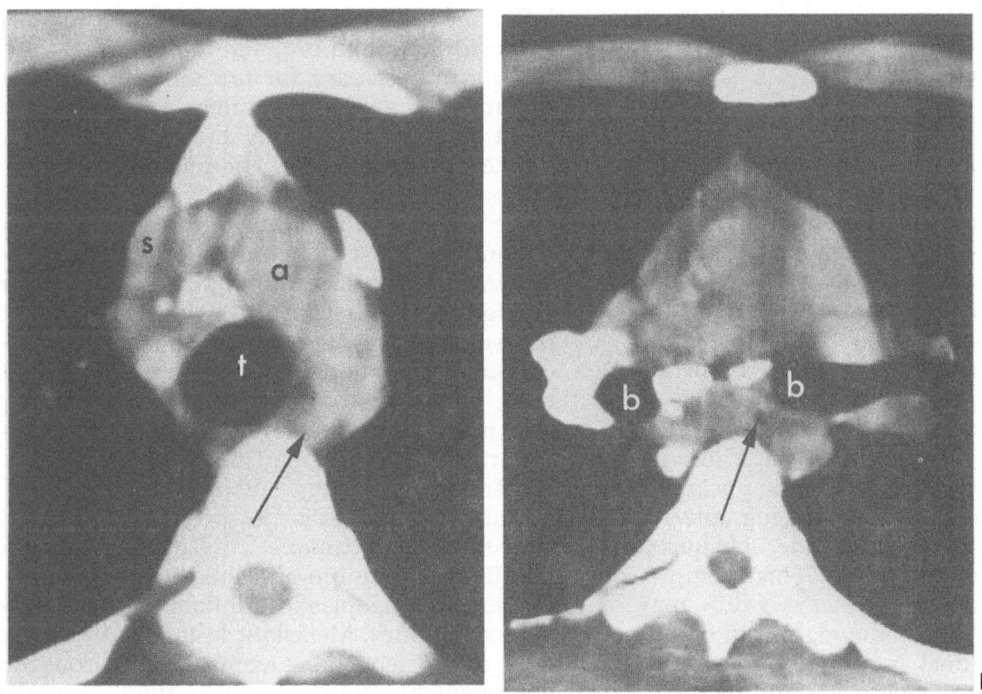

Fig. 4.18a,b. A 14-year-old boy with Hodgkin's disease who had received previous chemotherapy and radiotherapy. There is heavy calcification of the thymus and involved nodes in the mediastinum and right hilum. **a** Note the triangular calcification in the thymus. *s*, superior vena cava; *a*, aortic arch, *t*, trachea; *long arrow*, esophagus. **b** A scan performed just below the carina shows the main stem bronchi (*b*) and heavy calcification in subcarinal and right hilar nodes. The bulge to the right behind the superior vena cava in **a** and behind the right bronchus in **b** should always be considered abnormal and is usually due to enlarged nodes.

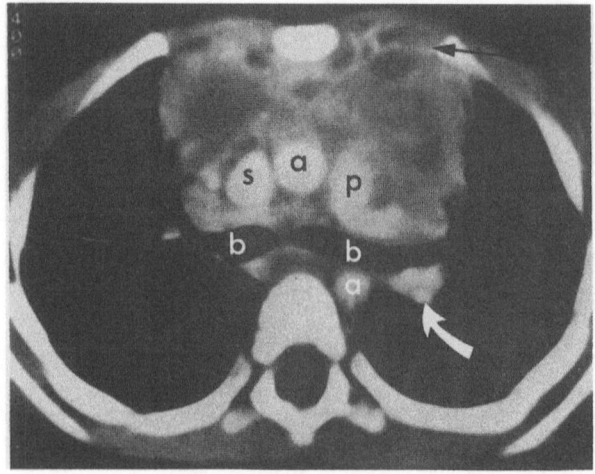

Fig. 4.19. A 6-month-old boy with anterior mediastinal mass caused by histiocytosis X. Scan performed during intravenous contrast injection shows a huge mass filling the anterior mediastinum and bulging to either side of the midline. The mass invades the anterior chest wall (*arrow*) on the left. This mass has extremely inhomogeneous attenuation values. *s*, superior vena cava; *a*, aorta; *p*, main pulmonary artery; *b*, major bronchi just below the carina; *curved arrow*, lower lobe branch of left pulmonary artery.

Leukemia in children rarely presents with a mediastinal mass such as enlargement of the thymus and pleural effusion. These features usually occur in patients with lymphomatous transformation, and mainly in those with T cell acute lymphocytic leukemia [26]. The changes noted in these masses on CT are similar to those present in patients with lymphoma.

Middle Mediastinum

In the pediatric age group, 25% of mediastinal tumors occur in the middle mediastinum. The main differential diagnosis includes lymphadenopathy and bronchopulmonary foregut malformations. Lymphadenopathy may be due either to inflammatory processes (see Fig. 4.20) or to malignant disease (metastatic, lymphoma, or leukemia; see Fig. 4.22). Bronchopulmonary foregut malformations include bronchogenic cysts, esophageal duplications (see Fig. 4.21), neurenteric cysts, and sequestration.

The nature and extent of these lesions can often be determined by their appearance on chest radiographs and esophagography. Occasionally, fluoroscopy and added oblique views may be helpful, and often CT may simply confirm the diagnosis. However, CT may be extremely useful in some regards in that it may provide additional information regarding the detailed extent of the lesion and its effects on adjacent great vessels and the airways. A mass in any of the mediastinal compartments may cause displacement, distortion, and compression of the major airway. The exact caliber of the airway can easily be assessed with CT, thus providing

the anesthetist with valuable information prior to any operative procedure.

The hila can be considered as part of the middle mediastinum as they contain the major bronchi and pulmonary vessels as they enter the lungs. Apart from enlarged vessels, masses in the hila are usually due to enlargement of nodes, which may be caused by either neoplasia or inflammation. When an unequivocal mass is noted in the hilum on plain radiographs, CT is usually unnecessary for further delineation of this mass. If an equivocal mass is present on a chest radiograph, it may be very difficult to define the mass on CT. The pulmonary vessels normally appear unexpectedly large in transverse sections in the hila, and even with intravenous contrast administration it may be extremely difficult to differentiate vessels from enlarged nodes that are not obviously larger than the surrounding vessels. For this reason, 55° oblique conventional tomograms are often of more help than CT in confirming or excluding hilar masses and should be used prior to CT [26].

Furthermore, CT may be of great value in characterizing lesions of the middle mediastinum when this is not possible with more conventional technique. Calcification in the middle mediastinum and hilar regions may be due to either neoplastic or inflammatory disease of lymph nodes. Metastatic lesions of the nodes caused by osteogenic sarcoma usually produce a homogeneous type of calcification, whereas inflammatory processes usually cause a more irregular or stippled type of calcification (Fig. 4.20). If the size of the calcification is small, it is impossible to differentiate between these two causes of calcification.

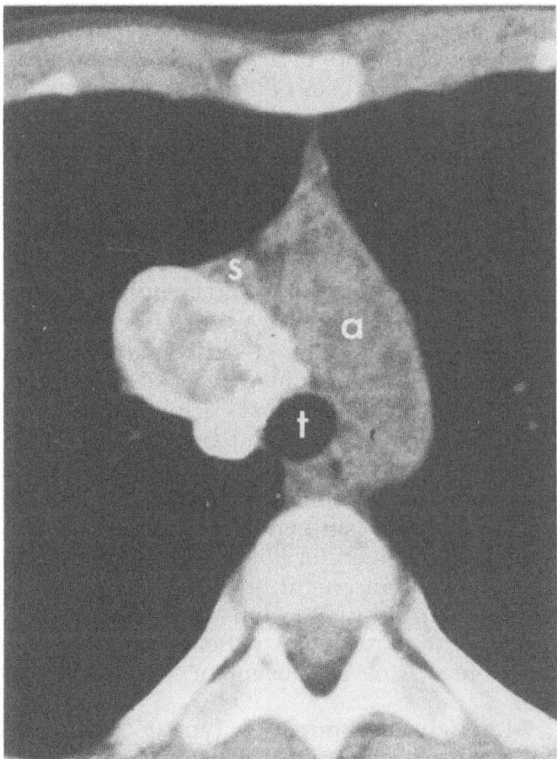

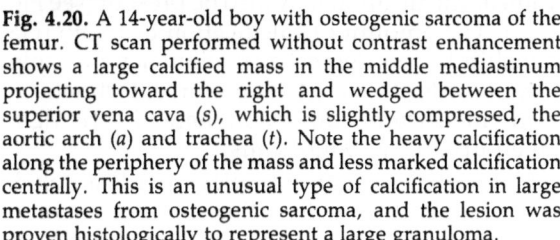

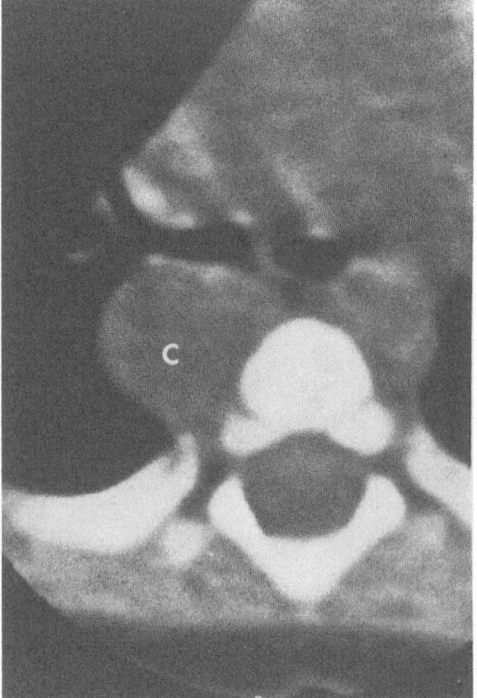

Fig. 4.20. A 14-year-old boy with osteogenic sarcoma of the femur. CT scan performed without contrast enhancement shows a large calcified mass in the middle mediastinum projecting toward the right and wedged between the superior vena cava (*s*), which is slightly compressed, the aortic arch (*a*) and trachea (*t*). Note the heavy calcification along the periphery of the mass and less marked calcification centrally. This is an unusual type of calcification in large metastases from osteogenic sarcoma, and the lesion was proven histologically to represent a large granuloma.

Bronchopulmonary foregut malformations show varying degrees of enhancement, depending on the size of the cystic component of the lesion. Bronchogenic cysts, esophageal duplications, and neurenteric cysts appear as large fluid-filled lesions, usually with only rim enhancement (Fig. 4.21). Associated vertebral anomalies may be seen with neurenteric cysts. Neurenteric cysts arise in the posterior mediastinum but may extend forward into the middle mediastinum. Lymphadenopathy may manifest as soft tissue masses within the middle mediastinum or hilar areas, having a nonspecific appearance and usually showing only a small degree of enhancement (Fig. 4.22). Scans performed during rapid bolus injection of intravenous contrast may help differentiate these masses from the adjacent vasculature of the mediastinum and hila.

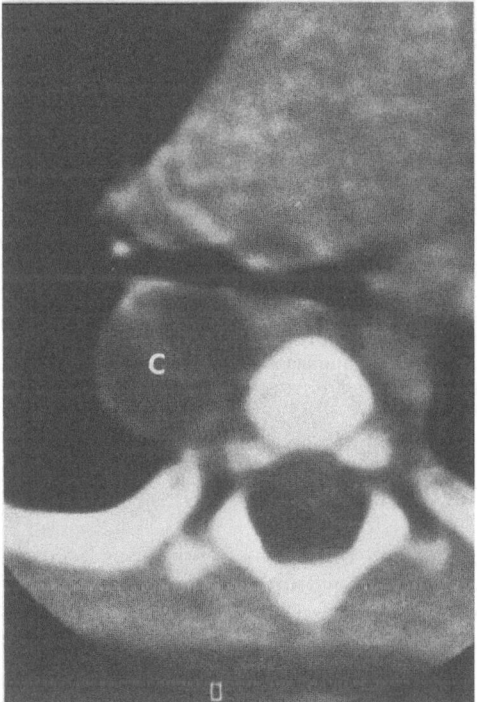

Fig. 4.21a,b. A 6-month-old girl with esophageal duplication cyst. Scans before (**a**) and after (**b**) intravenous contrast injection. The duplication cyst (*c*) is noted projecting from just behind the level of the carina in the middle mediastinum posteriorly toward the right. After intravenous contrast administration the central part of the cyst has failed to enhance, but a peripheral rim shows enhancement, particularly on the right, and represents the cyst wall.

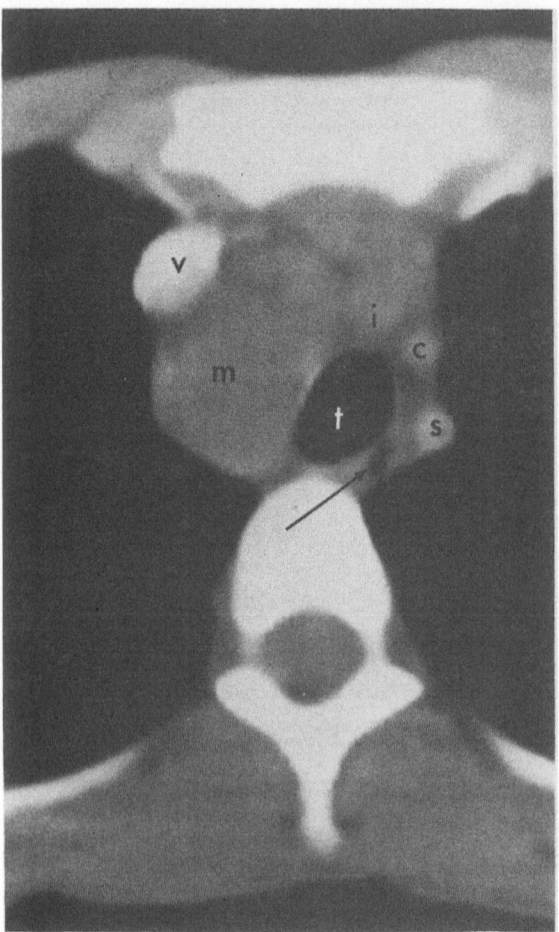

Fig. 4.22. A 16-year-old boy with previously resected hepatocellular carcinoma of the left lobe of the liver. CT performed during intravenous injection of contrast shows a large metastasis (*m*) between the superior vena cava (*v*) and trachea (*t*). There should be no convexity to the right in the outline of the mediastinum at this site. *i*, innominate artery; *c*, left common carotid artery; *s*, left subclavian artery; *long arrow*, esophagus.

Posterior Mediastinum

In children, 40% of mediastinal masses occur in the posterior mediastinum, and of these 95% are of neurogenic origin [26]. A posterior mediastinal mass in a young child should be considered a neuroblastoma until proved otherwise. Ganglioneuroblastomas and ganglioneuromas are much less common.

Neurogenic

Neoplasms arising in the sympathetic nervous system are discussed in detail in Chapter 10 (see p. 126). *Neuroblastoma* is the commonest tumor

of this group to occur in children, usually in those under 2 years of age. These lesions arise from the ganglion cells of the sympathetic chains on either side of the midline and orientate themselves in the vertical axis of the sympathetic nervous system, extending superiorly and inferiorly along the chain. Extension of the tumor may be seen into the mediastinum from the paravertebral sulci. The lesions may surround vascular structures and compress the airway. Because they arise posteriorly in the paravertebral sulci, the posterior margin of the mass is usually not outlined by air (see Figs. 4.23, 4.25, 4.26), but occasionally a lobulated tumor may extend anteriorly and may be separated from the posterior chest wall by a portion of the lung (see Fig. 4.24). These masses are usually smooth bordered and enhance occasionally in a homogeneous manner (Figs. 4.23–4.26). Inhomogeneous enhancement may be due to areas of necrosis within the lesion and may be particularly well seen in patients with ganglioneuroma. Rim enhancement has also been seen.

Although the commonest type of calcification has been described as speckled or punctate, curvilinear calcification may also be present (see Fig. 4.23). The amount of calcification bears no relationship to the degree of malignancy or benignity of the lesion or to the amount of technetium-99m methylene diphosphonate (^{99m}Tc-MDP) taken up during bone scans.

Computed tomography plays a critical role in the preoperative delineation of the extent of paravertebral thoracic neuroblastomas and also in their postoperative or post-therapeutic follow-up. CT metrizamide myelography documents extradural spread in 20% of children with neuroblastoma but no clinical neurological evidence of extradural spread or nerve compression. It is important that children with such extradural components to the mass have an initial decompression laminectomy prior to thoracotomy for removal of the mediastinal mass. The laminectomy prevents neurological morbidity related to bleeding from the residual extradural tumor. Because of this the CT study should be performed only after a small volume (2–7 ml) of metrizamide has been instilled into the subarachnoid space. This contrast outlines the dural sac and spinal cord exceptionally well on CT and delineates the presence or absence of extradural spread. Although the tumor may be shaped like a dumb-bell, with the extradural component causing cord compression, the extradural tumor will often extend for many segments beyond the

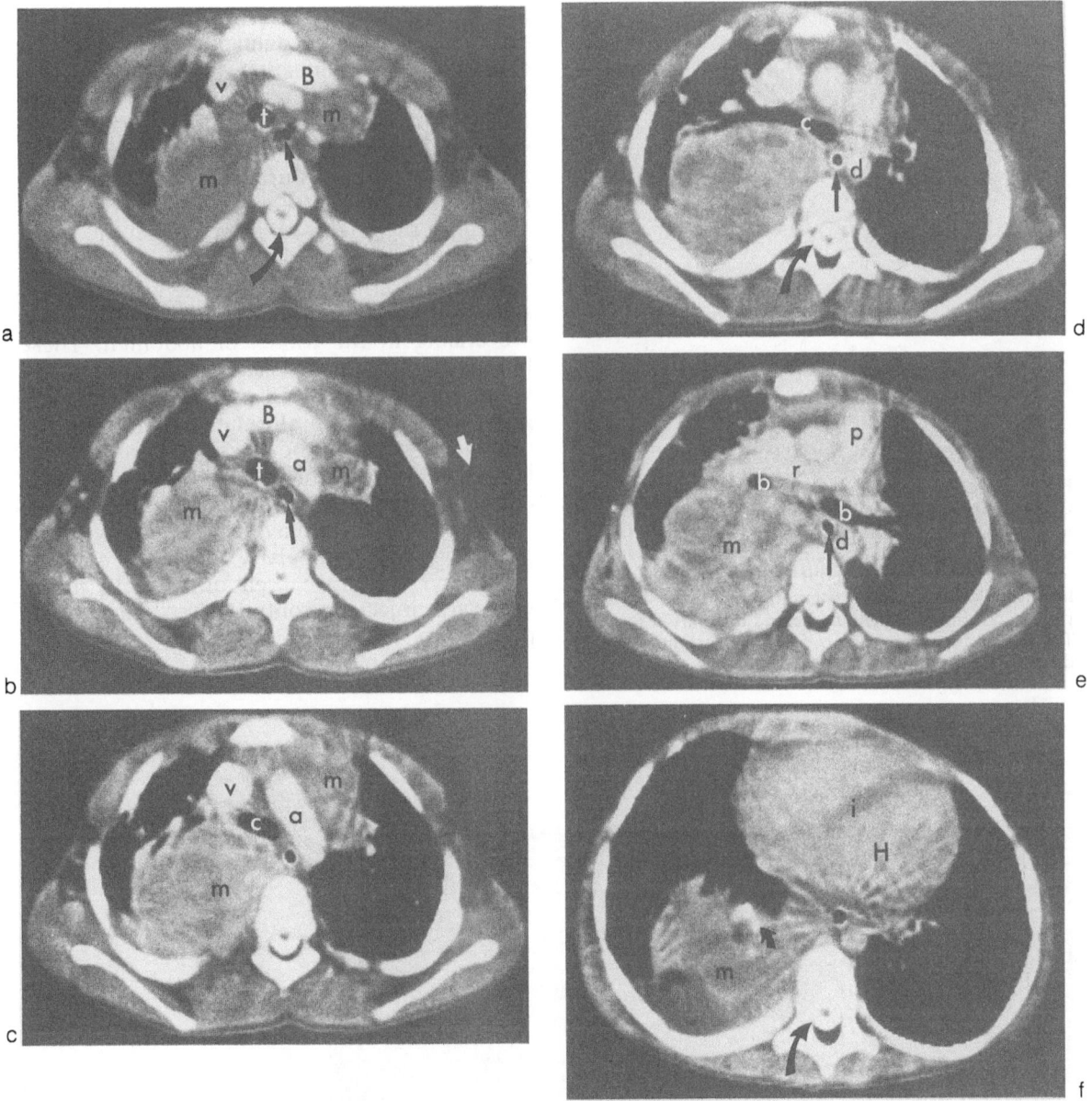

Fig. 4.23a–f. A 3-year-old boy with respiratory distress caused by a large thoracic neuroblastoma. All scans were performed after the injection of metrizamide intrathecally. The dural sac (*curved arrow*) is well outlined and shows no asymmetry or displacement to suggest intraspinal extension. These scans were performed during the injection of intravenous contrast material and the major vessels of the upper thorax have been well outlined. The mass (*m*) is easily seen in the right posterior mediastinum and its relationship to the vessels is easily visualized. A small amount of calcification (*short curved arrow*) is noted in **f**. Note that in the upper scans (**a–c**) the mass extends across the midline to bulge to the left of the mediastinum. *t*, trachea; *c*, carina; *b*, major bronchi; *short straight arrow*, feeding tube in esophagus; *a*, aortic arch; *d*, descending aorta; *v*, superior vena cava; *B*, brachiocephalic vein; *H*, heart; *i*, interventricular septum; *r*, right pulmonary artery.

level of the primary tumor as a sheet of cells displacing the subarachnoid space. Indeed, the area of maximal compression of the spinal cord may be at a distance several vertebral levels from the primary intrathoracic mass lesion. These changes are ideally demonstrated with CT.

The CT scan should be performed during a rapid bolus injection of intravenous contrast material in order that the vasculature of the mediastinum be outlined maximally (see Fig. 4.23). In this way the exact relationship of the mass to the major vessels of the mediastinum

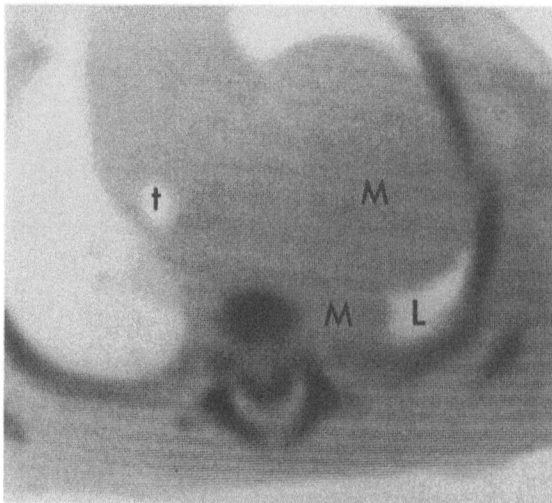

Fig. 4.24. A 6-week-old boy with respiratory tract infection. Chest radiograph revealed large left posterior mediastinal mass with tracheal shift. CT was performed after intrathecal injection of metrizamide. The mass (*M*) is noted extending forward from the left posterior mediastinal area. Note the large lobule of the mass extending anterolaterally with a portion of lung (*L*) extending behind this part of the mass. This is an unusual appearance for neuroblastoma. *t*, trachea displaced toward the right.

and the extension of the mass into the mediastinum will be best delineated. The study of choice in the delineation of thoracic neuroblastomas is thus a CT scan performed after prior injection of metrizamide into the subarachnoid space and with simultaneous bolus injection of intravenous contrast during scanning. This technique will demonstrate any extradural extension as well as the effects of the tumor on the mediastinal vasculature and airway.

It may be difficult to determine whether masses occurring at the thoracoabdominal junction are arising in the thorax or abdomen. These lesions are often neuroblastomas and the transverse axial images of CT may provide the surgeon with detailed information regarding the origin and extent of the mass [19]. Masses lying lateral to the diaphragmatic crura are intra-abdominal. Extension of such lesions deep to the crura into the chest may occur and is well displayed by CT, particularly when the azygous veins and aorta are well outlined by intravenously injected contrast (see Fig. 10.5a, p. 130).

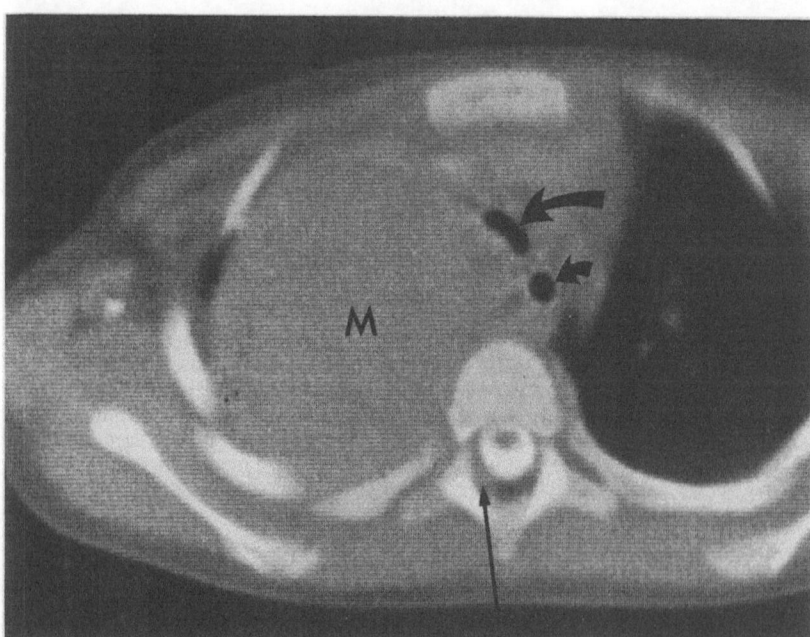

Fig. 4.25. A 2-year-old girl with thoracic neuroblastoma. Note the large mass (*M*) filling the right hemithorax. The carina (*long curved arrow*) is displaced forward and to the left. The esophagus (*short curved arrow*) is displaced forward and to the left. The scan was performed after the injection of intravenous contrast material, and the relationship of the mass to the vasculature cannot be well visualized. *Long straight* arrow shows intraspinal extension of tumor causing subtle asymmetry of the dural sac.

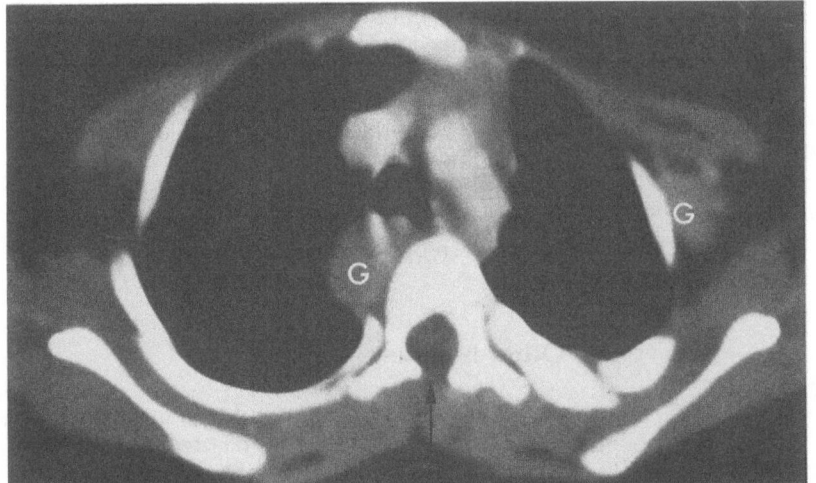

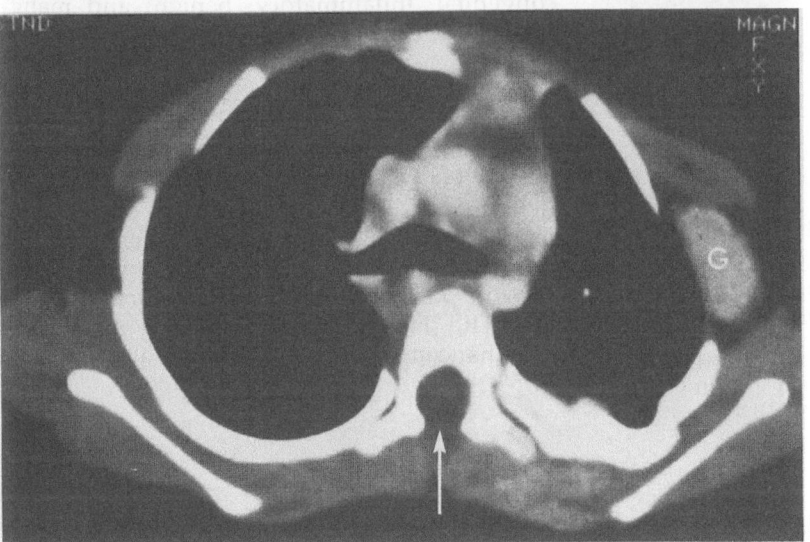

Fig. 4.26a,b. A 4-year-old girl with previously removed left cervicothoracic neuroblastoma with intraspinal extension. The laminectomy defect is noted posteriorly (*arrow*). Recurrent masses are noted in the right paravertebral area and left axilla (G). These lesions were thought to represent recurrent neuroblastoma and increased in size despite chemotherapy. Surgical removal of both masses showed the presence of benign ganglioneuroma with no recurrent malignant elements.

Ganglioneuroma may have the same appearance on CT as neuroblastoma (see Fig. 4.26). Indeed, some neuroblastomas may mature into the benign ganglioneuroma. We have seen two ganglioneuromas that have continued to grow. This growth, however, does not indicate the persistence of malignant disease, and the histology of such lesions should not be predicted from the CT appearances but rather by histological technique.

Pheochromocytomas of the chest are uncommon (Fig. 4.27); thus routine chest CT is not performed unless a lesion is suspected on a chest radiograph or unless the abdominal and pelvic CT reveals no lesion but there is still strong clinical and biochemical evidence of pheochromocytoma. We consider it wise to perform chest CT in the latter situation, although we are not aware of an instance in which the diagnosis of pheochromocytoma has been made on CT in the presence of a negative chest radiograph. In the rare cases of malignant abdominal pheochromocytoma, chest CT is of value in determining the presence or absence of metastatic disease in the lungs (see also Chap. 10, p. 135).

Neurofibromas of the nerves of the chest are very much less common in children than in adults. These lesions may occur in patients with

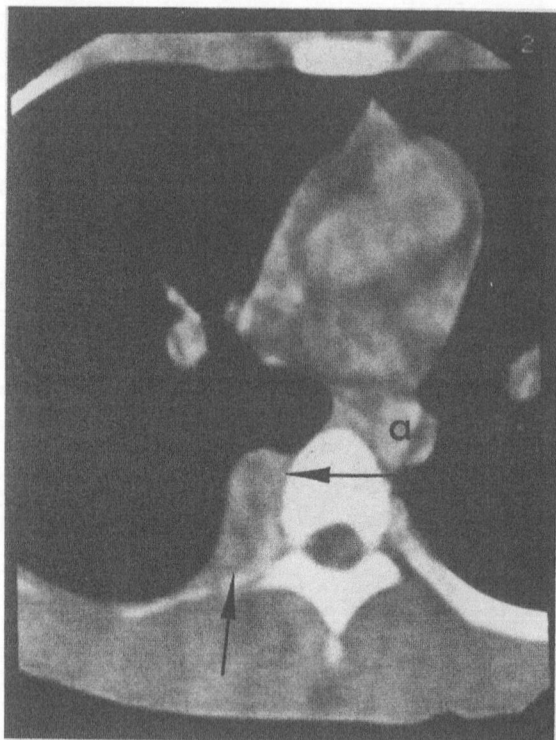

Fig. 4.27. A 17-year-old boy with previous abdominal pheo-chromocytoma. Patient presented again with hypertension and a chest radiograph showed a right paravertebral mass. This mass is delineated on CT (*arrows*). *a*, aorta. A further mass was noted in the left adrenal at this time. This patient is an example of a child with multiple recurrent pheo-chromocytomas but with no family history or associated endocrine syndrome.

Von Recklinghausen's disease and on CT have a somewhat nonspecific appearance (Fig. 4.28). Neurofibromatosis may also cause nodular swelling of the intercostal nerves which may appear as lobulated densities deep to the ribs (see Fig. 6.10, p. 76).

Neurenteric cysts may present in this compartment and appear as cystic structures. Their associated vertebral anomalies are easily seen.

Other Masses

At the Hospital for Sick Children in Toronto we have seen several rare lesions presenting as posterior mediastinal masses. These have included congenital, inflammatory, benign, and malignant neoplasms [9].

An unusual inflammatory process was seen in a neonate with staphylococcal osteomyelitis of a cervical vertebra which became dislodged and formed a large abscess in the posterior mediastinum (Fig. 4.29). Post-thoracotomy complications may also present as posterior mediastinal masses (Fig. 4.30). Congenital lesions such as bronchogenic cysts [23] (Fig. 4.31) very rarely present posteriorly, and pulmonary sequestrations [10] (Fig. 4.32) may show varying degrees of enhancement in the mass (see also Fig. 5.4, p. 58).

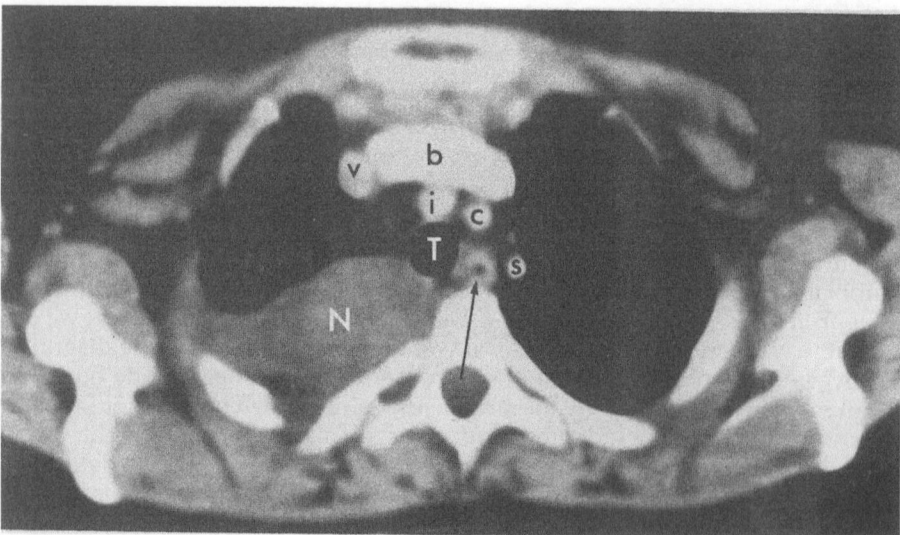

Fig. 4.28. A 17-year-old boy with neurofibromatosis and a large paravertebral neurofibroma (*N*). The enhancement of this lesion is a little inhomogeneous. *T*, trachea; *arrow*, esophagus; *v*, superior vena cava; *b*, brachiocephalic vein; *i*, innominate artery; *c*, left common carotid artery; *s*, left subclavian artery.

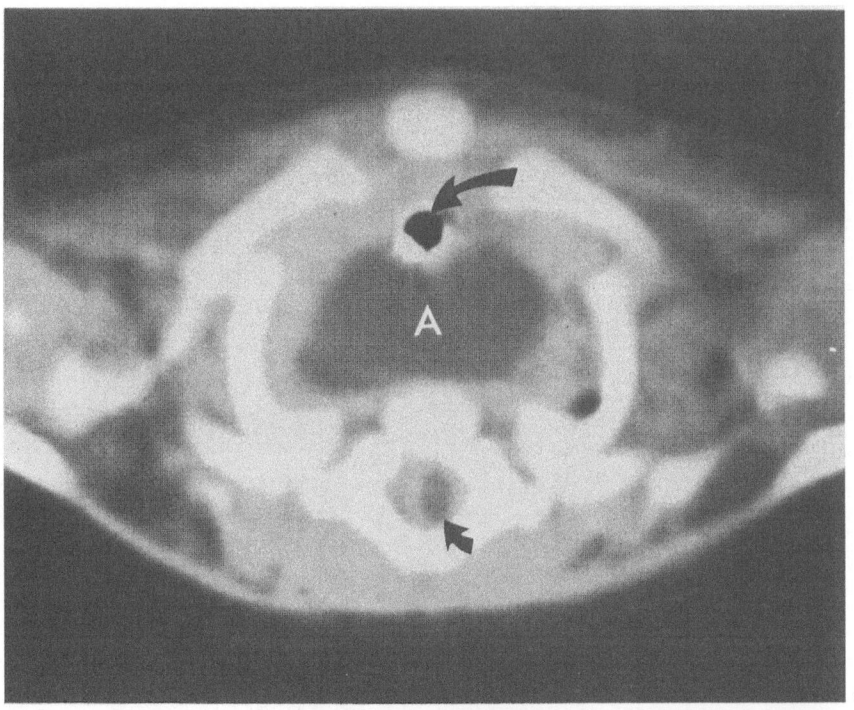

a

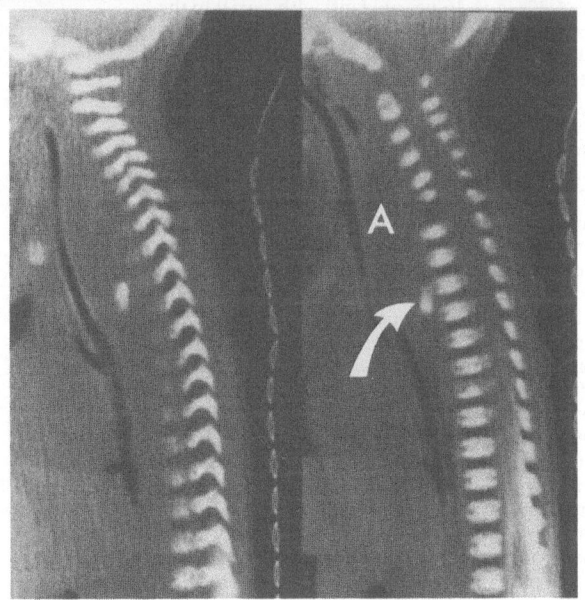

b

Fig. 4.29a,b. Neonate with severe respiratory distress and fever. **a** CT following intravenous injection of contrast material shows a large posterior mediastinal mass (*A*) that has failed to enhance and has displaced the trachea containing an endotracheal tube forward (*long curved arrow*). This large mass represents a large posterior mediastinal abscess which is almost filling the thoracic inlet. Note the asymmetry of the tissues in the spinal canal. The low attenuation mass on the left (*short curved arrow*) represents extension of the abscess into the spinal canal. **b** Direct sagittal views of the cervicothoracic spine show displacement of the trachea forward by the mediastinal abscess (*A*). The body of C–6 is smaller than normal, and there is a defect in the position where the body of C–7 should be. The *curved arrow* indicates the body of C–7, which has been displaced into this position as the result of the erosion and destruction from the abscess. The inflammatory process was considered to originate from an osteomyelitis involving the vertebral column.

Cellular hemangioma of infancy has a non-specific appearance (Fig. 4.33), and a lymphangioma (Fig. 4.34) had the typical appearances of a cystic fluid-filled mass. Metastatic disease may rarely present as a posterior mediastinal mass (Fig. 4.35). We have also seen lesions extending from adjacent areas into the posterior mediastinum and presenting as a posterior mediastinal mass; these have included hemangiomas of the chest wall and neoplasms of vertebral bodies, including Ewing's sarcoma, chondrosarcoma, and anaplastic sarcoma.

Any patient with a mediastinal mass who has either clinical or radiological evidence of extradural spread should be examined in the manner described above for the delineation of the extent

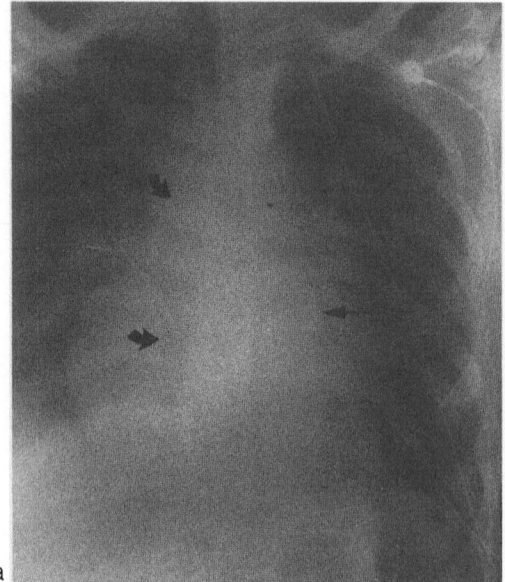

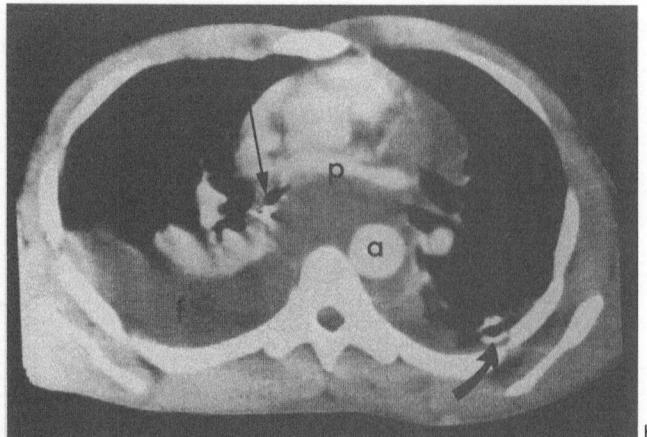

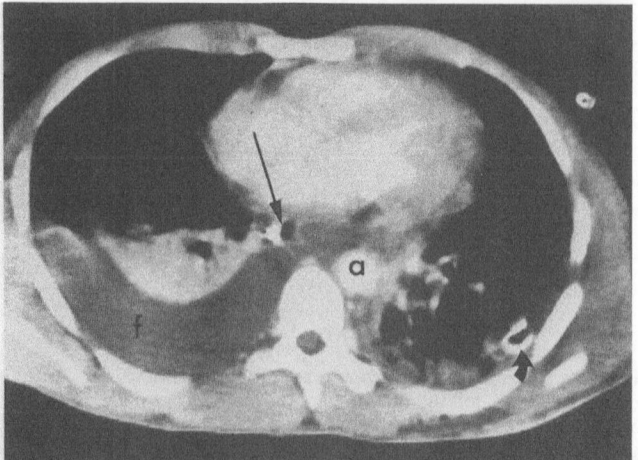

Fig. 4.30a–c. A 16-year-old girl with a graft to the descending aorta. **a** Postoperative chest radiograph shows a soft tissue mass in the posterior mediastinum extending to the left (*straight arrow*). The *short curved arrows* show the displacement of the nasogastric tube in the esophagus toward the right. It was felt that this might represent a large leak from the area of the graft and a CT was thus performed. **b, c** Scans performed during intravenous contrast injection delineate the position of the aorta (*a*), the nasogastric tube, and air filling the esophagus, which has been displaced anteriorly and to the right (*long arrow*). A large amount of fluid is present around the aorta in the posterior mediastinum, forming a mass which displaces the pulmonary veins (*p*) forward. Further fluid (*f*) is noted collecting in the pleural cavities, particularly on the right, and there is also some basal collapse. These transverse scans delineated the relationships of the structures in the mediastinum, provided useful clinical information, and excluded a leak from the graft. **d** Another example of the value of CT in the postoperative period. Following a Blalock–Taussig bypass for tetralogy of Fallot, a chest radiograph showed a left mediastinal mass. CT shows the mass to be a seroma (*s*) adjacent to the graft. Note right-sided descending aorta (*a*) and intercostal drain (*curved arrow*).

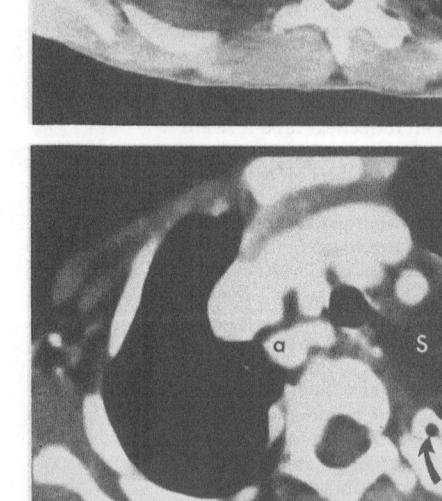

of neuroblastoma, i.e., with intrathecal metrizamide and bolus injection of intravenous contrast material. Indeed, in some patients in whom a mass lesion has been noted on plain radiographs as lying close to the vertebral column but in whom there has been no definite clinical or radiological evidence of extradural spread we have felt it prudent to perform the CT with metrizamide in the subarachnoid space as a precautionary measure.

ↄ

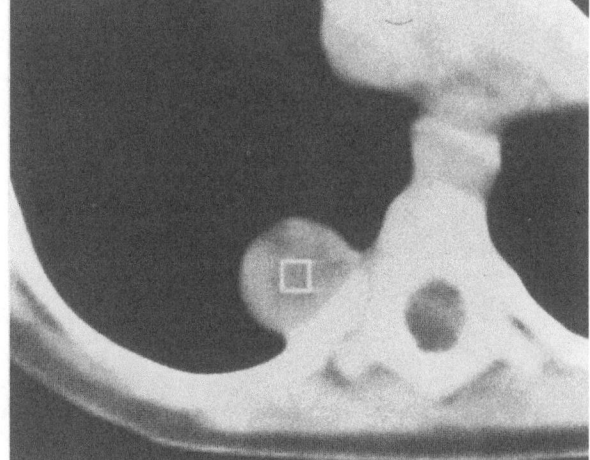

Fig. 4.31. A 2-year-old boy with bronchogenic cyst (*square cursor*). This cyst presented as a posterior mediastinal mass, which is a somewhat unusual position for these lesions.

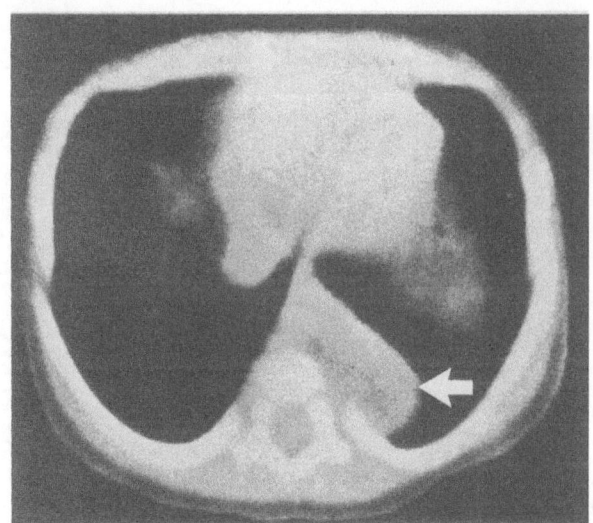

Fig. 4.32. Neonate with soft tissue mass in the left chest on a chest radiograph. This mass (*arrow*) was proven to represent a sequestration involving the lower lobe of the left lung.

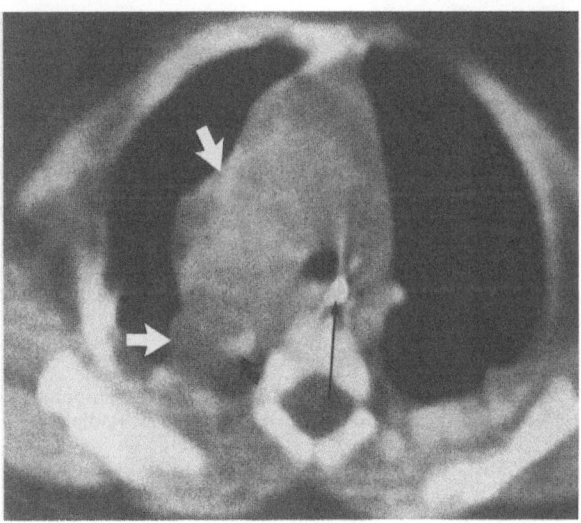

Fig. 4.33. A 15-month-old girl with respiratory distress caused by a large cellular hemangioma of infancy. The scan shows the large mass filling the posterior mediastinum ᴑn the right (*white arrows*). Posteriorly some calcification (*curved black arrow*) is present. Note the slight distortion of the trachea caused by the mass. *Long arrow*, feeding tube in esophagus.

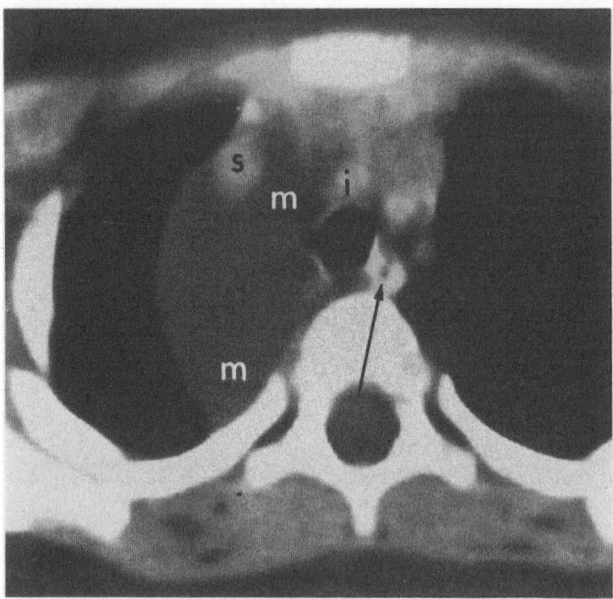

Fig. 4.34. A 3-year-old boy with right posterior mediastinal mass caused by a lymphangioma. CT performed during the intravenous injection of contrast material shows the mass (*m*) extending from the right posterior mediastinum forward between the superior vena cava (*s*) and the innominate artery (*i*). There is no enhancement in this lesion. *Long arrow,* esophagus to the left of the trachea.

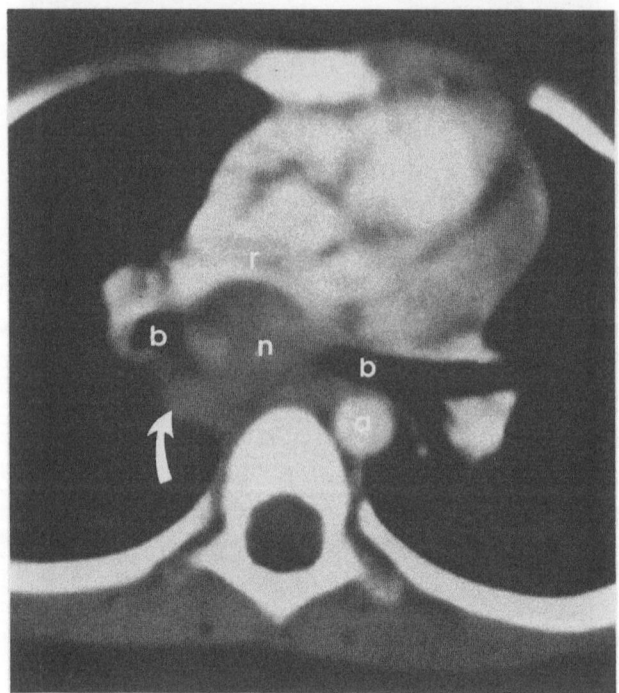

Fig. 4.35. A 2-year-old girl with a previously resected sacrococcygeal endodermal sinus tumor. Follow-up chest radiograph showed a right paravertebral mass. CT shows large metastatic mass in posterior mediastinal lymph nodes (*n*). These nodes lie below the carina and extend posteriorly on the right (*curved arrow*). *b*, major bronchi; *a*, aorta; *r*, right pulmonary artery, which is displaced forward by the mass.

References

1. Baron RL, Lee JKT, Sagel SS, Levitt RG (1982) Computed tomography of the abnormal thymus. Radiology 142:127–134
2. Baron RL, Lee JKT, Sagel SS, Peterson RR (1982) Computed tomography of the normal thymus. Radiology 142:121–125
3. Benjamin B, Cohen D, Glasson M (1976) Tracheomalacia in association with congenital tracheoesophageal fistula. Surgery 79(5):504–508
4. Berdon WE, Baker DH, Bordiuk J, Mellins R (1969) Innominate artery compression of the trachea in infants with stridor and apnea. Radiology 92:272–278
5. Berdon WE, Baker DH, Wung JT, Chrispin A, Kozlowski K, de Silva M, Bales P, Alford B (1984) Complete cartilage-ring tracheal stenosis associated with anomalous

left pulmonary artery: the ring-sling complex. Radiology 152:57–64

6. Berger PE, Kuhn JP, Kuhns LR (1980) Computed tomography and the occult tracheobronchial foreign body. Radiology 134:133–135

7. Brown BM, Oshita AK, Castellino RA (1983) CT assessment of the adult extrathoracic trachea. J Comput Assist Tomogr 7(3):415–418

8. Butz RO (1968) Length and cross-section growth patterns in the human trachea. Pediatrics 42(2):336–341

9. Chan HSL, Sonley MJ, Moes CAF, Daneman A, Smith CR, Martin DJ (1985) Primary and secondary tumors of childhood involving the heart, pericardium and great vessels. Cancer 56:825–836

10. Choplin RH, Siegel MJ (1980) Pulmonary sequestration: six unusual presentations. AJR 134:695–700

11. Cohen M, Hill CA, Cangir A, Sullivan MP (1980) Thymic rebound after treatment of childhood tumors. AJR 135:151–156

12. Dalal BI, Raju BS, Datta BN, Khatri HN (1978) Metastatic osteosarcoma of heart: report of a case and review of literature. Int J Cancer 15:84–86

13. Daneman A, Martin DJ, Chan HSL (1983) Cardiac metastases from osteosarcoma. A report of two cases. CT 7(1):41–43

14. Dunnick NR, Seibert K, Cramer HR (1981) Cardiac metastasis from osteosarcoma. J Comput Assist Tomogr 5:253–255

15. Effman EL, Fram EK, Vick P, Kirks DR (1983) Tracheal cross-sectional area in children: CT determination. Radiology 149:137–140

16. Ein SH, Friedberg J, Williams WG, Fearon B, Barker GA, Mancer K (1982) Tracheoplasty — a new operation for complete congenital tracheal stenosis. J Pediatr Surg 17(6):872–877

17. Fearon B, Whalen JS (1967) Tracheal dimensions in the living infant. Ann Otol Rhinol Laryngol 76:964–975

18. Fon GT, Bein ME, Mancuso AA, Keesey JC, Lupetin AR, Wong WS (1982) Computed tomography of the anterior mediastinum in myasthenia gravis. Radiology 142:135–141

19. Gaisie G, Oh KS (1983) Paraspinal interfaces in the lower thoracic area in children: evaluation by CT. Radiology 149:133–135

20. Gamsu G, Webb WR (1982) Computed tomography of the trachea: normal and abnormal. AJR 139:321–326

21. Griscom NT (1982) Computed tomographic determina-

tion of tracheal dimensions in children and adolescents. Radiology 145:361–364

22. Griscom NT (1983) Cross-sectional shape of the child's trachea by computed tomography. AJR 140:1103–1106

23. Heithhoff KB, Sane SM, Williams HJ, Jarvis CJ, Carter J, Kane P, Brennom W (1976) Bronchopulmonary foregut malformations. A unifying etiological concept. AJR 126(1):46–55

24. Hope JW, Borns PF, Koop CE (1963) Radiologic diagnosis of mediastinal masses in infants and children. Radiol Clin North Am 1:17–50

25. Johns AN (1981) Congenital tracheal stenosis. Int J Pediatr Otorhinolaryngol 3:157–161

26. Kirks DR, Korobkin M (1981) Computed tomography of the chest in infants and children: techniques and mediastinal evaluation. Radiol Clin North Am 19:409–419

27. Kirks DR, Fram EK, Vock P, Effmann EL (1983) Tracheal compression by mediastinal masses in children: CT evaluation. AJR 141:647–651

28. Kittredge RD (1981) Computed tomography of the trachea: a review. J Comput Assist Tomogr 5:44–50

29. Landing BH (1975) Syndromes of congenital heart disease with tracheobronchial anomalies. AJR 123(4):679–686

30. Liu P, Daneman A (1984) Computed tomography of intrinsic laryngeal and tracheal abnormalities in children. J Comput Assist Tomogr 8(4):662–669

31. MacDonald RE, Fearon B (1971) Innominate artery compression syndrome in children. Paper presented at meeting of American Broncho-esophagological Association, San Francisco, California, 26–27 May 1971

32. MacKenzie CF, McAslan TC, Shin B, Schellinger D, Helrich M (1978) The shape of the human adult trachea. Anesthesiology 19(1):48–50

33. Moore AV, Korobkin M, Olanow W, Heaston DK, Ram PC, Dunnick NR, Silverman PM (1983) Age-related changes in the thymus gland. AJR 141:241–246

34. Romeo MAA, Miller LG, Szeto PM (1982) Cardiac calcification from metastatic osteosarcoma. J Canad Assoc Radiol 33:113–115

35. Sagel SS, Stanley RJ (1982) Lung, pleura, pericardium and chest wall. In: Lee JK (ed) Computed body tomography. Raven, New York, pp 122–126

36. Seibert KA, Rettenmeir CW, Waller BF, Battle WE, Levine AS, Roberts WC (1982) Osteogenic sarcoma metastatic to the heart. Am J Med 73:136–141

Chapter 5

Lung Parenchyma

Introduction

In our experience in Toronto, the lungs and pleura of children who have had no previous thoractomy, chemotherapy, or thoracic radiation appear clear on CT. In the hilar regions the large arteries and veins are seen branching together with major bronchi as they enter the lung. The vessels normally appear unexpectedly prominent on transverse scans, and it may be extremely difficult, particularly in younger children, to differentiate these structures from enlarged hilar lymph nodes, even with intravenous contrast enhancement. The pulmonary vessels are usually the only normal structures that can be seen silhouetted against the low attenuation of the lung parenchyma. They branch several times and become progressively smaller as they course toward the periphery of the lung. It is impossible to differentiate veins and arteries in the peripheral lung fields. The vessels terminate before reaching the pleura. Occasionally, small normal subpleural lymph nodes may be seen and may mimic metastases (see Fig. 5.7).

In children, the pleura of the pulmonary fissures is not usually seen with 10- or 5-mm thick scans. However, the lung fields adjacent to the fissures are relatively avascular and one can identify the regions of the fissures by recognizing these avascular areas and following their course in adjacent scans (Fig. 5.1). In this way one is able to define the lobes and even segments of the lungs in transverse scans. A large avascular area in the mid portion of the right lung, roughly at the level of the carina, represents the region of the minor fissure (see also Fig. 5.5). Similar avascular areas are noted adjacent to accessory fissures (see Fig. 3.2, p. 24.)

Computed tomography is of value in delineating diffuse disease, nodules and mass lesions of the pulmonary parenchyma; indeed CT is able to detect small pulmonary nodules and early diffuse parenchymal disease when other more conventional techniques fail to do so. CT does have its limitations, however, with regard to pulmonary lesions, in that it may be difficult at times even with this modality to differentiate peripheral lung nodules and masses from lesions of the pleura or adjacent chest wall and mediastinum (see Figs. 5.12, 5.13; see also Fig. 6.5, p. 73).

As with other organs the attenuation of the lung may be recorded by CT. Ranges of attenuation for different portions of the lung parenchyma have been established in adults [3, 5]. The equivalent ranges of attenuation in children have a lower negative number, and it has been suggested that this distinction may be related to an increased amount of water content of the lungs in children [3]. In the transverse axial scans produced by CT, the more dependent portions of the lung have a greater attenuation because of the greater vascular flow to these areas. These changes in attenuation numbers can be altered by changing the position of the patient. The attenuation of both diffuse disease and nodules in lung parenchyma is of value in characterizing these lesions (see Figs. 5.9, 5.10, 5.12).

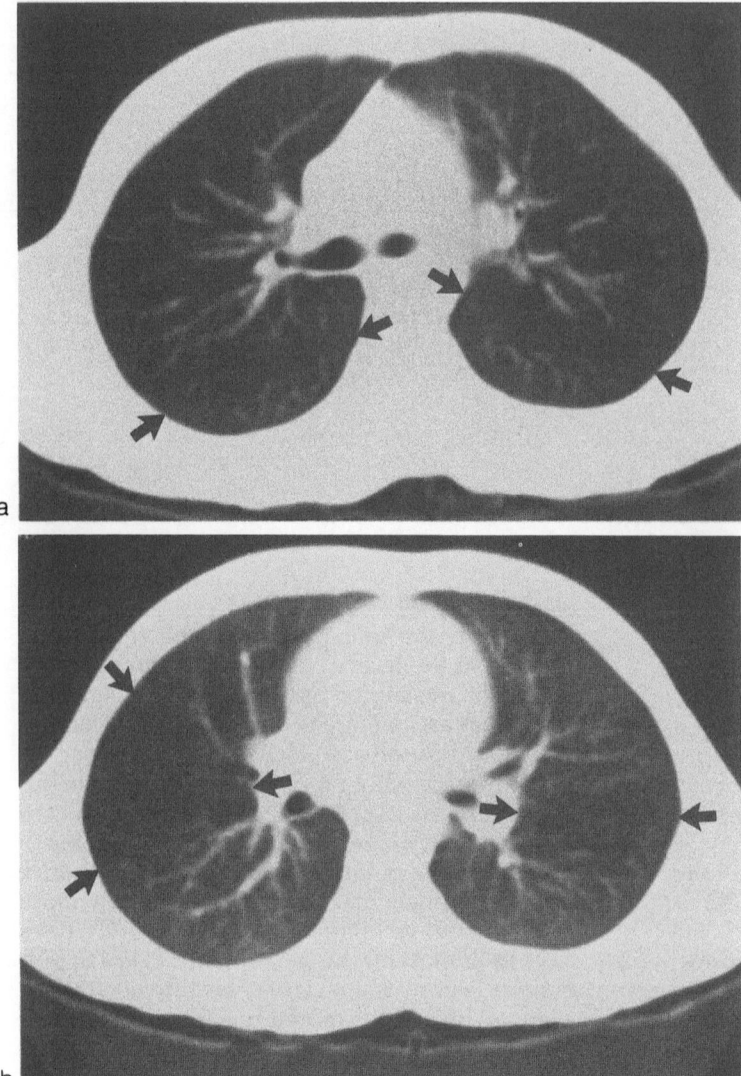

a

b

Fig. 5.1a,b. CT images illustrating normal lungs. Note the branching arteries and veins as they course through the lung fields. The most peripheral areas of lung are relatively avascular, as are the areas of lung adjacent to the fissures (*arrows*). Although the pleura of the fissures is not always visible, the regions of the fissures may be easily followed in each scan by following the relatively avascular areas (*arrows*). The region of the minor fissure on the right is represented by a large relatively avascular area in scan **b**, as the CT scan often passes directly through this almost transverse fissure. In **a** the vessels behind the level of the fissures are those in the apical segment of the lower lobes.

Diffuse Parenchymal Disease

Diffuse changes in the lung fields are usually diagnosed and followed with chest radiographs. CT is rarely used to assess diffuse lung disease in children, and the appearance of these diseases on CT is often nonspecific. However, the progression of severe diffuse disease is occasionally difficult to assess on chest radiographs. When important decisions, based on the progression of lesions, have to be made regarding a patient's treatment, CT may be helpful in determining subtle changes in the progression of a diffuse lung lesion. Although we have rarely used CT for this purpose, it has been of immense help in the few patients that we have followed in this way. These have included patients with histiocytosis and postradiation changes in the lungs (see Fig. 6.16, p. 80 and also Fig. 5.2).

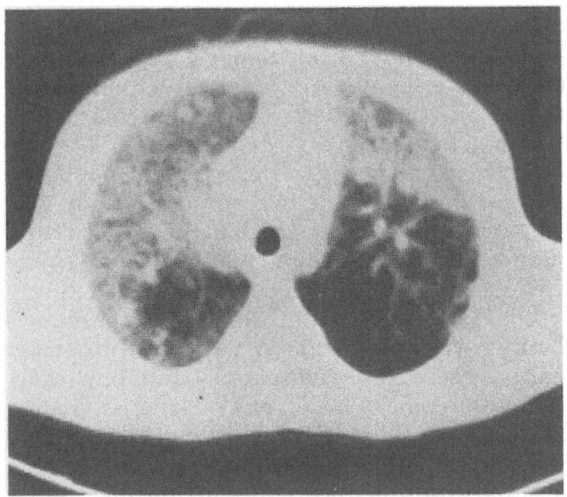

Fig. 5.2. A 12-year-old boy with alveolar proteinosis. This study was performed to assess the caliber of the trachea and bronchi so that sufficiently large tubes could be used for bronchial washouts. CT shows increased attenuation of the more diseased portions of the lung, especially anteriorly. The demarcation between the abnormal lung anteriorly and the more normal lung posteriorly is well seen on the left.

Minor changes in pulmonary parenchymal density on CT may well be useful in detecting, characterizing, and quantitating early lung disease which is not evident on conventional radiographs; however, this use of CT has not, as yet, been extensively made [3].

Mass Lesions

Most large mass lesions of the lung are metastatic in origin. In the late stages of metastatic disease, pulmonary lesions may grow to an enormous size (Fig. 5.3). These lesions are easily visualized on plain radiographs and can be followed simply in this way. Occasionally, CT may give useful information in these patients, particularly at the time of decision making regarding therapy. If a single large metastasis is seen on a chest radiograph, CT will be helpful in excluding other smaller lesions if thoracotomy excision is contemplated. Furthermore, CT is more accurate than plain radiography in following the progress of mass lesions and shows more subtle changes, which may be important when deciding how to adjust appropriate therapy.

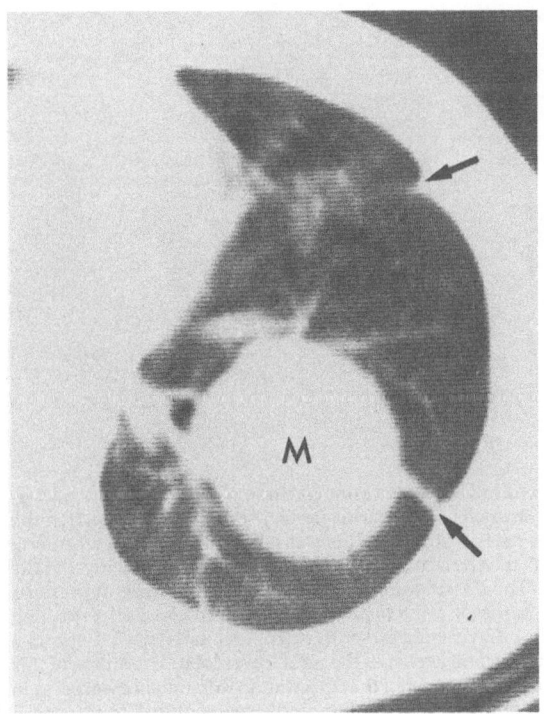

a

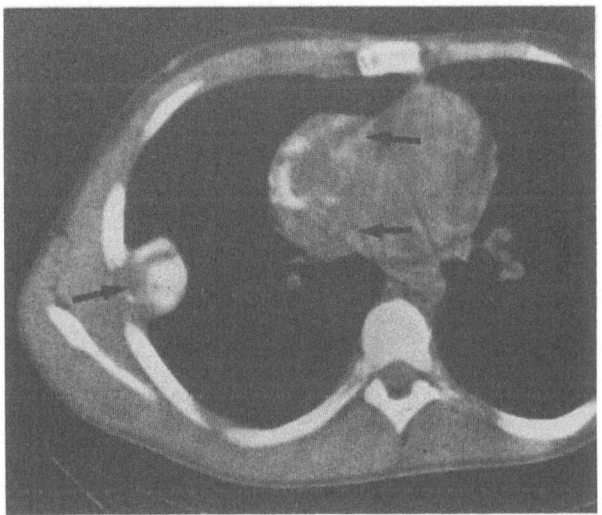

b

Fig. 5.3a,b. Pulmonary mass lesions from metastases from osteogenic sarcoma. Both patients were teenage boys with osteogenic sarcoma of the femur. **a** A large left pulmonary mass (*M*) is noted with linear densities (*arrows*) related to pleural and pulmonary changes from previous thoracotomy. **b** In this patient the metastases, which are adjacent to the chest wall and heart (*arrows*), are heavily ossified.

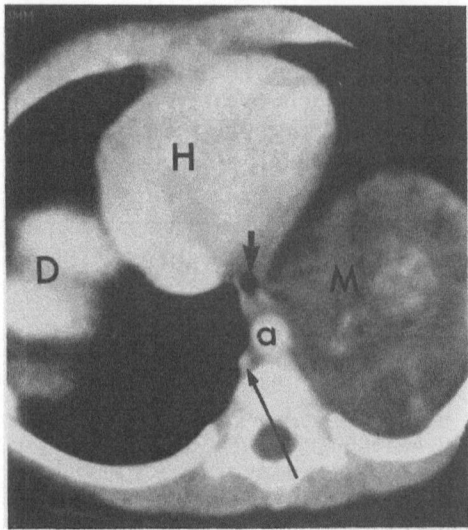

Fig. 5.4. A 7-day-old baby with left pulmonary mass (*M*). CT of the mass shows patchy enhancement. The mass was shown to be a large sequestration. *H*, heart; *D*, right hemidiaphragm; *a*, aorta; *long arrow*, azygous vein; *short arrow*, esophagus.

Primary mass lesions within the lung are rare and may be either congenital, e.g., sequestration (Fig. 5.4); inflammatory, e.g., acute pneumonia (Fig. 5.5), abscess (Fig. 5.6); granuloma; tuberculoma; neoplastic, e.g., lymphoma, plasmacytoma; vascular, e.g., arteriovenous malformation; or posttraumatic hematoma. CT may give valuable information regarding the exact site and nature of these lesions and may also reveal subtle changes during follow-up (Fig. 5.6).

Our experience with these types of lesions is limited. We have seen two patients with malignant disease (one lymphoma and one rhabdomyosarcoma) who developed large, cavitating masses within the lungs and two children with plasmacytoma. Plasmacytomas are benign lesions, and it is uncertain whether they represent neoplasms or inflammatory masses. Both lesions had a soft tissue attenuation with enhancement on CT but no evidence of calcification.

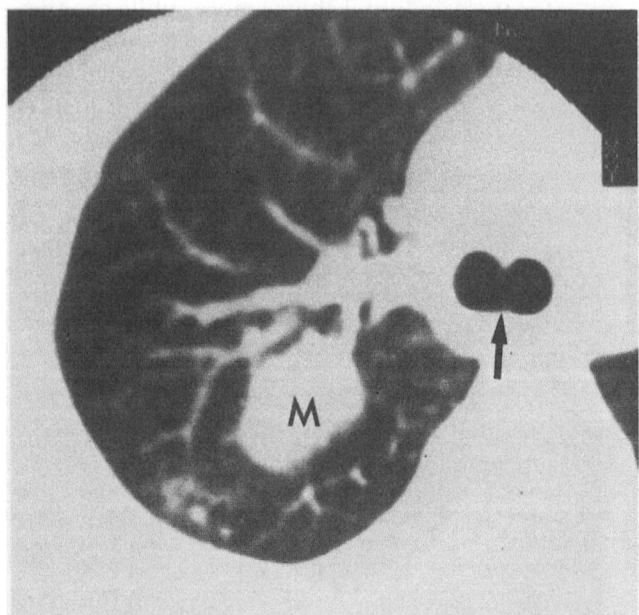
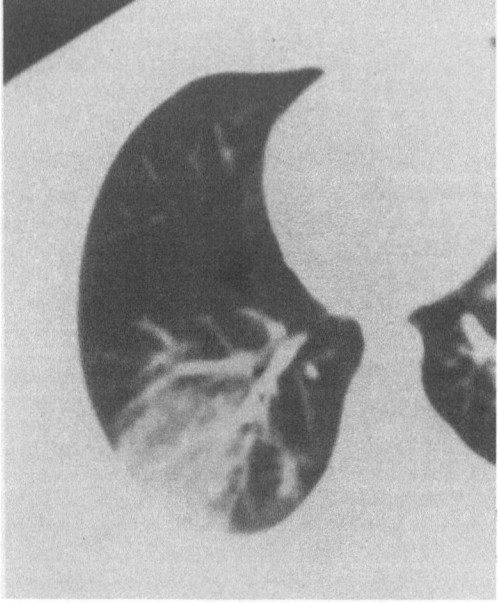

a   b

Fig. 5.5a,b. Mass lesions caused by inflammatory disease. **a** An 18-year-old boy with choriocarcinoma of the pineal gland was shown to have a mass in the right lung on chest radiograph. CT at the level of the carina (*arrow*) shows the mass (*M*) in the posterior portion of the right lung. The posteromedial aspect of this mass is straight. This was a helpful clue in determining that the mass was in the posterior segment of the right upper lobe as the straight posterior margin represents the level of the oblique fissure, although the pleura of this area cannot be seen. The vasculature posteromedial to the mass represents vasculature of the apical segment of the right lower lobe. A diagnosis of a mass pneumonia was made, and follow-up radiographs after antibiotic therapy showed complete resolution. **b** A 17-year-old girl with osteogenic sarcoma. CT shows a triangular area of inhomogeneous increased attenuation in the posterolateral aspect of the right lower lobe. The shape of this abnormal tissue and its distribution in adjacent superior and inferior scans suggested that this was an inflammatory process in the lateral basal segment of the right lower lobe. The avascular area of the oblique fissure can be seen anterior to this area.

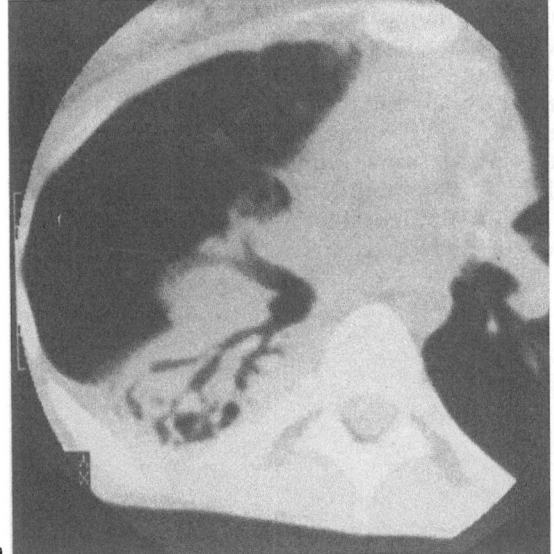

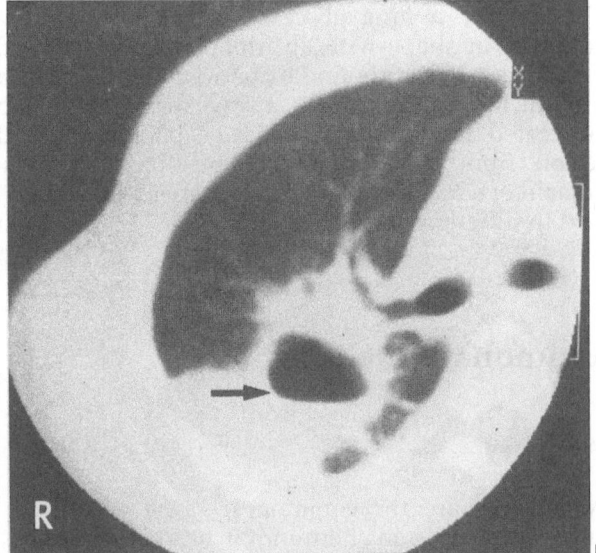

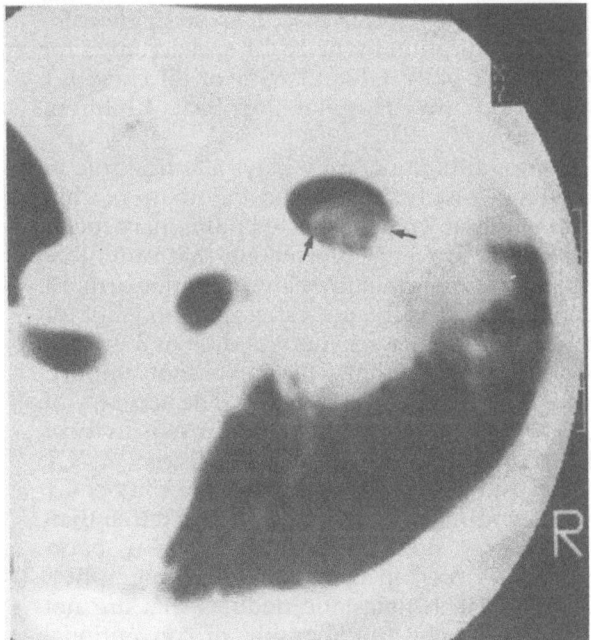

Fig. 5.6a–c. A 15-year-old girl with known Hodgkin's disease **a** CT shows a large area of soft tissue attenuation in the posterior aspect of the right lung with a well-marked air bronchogram pattern within this tissue. The findings are typical of consolidation. **b** Following therapy the volume of abnormal tissue has diminished, but an abscess cavity has developed with an air-fluid level (*arrow*). **c** A further follow-up study taken with the patient in the prone position shows that a solid filling defect (*arrows*) is present in the abscess cavity. This was proven histologically to represent a fungus ball.

Arteriovenous malformations may appear as enhancing masses within the lungs, and the feeding arteries and draining veins may be seen coursing to and from the lesion respectively on CT. Lung abscesses are rarely studied with CT, but this modality may be helpful in the delineation of the extent of lung abscesses and in following their progress. We have seen two patients who developed fungus balls within the abscess (see Fig. 5.6).

Computed tomography may be useful in differentiating peripheral pulmonary abscesses from pyopneumothoraces [5]. This differentiation is important as lung abscess is treated with postural drainage and antibiotics and empyema by thoracostomy tube. This differentiation may be extremely difficult with conventional radiography.

On CT, a pyopneumothorax usually has a sharp, smooth margin between the lesion and the lung. The technique of performing scans with the patient in different positions will reveal air-fluid levels of unequal length and may also reveal a change in configuration of the cavity.

Conversely, a lung abscess is usually more rounded in shape with an irregular thick wall and lacks a discrete boundary between the lesion and the lung. Occasionally, a very small amount of aerated lung may be visualized separating the lesion from the pleura. The air-fluid levels remain of equal length when the patient is scanned in different positions.

Pulmonary Nodules

Accuracy

Metastases are the commonest cause of pulmonary nodules in children. CT has been used extensively at our institution to evaluate the lungs for metastatic disease. It is the single commonest indication for body CT and accounts for 30% of all body CT and 60% of all chest CT studies at the Hospital for Sick Children, Toronto.

Computed tomography plays a critical role in the diagnosis, treatment and follow-up of children with known or suspected pulmonary metastases and provides information that cannot be obtained or determined by any other nonsurgical technique. CT is the most accurate modality for detecting whether a solitary nodule or a myriad of nodules are present. This is extremely important if resection is contemplated. The accuracy of CT is due to the intrinsically greater sensitivity of the CT system, the transverse display of CT scans, and the greater detection capability of CT (white nodules on a dark background rather than lighter gray nodules on a darker gray background as seen in conventional tomography). CT can detect metastatic nodules that are not apparent on chest radiographs or conventional tomography. This accuracy has been proven at our institution as well as elsewhere [2, 3].

It has been stated that pulmonary nodules as small as 2 mm in diameter may be detected in adults [5]. Our experience in children has shown that we have detected all lesions larger than 1 cm in size but have missed some lesions under 0.5 cm. This may be related to the thickness of the scans and the repeatability of the level of respiration during each scan.

In adults, this high sensitivity of detecting lung nodules on CT is associated with a low specificity. Of additional nodules detected by CT, 60% are benign [5]. However, in children

with malignant disease, our experience has been that 95% of all lung nodules detected on CT are malignant. Our review of the thoracotomies at our hospital for resection of lung nodules detected on CT show that in only five instances were the lesions found to be nonmalignant (Fig. 5.7). The nodule represented a granuloma in one, a subpleural lymph node in one, and an area of atelectasis in one. In the other two

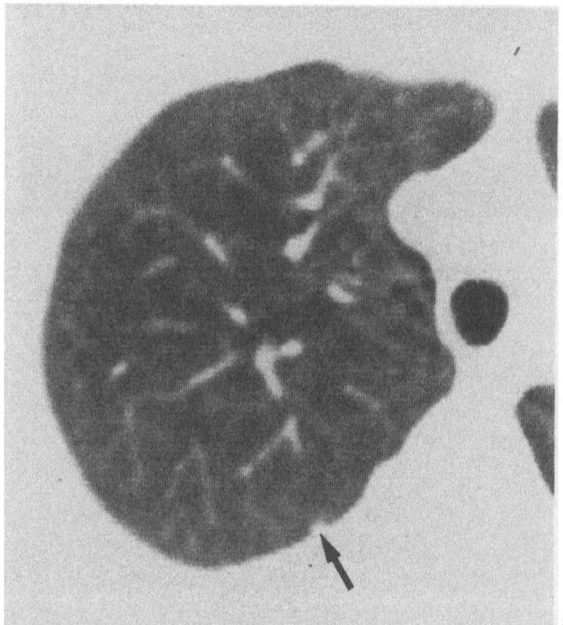

a

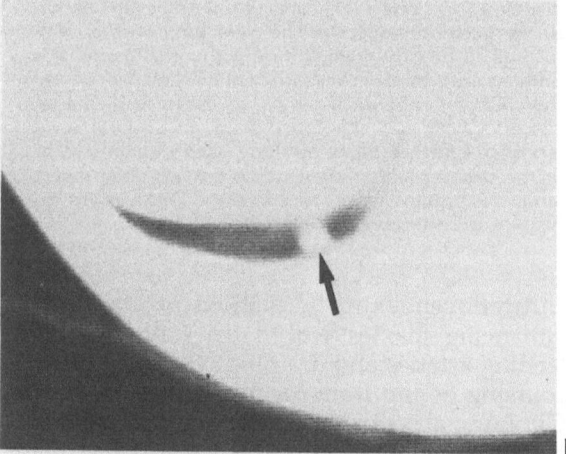

b

Fig. 5.7a,b. Examples of children with malignant disease and pulmonary nodules that were proven to be benign. **a** A 15-year-old boy with osteogenic sarcoma. Posterior nodule (*arrow*) was shown histologically to represent a normal small subpleural lymph node. **b** A 12-year-old boy with carcinoma of the colon. Posterior lung nodule (*arrow*) was shown to represent a granuloma of the lung.

patients, multiple lesions were detected on CT; these were pulmonary hamartomas in one (see Fig. 5.12) and nodules of fibrosis caused by bleomycin therapy in the other. Therefore, all pulmonary nodules detected in children with known malignant disease who have not had previous thoracotomy, chemotherapy, or radiation therapy should be considered malignant until proved otherwise, particularly if the nodule is peripheral or subpleural. In children treated with one of these modalities, densities in the lungs on CT may not all be metastatic and may be related to complications of therapy, other associated abnormalities, or unassociated lesions (see Figs. 5.11, 5.12).

A further limitation of CT is that one cannot determine whether a pulmonary nodule contains active neoplastic tissue or necrotic inactive fibrous tissue following chemotherapy. Resection of such nodules is necessary to determine the future course of therapy, since nodules that remain static in size following therapy may well be fibrous scars caused by a nonspecific reaction to chemotherapy-induced necrosis of neoplastic tissue. Despite these limitations, however, CT remains the most sensitive modality for the detection of metastatic disease of the lungs in children, and its specificity is higher than in adults.

Chest radiographs should always be reviewed before performing chest CT to evaluate the lungs for pulmonary metastases. There are two major reasons for this. First, if a myriad of pulmonary metastases are visualized on the chest radiograph, the CT study does not usually add significant further information. Secondly, it is impossible to diagnose metastatic disease within an area of collapsed or consolidated lung unless the metastases are ossified lesions from osteogenic sarcoma. If areas of collapse or consolidation are evident on the chest radiograph, it is better to defer the chest CT study until these have resolved.

Evaluation of the lungs for metastases is recommended whenever the information obtained from such a study will influence the type of therapy the patient receives. For this reason, CT should be performed at the time of initial presentation in all patients who have a tumor that has the propensity to metastasize to the lungs. Pulmonary metastases are most commonly found in children with sarcomas (Wilms' tumor, osteogenic sarcoma, Ewing's sarcoma, rhabdomyosarcoma, and undifferentiated soft tissue sarcomas); germ cell tumors (endodermal sinus tumors); and lymphoma. Other less common

tumors may also metastasize to the lungs and these include carcinomas arising in the adrenal and thyroid. Neuroblastoma and brain tumors do not commonly metastasize to the lungs during the early phases of the disease. Consequently, we have not routinely surveyed the lungs with CT in the search for metastases in patients with these lesions. We have, however, seen two patients with abdominal neuroblastoma with pulmonary and pleural lesions at the time of diagnosis.

At the time of initial presentation it is best to perform chest CT prior to a long general anesthetic or thoracotomy as these procedures occasionally cause areas of lung collapse and consolidation which may persist postoperatively (see Fig. 5.11); this may make accurate exclusion of metastases impossible and may lead to undue delay in the institution of the correct therapy. Follow-up chest CT is recommended at frequent intervals for early diagnosis of new metastases, as well as for following the response of previously documented lesions to treatment. Because time is at a premium in a large, busy institution, chest CT should be done more often in those patients with tumors that have a propensity for lung metastases and those in whom lung metastases have been documented previously. Follow-up chest CT is also important at any time when a decision has to be made regarding a possible change in a patient's therapy. The presence of new metastases or the resolution of previous lesions may significantly alter the type of subsequent therapy.

Appearances

Pulmonary metastases usually have a round or occasionally slightly oval shape and have relatively smooth margins (Fig. 5.8). They are usually found in the peripheral and subpleural areas of the lungs. The transverse axial display of CT makes this the ideal modality for visualizing these peripheral nodules, since it has the advantage over conventional tomography of permitting visualization of these nodules without superimposition of the bones, diagphragm, mediastinum, and vessels. Sites that are much better displayed for this reason are the posterior costophrenic sulci, lung apices, and the subpleural, retrocardiac, and retrosternal areas.

Less commonly, metastases may be located more centrally in the lung fields adjacent to the major pulmonary vessels and hila. CT is extremely useful in assessing the operability of

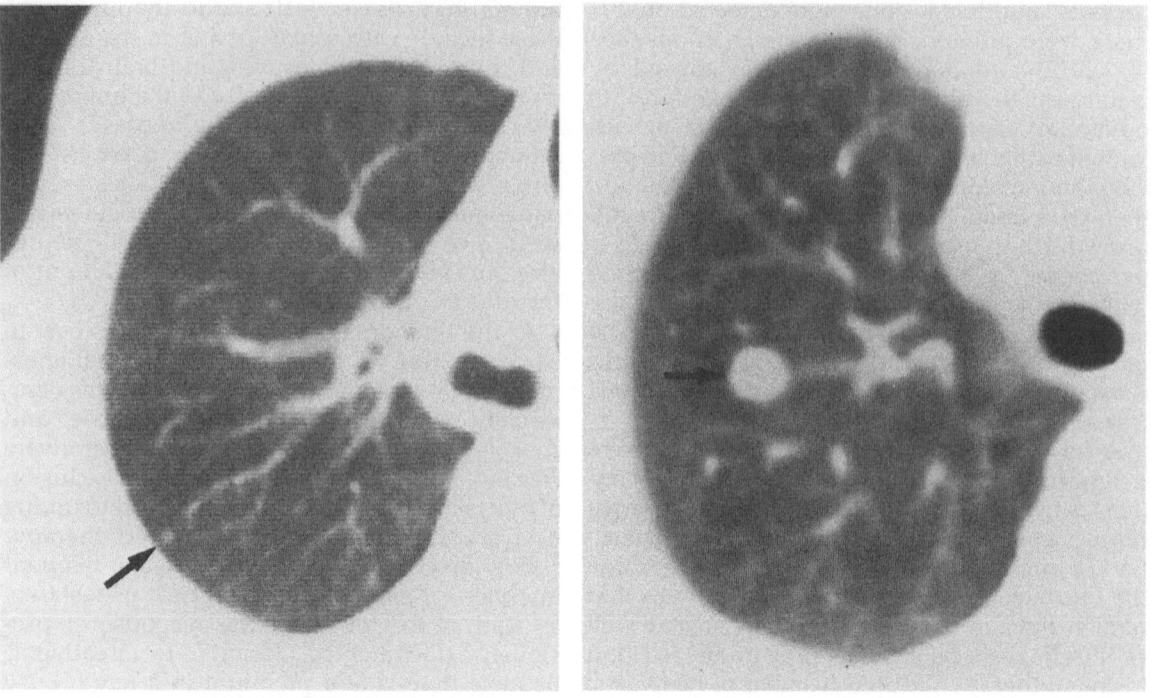

a   b

Fig. 5.8a,b. Usual appearance of metastases in the lung. **a** A 12-year-old girl with carcinoma of the thyroid and multiple pulmonary metastases. A small subpleural metastasis is illustrated in this image. **b** A 12-year-old boy with osteogenic sarcoma and a larger, more centrally placed, well-defined round metastasis (*arrow*).

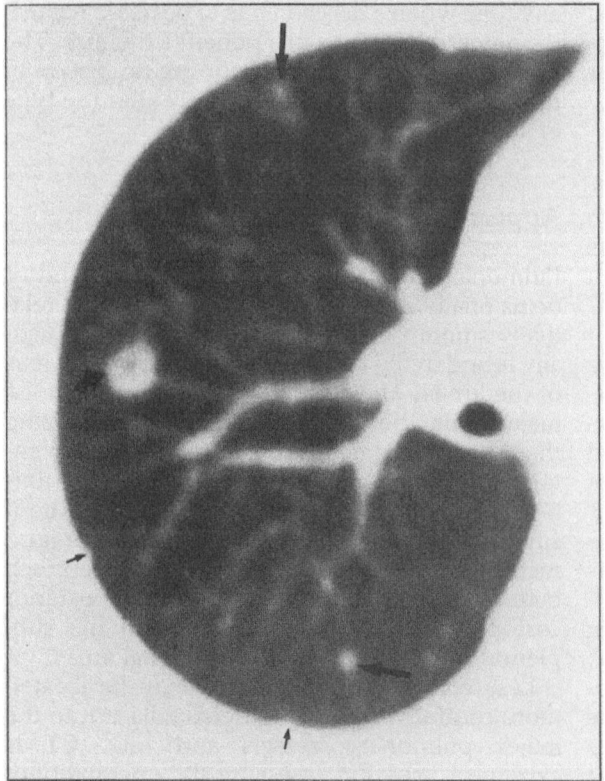

Fig. 5.9. A 12-year-old girl with osteogenic sarcoma and multiple metastases. (*Short straight arrows*, subpleural metastases; *longer straight arrows*, larger, more central metastases.) A larger metastasis is noted laterally (*curved arrow*). A central low attenuation area within this metastasis represents cavitation.

such lesions by accurately defining their relationship to the vasculature (Fig. 5.8b).

The vast majority of metastases have a homogeneous attenuation. Rarely, air within a metastasis may be due to cavitation (Fig. 5.9), and areas of high attenuation may be seen in ossified areas of metastases from osteogenic sarcoma (Fig. 5.10).

Occasionally, metastases may have a more irregular margin and shape (Figs. 5.10, 5.11) and may then simulate areas of inflammation, atelectasis, or fibrosis within the lungs. These pathological processes usually cause irregular, triangular, or linear densities on CT and are commonly found in children who have had a previous thoracotomy. Following a thoracotomy, densities with these shapes should be considered as postoperative changes within the lungs and pleura (Fig. 5.11); however, it is impossible to exclude the possibility of small areas of metastatic tissue within such densities. CT is valuable in following their progress. The benignity of such a lesion is confirmed if it remains static in size or resolves. Any new increase in size should be considered suspicious, and resection is necessary if a decision regarding a change in therapy is to be made based on the nature of such a lesion. Extremely rapid growth of a density in the lungs is usually associated with an inflammatory process but can be seen when there is sudden hemorrhage into the metastasis. This may also give the lesion an irregular outline on CT (see Fig. 5.10).

Rarely, a pneumothorax may be an unexpected finding in patients being scanned for metastases (see Fig. 6.15, p. 79). This is most commonly found in patients with osteogenic sarcoma but may be seen in patients with other types of sarcomas. The metastatic lesions causing the pneumothorax may be so small that they cannot be detected on CT.

At the Hospital for Sick Children, Toronto, we have had the opportunity to study four patients with lung nodules in whom the lung adjacent to the nodule showed slight expansion, with areas of higher negative attenuation values than the surrounding normal lung. These areas have been interpreted as representing focal emphysema, probably related to partial obstruction of a small bronchiole by the nodule. The nodules in these four patients were pulmonary hamartomas (Fig. 5.12), lymphoma, and metastases from rhabdomyosarcoma and osteogenic sarcoma. Pneumothoraces developing in association with pulmonary nodules are thought to develop as a result of either focal emphysema adjacent to the nodules or cavitation within the nodule [1]. Of the patients that we have studied with cavitation within metastases or focal emphysema associated with metastases, none have developed pneumothoraces.

Technique

When performing chest CT for the evaluation of metastatic disease of the lungs the entire chest should be scanned. The superior and inferior limits of the field to be scanned should be chosen from the frontal or lateral computed radiograph and must include the most superior limits of the lung apices and the inferior extent of the costophrenic sulci. A common mistake is to underestimate the inferior extent of the costophrenic sulci on the frontal radiograph; it is easier to assess on the lateral view. Intravenous contrast enhancement is not necessary for the study. Adjacent 1-cm thick scans are performed through the entire area. In infants, 5-mm thick scans can be used. Before starting the study, patients that can cooperate should be instructed how to breathe, namely to take in a maximal breath and hold the breath at the same level for each scan. Occasionally, one has to reinstruct the patient how to breathe after the first scan has been performed in order that they may perfect the technique and help the technician obtain an optimum study. In younger children that cannot cooperate or in those that are sedated, scans are performed during quiet respiration. In those rare instances where patients are being scanned under general anesthetic, the anesthetist can be instructed how to inflate the lungs to the same level for each scan.

Before the patient is allowed to leave the CT room each scan should be checked and viewed at variable window settings that will allow visualization of not only the lungs but also all the other structures of the chest. In this way, lesions of the rib cage and the mediastinum that may not be obvious on previous chest radiographs may be diagnosed. Further scans can be obtained if required. There are many reasons why further scans may be necessary at the end of such studies. First, the entire chest may not have been scanned because of a faulty choice of scan field from the computed radiograph. This commonly occurs when the lowermost extension of the costophrenic sulci has been underestimated. Individual scans should be redone if a patient has moved or breathed excessively during a particular exposure. Not infrequently, patients may be

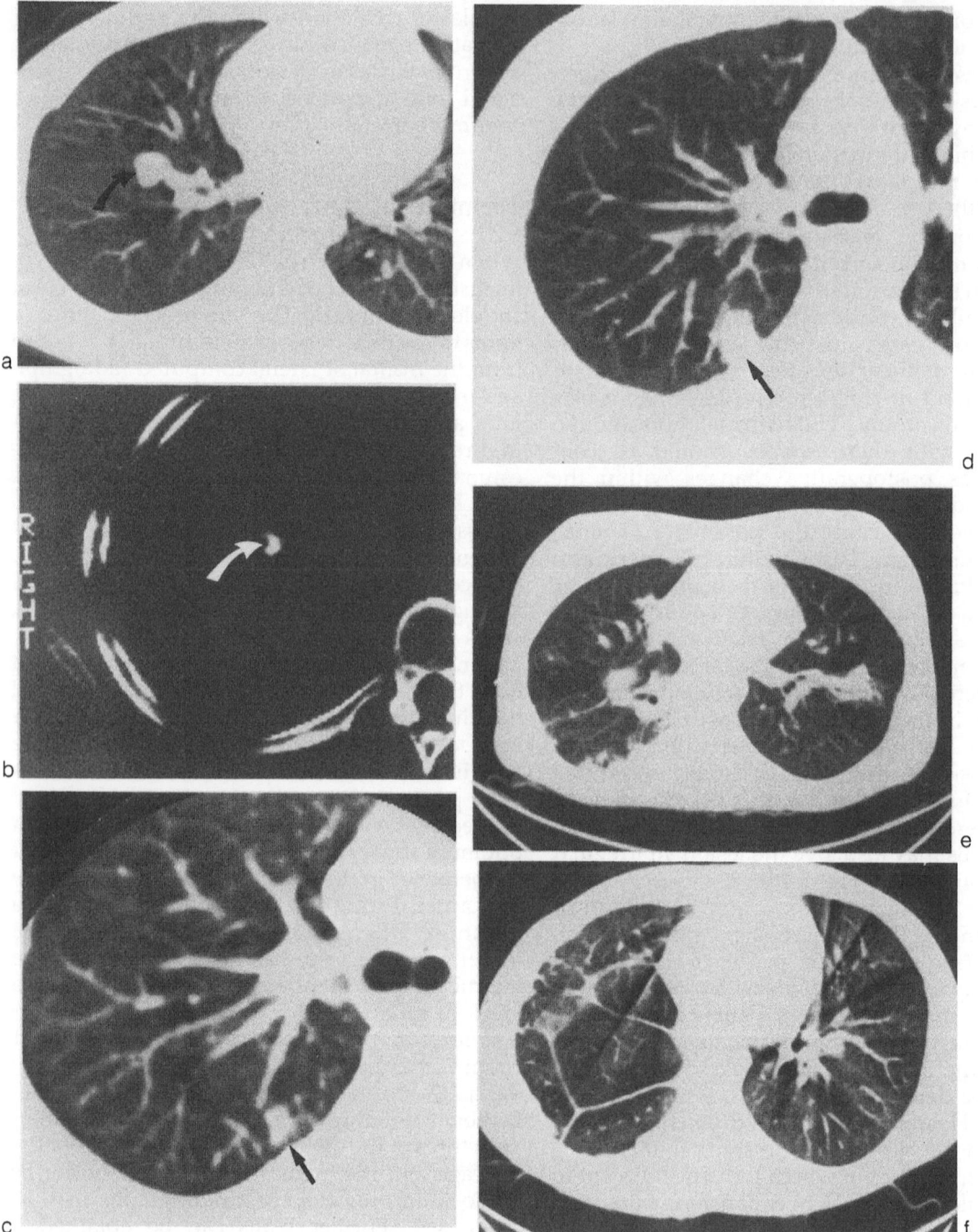

Fig. 5.10a–f. A 15-year-old boy with osteogenic sarcoma. **a** CT shows a rounded metastasis (*curved arrow*) centrally placed adjacent to the larger vessels. Occasionally, it may be difficult, even with intravenous contrast injection, to differentiate metastases from the large hilar and pulmonary vessels. **b** Viewing the same image as in **a** with a narrow window, shows that the lesion is heavily ossified. This is an extremely useful technique when attempting to differentiate metastases from vessels in patients with osteogenic sarcoma, as the metastases often have a malignant ossification. **c** Following a right lobectomy a follow-up study 1 year later shows an irregularly shaped subpleural lesion (*arrow*). Because of the irregular shape and the previous thoracotomy it was felt that this could represent postoperative changes, but a follow-up study 1 month later (**d**) shows that the lesion has enlarged. Histologically this was proven to be a metastatic nodule with extensive hemorrhage in the lesion. **e,f** Following further bilateral thoracotomies there are extensive changes in both lung fields. Some of these are subpleural (on the right in **e**), and others are more centrally situated because of areas of collapse and old consolidation. Linear densities noted on the right in the lower part of the lung represent areas of collapse or fibrosis.

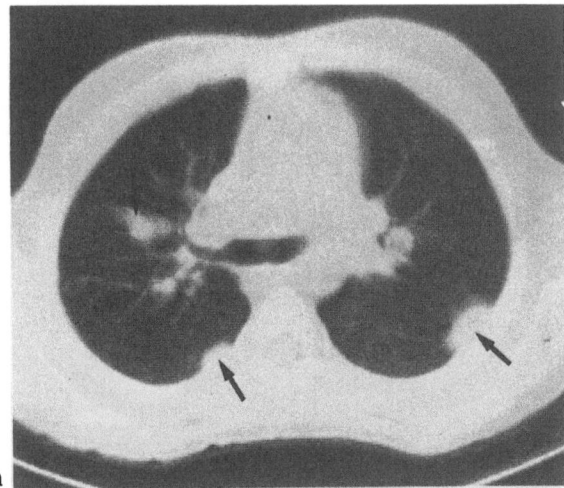

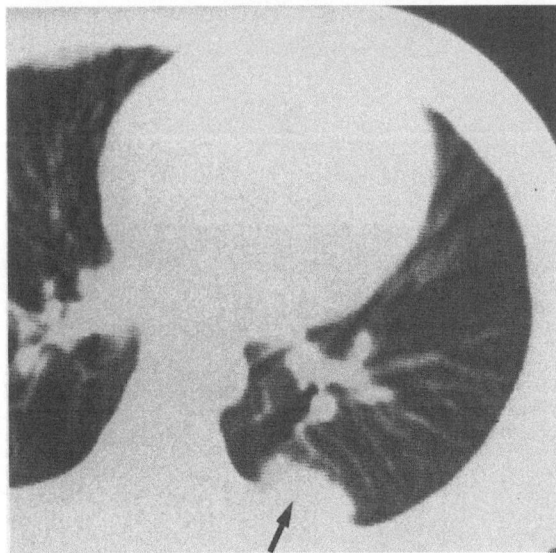

Fig. 5.11. a A 14-year-old boy with previous Ewing's sarcoma. Note the central and subpulmonary metastases (*arrows*). These are somewhat irregular in outline and oval in shape. **b** A 4-year-old boy with previous left thoracoabdominal operation for resection of a large Wilms' tumor. CT shows an oval-shaped lesion on the left with irregular outline (*arrow*). The CT was performed a few weeks after the operation, and this lesion was thought to be postoperative in nature but could not really be differentiated from those lesions illustrated in **a**. A follow-up of this patient showed that the lesion disappeared completely; it probably represented subpleural or loculated pleural hemorrhage.

unable to inflate their lungs to the same level of inspiration for each scan, and because of this some scans may be out of sequence. Further scans of the area that is considered to have been inadequately scanned should be obtained, after reinstructing the patient to breathe to the same level. If rescanning is not performed, lesions of more than 1 cm in size may be missed. Further scans with the patient in a different position may also be necessary to help in the differentiation of pulmonary vessels from metastatic disease.

Differentiation from Vessels

Pulmonary vessels seen end-on as they pass through a scan slice appear as rounded densities, and it may be difficult to differentiate these from metastatic nodules. The pulmonary vessels are largest in the hilar regions and become progressively smaller as the vessels course out into the lung fields and branch. The vessels do not pass all the way to the periphery of the lung or to the level of the fissures, and a small band of relatively avascular lung parenchyma is noted around the peripheral portions of the lung fields and along the regions of the fissures. Rounded nodules in these areas that are relatively avascular should be considered as metastatic disease, since the size of these lesions, even when small, is usually out of proportion to that of the closest adjacent vessels. When such densities are visualized in these portions of the lung, the diagnosis of metastases can usually be made with confidence. When these densities occur in the more vascular portions of the lung, however, the differentiation is much more difficult.

Kuhns has described the "twinkling star" effect around vessels [4]. This description refers to artifactual lines which radiate from the vessel and are due to pulsation within the vessel. The presence of this effect around a density confirms that the density is in fact a vessel. These artifacts are not associated with pulmonary metastases.

A number of techniques can be employed to help differentiate vascular structures from metastases when the "twinkling star" effect is not obvious and when the suspicious densities lie adjacent to the other vessels. Firstly, we have found the use of the cursor extremely helpful. The cursor may be placed adjacent to the suspicious density, and then, while leaving the cursor in position, the scans above and below are viewed. If the lesion is part of the vessels of the lungs, the cursor will be noted to lie adjacent to further densities, which may indeed be longitudinal in the adjacent cuts. This appearance confirms that the density is part of the vasculature of the lung. If no such vessels course toward the suspicious lesion in adjacent cuts, then one can be more confident that one is dealing with a metastasis.

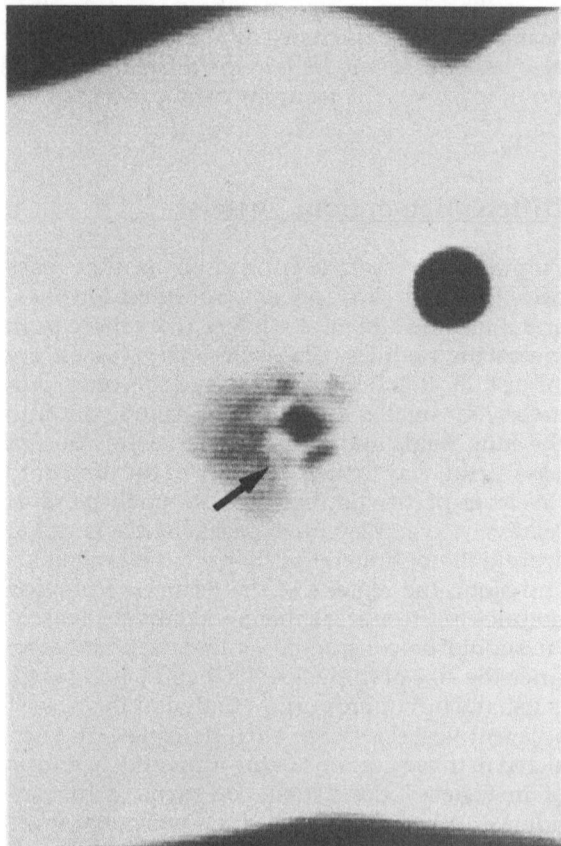

a

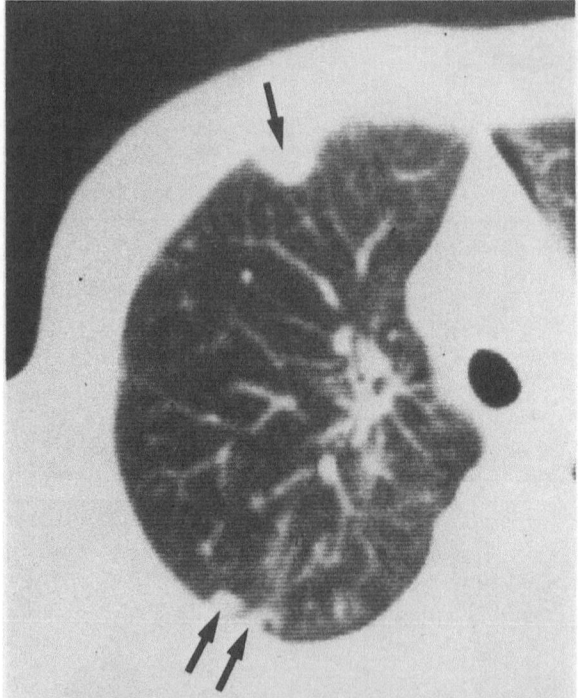

b

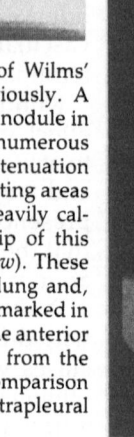

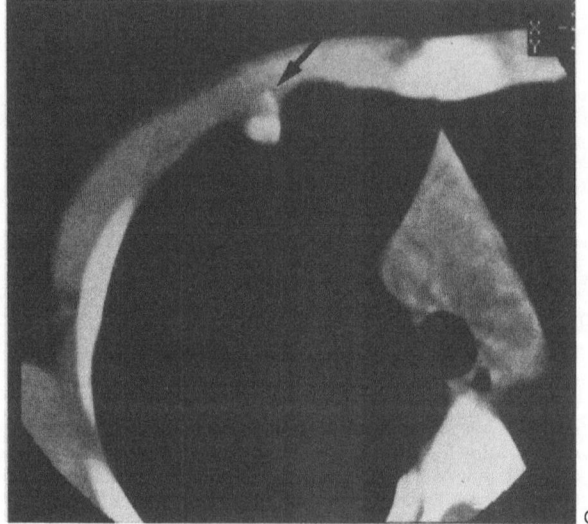

c

Fig. 5.12a–c. A 14-year-old boy with a history of Wilms' tumor and pulmonary metastases 10 years previously. A follow-up chest radiograph at this time revealed a nodule in the upper portion of the right lobe. CT shows numerous nodules (*arrows*). **a** Two loculi of more negative attenuation are noted medial to the nodule, probably representing areas of focal emphysema. **b** The anterior nodule is heavily calcified, as shown in scan **c**. Note the relationship of this nodule to the anterior end of the adjacent rib (*arrow*). These lesions were all found to be hamartomas of the lung and, although they were present bilaterally, were more marked in the right upper lobe. Compare the appearance of the anterior nodule, particularly in **c**, to the exostosis arising from the anterior end of the rib illustrated in Fig. 6.5. This comparison illustrates how difficult it may be to differentiate extrapleural from intraparenchymal lesions.

Secondly, viewing the lung fields at narrower window widths may help to determine whether there is any calcification within the suspicious density. The presence of calcification within such a density would be in keeping with either an inflammatory process or lesions related to osteogenic sarcoma that have ossified (see Fig. 5.10).

Thirdly, the position of the patient may be changed. If the lesion is in the posterior portion of the lung field, the lungs may be rescanned at the same level with the patient prone. Changes in gravity will make vessels in the region drain and become smaller, but metastases will stay the same size. When changing the position of the patient, the scan with the questionable lesion

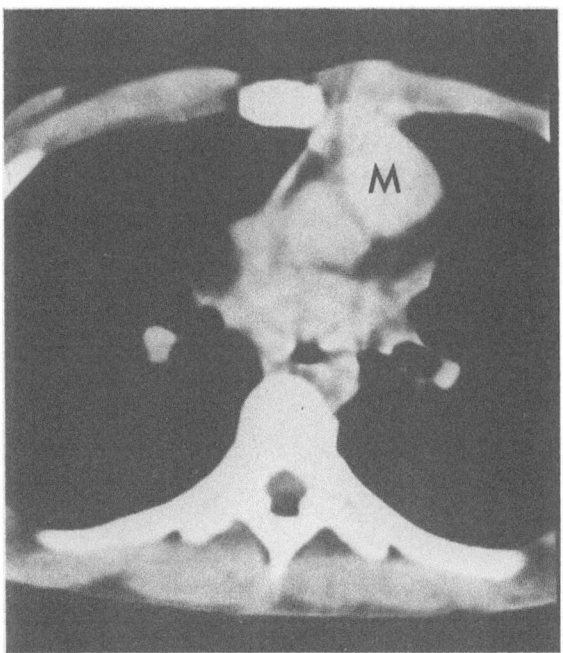

Fig. 5.13. A 10-year-old boy with metastasis from an osteogenic sarcoma. The metastatic lesion (*M*) lies anteriorly and may be mistaken for a mediastinal metastasis. This would be an unusual site for a metastasis without lung involvement. At operation the lesion was found to lie in the anterior portion of the left lung. This image also illustrates the difficulty in differentiating mediastinal from peripheral pulmonary nodules.

References

1. Daneman A, de Silva M (1978) Cyst formation and cavitation in pulmonary metastases from Wilms' tumor. Pediatr Radiol 7:4–6
2. Kirks DR, Korobkin M (1980) Computed tomography for chest examinations. Pediatr Ann 9:192–199
3. Kirks DR, Korobkin M (1981) Computed tomography of the chest wall, pleura and pulmonary parenchyma in infants and children. Radiol Clin N Am 19:421–429
4. Kuhns LR, Borlaza G (1980) The "twinkling star" sign. Radiology 135:763–764
5. Sagel SS (1983) Lung, pleura, pericardium and chest wall. In: Lee JKT, Sagel SS, Stanley RJ (eds) Computed body tomography. Raven, New York, pp 55–98

must first be posted on the original scout radiograph. After the position of the patient has been changed, it is best to repeat the computed radiograph and choose exactly where the slice should be taken, referring again to the original computed radiograph, because the position of the patient may have changed in relationship to the table. Furthermore, as the position of the patient changes, the position of the viscera of the chest and the relationships of the lung to the adjacent mediastinum alter. When viewing the second scan in the new position one should check that the anatomy of the chest wall, mediastinum, and pulmonary vasculature corresponds to the anatomy of the original scan as closely as possible. If not, further scans above or below this level should be taken, depending on how the anatomy has changed. If attention is not paid to the changes in anatomy, fallacious results may be obtained. If a questionable lesion is found in the lateral decubitus, the patient should be placed in position with the questionable side superior, so that the vessels in that part of the lung become small as the result of gravity.

Chapter 6

Chest Wall and Pleura

Introduction

For the purposes of description, the chest wall may be divided into its various components:

1. Superficial soft tissues, including skin, subcutaneous tissues, and muscle
2. Bones including ribs, sternum, scapulae, clavicles, and thoracic spine
3. Extrapleural tissues
4. Pleura

At the Hospital for Sick Children, Toronto, delineation of a lesion of the chest wall and pleura accounts for only 10% of all chest CT examinations, but at Duke University, North Carolina, it has been reported as accounting for 29% of 108 children undergoing chest CT [7, 8]. Most children having CT examinations to delineate lesions of the chest wall and pleura have mass lesions which are either suspected or confirmed on clinical examination or on a chest radiograph. The chest wall and pleura are the rarest sites for mass lesions of the chest in children, and few series have been published [5, 7, 9].

In 1984, Donoghue et al. [4] reviewed the clinical and radiological features of 39 children with 40 chest wall masses at the Hospital for Sick Children, Toronto during the 5½-year period of 1979–1984, inclusive. In several patients the lesions were found during a CT study that was being performed to screen the lungs for metastatic disease. There were 21 males and 18 females, and the age range at the time of presentation was 8 months to 20 years (mean age 10.3 years). Lesions were found in the skin and subcutaneous tissues (benign 6, malignant 4), bony thorax (benign 11, malignant 13), and extrapleural tissues (benign 2, malignant 4). The details are summarized in Table 6.1.

The review confirmed that plain radiography supplied sufficient information for correct management for most benign lesions, particularly those of bony origin. Radionuclide scans are sensitive but are nonspecific. CT was found to be useful in the majority of chest wall masses as it can demonstrate the exact site of origin and extent of the mass. This information is particularly important when large pleural effusions and pulmonary consolidations are present, obscuring the limits of the mass on plain radiography. CT shows the various soft tissue components and bone without overlap in greatest detail and may give valuable information regarding the tissue character of the lesion, which may not be evident on plain radiographs. This information is crucial when planning surgical and radiation therapy. Chest CT is mandatory in all malignant chest wall tumors in order to assess the lungs for metastases, because these may not be visualized on chest radiographs. CT is particularly helpful in evaluating the response of

Table 6.1. Chest wall lesions, the Hospital for Sick Children, Toronto, 1979–1984

Superficial soft tissues	
Benign tumors:	
aggressive fibromatosis	2
hemangiomas	2
cystic hygroma	1
stitch granuloma	1
Malignant tumors:	
undifferentiated sarcoma	1
malignant Schwannoma	1
Ewing's sarcoma	1
metastatic osteosarcoma	1
Bone lesions	
Benign lesions:	
exostoses	9
enchondroma	1
osteomyelitis	1
Malignant lesions:	
Ewing's sarcoma	4
osteosarcoma	4
parosteal osteosarcoma	1
undifferentiated sarcoma	1
metastatic rhabdomyosarcoma	1
malignant lymphoma	1
metastatic angiosarcoma	1
Extrapleural lesions	
neurofibromatosis	1
eosinophilic granuloma	1
embryonal rhabdomyosarcoma	1
malignant lymphoma	1
anaplastic small cell tumor	1
leukemic infiltration	1

malignant tumors to chemotherapy and/or radiotherapy prior to surgical resection and for postoperative follow-up for the detection of early recurrence. Angiography (performed in only two of our patients) is only occasionally necessary as an aid to the surgeon in preoperative planning of excision of large masses. Myelography (performed in only one of our patients) is mandatory if there is a suspicion of intraspinal extension. Sonography is occasionally useful for the detection of pleural effusions, particularly if these are to be tapped. Diaphragmatic movement can also be assessed with sonography if direct extension into the diaphragm or phrenic nerve is suspected clinically. Conventional tomography is rarely of any help as the beam may not be tangential to the bulk of the mass.

For a more detailed description and further illustrations of the CT appearances of the bone and soft tissue lesions discussed in this chapter the reader is referred to Section V: Musculo-skeletal System.

Superficial Soft Tissues

Masses in this compartment may arise from any of the components of the soft tissues such as fat, vessels, nerves, fibrous tissue, or muscles [7, 8]. Most of these lesions are benign (see Table 6.1), and malignant sarcomas are rare. The more commonly encountered lesions clinically include hemangiomas (Fig. 6.1) [10], lymphangiomas, and lipomas. Many of these lesions do not require extensive radiological work-up for adequate therapy, but it is important to delineate the extent of larger lesions preoperatively. At the Hospital for Sick Children, Toronto, our experience also includes two patients with aggressive fibromatosis of the chest wall [2, 6] (Figs. 6.2, 6.3; see also Chap. 21, p. 321).

It has been stated by Franken et al. [5] that the radiographic study of visible subcutaneous masses is generally unrewarding. Kirks et al. [7] have stated that meticulous fluoroscopy and oblique radiographs can usually determine if a mass is limited to soft tissues and that CT has a very limited role in the evaluation of such lesions. CT added essential information, particularly with regard to the exact extent of eight of the ten masses in the superficial soft tissues that we studied (see Figs. 6.1–6.3). Our study [4] showed that CT was extremely helpful in delineating the more detailed anatomical extent of lesions that have poorly defined margins clinically (see Fig. 6.2) and also very large lesions, particularly if there is a suggestion on plain radiographs that there is extension into the thoracic cavity. CT is also invaluable in defining the lesion and its anatomical relationships in areas of complex anatomy or areas that are difficult to evaluate clinically, such as the axilla, where we have seen several lesions originate (see Fig. 6.2) or metastasize (see Fig. 22.14, p. 342).

Bony Thorax

Masses involving the bony thorax may be due to either generalized or focal bony disease [7, 8]. Generalized bony diseases such as fibrous dysplasia and neurofibromatosis rarely require evaluation with CT. Focal bony lesions may be either benign or malignant and may be primary or secondary. The lesions that we have studied are

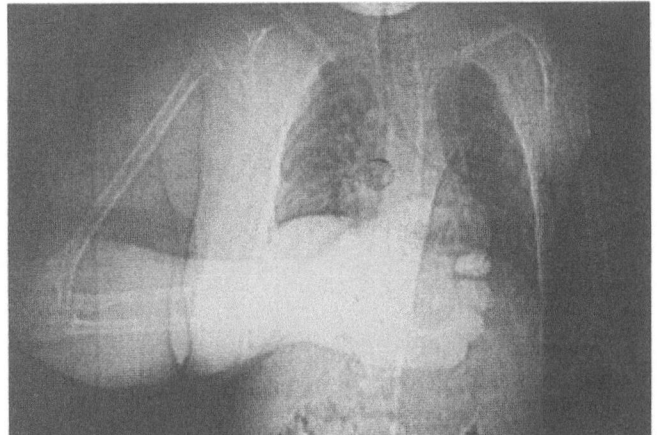

a

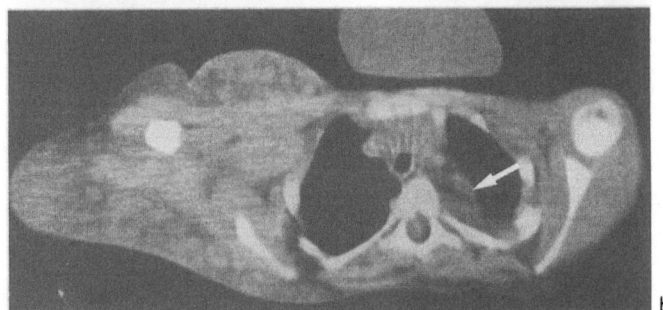

b

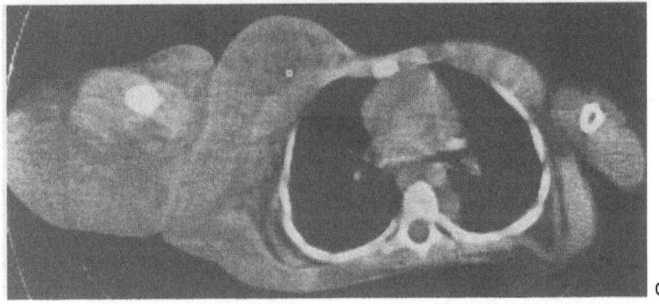

c

Fig. 6.1a–c. A 5-year-old boy with large hemangioma. **a** Scout film shows enlargement of the soft tissues of the right upper limb and chest wall. **b**, **c** Scans performed after the intravenous injection of contrast material show an inhomogeneous soft tissue lesion involving the superficial tissues of the right upper extremity and chest wall. The patchy attenuation values are related to the vast amount of fatty material between the enhancing components of the hemangioma. The muscles are not involved. Note a separate hemangioma in the left paravertebral area (*arrow*). This CT examination was extremely useful in delineating the tissues involved with the hemangioma for the planning of the correct plastic surgery.

listed in Table 6.1 and illustrated in Fig. 6.4–6.9. CT is rarely of any use in the further delineation of infective processes in the bone (Fig. 6.4), and the changes observed may often be nonspecific. The commonest benign lesion that we have studied with CT is exostosis of the thoracic wall (Fig. 6.5; see also Fig. 22.3, p. 332, and Fig. 23.2, p. 367). Enchondromas of the ribs are less commonly encountered (Fig. 6.6).

Malignant lesions of the bony thorax are somewhat more common than benign lesions (see Table 6.1). These include both osteogenic sarcomas (Fig. 6.7) and Ewing's sarcoma (Fig. 6.8; see also Fig. 22.17, p. 343), which is reported in the literature as being the commonest primary malignancy of the chest wall [1, 7]. Metastatic disease of the chest wall is better assessed with radionuclide scans and conventional radiographs. Nevertheless, all children undergoing chest CT examinations should have the images viewed with a wide and narrow window centered at bone and lung attenuation to enable assessment of all structures (see Chap. 3, p. 22); thus a complete study can be performed. The incidental finding of metastatic disease in this way is not common, however (Fig. 6.9).

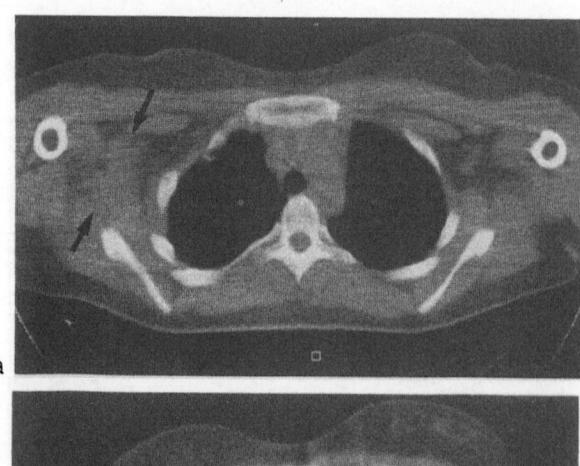

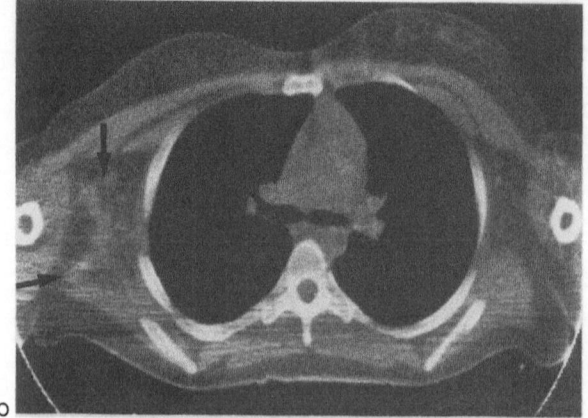

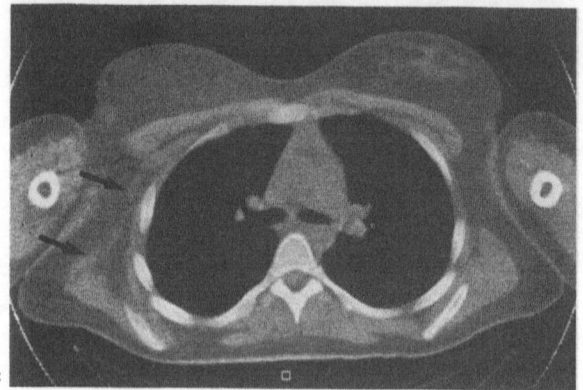

Fig. 6.2a–c. A 15-year-old girl with aggressive fibromatosis of the right axilla and chest wall. Scans performed without contrast enhancement show irregular increased soft tissue (*arrows*) in the right axilla in **a** and extending down the lateral chest wall in **b** and **c**. This tissue is invading the adjacent fat and distorts the adjacent muscles. This CT examination was extremely useful in delineating the exact extent of this lesion as it was ill defined and difficult to evaluate clinically. (Campbell et al. 1983 [2])

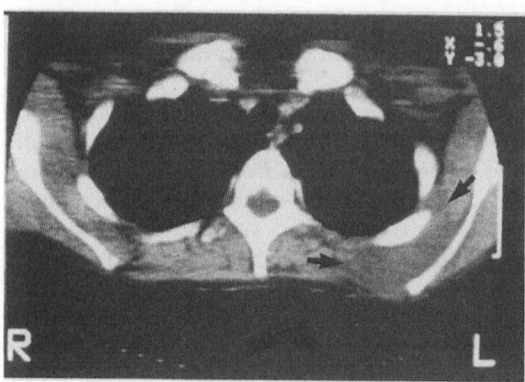

Fig. 6.3. A 13-year-old boy with aggressive fibromatosis of the posterior chest wall deep to the left scapula. Scan without contrast enhancement shows a soft tissue mass (*arrows*) deep to the left scapula, extending toward the axilla and medial to the vertebral margin of the scapula. The mass displaces the scapula posteriorly and has a lower attenuation value than the adjacent muscle. This scan was particularly useful in delineating the extent of the lesion toward the axilla preoperatively. (Campbell et al. 1983 [2])

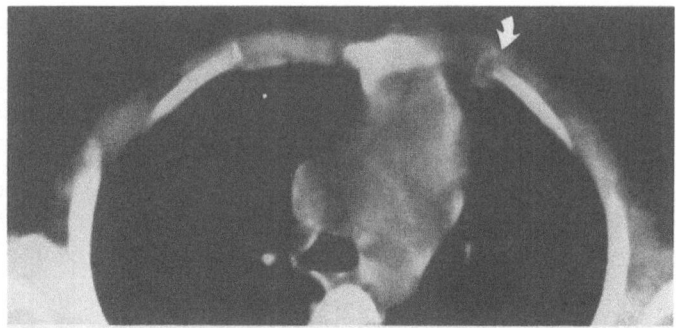

Fig. 6.4. A 6-year-old boy with leukemia and a tender mass at the third costochondral junction on the left. CT shows irregularity and destruction of the anterior end of the left third rib (*curved arrow*). Note the adjacent soft tissue swelling and compare these findings with those of the normal right side. The changes noted here are nonspecific and represent an osteomyelitis.

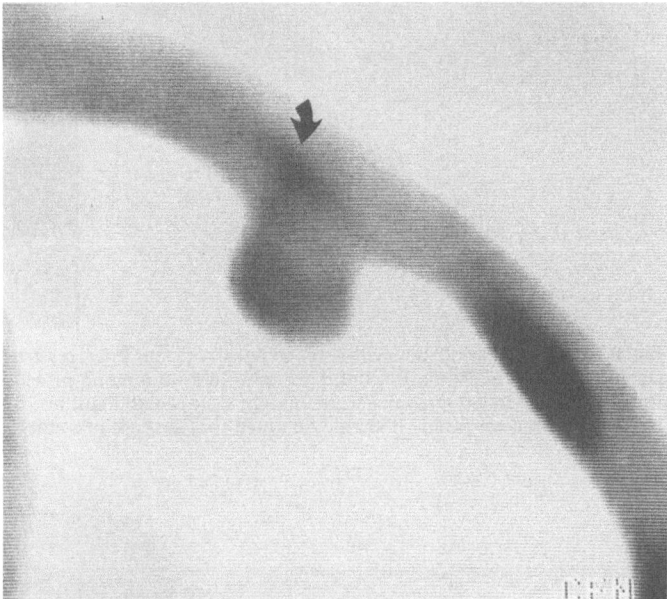

Fig. 6.5. A 5-year-old boy with exostosis of the deep aspect of the left fifth rib anteriorly. Note the relationship of this lesion to the anterior end of the rib (*curved arrow*). The lesion shows calcification in its deepest aspect. The margins of the lesion do not show obtuse angles even though this lesion has extended from an extrapleural site. Differentiation between the extrapleural lesion illustrated in this figure and the intrapulmonary hamartoma adjacent to a rib end in Fig. 5.12 is impossible.

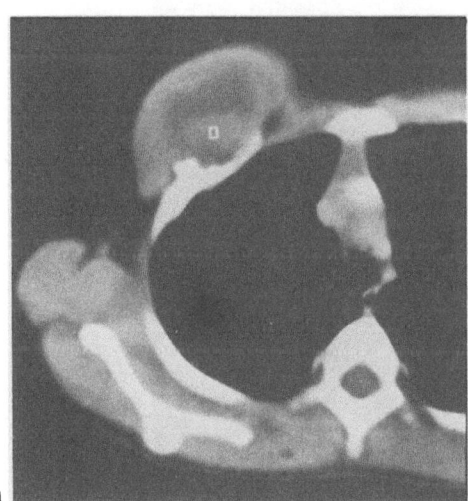
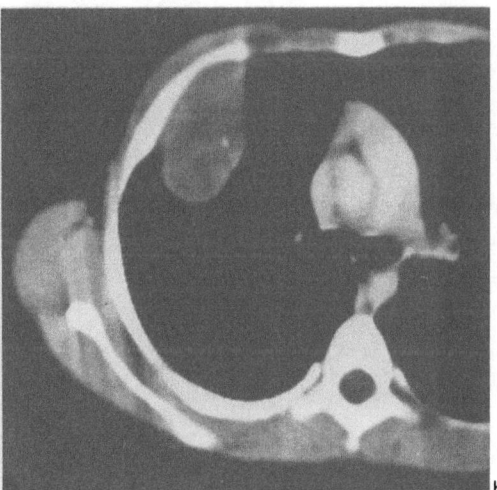

a
b

Fig. 6.6a,b. A 9-year-old girl with an enchondroma of the anterior end of the right second rib. Note the external (a) and internal (b) extension of this mass and the irregularity of the involved rib. Scans have been performed following the intravenous injection of contrast material and show the inhomogeneous attenuation of this lesion.

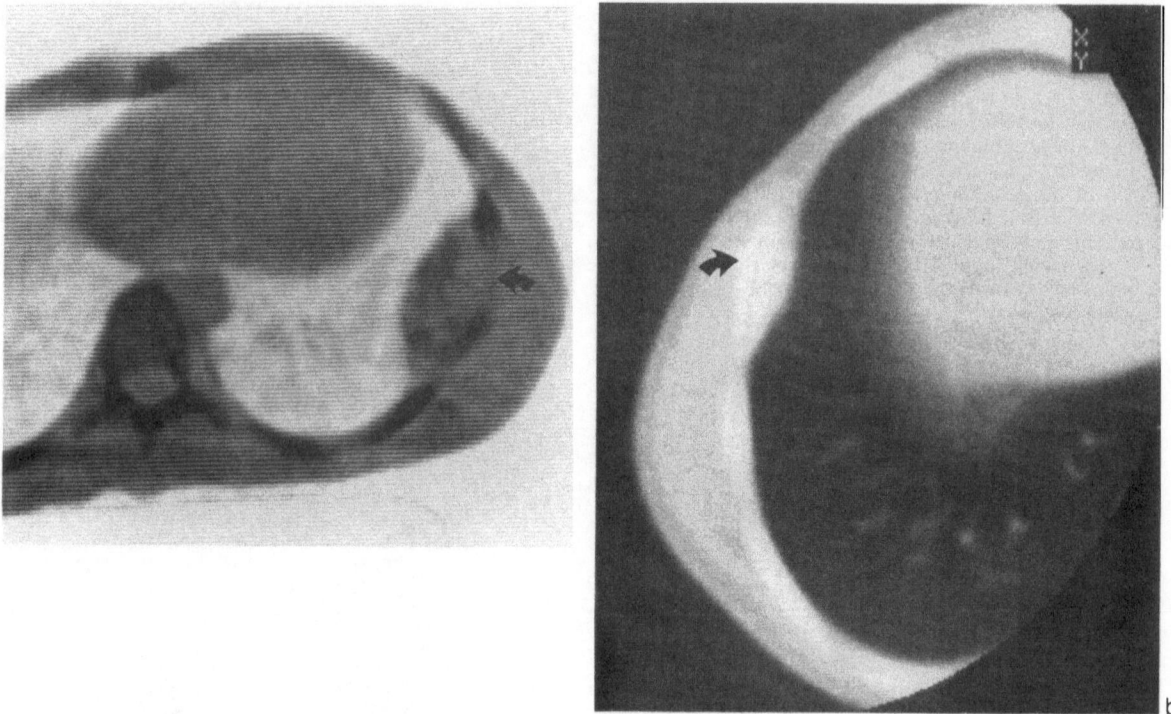

Fig. 6.7. a An 18-year-old boy with osteogenic sarcoma of rib (*curved arrow*). **b** A 17-year-old boy with parosteal sarcoma of right seventh rib (*curved arrow*). Both of these boys had undergone previous chest radiation for metastatic disease from Wilms' tumor. The illustrated sarcomas were thought to be radiation induced. In each case the character of the lesion was impossible to evaluate on these scans. It should be noted that absence of a soft tissue mass (**b**) does not exclude malignancy.

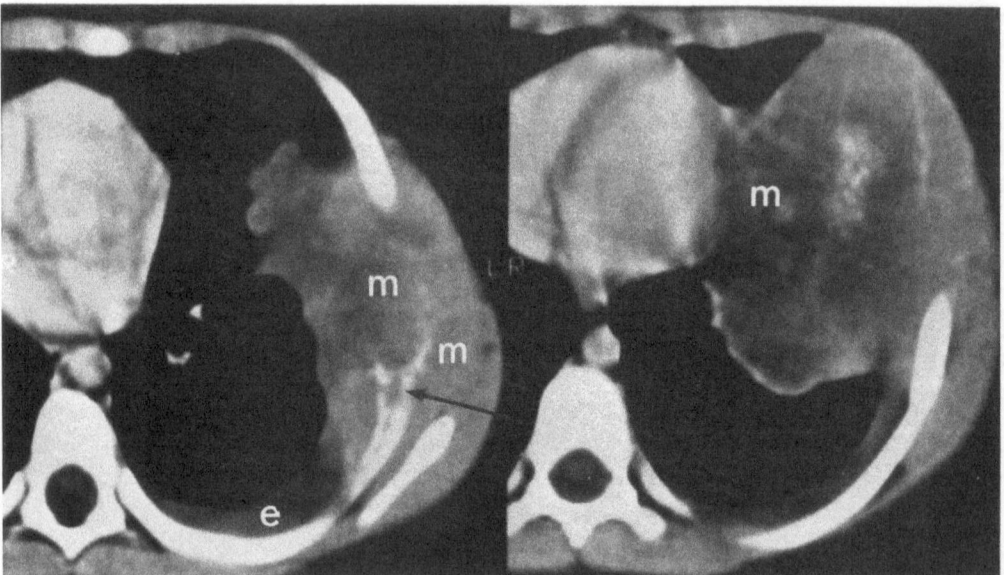

Fig. 6.8. A 4-year-old girl with huge Ewing's sarcoma of left sixth rib. Scans performed after intravenous contrast administration show an inhomogeneous attenuation of the mass. There is an associated pleural effusion which made evaluation of the extent of the mass impossible on plain radiographs. The mass extends up to the pericardium medially, and it is difficult to judge whether the pericardium is infiltrated or not. *m*, mass; *arrow*, rib destruction; *e*, pleural effusion.

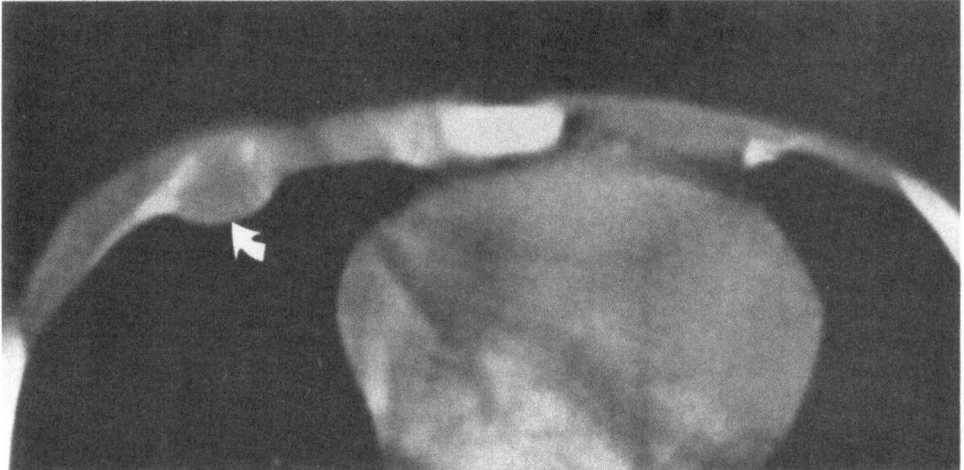

Fig. 6.9. A 10-year-old boy with pelvic rhabdomyosarcoma. Chest CT reveals a metastasis in the anterior end of the right sixth rib (*curved arrow*). It was difficult to appreciate the presence of this lesion on a plain chest film. For this reason, all children undergoing chest CT for the detection of pulmonary metastases should have the images viewed with a wide and narrow window setting in order to assess the soft tissues and bones.

Conventional radiography remains the cornerstone for the evaluation and characterization of lesions of the bony thorax and provided sufficient information for correct management in 10 of our 24 patients (osteochondromas 8, sarcomas 2). In the definition of bone lesions of the chest, CT has two drawbacks. Firstly, it is as difficult to characterize bone lesions with CT in this region, as it is elsewhere in the body. Secondly, the ribs take an oblique course in the chest, and thus only a small portion of each rib is visualized in each transverse scan. Because of these limitations CT does not provide much extra information regarding the character of a bone lesion itself, compared with conventional radiography (see Figs. 6.4–6.7). Absence of a soft tissue mass adjacent to a focal bone lesion does not rule out malignancy (see Fig. 6.7b). Oblique radiographs were more helpful in confirming the malignant character of the lesion in two patients.

Extrapleural Tissues

The lungs extend peripherally to the chest wall and lie immediately deep to the inner surface of the ribs on CT. The extrapleural soft tissues lie external to the parietal pleura. Deep masses of the chest wall involving the extrapleural intra-thoracic tissues may be difficult to assess with conventional radiography as the X-ray beam may not be tangential to the mass [7, 8]. The cross-sectional anatomical display on CT is often useful to delineate these lesions further.

Extrapleural masses in children are usually caused by extension of skeletal (see Figs. 6.5, 6.6), mediastinal, or soft tissue lesions. Even with high-resolution scans, it may be difficult to differentiate lesions extending into the extrapleural space from very peripheral subpleural lung lesions. An illustration of this point is made by comparing Fig. 6.5, showing an exostosis of a rib, with Fig. 5.12 (see p. 66), illustrating a hamartoma of the lung lying adjacent to the anterior end of a rib.

Masses arising in the extrapleural space are rare in children and are less commonly benign than malignant. We have studied one boy with neurofibromatosis [3] (Fig. 6.10). Lobulated densities deep to the ribs were considered to be due to fusiform enlargement of the intercostal nerves (see also Chap. 21, p. 319). Malignant metastases from lymphoma and leukemia are also uncommon in the extrapleural space (Fig. 6.11). The commonest primary malignant lesion arising in the extrapleural tissues is rhabdomyosarcoma, which usually appears as a soft tissue mass without calcification or obvious bone destruction (Fig. 6.12). These lesions may enhance in an irregular manner and occasionally may mimic an empyema.

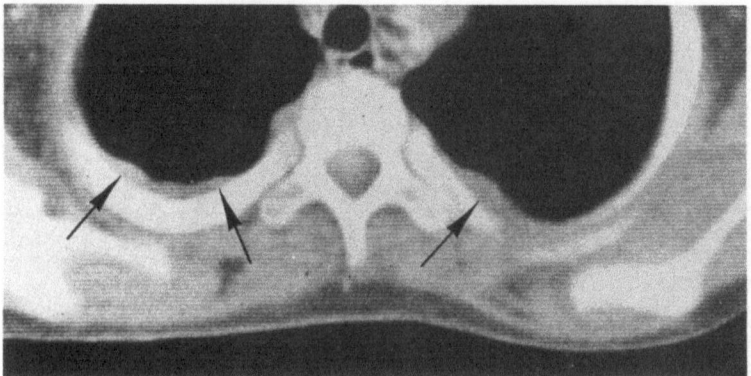

Fig. 6.10. A 13-year-old boy with neurofibromatosis. Chest CT was performed in the search for pulmonary metastases from a malignant Schwannoma which had been removed from the calf. Nodular soft tissue densities (*arrows*) deep to the inner aspect of the ribs are due to fusiform enlargement of intercostal nerves. This is the same patient shown in Fig. 21.7 (Daneman et al. 1983 [3])

Pleura

Incidental pleural abnormalities are rarely found in children, in contrast to their frequent detection in adults on CT. Even with fast, high-resolution scans the pleural fissures are not often visualized in children when 10- or 5-mm thick scans are used. Because the lung field adjacent to the fissures is relatively avascular, the anatomical regions of the fissures are usually easy to locate even in very young children by observing the pattern of avascular areas in the lung fields (see Fig. 5.1, p. 56; see also Fig. 3.2, p. 24). By following these areas in adjacent scans one can follow the major and minor fissures with ease. Not uncommonly a scan taken directly through

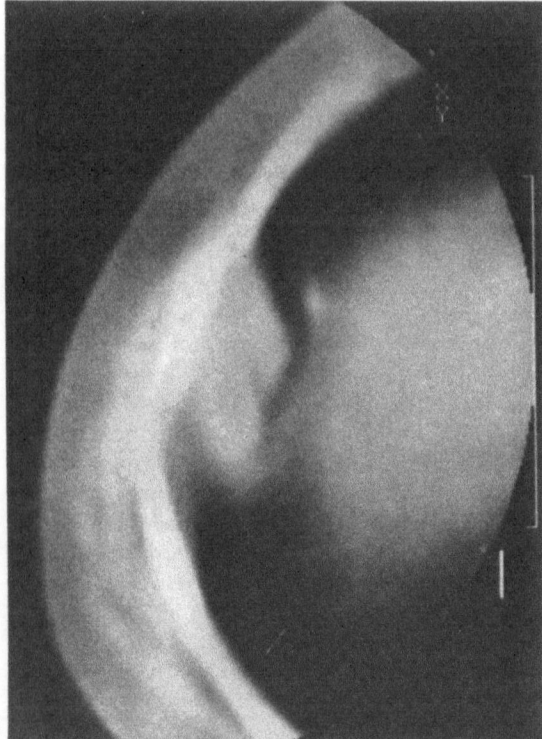

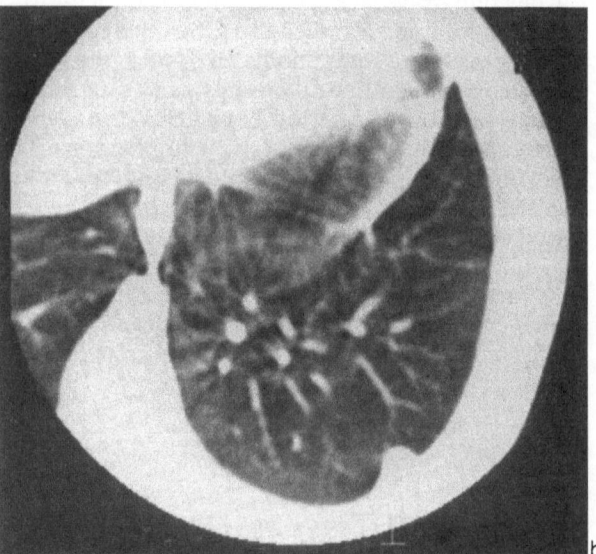

Fig. 6.11a,b Extrapleural malignant deposits in leukemia (**a**) and lymphoma (**b**). Note the variation in shapes of these deposits.

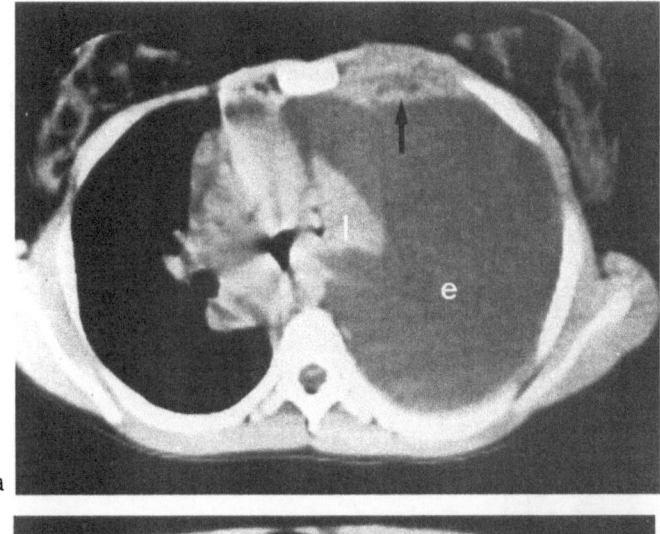

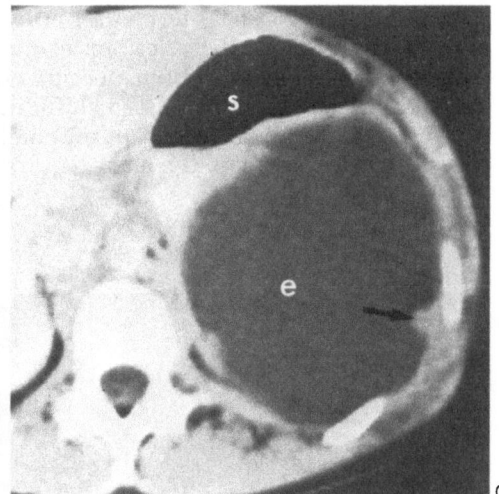

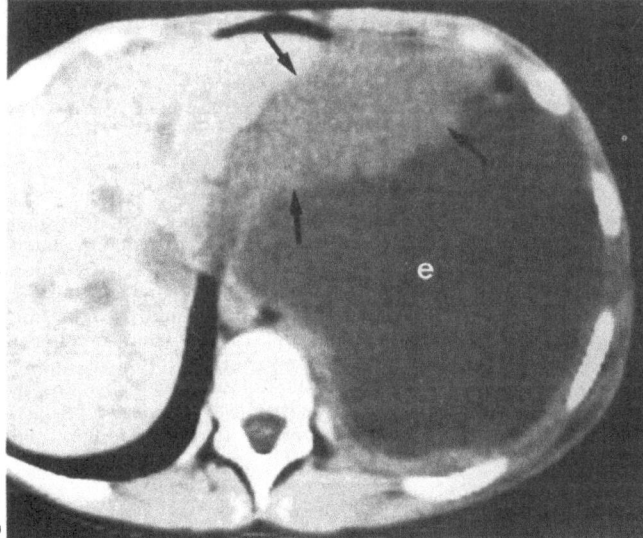

Fig. 6.12a–c. A 15-year-old girl with embryonal rhabdomyosarcoma. A large left pleural effusion (*e*) is noted in all images. **a** The lung (*l*) is collapsed and lies adjacent to the mediastinum. **b** A mass (*arrows*) is noted in the anterior chest wall on the left and extends posteromedially. **c** A further extrapleural deposit (*arrow*) is noted laterally. This CT study was extremely useful in delineating the exact extent of the extrapleural rhabdomyosarcoma and the metastasis laterally, as well as giving information regarding the underlying lung. The large pleural effusion made delineation virtually impossible on the chest radiographs. Note the mediastinal shift in **a** and the appearance of the pleural effusion in **c**, where the diaphragm has been inverted and the pleural fluid posterolateral to the stomach (*s*).

the level of the minor fissure on the right will reveal a large avascular area of the right lung which may appear somewhat unusual but is a normal finding as the minor fissure is almost horizontal and parallels the plane of the scan (see Fig. 5.1, p. 56).

Conventional radiographs remain the primary procedure for the detection of pleural effusion and pneumothorax. However, these abnormalities are easily visualized on CT, and the fissures become readily visible even when only a small amount of fluid or air collects within the pleural space of the fissure.

In patients with known malignant or inflammatory disease or thoracoabdominal trauma, CT may reveal small pleural fluid collections which may not be evident on plain chest radiographs.

Pleural effusions appear as nonenhancing soft tissue densities internal to the chest wall and may extend into the fissures of the lungs. Scanning the patient in different positions may determine whether the fluid collections are loculated or free in the pleural cavity. Attenuation values may not be specific enough to distinguish the composition of various types of pleural fluid collections. Although differences in attenuation values are usually helpful in differentiating loculated pleural fluid from soft tissue pleural or extrapleural masses, occasionally this differentiation is not possible. We have used sonography extensively and successfully to differentiate pleural fluid collections from solid mass lesions. The echo pattern of the fluid may be helpful in determining the composition of the fluid.

In the presence of large pleural effusions it may be difficult to assess lesions of the chest wall, lung, and mediastinum on conventional radiographs. CT is particularly helpful in these instances as the transverse scans and high-density resolution display the various structures without overlap, and thus the extent of disease is extremely well illustrated (see Figs. 6.8, 6.12, 6.13). Large effusions may cause complete collapse of underlying lung (Figs. 6.12, 6.13) and mediastinal shift toward the opposite hemithorax.

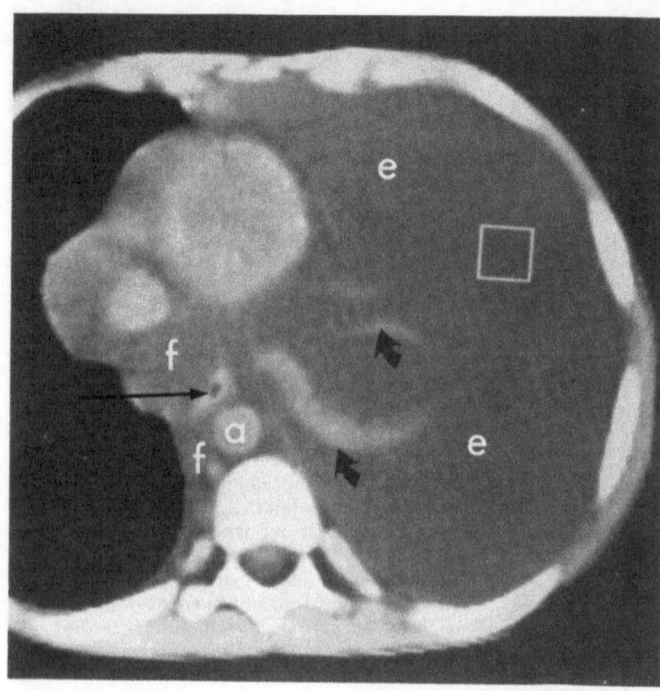

Fig. 6.13. A 12-year-old girl with congenital lymphangiomatosis. The patient presented with respiratory distress, and her chest radiograph revealed a large left pleural effusion. CT shows a large amount of fluid (*e*) filling the entire left pleural cavity. Fluid of similar attenuation (*f*) is also noted in the mediastinum. This is the chest CT of the patient illustrated in Fig. 17.7. *a*, aorta; *long arrows*, esophagus; *curved arrows*, portions of collapsed lung.

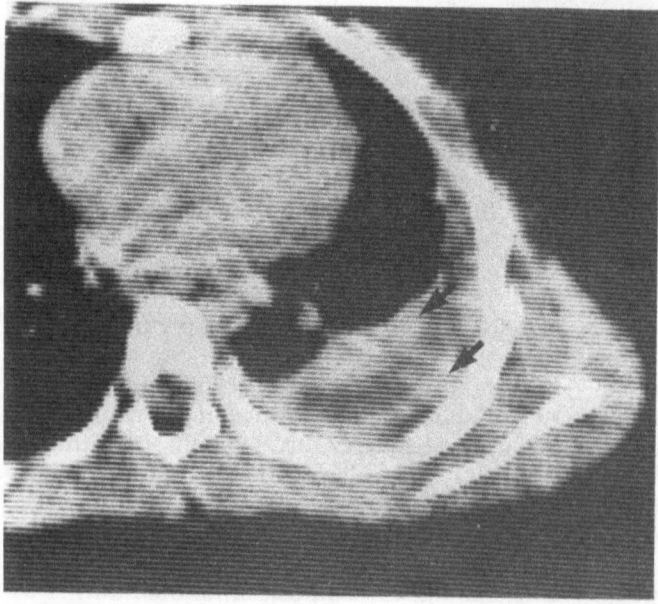

Fig. 6.14. A 10-year-old boy with left empyema following pneumonia. The pleural reaction shows enhancement peripherally (*arrows*), caused by vascular inflammatory tissue, and no enhancement centrally because of the presence of pus.

Loculated empyema may mimic a chest mass on plain films or CT. Following intravenous injection of contrast material the empyema may enhance peripherally on CT (Fig. 6.14). Occasionally, extrapleural tumors with central necrosis may have a similar appearance on CT following intravenous contrast enhancement. CT may also be useful in the differentiation of loculated empyema from peripheral lung abscess [7].

Pneumothoraces appear as air collections around the lung. The visceral pleura is easily visualized as separating the underlying lung from the surrounding pneumothorax, which has an attenuation coefficient of even higher negative values than normal lungs (Fig. 6.15). Small pneumothoraces may occasionally be found as unexpected findings in children undergoing chest CT for trauma or in the search for pulmonary metastases. This may occur, for example, in patients with osteogenic sarcoma. In these patients the underlying metastases causing the pneumothorax may be so small that they are not visible on CT.

Moreover, CT may show small pleural lesions at an earlier stage than conventional radiographs and it is also of value in evaluating pleural mass lesions when conventional radiographs fail to delineate these lesions adequately in profile. Pleural mass lesions may be inflammatory (such as postoperative complications or empyema), or malignant, when they are usually metastases. The commonest densities seen adjacent to the inner aspect of the chest wall on CT in children are usually related to a previous thoractomy. The more irregular oval or rounded lesions may represent areas of focal hemorrhage, fluid collection, or inflammatory masses, and it may be impossible to distinguish whether these densities are extrapleural, pleural, or subpleural intrapulmonary in location (see Fig. 6.5; see also Fig. 5.12, p. 00). Their irregular outline usually differentiates these lesions from metastases, which usually have a smoother outline and are more rounded. Pleural metastases can occasionally have a somewhat unusual shape and may be oval or cylindrical. If such densities are noted on CT as new lesions several months after a thorac-

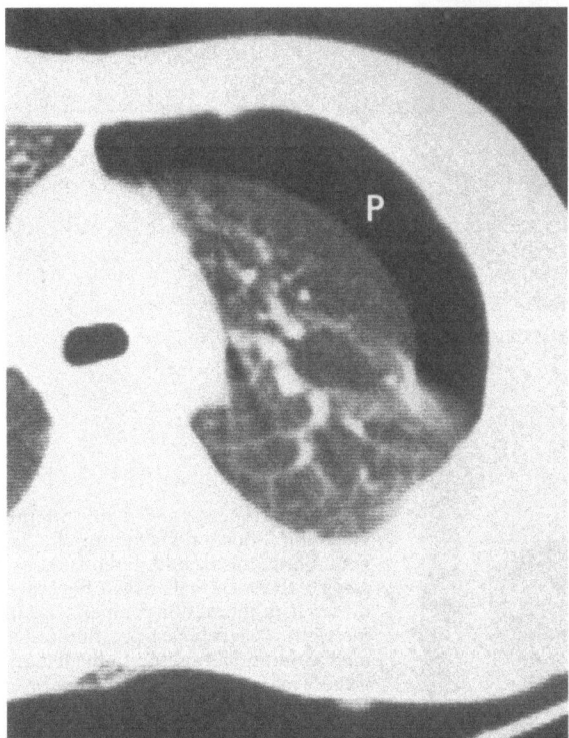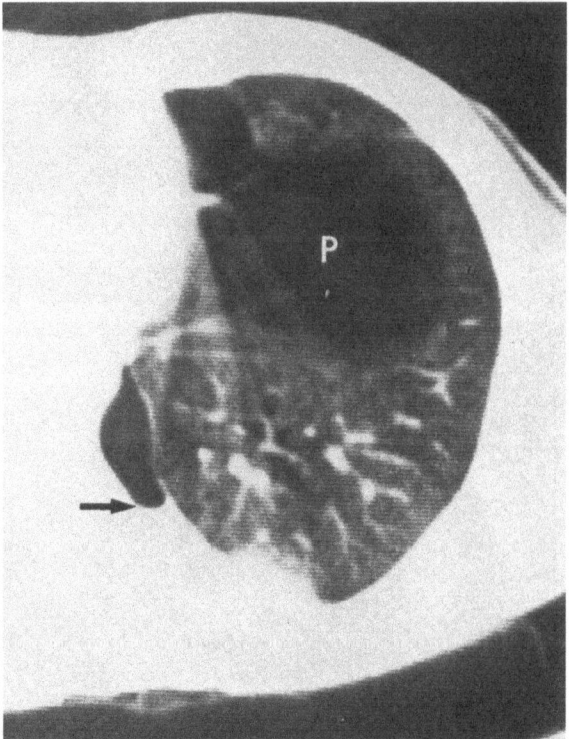

a b

Fig. 6.15a,b. A 14-year-old boy with osteogenic sarcoma and left pneumothorax. **a** Scan shows pneumothorax (*P*) anterolaterally. **b** More inferiorly, pneumothorax is noted below the lung (*P*), and a loculated hydropneumothorax is present medially with an air-fluid level (*arrow*). The pneumothorax has a higher negative attenuation value than the normal pulmonary parenchyma. A faint white line, the visceral pleura, separates the lung and pneumothorax anterolaterally in **a** and posteromedially in **b**. It cannot be seen more centrally in **b** as this area is sectioned tangentially.

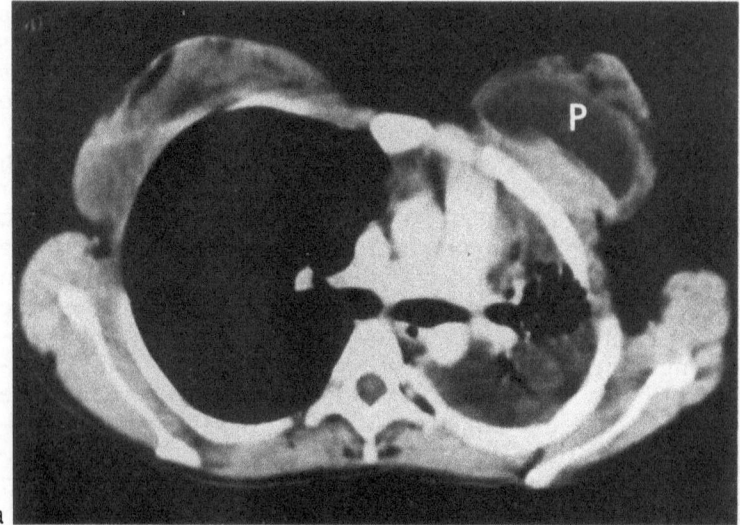

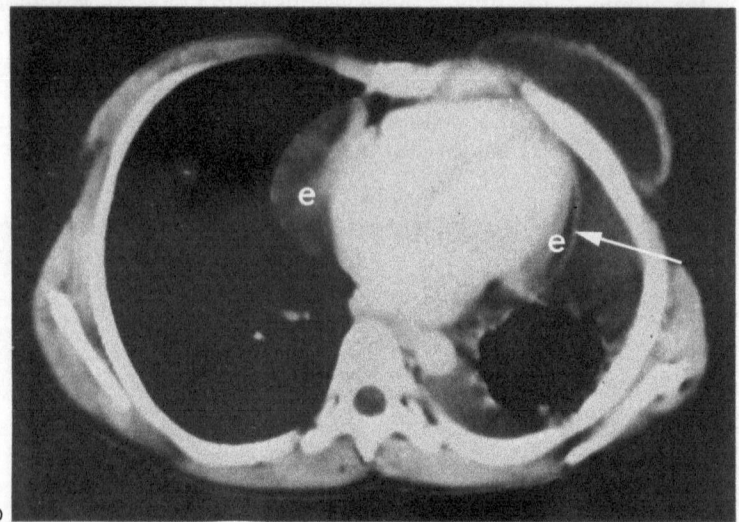

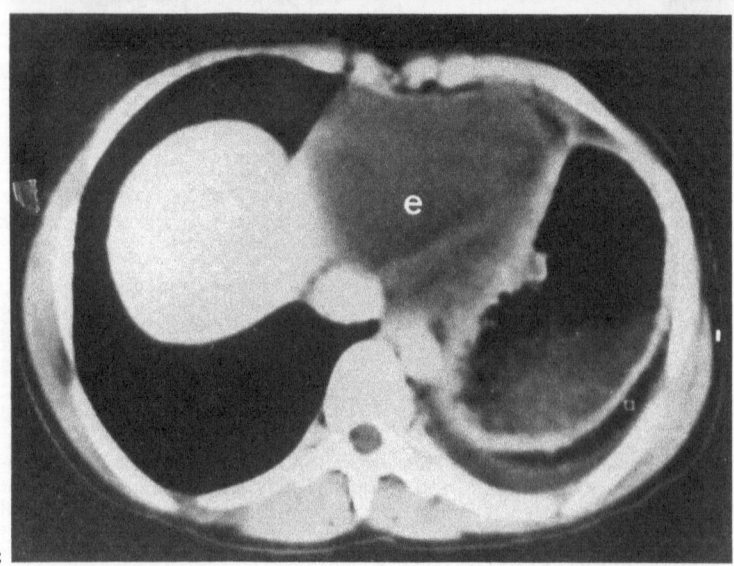

Fig. 6.16a–c. A 16-year-old girl with previous high-dose radiation to the left hemithorax for an undifferentiated sarcoma of the chest wall. **a** Note how small the left hemithorax is in comparison with the right. *P*, left breast prosthesis. The mediastinum has shifted to the left and there is marked scarring and an air bronchogram pattern in the left lung. A pleural reaction is noted and in **b** it is separated from the pericardial effusion (*e*) by the pericardium (*arrow*), which has enhanced following intravenous contrast administration. **c** A large collection of pericardial fluid is noted below the heart (*e*).

tomy, they should be considered as metastatic lesions until proved otherwise. If lesions with these shapes are present on immediate post-thoracotomy scans they should be considered as postoperative changes and can be followed, if necessary, by CT at 6-weekly intervals until they have resolved. Other triangular or linear densities adjacent to the chest wall probably represent areas of postoperative fibrosis and atelectasis within the lung.

Postradiation Changes

Children with bony or soft tissue sarcomas of the chest wall usually receive high-dose radiation to the chest as part of their treatment protocol. This radiation is usually given to all or most of the involved hemithorax. Such high-dose radiation causes profound scarring and growth retardation of the thoracic structures in the radiation field. The resultant deformity in the thoracic wall, scarring of the underlying lung, and concomitant ipsilateral mediastinal shift make postradiation plain chest radiographs in these children extremely difficult to interpret. Local recurrent mass lesions and underlying pulmonary metastases are exceedingly difficult to appreciate on these chest radiographs. We have performed CT repeatedly as follow-up studies in eight patients with such deformities at the Hospital for Sick Children, Toronto. The transverse CT scans depict the various components of the hemithorax without overlap and make evaluation of the chest wall and underlying lung very much easier than conventional radiography (Figs. 6.16, 6.17).

The main features noted in the hemithorax of patients who have received high-dose radiation to the chest are: marked deformity of the chest wall with diminution in the size of the hemithorax compared with the opposite hemithorax; marked scarring and consolidation of the underlying lung with a well-marked air bronchogram pattern; varying degrees of pleural reaction; and varying degrees of pericardial effusion (Figs. 6.16, 6.17).

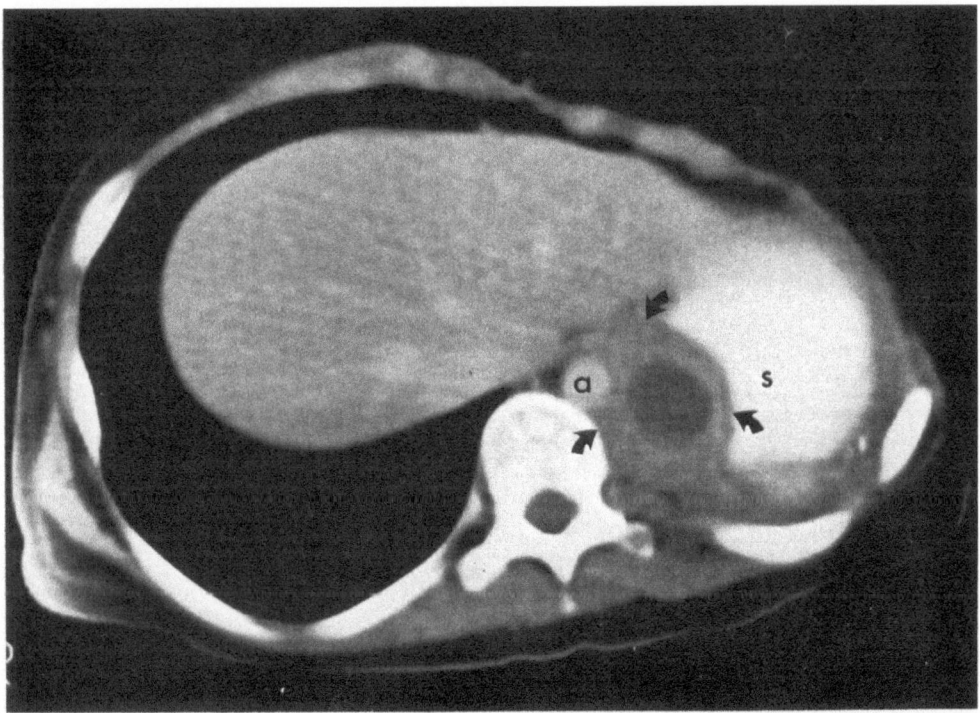

Fig. 6.17. A 16-year-old girl with previous high-dose radiation to the chest for a Ewing's sarcoma of the left eighth rib. CT scan through the lower chest shows that the left hemithorax and upper abdomen are much smaller than the right. A soft tissue mass is noted medially and represents recurrent paravertebral tumor (*arrows*). This indents the stomach (*s*). *a*, aorta. The mass was not appreciated on the plain chest radiograph.

Following intravenous contrast administration the various components can be visualized better, and the nonenhancing pleural and pericardial reactions can be differentiated from the underlying lung and any recurrent masses. Even with this technique, however, it is impossible to visualize extremely small metastatic disease in the lung that has been severely scarred with radiation changes (Fig. 6.16a).

It should be stressed that children who have received lower dose radiation for malignant disease may develop secondary radiation-induced neoplasms [11] of the chest wall and thyroid gland. These may be benign (see Fig. 22.3, p. 332, and Fig. 23.20, p. 352) or malignant (see Fig. 6.7).

References

1. Askin FB, Rosal J, Sibley RK, Dehner LP, McAllister WH (1979) Malignant small cell tumor of the thoracopulmonary region in childhood. Cancer 43:2438–2451
2. Campbell AN, Chan HSL, Daneman A, Martin DJ (1983) Aggressive fibromatosis in childhood. CT 7:109–113
3. Daneman A, Mancer K, Sonley M (1983) CT appearance of thickened nerves in neurofibromatosis. AJR 141:899–900
4. Donoghue VB, Daneman A, Chan HSL, Qualman SJ (1985) Chest wall masses in children. Paper presented at Meeting of the European Society for Paediatric Radiology, Glasgow, 1985
5. Franken EA, Smith JA Jr, Smith WL (1977) Tumours of the chest wall in infants and children. Pediatr Radiol 6:13–18
6. Hudson TM, Vandergriend RA, Springfield DS, Hawkins IF, Spanier SS, Enneking WF, Hamlin DJ (1984) Aggressive fibromatosis: evaluation of computed tomography and angiography. Radiology 150:495–501
7. Kirks DR, Korobkin, M (1980) Chest computed tomography in infants and children. An analysis of 50 patients. Pediatr Radiol 10:75–82
8. Kirks DR, Korobkin, M (1981) Computed tomography of the chest wall, pleura and pulmonary parenchyma in infants and children. Radiol Clin North Am 19:421–429
9. Leitman BS, Firooznia H, McCauley DI, Ettenger NA, Reede DL, Golimbu CN, Rafii M, Naidich DP (1983) The use of computed tomography in evaluating chest wall pathology. CT 7:399–405
10. Liu P, Daneman A, Stringer DA, Smith CR (1984) CT appearance of hemangiomas and related lesions of soft tissues in childhood. (Submitted for publication)
11. Moyes J, Chan HSL, Daneman A (1984) Second tumours in children with previously treated malignancy. (Unpublished data)

Chapter 7

Technique

Introduction

The general approaches to CT technique apply to the abdomen and pelvis as they do elsewhere in the body and have been outlined in detail in Chapter 2. Certain specific points require stressing. These involve the administration of oral and intravenous contrast material for scanning technique. The vast majority of scans of the abdomen and pelvis are performed to delineate mass lesions or in follow-up after surgery or radiotherapy. It is extremely important to have the bowel and vasculature opacified in order to delineate the extent of these lesions and exclude recurrences accurately.

Gastrointestinal Contrast Material

The stomach and small intestine are usually filled with varying amounts of fluid and gas (see Figs. 7.2, 7.3). Any portion of this part of the gastrointestinal tract may simulate a soft tissue mass lesion on CT when filled completely with fluid and may even masquerade as an abscess when filled with fluid and air. Filling of the stomach and small bowel with dilute oral con-

trast material is mandatory in order to avoid confusion. Our approach has been to give the child the necessary amount of oral contrast material 30–45 min prior to scanning. Usually this ensures adequate filling of all distal small bowel loops. The distal large bowel does not often simulate a mass lesion as it is usually filled with formed stool and air. If it does pose a problem, a small amount of contrast may be injected into the distal large bowel via a Foley catheter placed in the rectum. The reader is referred to Chapter 17, p. 273 and Fig. 15.10, p. 232, for further information.

The contrast material used to opacify the gastrointestinal tract is 5 ml Gastrografin in 180 ml (6 oz) of fluid. Dilution of the Gastrografin with fruit-flavoured drinks helps to camouflage its taste. The volume of contrast administered to a child will vary depending on the child's size and also whether the upper abdomen or lower pelvis are to be examined. Larger quantities are required to outline the small bowel in the pelvis. Neonates require approximately 50 ml of diluted contrast to fill the stomach and upper gastrointestinal tract and 100 ml to opacify the small bowel. Young children require 360 ml (about two 6-oz cups) and older children 720 ml (four cups) to opacify the small bowel adequately. If patients are to be sedated, or if they refuse to drink the contrast material, a feeding tube is placed with its tip in the stomach and the correct volume of contrast is administered.

Intravenous Contrast Material

When examining the soft tissues of the abdomen we routinely perform scans during rapid bolus injection of intravenous contrast material. We administer 2–3 ml/kg, Hypaque Sodium 60% depending on the size of the patient and the size of the area to be examined. The vascular anatomy of the upper abdomen is particularly complex, and adequate studies of this area cannot be performed unless the vessels are adequately outlined with intravenous contrast material. The vasculature of the lower pelvis is less complex, and scans in this area may be performed after the injection of contrast material as this will be sufficient to delineate the vessels, ureters, and bladder. When scans are performed to evaluate small lesions within the kidneys, only 1 mg/kg Hypaque Sodium is necessary as larger quantities may cause some artifact and obscure the small lesions. We have found it useful to administer intravenous contrast material for examinations of the pelvis and have not found that the density of the bladder causes too much artifact when filled with contrast administered in the abovementioned doses. Intravenous contrast is not required for scans that are performed only for the purpose of detecting calcification or for the assessment of osseous lesions.

Scan Technique

Scans of the abdomen and pelvis are usually done with the patient in the supine position and adequately immobilized. Patients may be moved into other positions if they are uncomfortable lying supine or if one is attempting to determine whether fluid is loculated or free.

It is essential to obtain an initial anteroposterior computed radiograph from which one can choose the intended slices (Fig. 7.1). Adjacent scans, 1 cm thick, are performed over the area of interest; additional scans may be required to cover more distant extensions of mass lesions. Scans 5 mm thick may be required for adequate delineation of the adrenals or for small lesions. Occasionally, certain areas may have to be reexamined if one is unsure whether a structure is indeed a mass or unopacified loops of bowel (Figs. 7.2, 7.3). Digital radiographs at the end of the study may show the relationship of a mass to the urinary tract. This technique saves the child an extra injection of contrast and radiation if a formal excretory urogram is requested by a clinician.

All scans should be carefully monitored and all images viewed at multiple window settings in order to achieve optimum assessment of all structures in the scan field.

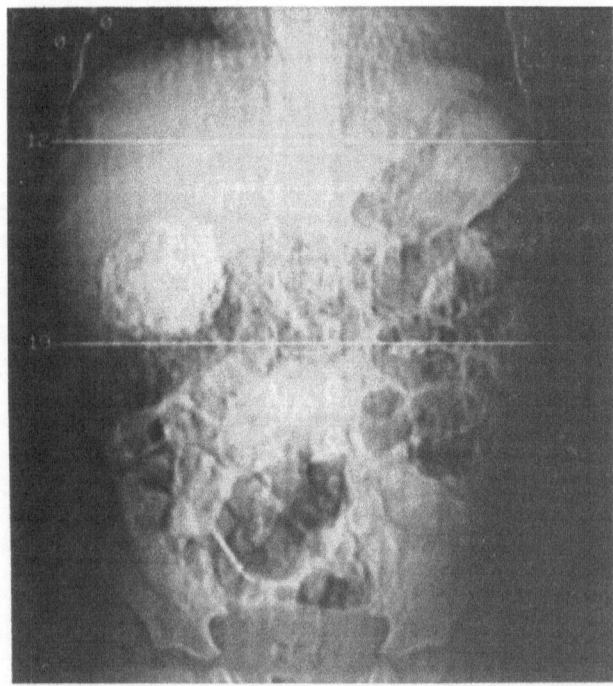

Fig. 7.1. Computed radiograph of patient with previously treated right Wilms' tumor. A heavily calcified mass is noted in the region of the right upper quadrant. From the axial scans the limits of the lesion were noted to be on scans *12* and *19*. These two lines have been posted on the scout radiograph to delineate the limits of the lesion.

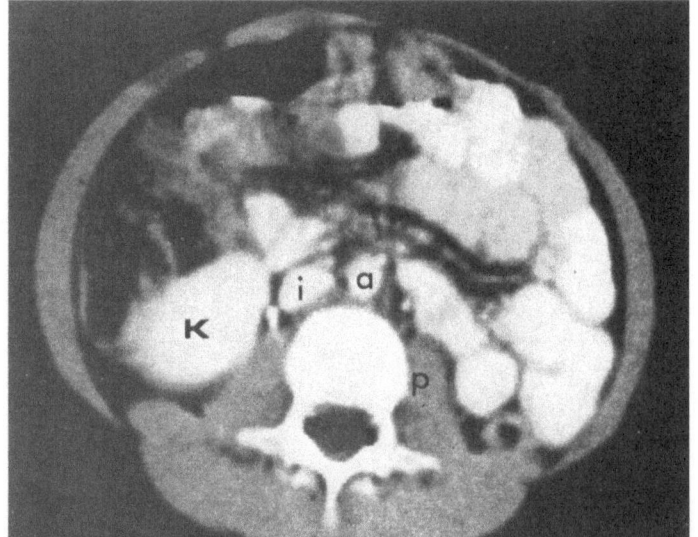

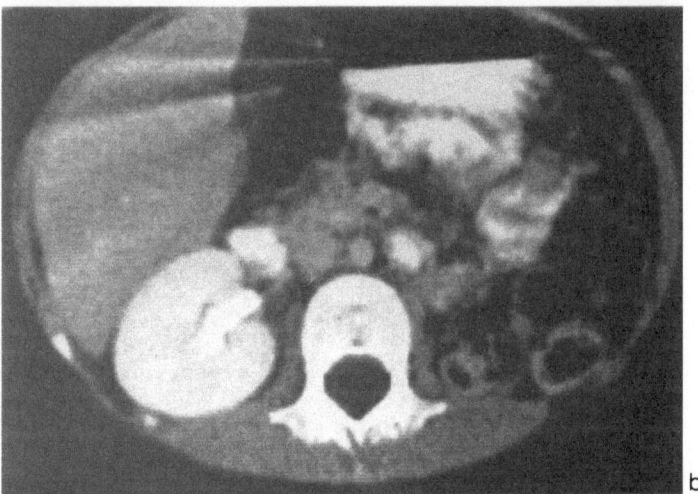

Fig. 7.2a. Example of excellent opacification of the small bowel with dilute oral water-soluble contrast material. Note the densely opacified small bowel loops in the left flank following a left nephrectomy. This appearance adequately rules out any local recurrence. *K*, kidney; *i*, inferior vena cava; *a*, aorta; *p*, psoas muscle. **b** Following left nephrectomy the large bowel has filled the left renal fossa. This has not been opacified with contrast, but the presence of gas and stool within the bowel makes exclusion of a mass lesion easy. **c** Following left nephrectomy small bowel loops fill the left flank. Some of these have been well filled with contrast, but others more posteriorly (*B*) have not filled well. These may masquerade as a recurrent lesion. However, in a delayed scan (**d**) these small bowel loops have filled well with contrast and have excluded the presence of a mass. Images **c** and **d** illustrate the value of delayed scans when the bowel is not opacified and a local recurrence is suspected. (*Fig. 7.2d overleaf*)

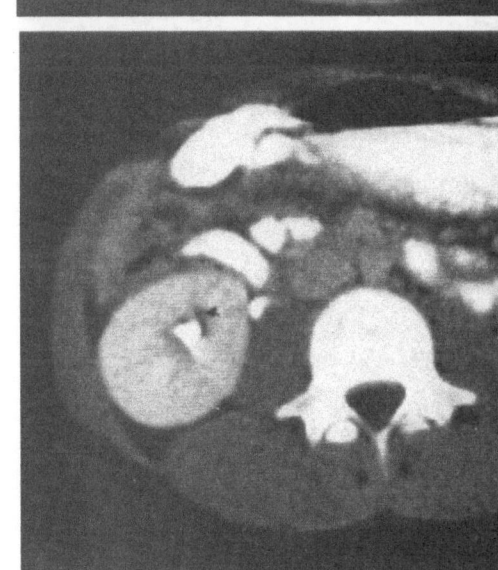

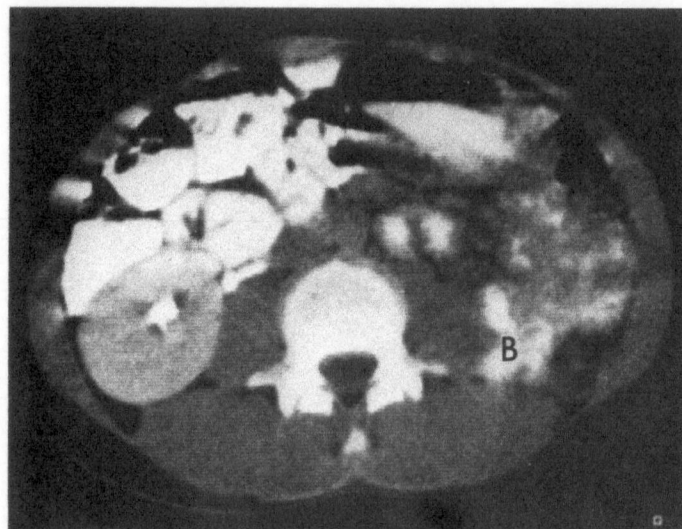

Fig. 7.2d

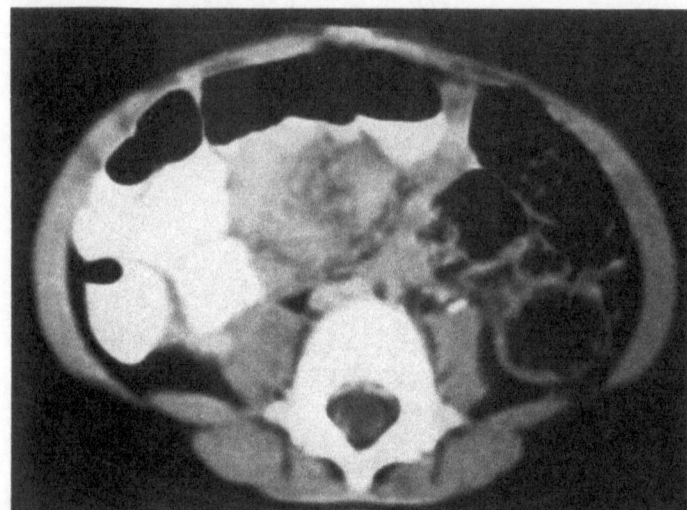

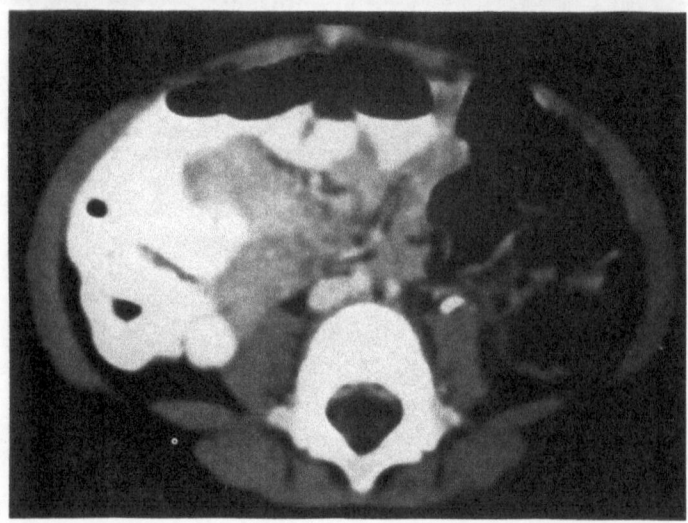

Fig. 7.3a,b. Scans performed as a follow-up in a patient who had a previous resection of a huge right renal clear cell carcinoma. In **a** a large mass is present in the central portion of the abdomen, simulating the presence of a local recurrence. However, in a delayed scan (**b**) the shape of this area has changed dramatically, indicating that this area is merely occupied by bowel loops that have filled poorly with contrast. This illustration demonstrates strikingly the value of delayed scans in excluding recurrent disease. Even if the involved loops have not filled with contrast, a change in the fluid, contrast, or gaseous content of these loops will help to exclude a recurrence.

Chapter 8

Retroperitoneum

Introduction

Prior to the advent of CT and sonography the delineation of anatomical structures and their relationship to pathological processes in the retroperitoneal region was extremely difficult. Adequate assessment of the retroperitoneal area often required the use of multiple, difficult, and invasive procedures and involved a high radiation dose. These procedures included excretory urography with nephrotomography, angiography, venography, lymphangiography, and retroperitoneal carbon dioxide insufflation. Although sonography is an excellent noninvasive modality to delineate the retroperitoneum of the upper abdomen and lower pelvis, it has the disadvantage of not being able to assess adequately the retroperitoneum of the mid abdomen and upper pelvis because of overlying bowel gas in many patients.

We have found CT to be the single most reliable and accurate modality in the assessment of the entire retroperitoneal area. Although it is our modality of choice in the examination of this region, the paucity of fat in children makes visualization of structures in this area naturally poor because of the low contrast between the structures. Adequate delineation of anatomical structures and pathological processes depends on the adequate opacification of bowel, achieved by administering oral contrast material, and the adequate opacification of the vasculature, achieved by doing scans during injection of intravenous contrast material. Nowhere in the abdomen is meticulous attention to technique more important.

Adequate visualization of these structures is not only important in the delineation of primary diseases in the retroperitoneum but also in the delineation of disease adjacent to the retroperitoneum. Indeed, adequate visualization of structures in the retroperitoneum is the key to obtaining a successful and meaningful study in most examinations of the abdomen. The commonest reason for doing CT is to define structures and viscera of the retroperitoneum, and this accounts for over 40% of all body CT examinations performed at our institution.

This chapter will deal with the pathology involving the lymph nodes, sympathetic nervous system, soft tissues, and vasculature of the retroperitoneum. Lesions of important retroperitoneal viscera including the pancreas, adrenals, and kidneys will be dealt with separately in Chapters 9, 10, and 11, respectively.

Anatomy

The retroperitoneum is that space lying posterior to the posterior parietal peritoneum. Its posterior limit is the transversalis fascia. The space contains the great vessels and their major branches, the psoas muscles, sympathetic nerve chains, lymph nodes and pancreas, kidneys, and adrenals.

The retroperitoneal area can be subdivided into three compartments; however, this has very much less value for the interpretation of scans of the abdomen in children than it has in adults.

1. The anterior pararenal space lies between the posterior parietal peritoneum and the anterior renal fascia. It contains the pancreas, retroperitoneal portion of the descending duodenum, and descending and ascending colon.

2. The perirenal space lies between the anterior and posterior renal fascia and contains the kidneys and adrenals. Extension of this space to the midline includes the major vessels in this space.

3. The posterior pararenal space lies between the posterior renal fascia and the fascia transversalis and contains no vital structures.

In the upper abdomen the pancreas, adrenals, and kidneys are easily visualized (Fig. 8.1). The kidneys are separated from the vertebral bodies by the psoas muscles. The crura of the diaphragm are well visualized and are usually asymmetrical in thickness. The right crus is often thicker and may be quite irregular in outline (Fig. 8.2; see also Fig. 14.1, p. 210). As the crura descend anterior to the vertebral bodies they separate the inferior vena cava and aorta respec-

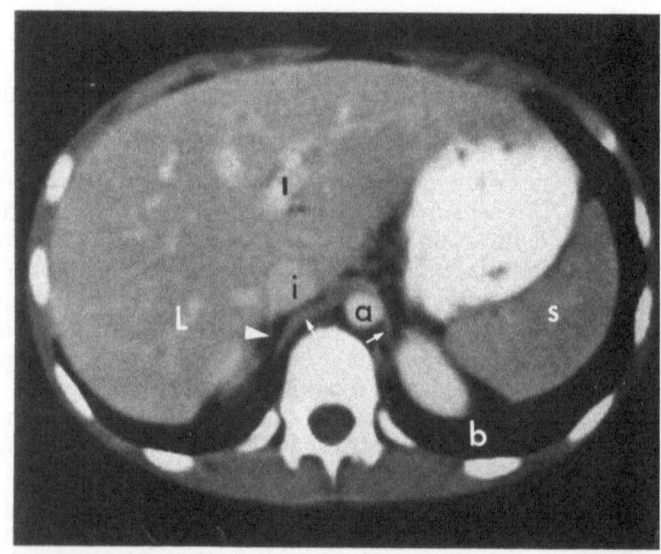

a

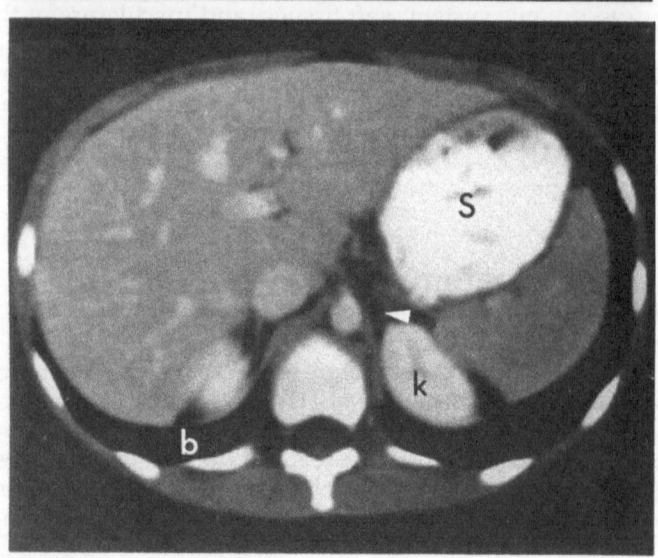

b

Fig. 8.1a–g. Scans of the upper abdomen in a 10-year-old boy performed after the ingestion of dilute water-soluble contrast material and during the intravenous injection of contrast material. In all scans the liver (L), stomach (s), kidneys (k) and spleen (s) are easily seen. The pancreas (p) is seen in scans c–f: the tail in c, the body in d and the head in e and f. *Small black arrow*, common bile duct in posterior portion of pancreatic head in f. In scans a–c the adrenals (*small white arrowhead*) are seen, as well as the lung bases (b). g, gallbladder; a, aorta, i, inferior vena cava; c, colon; j, poorly opacified jejunum; d, poorly opacified duodenum. The second portion of the duodenum lies to the right of the pancreatic head in d–f, and the third part of the duodenum (*small black arrowheads*) crosses the midline in front of the aorta and inferior vena cava and behind the superior mesenteric artery and vein (*curved arrow*) in g. *Small white arrows*, diaphragmatic crura. The left branch of the

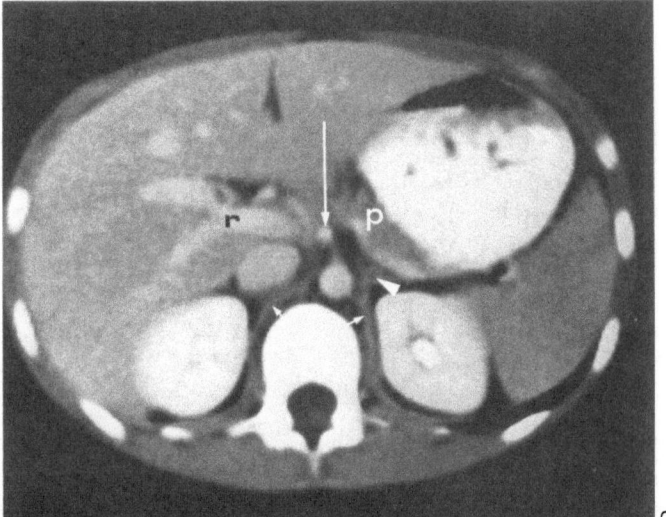

c

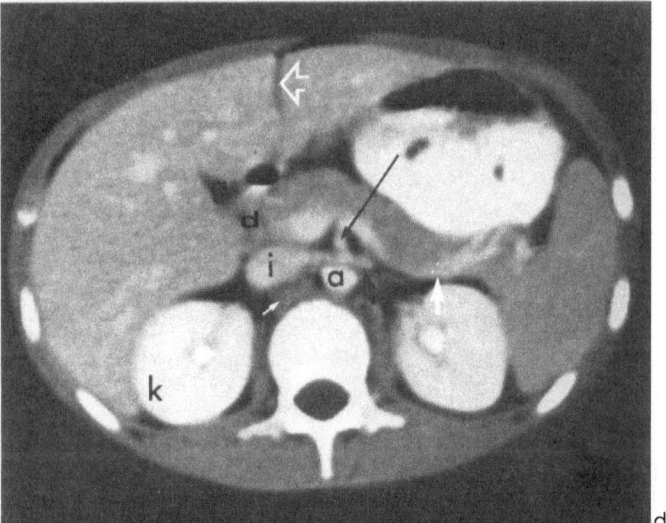

d

Fig. 8.1. (*continued*)
portal vein (*l*) is seen in a more cranial scan in
a than the right branch (*r*) which is seen in scan
c. The celiac artery bifurcates (*long white arrow*)
into the hepatic artery, passing in front of the
portal vein, and the splenic artery, passing
behind the pancreatic tail in scan **c**. In scan **d** the
splenic vein (*short white arrow*) passes from the
spleen behind the pancreas toward the right.
The left renal vein (*short black arrow*) lies
between the aorta *a* and the superior mesenteric
artery (*long black arrow*). *Open white arrow*,
falciform ligament in liver. Note the paucity of
fat in the retroperitoneum. Without the administration of oral and intravenous contrast the
retroperitoneal structures would not have been
easily distinguished. Note the short right renal
vein (*white arrowhead*) and left renal artery and
vein (*black arrowhead*) in **e**. The ureters (*curved
black arrows*) are seen in scan **g** anterior to the
psoas (*m*) muscle.

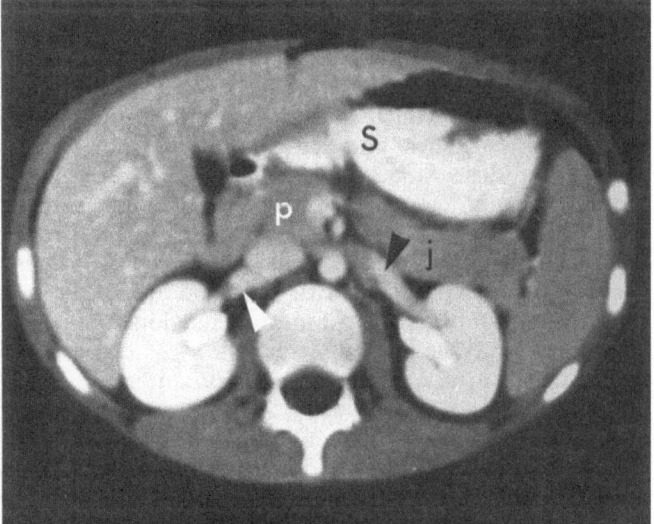

e

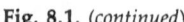

Fig. 8.1. (*continued*)

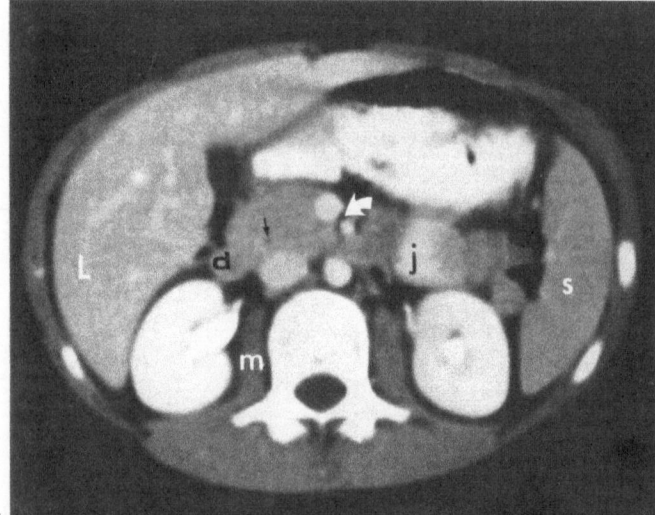

f

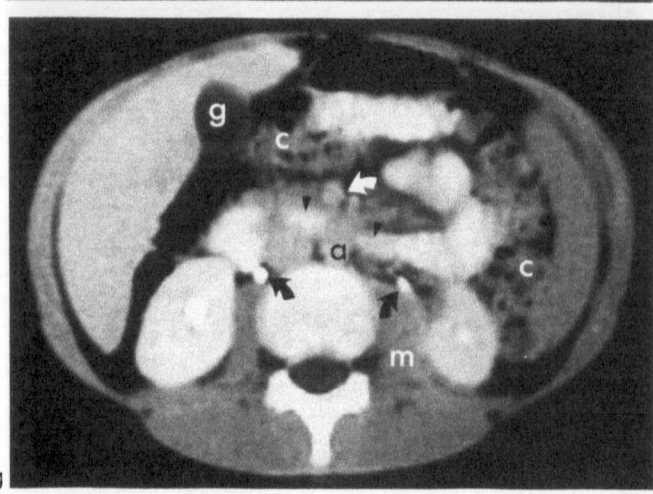

g

tively from the anterior surface of these bones. The thickness of the crura in these positions is quite variable and should not be mistaken for lymphadenopathy. Following these structures in adjacent scans will usually help to differentiate a normal thick and irregular crus from enlarged nodes. Adjacent to the aorta in the retrocrural area are the azygous and hemiazygous veins (see Fig. 10.4, p. 129) which enhance with contrast administration. These should not be confused with enlarged nodes caused by lymphoma or tumor extension in neuroblastoma (see Fig. 10.5, p. 130).

The celiac artery is the first major anterior branch to arise from the aorta as it enters the abdomen behind the crura of the diaphragm. During rapid bolus injection of contrast material the celiac artery may often be seen branching into the splenic artery, which courses to the

splenic hilum above the body of the pancreas, and the common hepatic artery, which courses to the right into the porta hepatis anterior to the main portal vein (see Figs. 8.1, 8.6). The next major anterior branch of the aorta is the superior mesenteric artery, which courses forward to meet the superior mesenteric vein to the left of the head of the pancreas (see Fig. 8.1). The third major anterior branch of the aorta is the inferior mesenteric artery and is not as constantly visualized as the previous two anterior branches. The renal arteries are the major lateral branches of the aorta and course toward the hilum of each kidney. The right renal artery passes behind the inferior vena cava. If there is paucity of retroperitoneal fat it may be difficult to distinguish these arteries from the renal veins and renal pelvis without the use of intravenous contrast material.

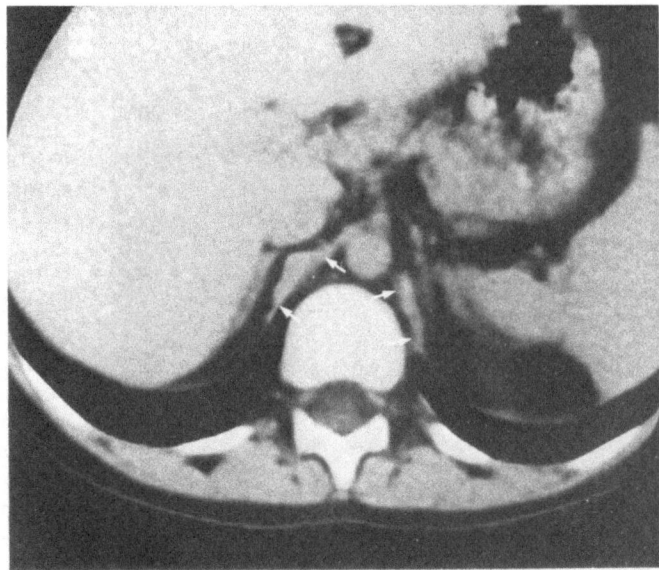

Fig. 8.2. Upper abdominal scan in a 12-year-old boy shows asymmetry and irregularity of the diaphragmatic crura (*white arrows*). The right crus is bigger than the left.

As it courses toward the right atrium the inferior vena cava lies anterior to the level of the aorta in scans of the upper abdomen. Even without contrast administration hepatic veins may be easily visualized as they drain into the upper inferior vena cava (see Fig. 8.1). Below the level of the liver the inferior vena cava lies to the right of the aorta and both vessels can be traced inferiorly anterior to the vertebral bodies. The renal veins lie anterior to the renal arteries as they course toward the inferior vena cava. The right renal vein is often extremely short as the inferior vena cava lies in close proximity to the right renal hilum. The left renal vein has a longer course as it passes toward the inferior vena cava in the angle between the aorta posteriorly and the superior mesenteric artery anteriorly (Fig. 8.3; see also Fig. 9.3, p. 110).

The inferior vena cava often has a tear-drop shape in cross section at the point where the left renal vein drains into it. Scans performed during rapid bolus injection of contrast into a vein on the dorsum of a foot will show dramatic enhancement of the inferior vena cava. Unopacified blood draining into the inferior vena cava from the renal veins does not mix immediately with the opacified caval blood. The stream from each renal vein appears as a large filling defect within the inferior vena cava (Fig. 8.4). It is extremely

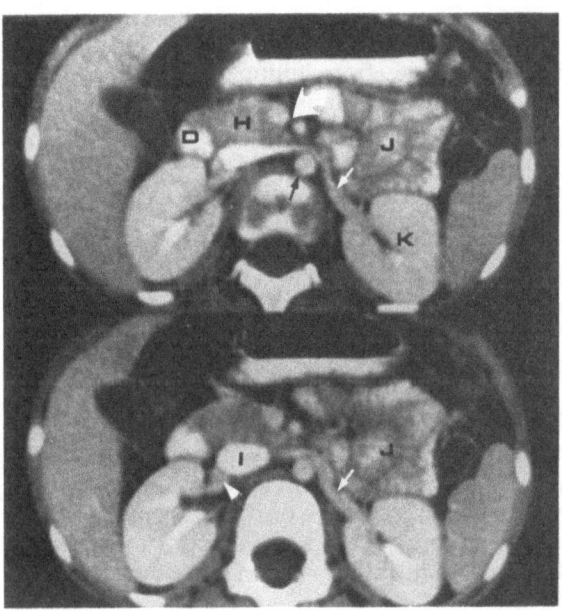

Fig. 8.3. Upper abdominal scans performed after the oral ingestion of dilute water-soluble contrast and during the intravenous injection of contrast material into a vein on the dorsum of the foot. Note the dense opacification of the inferior vena cava (*I*), which is more densely opacified than the other vessels. The left renal vein (*small white arrows*) passes from the left kidney (*K*) in front of the aorta (*small black arrow*) toward the inferior vena cava. Note the short right renal vein (*white arrowhead*) and the defect of opacification in the inferior vena cava on the right in the *upper* scan caused by the flow from the right venal vein. The pancreatic head (*H*) lies anterior to the inferior vena cava between the opacified second portion of the duodenum to the right (*D*) and the superior mesenteric artery and vein (*curved white arrow*) to the left. *J*, jejunum.

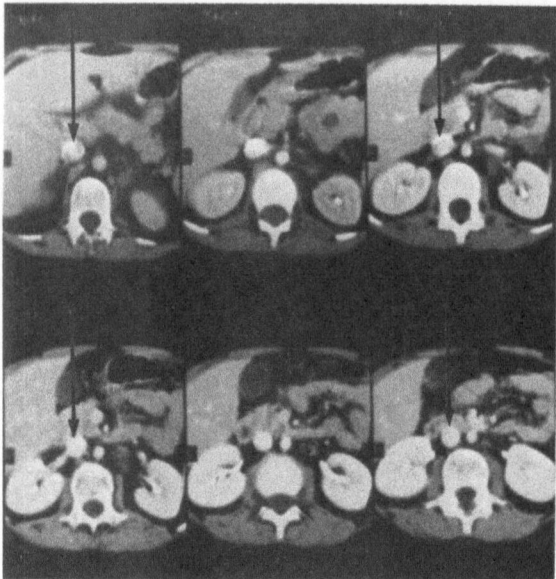

Fig. 8.4. Scans of the upper abdomen during intravenous injection of contrast into a vein on the dorsum of a foot shows opacification of the inferior vena cava (*arrow*). In the *upper scans* filling defects in the inferior vena cava are related to flow of unopacified blood from the kidneys into the cava. Note the junction with the inferior vena cava of the left renal vein in the *upper middle scan* and the right renal vein in the *lower left scan*. The *lower scans* below the level of the renal veins show homogeneous opacification of the inferior vena cava without flow defects.

important to differentiate these defects caused by blood flow from filling defects within the inferior vena cava caused by intravenous tumor growth from neoplasms of the kidney or adrenal. If it is uncertain what these defects represent, delayed scans can be obtained, at which time there will be a more even distribution of contrast in the vascular system and these defects will no longer be visualized. Sonography is extremely useful in the delineation of tumor spread into the inferior vena cava from the above-mentioned neoplasms.

The splenic vein passes from the splenic hilum behind the tail and body of the pancreas toward the neck of the pancreas, where it joins the superior mesenteric vein to form the main portal vein (see Fig. 8.1). The portal vein courses superiorly, anteriorly, and to the right to the porta hepatis behind the common bile duct and hepatic artery.

In the lower abdomen at the level of the fourth lumbar vertebra the aorta bifurcates into the two common iliac arteries (see Fig. 15.4, p. 224). Scans at this level will show three vessels in cross section with the two common iliac arteries lying to the left of the inferior vena cava. The two common iliac veins join to form the inferior vena cava below the level of the aortic bifurcation (see Fig. 15.4). The left common iliac vein passes behind the right common iliac artery as these vessels enter the pelvis. In younger children, it may be extremely difficult to visualize the common iliac vessels individually at this level because of the lack of retroperitoneal fat. The common iliac arteries lie anterior to the common iliac veins as they pass inferiorly medial to the psoas muscle. In the lower parts of the pelvis the external iliac arteries come to lie a little more lateral than the external iliac veins. The caliber of the inferior vena cava and iliac veins varies greatly and there is often asymmetry between the two iliac veins. Their caliber is also influenced by the various phases of respiration.

Normal ureters are difficult to visualize in the retroperitoneum and pelvis but when dilated they may be visualized as rounded fluid-filled structures. After intravenous contrast administration the ureters will be readily visualized as they fill with contrast material and are noted to lie anterior to the psoas muscle (see Fig. 8.1; see also Fig. 15.4, p 224). Slight asymmetry in their course and caliber can be accepted as a normal finding if no mass lesions are visualized. The caliber of the ureters may appear unduly large when filled with contrast. In part, this is the effect of the presence of contrast within the ureter but may also be due to peristaltic activity and may thus be transient. Because of this activity a ureter may well not be visualized in a particular image despite intravenous contrast administration. If there is any doubt about the caliber of a ureter, a digital radiograph should be obtained at the end of the examination to display the entire renal collecting system. If this is not available, a plain abdominal radiograph will suffice.

The sympathetic nervous system consists of two chains, one on either side of the midline. In the lumbar region each chain consists of four ganglia connected by nerve fibers. Each chain connects with the thoracic segments of the chain behind the medial lumbocostal arch of the diaphragm and with the sacral segments behind the internal iliac artery. The chains lie in the groove between the psoas muscles and the vertebral bodies.

Pathology

Lymph Nodes

Introduction

In children, CT is used specifically to evaluate the retroperitoneal lymph nodes, most commonly in patients with Hodgkin's disease and in boys with testicular tumors. The retroperitoneal nodes are always assessed in patients with other intra-abdominal neoplastic masses. Children with dysgammaglobulinemia may also develop enlarged retroperitoneal nodes, and we have used CT on rare occasions to follow the response of these nodes to therapy.

Computed tomography of the abdomen and pelvis is used as the initial modality to detect lymphadenopathy in the above-mentioned patients because lymphangiography is more invasive, often difficult to perform in children, and uncomfortable for the patient. It is also limited to delineating disease in nodes in the pelvis and mid abdomen only [3, 5]. CT, however, delineates all lymph node areas of the abdomen and pelvis as well as displaying valuable information regarding the liver, spleen, kidneys, and bowel. The drawback of CT is that it cannot demonstrate architectural abnormality in normal-sized nodes.

Size

In adults, normal-sized nodes are commonly seen in the retroperitoneum on CT [5]. Nodes under 1 cm in size are considered normal and those above 1.5 cm are generally considered abnormal. Nodes between 1 and 1.5 cm in size are considered equivocal [5]. In children, normal-sized nodes have been said to be rarely visible in the retroperitoneum on CT [1, 6, 7]. However, with high-resolution scanners and with strict attention to technique, small, normal-sized nodes only a few millimeters in size can occasionally be visualized, particularly in older children (see Fig. 8.1).

Enlargement of retroperitoneal nodes is seen most commonly in children with Hodgkin's disease (Fig. 8.5) but is also often seen as a result of metastatic disease from other neoplasms, such as Wilms' tumor, neuroblastoma, and testicular tumor. Enlarged nodes may also be seen in chil-

dren with inflammatory processes, sinus histiocytosis, and pseudolymphoma in immunodeficient children [1, 11] (Fig. 8.6). The CT appearances of the nodes in these various conditions is nonspecific. Calcification may be seen in lymph nodes involved with metastatic neuroblastoma (see Fig. 10.5, p. 130) or in children with Hodgkin's disease who have been treated with chemotherapy or radiation therapy (see also Fig. 4.18, p. 41). Retroperitoneal fibrosis may cause masses simulating lymphadenopathy, but this is very rare in children [1].

Attenuation

When retroperitoneal lymph nodes are visualized their attenuation value is that of soft tissues. Following intravenous contrast administration, lymph nodes do indeed enhance. The enhancement can be particularly well appreciated if the nodes are pathologically enlarged (Fig. 8.6). This is seen not only with enlarged retroperitoneal and pelvic nodes but also with nodes in the neck and mediastinum.

Increased attenuation of lymph nodes is found in children on chronic blood transfusion programs, when excess iron is deposited in nodes, which then become enlarged (Fig. 8.7). Not only retroperitoneal nodes are involved, but also other groups of nodes in the abdomen. The iron gives the node an irregular patchy increase in attenuation (see also Fig. 9.4, p. 110, and Fig. 13.6, p. 202).

Abdominal CT scans performed following lymphangiography show increased attenuation of retroperitoneal and pelvic lymph nodes caused by the presence of lipiodol in the nodes (Fig. 8.8). Although lymphangiography may reveal filling defects in a group of nodes, these defects will not be appreciated on CT if some lipiodol has entered the node. The presence of lipiodol within a lymph node diminishes the accuracy in assessing nodal size on CT as the presence of this contrast material tends to make the node appear larger than its true size. It is therefore difficult to follow patients with lymphoma by using CT in this way. Lipiodol remains in lymph nodes for a variable length of time and may be visible on CT when it is no longer evident on plain radiograph.

At the Hospital for Sick Children, Toronto, we have had the opportunity to study two children with congenital lymphedema. In both cases abdominal CT following lymphangiography

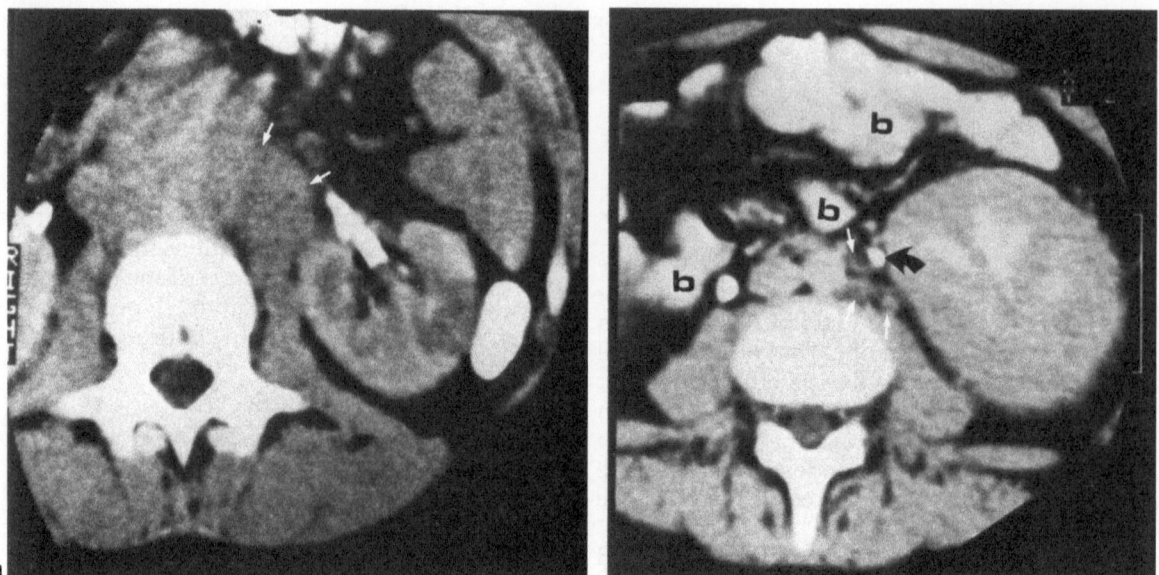

Fig. 8.5a,b. Scans through the abdomen in a 12-year-old boy with Hodgkin's disease. **a** At the time of diagnosis, enlarged retroperitoneal lymph nodes are evident (*small white arrows*) but cannot be separated from the retroperitoneal vessels, as the scan was performed after rather than during the injection of intravenous contrast medium. The low-density areas within the renal parenchyma on the left represent lymphomatous infiltration of the kidney. **b** Twelve months following diagnosis a scan performed during the intravenous injection of contrast medium outlines the retroperitoneal vasculature well. The retroperitoneal lymph nodes are very much smaller (*small white arrows*). The kidney on the left is markedly enlarged at this time, because of infiltration of the entire kidney. The ureters (*curved black arrow*) and bowel (*b*) are well opacified. (Daneman et al. 1982 [3])

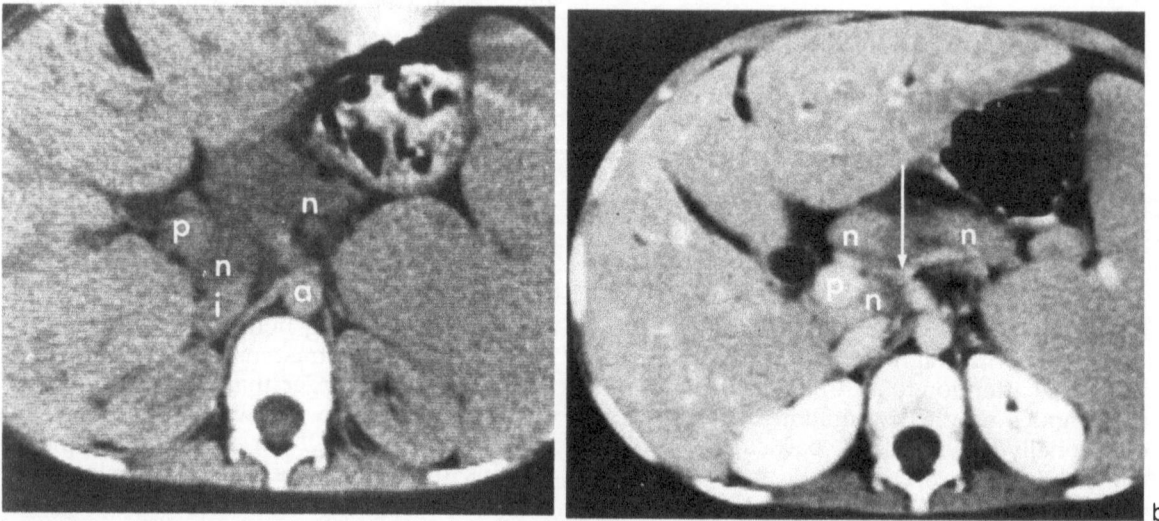

Fig. 8.6a,b. Scans of the upper abdomen in a 10-year-old boy with dysgammaglobulinemia before (**a**) and during (**b**) intravenous contrast administration. **a** Enlarged retroperitoneal lymph nodes (*n*) are seen anterior to the inferior vena cava (*i*) and aorta (*a*) and to the left of the portal vein (*p*). **b** The nodes (*n*) are noticed to enhance in comparison with the previous scan when images are taken with the same window setting. *Long arrow,* bifurcation of celiac artery into splenic artery to the left and hepatic artery to the right, passing in front of the portal vein. This is the same patient that is illustrated in Figs. 9.3 and 13.8.

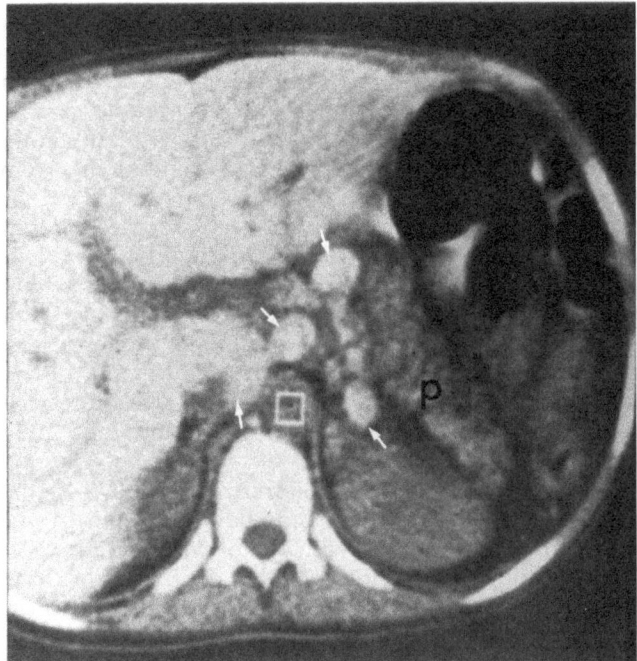

Fig. 8.7. A 15-year-old boy with thalassemia major. There is increased attenuation of lymph nodes (*small arrows*) in the retroperitoneum and porta hepatis. Note the increased attenuation in the liver and in the pancreas, which is extremely lobulated (*p*).

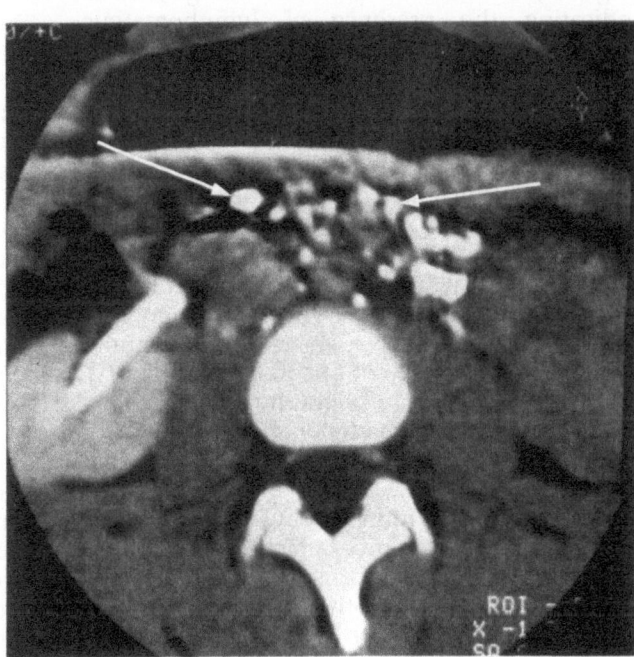

Fig. 8.8. A 15-year-old girl with congenital lymphedema of the legs. CT scan after a lymphangiogram shows increased attenuation of lymph nodes in the retroperitoneum and mesentery (*arrows*) because of the contrast from the lymphangiogram. This extensive filling is not normally seen and is related to the abnormal channels.

revealed a bizarre collection of lipiodol in many abdominal lymph node groups. The pattern simulated the presence of a mass lesion in the retroperitoneum as the cause for the lymphedema (Fig. 8.8). These two examples further underline the difficulties in assessing the size and config-uration of lymph nodes that are filled with lipiodol. In another child with congenital lymphangiomatosis lipiodol was noted to pass from the retroperitoneal nodes into lymphangioectatic spaces within the adjacent lumbar vertebrae.

Neoplasms

Lymphoma The value of CT and its accuracy relative to lymphangiography in the assessment of retroperitoneal lymph node involvement in Hodgkin's disease has been well documented in adults [5]. Two series have been reported describing the value of CT in childhood lymphoma [6, 13]. In only one of the studies reported by Tschappeler [13] a small group of patients with enlarged retroperitoneal nodes had both CT and lymphography. CT demonstrated more extensive lymphadenopathy in the high para-aortic area than was noted on lymphangiography.

At the Hospital for Sick Children, Toronto, we have used CT of the chest and abdomen extensively to stage children with lymphoma before therapy and during follow-up [3]. It has been our policy not to perform lymphangiography on those children who have obvious unquestionable enlarged retroperitoneal nodes on CT (Fig. 8.9). We have accepted this enlargement as indicating the presence of lymphomatous involvement, as the possibility that these nodes represent benign disease is small. Bipedal lymphangiography has been performed, however, in those children in whom the retroperitoneum appears normal on CT or in whom there is questionable lymphadenopathy.

In 1983, Daneman et al. [3] reported the findings in 17 patients with Hodgkin's disease from our institution who had lymphangiography following an abdominal CT which had been considered normal. This was done in an attempt to evaluate the accuracy of apparently normal CT (in relationship to lymphography) in delineating the absence of lymphadenopathy in the retroperitoneum. Since that time we have studied four further patients. CT and lymphangiography were performed within 10 days of each other. Routine laparotomy and examination of abdominal nodes was only performed in stage I patients at our institution, as all other patients in the past have been treated with combination chemotherapy and low-dose extended field radiotherapy [4]. In 86% of our 21 patients there was excellent correlation between the CT and lymphangiographic findings. In 17 of these no abnormality was detected in either study. In one patient enlarged nodes were evident anterior to the right sacroiliac joint in both studies, which otherwise revealed no abnormality in the remainder of the abdomen.

In another patient CT revealed the presence of lymphadenopathy in the para-aortic area at the level of the second lumbar vertebra. These nodes were not filled with contrast on lymphangiography, which otherwise confirmed the absence of disease elsewhere.

Lymphangiography revealed the presence of pelvic lymphadenopathy in two patients in whom the CT was initially interpreted as being normal. In one of these patients (aged 6 years) the enlarged nodes enhanced dramatically on CT (70–80 HU) during the injection of intravenous contrast material. These nodes had been interpreted as representing bowel loops filled with contrast. In the second patient (aged 3 years) the abnormal nodes in the pelvis were extremely small and were only appreciated on the CT scan in retrospect.

In Hodgkin's disease, involved nodes may be normal in size or only slightly enlarged [5]. Because CT cannot display architectural abnormalities in normal-sized nodes [5, 6], it has been suggested that despite the small percentage of false negative interpretations [5], it is prudent to perform lymphangiography in both adults and children with Hodgkin's disease, even if the abdominal CT is normal. From our findings in our 21 patients we consider that if strict attention is paid to technique the number of false negative interpretations of the CT examination will be extremely small. However, we recognise that our series is small and the findings are preliminary. We have continued to use lymphangiography, particularly in younger children who have an apparently normal abdominal CT. However, with our newer 2-s scanner we have become more confident in excluding enlarged nodes in even very young children. In children over 10 years of age, a negative CT scan is probably adequate. It is reassuring that none of the patients in our series have shown evidence of new intra-abdominal disease or recurrence. At institutions where lymphangiography is not per-

---

Fig. 8.9a,b. A 14-year-old boy with Hodgkin's disease, with large retroperitoneal and splenic hilar lymphadenopathy (*long arrows*) and also splenic involvement (*small arrows*). Scans were performed after the ingestion of dilute meglumine diatrizoate and during the intravenous injection of contrast medium. The retroperitoneal vasculature and bowel are well delineated. *i*, inferior vena cava; *a*, aorta; *curved arrow*, superior mesenteric artery and vein; *open arrow*, renal vein; *b*, bowel; *p*, pancreas. (Daneman et al. 1982 [3])

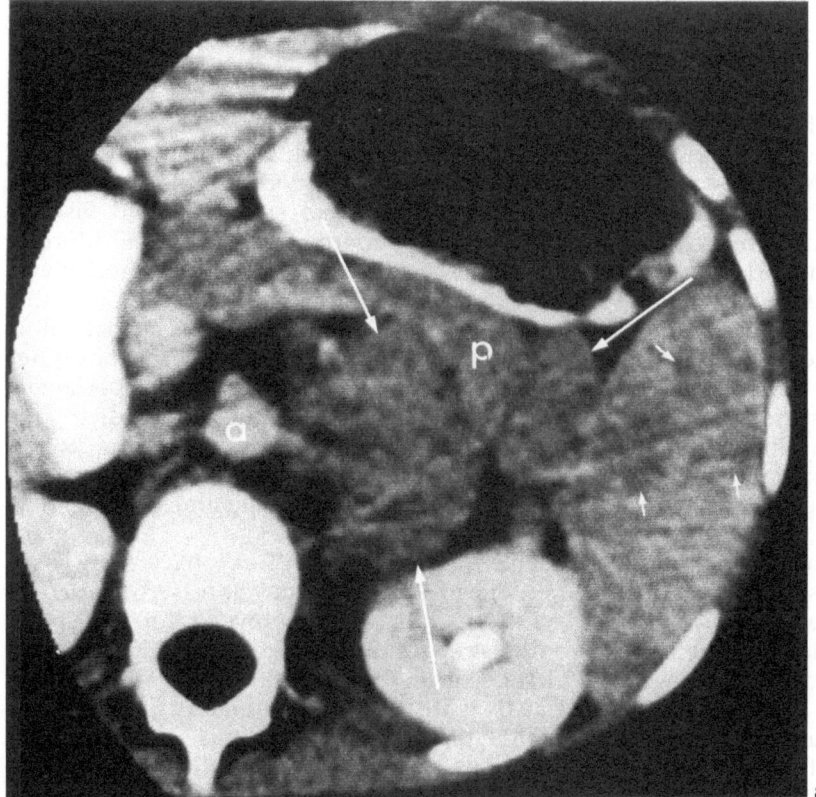

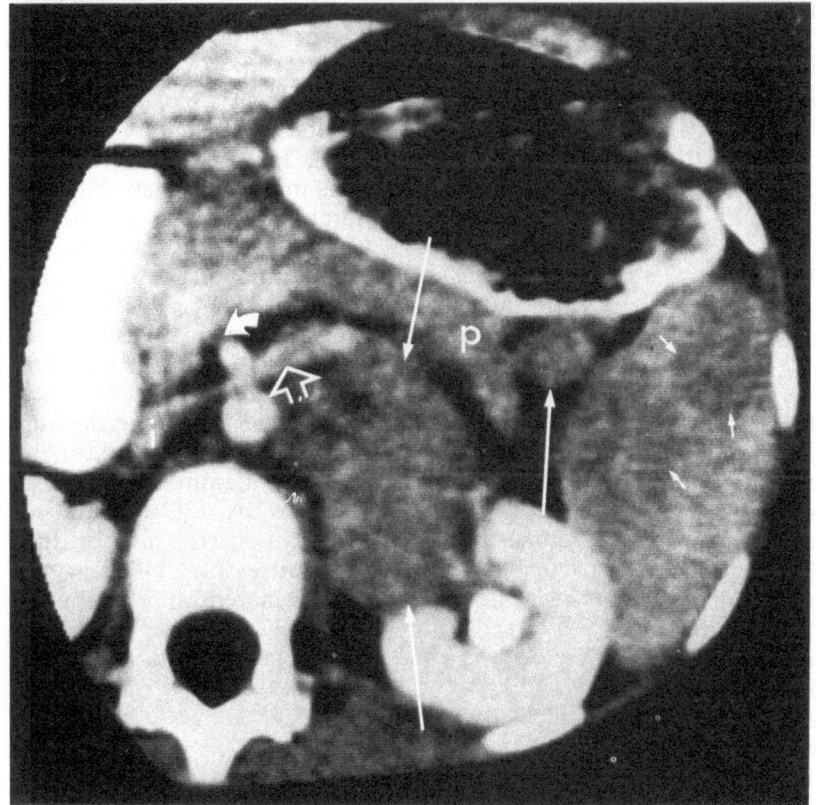

formed, a staging laparotomy is necessary following a normal CT, if the findings will alter management.

Other Neoplasms 6x28.6In children, testicular tumors usually occur in infancy and early childhood and account for 1%–2% of all solid neoplasms in this age group. The most common lesions are endodermal sinus tumors, which have a relatively good prognosis [1]. We have relied on CT of the upper abdomen in these children to evaluate the retroperitoneal nodes for metastatic disease and occasionally have found lymph node enlargement. We have accepted this as representing metastatic disease and have not performed lymphangiography in any of these very young patients. Lymphangiography is performed in older boys, however, if CT shows no abnormality.

The retroperitoneal lymph nodes are routinely evaluated in all children with solid intra-abdominal neoplasms as these neoplasms may all metastasize with varying frequencies to the lymph node chains. These lesions include all malignant renal (see Fig. 11.18, p. 164), hepatic, and adrenal neoplasms, as well as neuroblastoma (see Fig. 10.5, p. 130), and rarely from neoplasms in the lower limbs (Fig. 8.10). In the presence of extremely large primary tumors the enlarged involved lymph nodes may lie so close to the primary tumor that it is often difficult to appreciate that they represent enlarged metastatic nodes rather than a nodule of the primary lesion (see Fig. 11.18, p. 164). This is particularly true with large neuroblastomas.

Sympathetic Nervous System

Neoplasms

The sympathetic nervous system chains extend on either side of the vertebral column from the base of the skull down to the sacrum. Tumors of chromaffin tissue such as neuroblastoma, ganglioneuroma, and pheochromocytoma may thus occur anywhere along the length of these chains as well as in the adrenal medulla. For the sake of conciseness, these lesions are discussed in detail together in the section on neoplasms of the adrenal medulla and sympathetic nervous system in Chapter 10 (see p. 126). Suffice it to say here that CT is the modality of choice in the delineation of these lesions at the time of diagnosis and in follow-up.

Soft Tissues

Inflammation

In children, CT is much less commonly used to define inflammatory processes than neoplasms of the retroperitoneal structures and viscera. However, the superb anatomical detail afforded by CT has made this an invaluable modality in the delineation of inflammatory processes in this compartment. CT has provided crucial information that could not be obtained with any other modality in several patients with retroperitoneal inflammatory disease that we have studied. This has been confirmed in a study involving 28 children by Berger et al. [1]. Examples of patients that we have studied are illustrated in Fig. 8.11 and Fig. 11.10, p. 155.

Like others [1, 11, 12], we have seen retroperitoneal abscesses develop secondarily to spinal operations, osteomyelitis of the spine, and disc space disease (Fig. 8.11). Inflammatory changes in the psoas muscle may also be associated with renal inflammatory disease (see Fig. 11.10, p. 155). Adjacent retroperitoneal abscesses may be seen in the postoperative period or as a result of inflammatory bowel lesions such as appendicitis and Crohn's disease.

Early inflammation in the psoas muscle may be associated with a hypervascular area that enhances greatly after intravenous contrast administration (see Fig. 11.10, p. 155). The psoas and adjacent muscles may become swollen and tissue planes obliterated because of the inflammatory process. Abscess formation is suggested when areas of lower attenuation develop within the muscle. The presence of gas within these lesions confirms the diagnosis [10]. Abscesses may have circumferential contrast enhancement, and in longstanding cases calcification may be evident [10]. Associated bone destruction and disc space irregularity may indicate the primary etiology of the inflammatory process. Occasionally, based on the CT appearances alone the diagnosis of an abscess may be difficult, as similar appearances may be seen with necrotic neoplasms, hematomas, and muscle infarcts [12].

Hematomas

There has been no large series of patients with retroperitoneal hematomas described in the CT

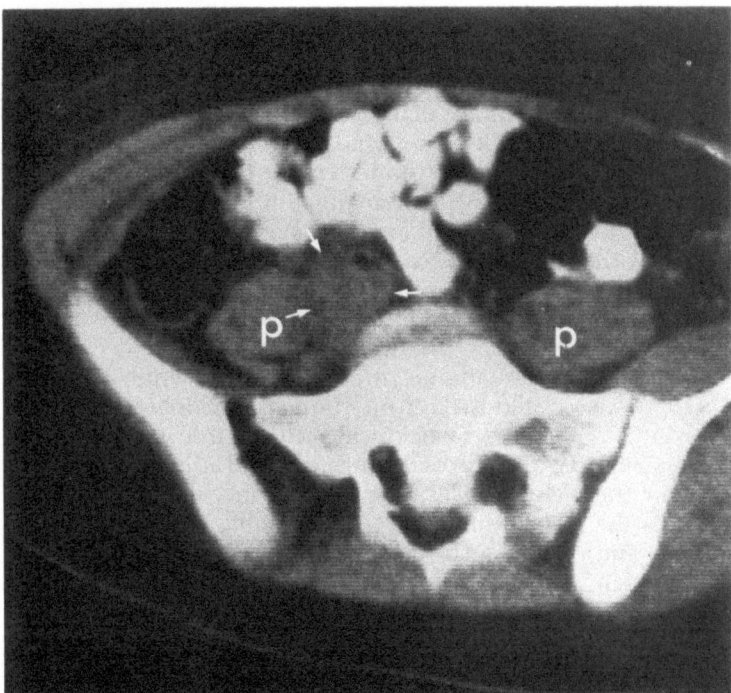

Fig. 8.10. Enlarged retroperitoneal lymph nodes (*arrows*) on the right in a 15-year-old girl with an osteogenic sarcoma of the lower right femur. *p*, psoas muscles.

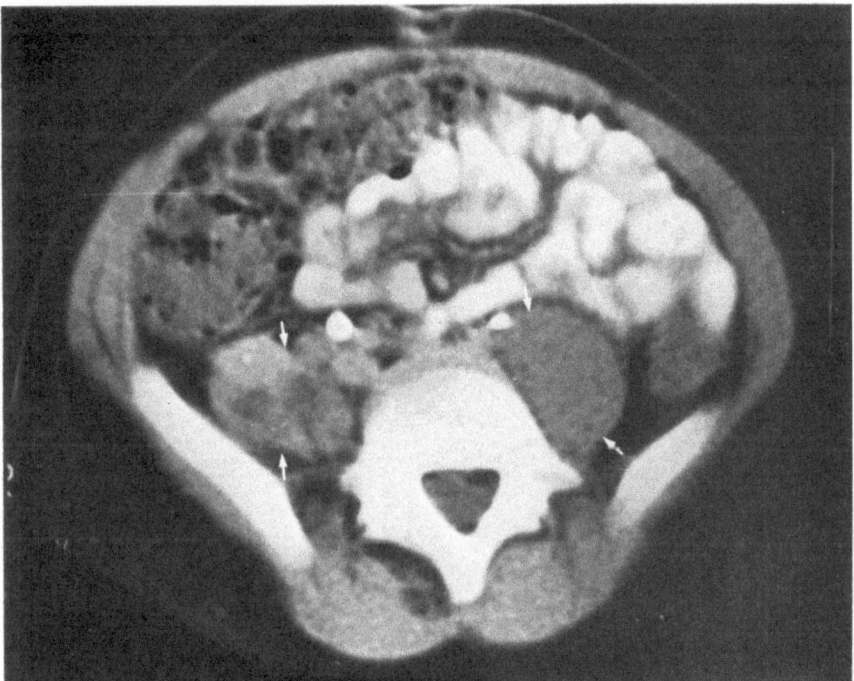

Fig. 8.11. Inflammatory changes in the right psoas muscle are related to infection from a previous spinal operation. The psoas muscles are outlined by the *white arrows*. Low attenuation within the right psoas is related to inflammatory changes, and the area of calcification anteriorly is due to chronic inflammation.

literature. Retroperitoneal hematomas may be diffuse or focal and may occur following severe trauma (Fig. 8.12); however, they may also be associated with hemorrhage into the psoas muscle in patients with hemophilia. Although CT is the most accurate modality in the delineation of hematomas in this anatomical compartment, we have used sonography successfully to assess the psoas muscles in patients with hemophilia.

Neoplasms

Both benign and primary and secondary malignant soft tissue neoplasms may occur in the retroperitoneum, but these are rare. CT is the most valuable modality in characterizing and defining the extent of these lesions. Benign lesions, including lymphangiomas [9], hemangiomas, neurofibromas (see Fig. 17.9, p. 272), and teratomas are occasionally encountered. These may extend into the posterior abdominal wall, into the mesentery, and surround the bowel. In fact, calcification may be noted in teratomas on CT, and hemangiomas may have enhancing spaces.

round the bowel. In fact, calcification may be noted in teratomas on CT, and hemangiomas may have enhancing spaces.

Primary malignant soft tissue lesions that we have encountered in the retroperitoneum include an endodermal sinus tumor in one patient and a malignant fibrous histiocytoma (Fig. 8.13) in another. We have also seen a large metastatic rhabdomyosarcoma in this region. The CT findings of these malignant lesions are, to a large extent, nonspecific. The masses usually enhance and often have necrotic areas with low attenuation centrally. In 1983, Stanley [12] illustrated two retroperitoneal rhabdomyosarcomas. In one case, calcification within the mass and extension of the mass around adjacent structures gave the lesion an appearance indistinguishable from that of a neuroblastoma. In the other case a large cystic component was associated with the mass.

Intraspinal extension may occur with any of these types of lesions but is much less common than with neuroblastomas. Tumors arising from the vertebrae and paraspinal muscles may project into the retroperitoneal space, but this is uncommon. However, Stanley [12] has described Ewing's sarcoma invading the retroperitoneal space.

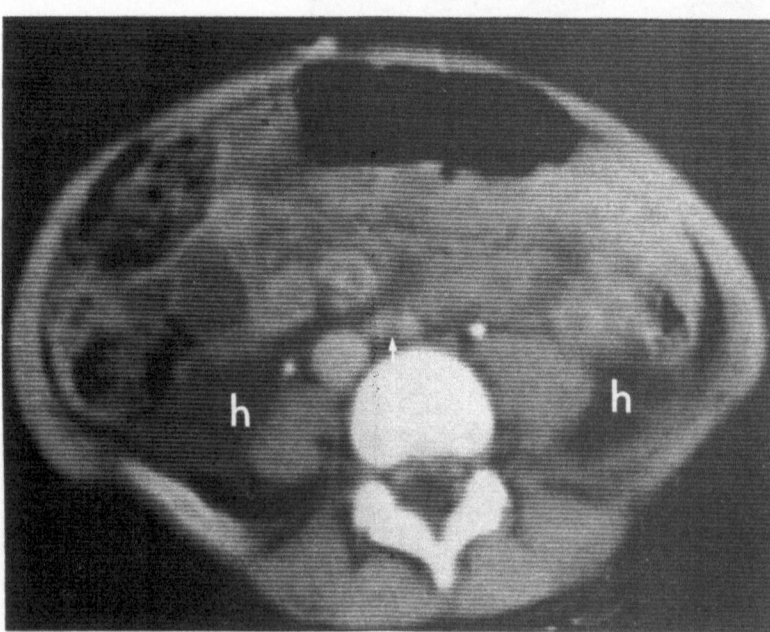

Fig. 8.12. Scan performed just below the level of aortic bifurcation (*small arrow*) shows retroperitoneal hemorrhage (*h*) in this patient following a motor vehicle accident.

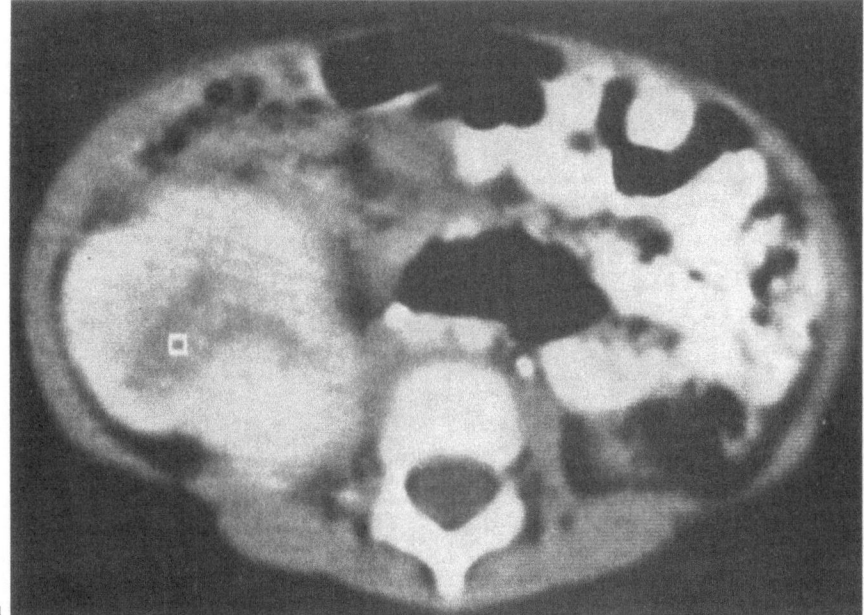

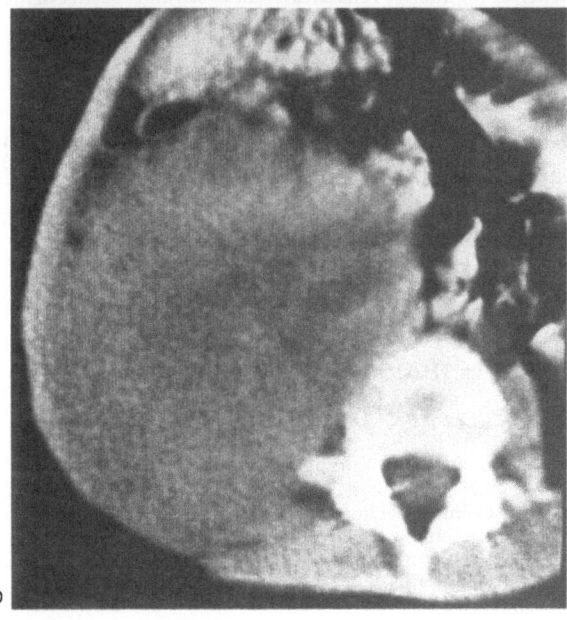

Fig. 8.13a,b. Examples of retroperitoneal malignant masses. **a** The right-sided mass is a malignant fibrous histiocytoma with a poorly vascularized central area (*cursor*). **b** The mass represents a metastasis from a rhabdomyosarcoma of the ear. The appearances of these lesions are nonspecific.

Blood Vessels

Arterial disease is a rarity in the pediatric age groups. The CT findings of an aortic aneurysm in one child were reported by Boldt and Reilly in 1977 [2].

Abnormalities of the retroperitoneal veins are more commonly noted but are still rare. Venous variations such as azygous or hemiazygous continuation of the inferior vena cava can easily be visualized (Fig. 8.14). These structures may simulate lymph node enlargement if the anatomic anomaly is not investigated by following these vessels into adjacent superior and inferior scans. Further scans with intravenous contrast administration or sonography will help to delineate the vascular nature of these structures. Dilatation of the portal venous system together with dilatation and tortuosity of retroperitoneal collaterals may be visualized in patients with portal hypertension (see Fig. 9.11, p. 118).

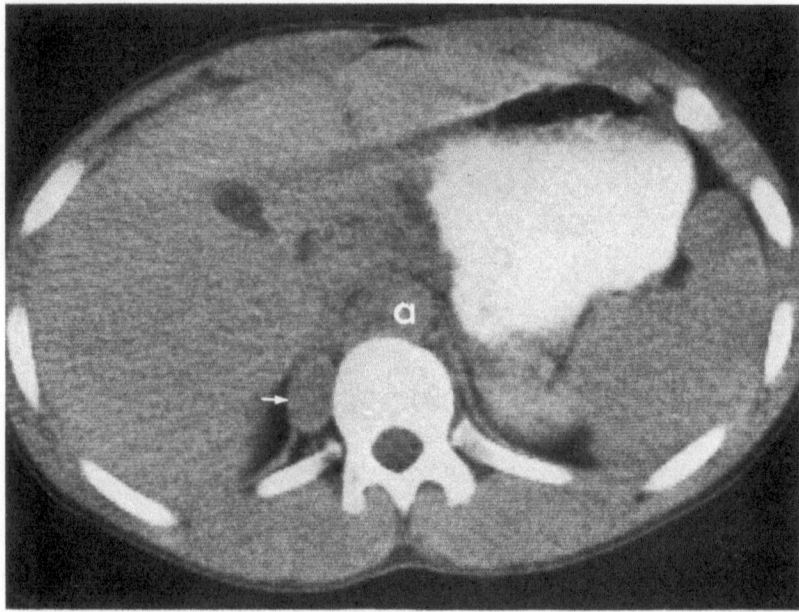

Fig. 8.14. Scan of the upper abdomen shows an azygous continuation of the inferior vena cava (*small arrow*) and absence of the inferior vena cava more anteriorly. The aorta (*a*) is easily seen.

Neoplasms such as Wilms' tumor and renal and adrenal carcinomas may extend into the veins draining these organs and grow up the inferior vena cava into the heart (see Fig. 4.9, p. 35, and Fig. 11.22, p. 167). Intravenous tumor thrombi may well calcify and are thus easily seen on CT. They appear as filling defects within the veins in scans performed after intravenous contrast enhancement (see Fig. 11.22b, p. 167). Following chemotherapy the tumor thrombus in the renal vein or inferior vena cava may be seen to calcify (see Fig. 11.22c, p. 167) or become necrotic (see Fig. 11.15, p. 162). These tumor defects should not be confused with flow pattern defects in the inferior vena cava, which are most commonly seen just above the entrance of the renal veins into the inferior vena cava (see Fig. 8.4). The effects of renal venous thrombosis have been diagnosed on CT after intravenous contrast administration [6] (see also Fig. 11.7, p. 152).

Nonpalpable Testis

Nonpalpable testes are usually located in the inguinal area and very rarely in the abdomen [8, 14, 15]. We have used sonography and CT successfully for locating undescended testes that are present in the inguinal area. We have not been able to locate a testis in the retroperitoneal area with CT in patients with undescended testes in whom no testis can be located in the inguinal area (see Chap. 15, p. 240).

References

1. Berger PE (1982) Computerized tomography in gastrointestinal imaging in pediatrics. In: Franken EA (ed) Gastrointestinal imaging in pediatrics. Harper and Row, Philadelphia, pp 490–529
2. Boldt DW, Reilly BJ (1977) Computed tomography of abdominal mass lesions in children. Radiology 124: 371–378
3. Daneman A, Martin DJ, Fitz CR, Chan HSL (1982) Computed tomography and lymphogram correlation in children with Hodgkin's disease. CT 7:115–122
4. Jenkin D, Chan H, Freedman M (1982) Hodgkin's disease in children: treatment results with MOPP and low dose, extended-field irradiation. Cancer Treat Rep 66:949–959
5. Korobkin M (1981) Computed tomography of the retroperitoneal vasculature and lymph nodes. Semin Roentgenol 16:251–267
6. Kuhn JP, Berger PE (1980) Computed tomographic imaging of abdominal abnormalities in infancy and childhood. Pediatr Ann 9:200–209
7. Kuhns LR (1981) CT of the retroperitoneum in children. Radiol Clin North Am 19:495–501
8. Lee JKT, McClennan BL, Stanley RJ (1980) Utility of com-

puted tomography in the localization of the undescended testis. Radiology 135:121–125

9. Leonidas JC, Brill BW, Bhan I (1978) Cystic retroperitoneal lymphangioma in infants and children. Radiology 127:203–206

10. Mendez G, Isikoff MB, Hill MC (1980) Retroperitoneal processes involving the psoas demonstrated by computed tomography. J Comput Assist Tomogr 4:78–82

11. Siegel MJ, Balfe DM, McClennan BL, Levitt RG (1982) Clinical utility of CT in pediatric retroperitoneal disease. AJR 138:1011–1017

12. Stanley P (1982) Computed tomographic evaluation of the retroperitoneum in infants and children. CT 7:63–75

13. Tschappeler H (1980) Computed tomographic imaging of abdominal abnormalities in infancy and childhood. Pediatr Ann 9:200–209

14. Wolverson MK, Jagannadharao B, Sundaram M (1980) CT in localization of impalpable cryptorchid testes. AJR 134:725–729

15. Wolverson MK, Houttuin E, Heiberg, E, Sundaram M, Shields JB (1983) Comparison of computed tomography with high-resolution real-time ultrasound in the localization of the impalpable undescended testis. Radiology 146:133–136

Chapter 9

Pancreas

Introduction

Prior to the introduction of sonography and CT, delineation of the pancreas was extremely difficult and visualization often relied on indirect techniques such as barium studies and invasive techniques such as angiography, endoscopic retrograde cholangiopancreatography, and percutaneous transhepatic cholangiography. In children, the pancreas is usually visualized with ease on sonography. This is the modality of choice in the investigation of children suspected of having pancreatic pathology, particularly pancreatitis and pseudocysts. Some children with pancreatitis or abnormalities of the pancreatic duct and lower common bile duct (e.g., choledochal cyst) may require endoscopic retrograde cholangiopancreatography or percutaneous transhepatic cholangiography following sonography to delineate disease processes in this area more adequately.

The need to use CT to define the pancreas in children is rare. At our institution, as well as elsewhere [3], well under 1% of all body CT scans in children are performed specifically to evaluate the pancreas. CT of the pancreas in children is limited to those uncommon instances where the pancreas or pseudocyst is inadequately delineated by sonography, to the delineation of large pancreatic tumors, and to patients suspected of having occult secretory lesions of the pancreas [11]. CT may also be useful in the assessment of fatty replacement of the pancreas in patients with cystic fibrosis [8]. Both sonography and CT can reveal the effects of pancreatic lesions on the intra- and extrahepatic bile ducts and pancreatic duct.

Despite the limited use of CT in pediatric pancreatic pathology, a thorough understanding of pancreatic anatomy and the relationship of the normal pancreas to adjacent viscera and vessels is vitally important for the interpretation of all CT scans of the upper abdomen. This is because scans are commonly performed through the area of the pancreas in children with abdominal tumors, blunt abdominal trauma, and suspected abdominal inflammatory processes. Without this understanding, interpretation of these scans becomes guesswork.

Anatomy

The pancreas is a curved, band-shaped organ lying obliquely or transversely across the upper abdomen (Fig. 9.1; see also Fig. 8.1 p. 90). In children, the outline of the gland may be difficult to visualize in scans performed without oral and intravenous contrast enhancement because of the relative lack of retroperitoneal fat. When visible, the edges of the gland are usually smooth in younger children. The attenuation of the gland is homogeneous and is somewhat less than that of the normal liver. In older teenagers and young adults, the gland has a more lobulated outline, and the attenuation is a little more inhomogeneous because of the increased

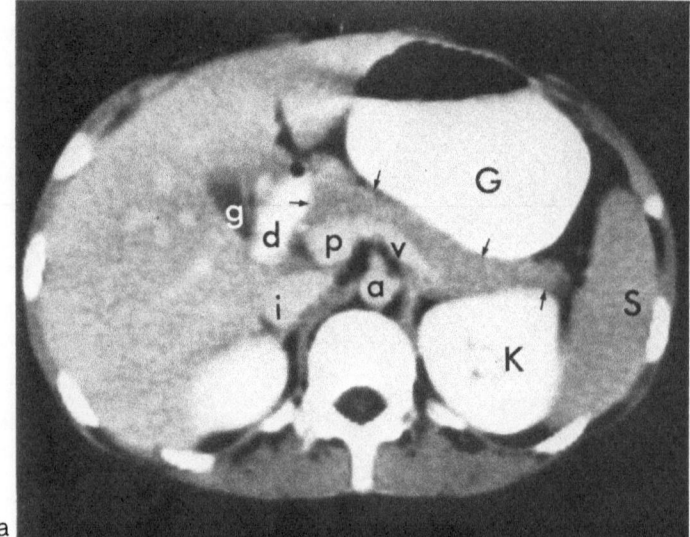

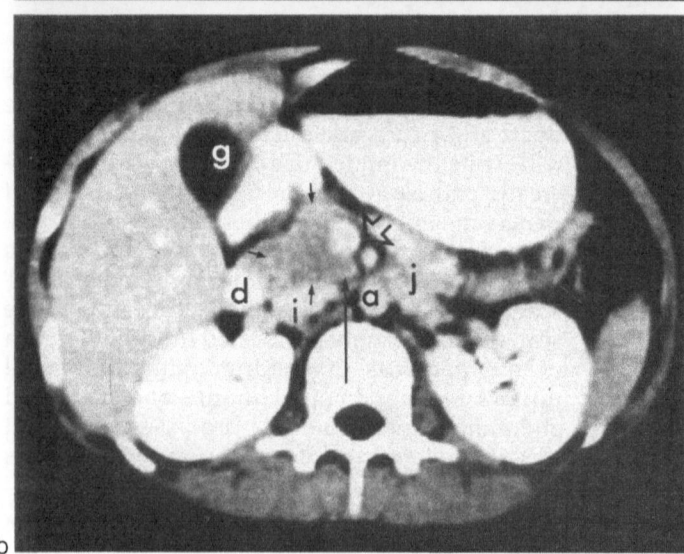

Fig. 9.1a,b. Normal pancreatic anatomy. Scans during intravenous contrast administration and after oral contrast ingestion. **a** CT scan shows pancreatic body and tail (*arrows*). Note tail lying between stomach (*G*) and left kidney (*K*) directed toward the spleen (*S*). Splenic vein (*v*) lies behind pancreatic body. *a*, aorta at origin of superior mesenteric artery; *p*, portal vein; *i*, inferior vena cava; *g*, gallbladder; *d*, duodenum. **b** Scan 1 cm below **a** shows pancreatic head (*small arrows*). Note relationship of head to second portion of the duodenum (*d*), superior mesenteric vein and artery (*open arrow*), and inferior vena cava (*i*). *Long arrow* indicates uncinate process passing behind the superior mesenteric vein. *j*, jejunum.

amount of fatty septa in the gland. Minimal changes in pancreatic attenuation have little diagnostic significance. A marked increase in the attenuation of the gland caused by excess iron deposition is seen in children receiving chronic blood transfusions, e.g., beta thalassemia (see Fig. 9.4). A marked decrease in attenuation is present in the late stages of cystic fibrosis where the pancreas is replaced by fat (see Fig. 9.11). Rarely, areas of increased attenuation may be due to calcification in patients with cystic fibrosis (see Figs. 9.12, 9.13).

If the pancreas lies transversely across the abdomen, the entire gland may be visualized in one slice. However, more commonly, the pancreas lies with varying degrees of obliquity across the abdomen, with the tail lying more cranial than the pancreatic body and head. Depending on the degree of obliquity, the thickness of the CT slices, and the size of the patient, several slices (3–5) may be necessary to demonstrate the entire gland. In this situation, only varying amounts of different portions of the gland will be visualized on each slice (Fig. 9.1).

Relationships

The most cranial slice shows the tail of the pancreas directed toward the hilum of the spleen on the left, lying posterior to the stomach and anterior (occasionally anterolateral) to the left kidney (Fig. 9.1). The next more caudal slice shows the body of the pancreas lying anterior to the splenic vein and the origin of the superior mesenteric artery from the aorta and posterior to the gastric antrum. Between the anterior surface of the pancreas and stomach is the potential space of the lesser sac, which occasionally may be filled with fluid in patients with ascites (see Fig. 17.6, p. 270). The third and fourth portions of the duodenum lie inferior to the body and tail of the pancreas, crossing from right to left between the inferior vena cava and aorta posteriorly and the superior mesenteric artery and vein anteriorly (see Fig. 8.1g, p. 92).

A bulbous dilatation at the right extremity of the splenic vein represents the confluence of this vein with the superior mesenteric vein to form the portal vein. This lies posterior to the neck of the pancreas. The pancreatic head and uncinate process may only be visualized in the next more caudal slice (see Figs. 9.1, 9.4, 9.12; see also Fig. 8.3, p. 93). The distal part of the gastric antrum lies anterior to, and the proximal portion of the duodenum to the right of, the pancreatic head. The superior mesenteric vein and artery lie just to the left of the pancreatic head as they enter the mesentery. The uncinate process, if prominent, extends from the posteromedial aspect of the head and lies posterior to these vessels (Fig. 9.1; see also Fig. 8.3, p. 93). The inferior vena cava

lies posterior to the head. The pancreatic duct and common bile duct are not commonly visualized in normal children (Fig. 9.2). When dilated the pancreatic duct may be readily visualized (Fig. 9.3).

Size

The dimensions of the pancreas vary depending on the age of the patient. Ranges for normal measurements of the pancreas in children have not been estimated on CT, and the diagnosis of enlargement is thus subjective. This has been done, however, using sonography, and these measurements should be helpful in assessing pancreatic size on CT [5]. Measurements in 80 children on sonography by Coleman et al. [5] revealed the following measurements: pancreatic head 1–2 cm; body 0.4–1 cm; tail 0.8–1.8 cm.

In unenhanced scans, the pancreas may appear to be larger than its true size as it merges imperceptibly with the surrounding vessels, stomach, duodenum, and jejunum because of the relative lack of surrounding fat. Adequate opacification of the splenic vein, stomach, and duodenum will reveal the true thickness of the pancreatic body and tail (Fig. 9.5). Unopacified loops of jejunum or splenic vessels may appear as pancreatic or left adrenal pseudomasses. The splenic vein lies between the pancreatic tail anterolaterally and the left adrenal gland posteromedially. If retroperitoneal fat is lacking, the pancreatic body and tail may simulate a left adrenal mass if the splenic vein is not adequately opacified with contrast material (Fig. 9.5).

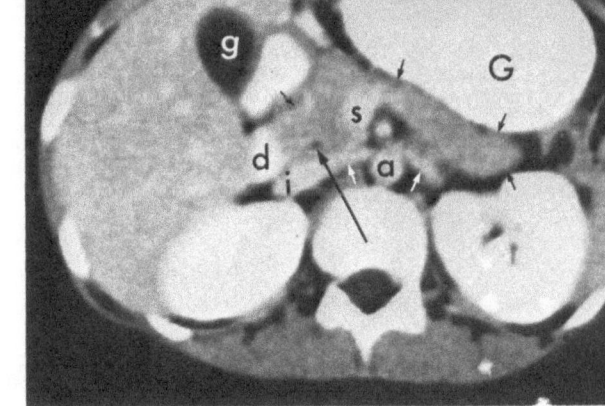

Fig. 9.2. Normal pancreatic anatomy in an 11-year-old boy. Scan shows pancreatic head, body, and tail (*small arrows*). *Long arrow* indicates normal-caliber common bile duct in posterior aspect of head. *i*, inferior vena cava; *a*, aorta; *s*, superior mesenteric vein; *d*, duodenum; *g*, gallbladder; *G*, stomach. Note left renal vein (*small white arrows*) passing from left kidney between superior mesenteric artery and aorta to join inferior vena cava.

Fig. 9.3a,b. A 10-year-old boy with hypogamma-globulinemia. Scan **a** shows pancreatic body and **b** shows head and neck (*white arrows*). Note dilatation of pancreatic duct (*small arrows*) and common bile duct (*open arrow*). Note slight dilatation of intrahepatic ducts. The cause for the duct dilatation is uncertain but has been considered to be due to excess of lymphoid hyperplasia in the duodenum. This is the same patient illustrated in Figs. 8.6 and 13.8. *G*, stomach; *s*, splenic vein; *v*, superior mesenteric vein; *i*, inferior vena cava at entrance of renal veins; *a*, aorta; *d*, duodenum.

▼

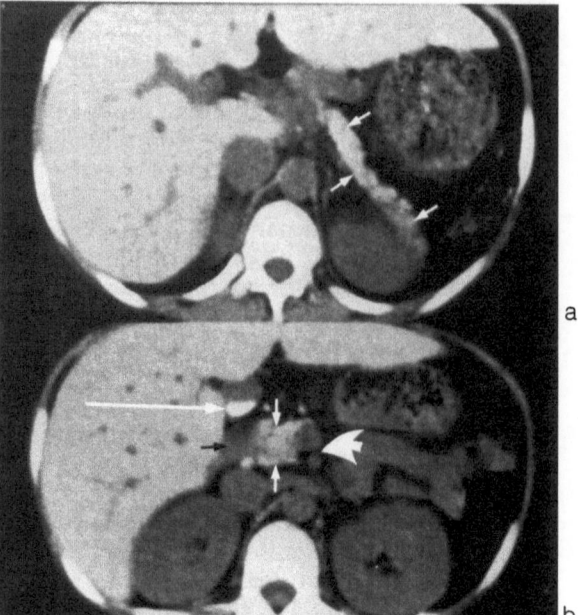

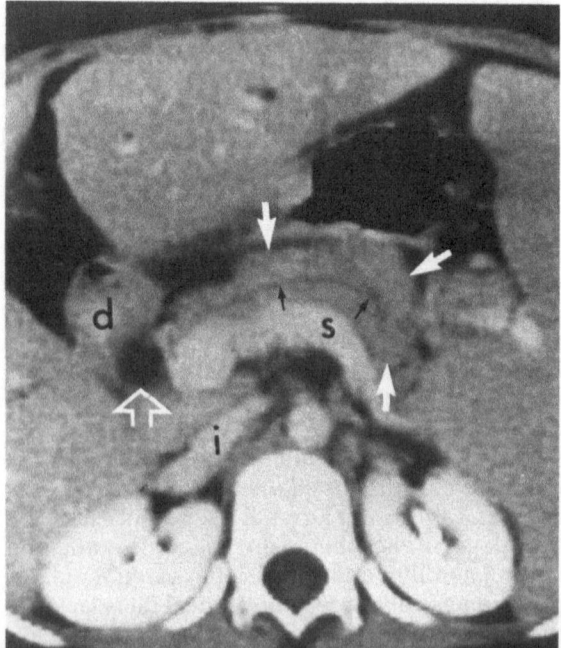

Fig. 9.4a,b. An 18-year-old boy with thalassemia. Scans performed without intravenous or oral contrast administration. The pancreatic body (**a**) and the head (**b**) are easily visualized (*small white arrows*) because of the increased attenuation caused by iron deposition. Note also the increased attenuation of the liver and the gallstones (*long arrow*). *Small black arrow*, second part of duodenum; *curved white arrow*, between superior mesenteric vein and artery.

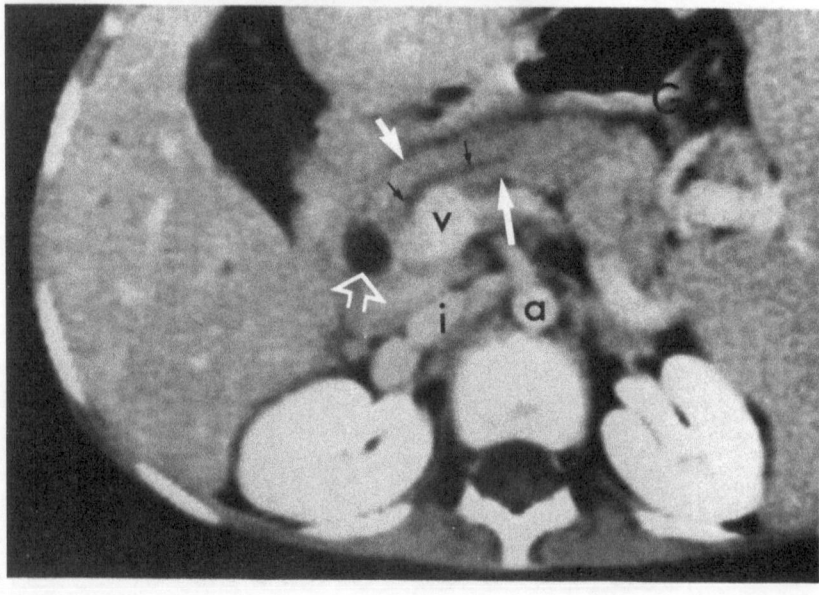

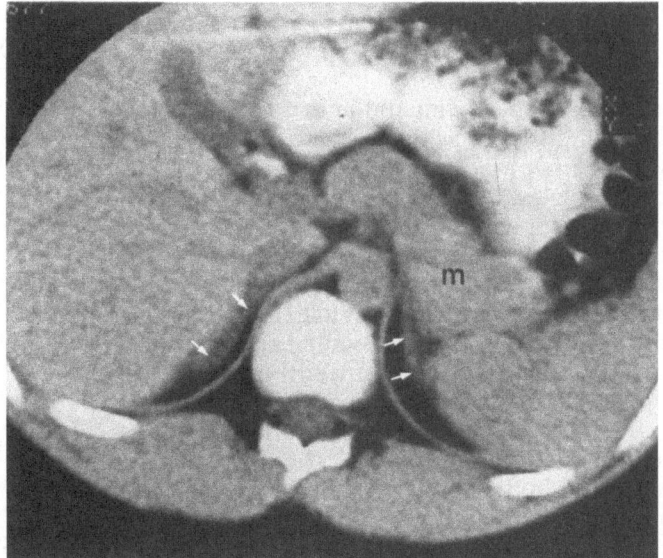

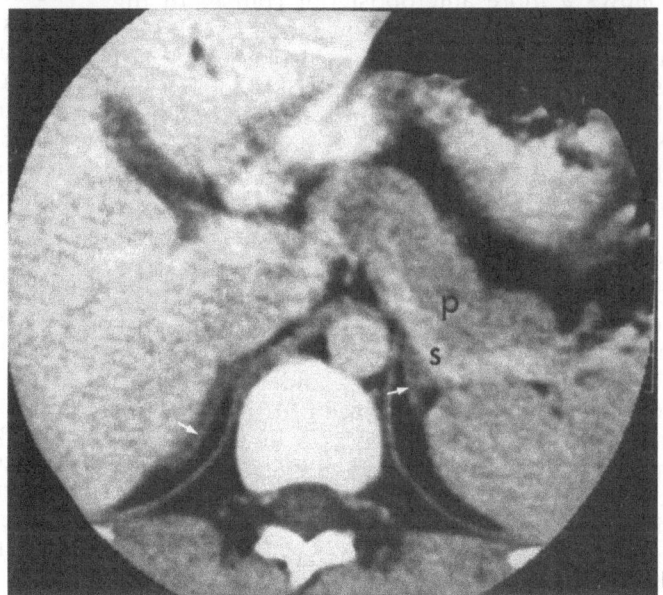

Fig. 9.5a,b. A 16-year-old boy with Cushing's syndrome. Both scans were performed after oral contrast ingestion. Scan **a** was performed before and **b** during intravenous contrast administration. Normal adrenals are easily visualized in both scans (*small arrows*). It is difficult, however, to exclude a soft tissue mass (*m*) in the lateral aspect of the left adrenal in scan **a**. However, in scan **b**, contrast outlines the splenic vein (*s*). This enables one to differentiate the left adrenal from the pancreas (*p*) and reveals the true dimensions of the pancreatic body and tail. They appear large in **a** and may masquerade as an adrenal mass or pancreatic enlargement in scans done without contrast enhancement.

When the various portions of the pancreas are visualized on separate slices (as described above), the pancreatic head may simulate a retroperitoneal mass. This may be a source of great confusion to anyone unfamiliar with this normal anatomical appearance and may lead one into a major pitfall in abdominal CT. Opacification of the superior mesenteric artery and vein, the inferior vena cava, and portal vein with intravenous contrast material, and the duodenum with dilute oral contrast material will reveal the true dimensions of the pancreatic head (see Fig. 9.1). The superior mesenteric vein is larger than the superior mesenteric artery and lies slightly anterior and to the right of the artery — both to the left of the pancreatic head and anterior to the uncinate process. These normal anatomical relationships are a characteristic constant finding. Meticulous attention to technique, as described above, is thus crucial for the adequate delineation of the pancreas; in this way the gland will be well outlined in the vast majority of children.

Displacements

In the presence of an abdominal mass and also following the resection of such masses, with or without nephrectomy, the pancreas and adjacent vessels are often displaced in a characteristic manner depending on the site of the mass or the type of resection. Knowledge of these characteristic displacements of the pancreas and adjacent vessels are of great help in determining the site of origin of an abdominal mass as well as in the exclusion of recurrent masses post-operatively, particularly on the left.

In the presence of retroperitoneal and posterior hepatic masses on the right, the pancreatic head and body are usually displaced anteriorly and to the left (see Fig. 10.3, p. 127, and Fig. 11.22, p. 167). The splenic vein in this situation follows a more anteroposterior course. In the presence of left retroperitoneal masses, the tail and body of the pancreas are displaced forward (see Fig. 10.4, p. 129, and Fig. 11.19, p. 165). In this situation, it is difficult to define the entire pancreatic body. Masses superior or inferior to the pancreas will displace the gland inferiorly or superiorly, respectively.

Resection of large, left retroperitoneal masses combined with nephrectomy causes the pancreatic tail to drop into the left renal fossa together with some jejunal loops. In this situation, the pancreatic body and tail lie adjacent to the psoas muscle medially and some jejunal loops laterally. The presence of the tail in this position may masquerade as a local recurrent mass on a particular slice (Fig. 9.6). Serial, adjacent, inferior slices will show that this soft tissue density is continuous with the remainder of the body of the pancreas passing anteriorly toward the midline.

Following the removal of a right retroperitoneal mass and nephrectomy, the pancreatic head does not usually become displaced to the right and posteriorly to the same extent as the tail does on the left.

Pathology

Pancreatitis

In children, pancreatitis may be caused by trauma, viral infections (e.g., mumps), hyper-lipidemia, drugs (e.g., L-asparaginase, steroids), or may be on a familial basis, or idiopathic [17]. The commonest complication of pancreatitis is pseudocyst formation. This is the result of escape of secretions from the pancreas and their dissection into surrounding tissues, with the production of masses of necrotic tissue. This most commonly occurs in the lesser sac but may occur less commonly elsewhere in the retroperitoneum or even the mediastinum. Other complications include suppuration and abscess formation in the pancreas.

The diagnosis of pancreatitis and pseudocyst formation may be suggested on plain films. Like others, we have used sonography very successfully in the evaluation of the pancreas in children with known or suspected pancreatitis. In acute pancreatitis, the pancreas may appear enlarged and have decreased echogenicity. Pseudocysts complicating pancreatitis are easily diagnosed and followed with sonography. They appear as well-defined, rounded, fluid-filled structures that may be totally echo free or may contain echogenic debris.

Our experience with the appearance of pancreatitis on CT in children is extremely limited, and the literature on this topic almost nonexistent, because of the success of sonography in this entity. CT need only be used if the pancreas or a suspected pseudocyst are not well visualized on sonography because of overlying bowel gas, or if the pseudocyst is so large that delineation of the anatomy cannot be made adequately with sonography (Figs. 9.7, 9.8).

In pancreatitis the pancreas may appear enlarged, with very unsharp margins caused by adjacent edema. Pseudocysts appear as fluid-filled cystic masses. Berger [3] has indicated that the CT signs of uncomplicated pancreatitis in adults may not be referable to children, and, although CT may be of value in complicated pancreatitis demonstrating pseudocysts and pancreatic abscesses, it may be difficult to differentiate these two entities based on the CT findings.

Trauma

Trauma is the commonest cause of pancreatitis and pseudocyst formation in early childhood [3]. It should always be remembered that these entities may well be the presenting feature in abused children. Occasionally, the traumatic incident may in fact be mild and the symptoms and signs nonspecific.

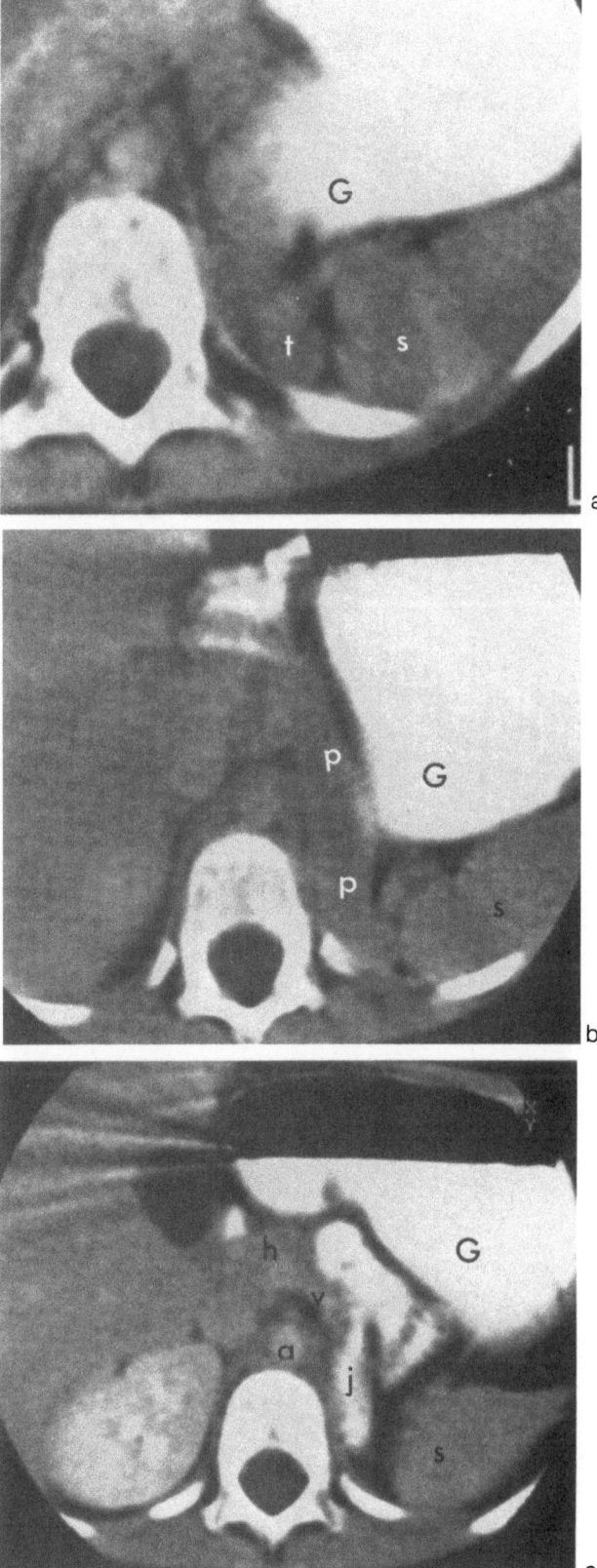

Fig. 9.6a–c. A 6-year-old girl with previous left nephrectomy for Wilms' tumor. Follow-up CT examination shows pancreatic tail (*t*) lying in left renal bed in scan **a**. In this scan the tail may masquerade as a mass of recurrent tumor. However, in a scan 1 cm below (**b**), this pseudomass is noted to be continuous with the remainder of the pancreatic body (*p*). One scan lower (**c**) shows jejunum (*j*) lying in the renal bed and the pancreatic head (*h*). *G*, stomach; *s*, spleen; *a*, aorta; *v*, splenic vein.

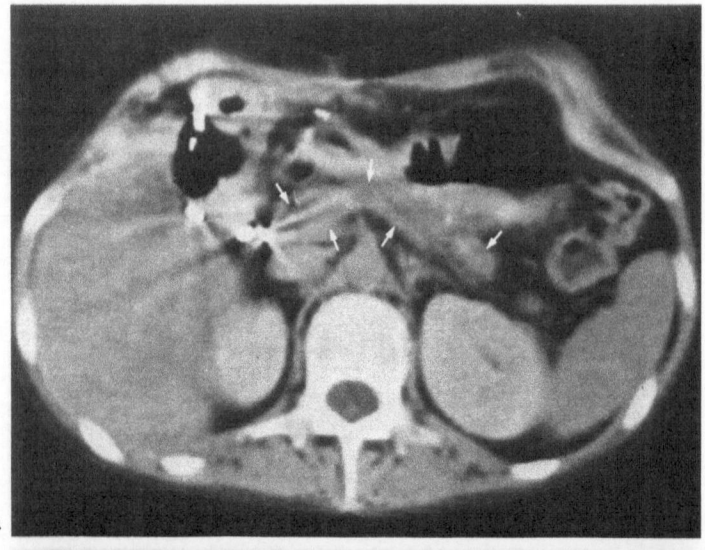

a

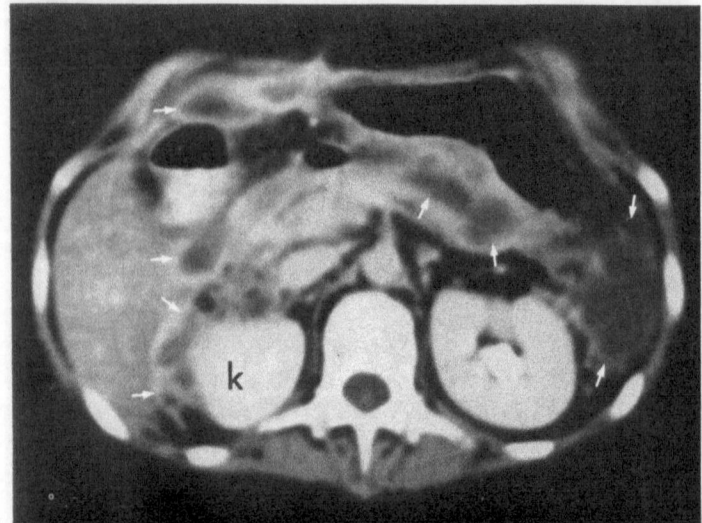

b

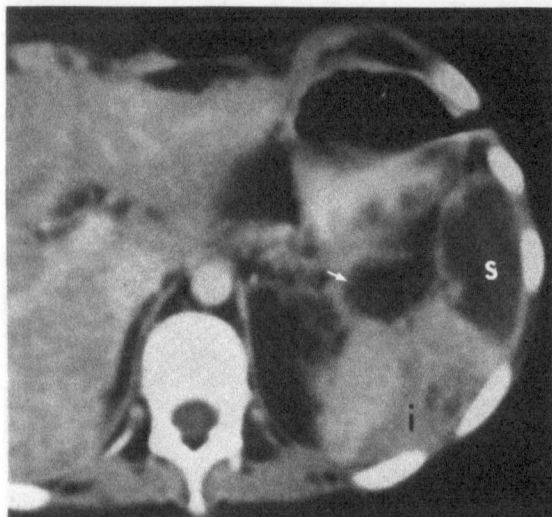

c

Fig. 9.7a–c. A 16-year-old girl with chronic pancreatitis. Scan **a** shows pancreas (*small arrows*) to be extremely thin. Artifacts are from feeding tubes. **b** Following distal pancreatectomy extensive pseudocyst formation (*small arrows*) is noted during an episode of recurrent acute pancreatitis. These pseudocysts represent extensive dissection of pancreatic secretions along tissue planes with inflammatory fluid collection. This is noted around the anterior aspect of the right kidney (*k*) and also in the anterior aspect of the spleen (*s*) and mesentery in scan **c**. A triangular low-attenuation area within the spleen (*i*) was thought to represent an infarct.

Fig. 9.8a–c. An 8-year-old boy with blunt abdominal trauma.
a Scan on admission shows hematoma in the left lobe of the
liver (*arrows*). A pancreatic pseudocyst (*open arrows*) is noted
between the stomach (G) and spleen (s). **b** Three weeks later
the pseudocyst (*open arrows*) has increased in size. Ascites (*a*)
is also noted. *p*, pancreatic head; *l*, liver; *s*, spleen. **c** Following drainage of the pseudocyst. Drains (*white arrows*) are
noted in pseudocyst, which has collapsed. The pancreas
(*small arrows*) can be seen easily. A large fluid collection (*f*) is
now present anterior to the stomach (G). This patient illustrates the value of CT in differentiating various fluid collections within the abdomen when sonography fails to do so.

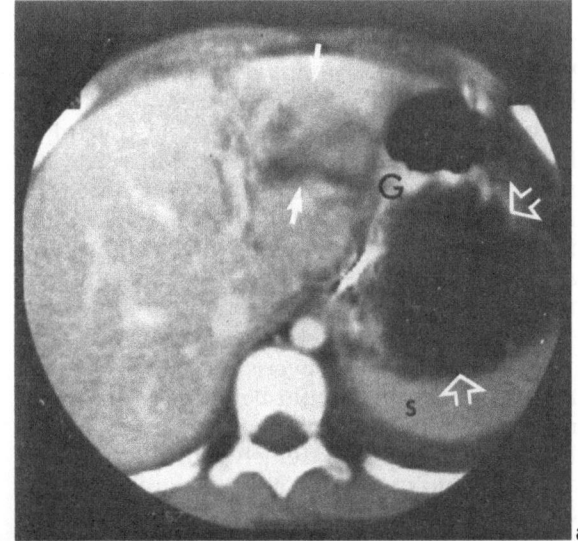

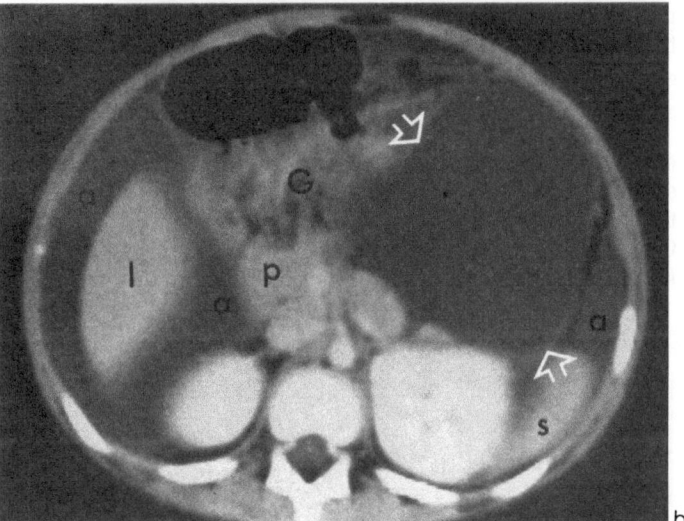

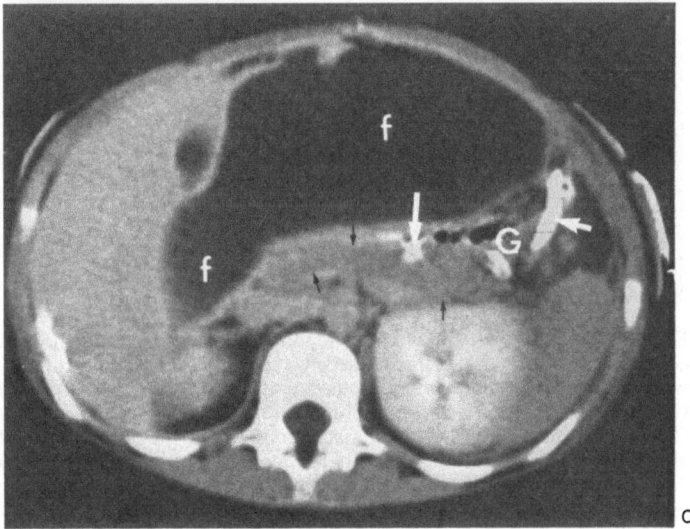

Sonography and CT are of value in the evaluation of the abdominal viscera in children with blunt abdominal trauma. Both modalities will help define the severity and extent of injuries, which may be unexpected, and are useful in follow-up. In contrast, radionuclide scans are not organ specific. CT and sonography are thus useful modalities in establishing the status of the intra-abdominal viscera following trauma and are helpful in determining which children require laparotomy for therapeutic rather than diagnostic reasons.

In the absence of severe abdominal tenderness, sonography should be used as the initial modality in the assessment of pancreatic injury. However, it may be extremely difficult to delineate the gland in the presence of significant tenderness or if the gland is obscured by overlying bowel gas caused by ileus, which often accompanies significant abdominal trauma. CT is useful in these situations as the pancreas can be adequately visualized even if the patient has tenderness and a large amount of bowel gas.

Pancreatic injuries are much less commonly seen on CT than injuries involving the liver, spleen, or kidneys. Pancreatic laceration or trans-section has been documented by CT [3]. CT is also very helpful in differentiating various fluid collections in the abdomen in children with complex intra-abdominal injuries, when sonography is unable to achieve this (Fig. 9.8).

Neoplasms

Pancreatic carcinomas and adenomas in the pediatric age group are rare and account for less than 1% of cancer deaths in children. These lesions can be classified as functioning and non-functioning lesions [10, 13].

Nonfunctioning lesions

The nonfunctioning tumors are adenocarcinomas [10, 13, 18], which have characteristic morphological features both at light microscopic and ultrastructural levels that permit their identification and separation from islet cell tumors [6, 18]. We have seen a pancreatic adenocarcinoma in a neonate — the youngest patient reported with such a lesion [16]. The CT and sonographic studies accurately demonstrated the local extent of the lesion (Fig. 9.9). The macroscopic features of the tumor could be inferred by both modalities. The mixed echogenicity on sonography and the inhomogeneous attenuation on CT

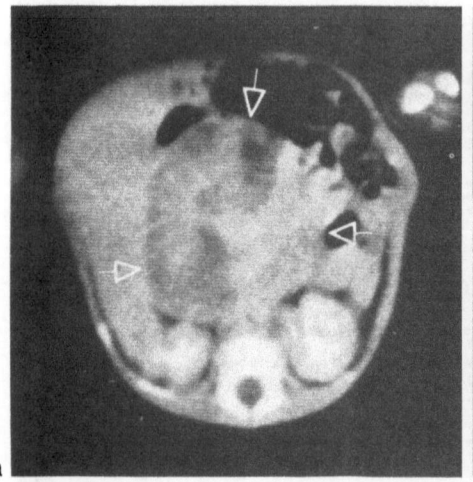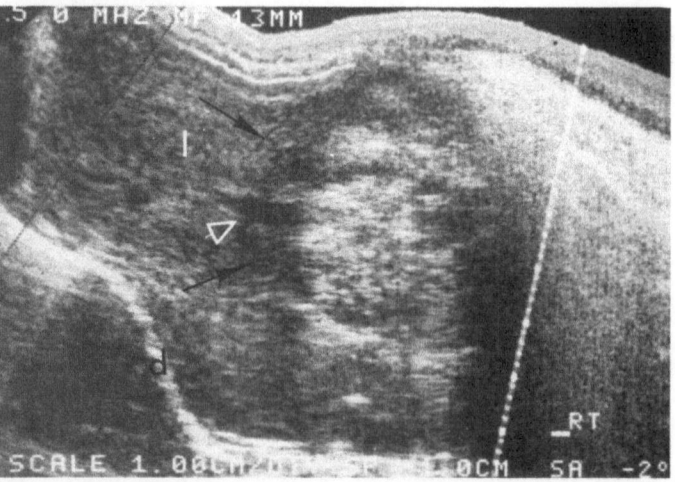

a   b

Fig. 9.9a,b. A 3-week-old boy with adenocarcinoma of pancreatic head. **a** CT scan of the abdomen following intravenous contrast enhancement. A large rounded mass (*open arrows*) extends from the retroperitoneum almost to the anterior abdominal wall. The mass has an inhomogeneous attenuation which reflects the cystic and hemorrhagic areas found on section of this tumor. No calcification is present. (Photograph courtesy of Dr. McIntyre, McKellar General Hospital, Thunder Bay, Ontario, Canada). **b** A longitudinal abdominal sonogram 1 cm to the right of the midline. The portal vein (*white open arrow*) is intimately associated with the posterior aspect of the echogenic mass (*black arrows*), suggesting that the mass is in the pancreatic head. This relationship may have been better delineated on CT had scans been performed during intravenous contrast injection. Neither CT nor sonography delineated the remainder of the pancreas clearly. *l*, liver; *d*, diaphragm. (Robey et al. [16])

(both before and after intravenous contrast administration) reflected the cystic and hemorrhagic areas found on resection of the tumor. This appearance is characteristic of adenocarcinomas but unusual in islet cell tumors [2]. Sonography accurately defined the relationship of the mass to the adjacent vessels; its intimate relationship to the anterior surface of the portal vein strongly suggested the presence of a lesion in the head of the pancreas (Fig. 9.9).

The first case of adenocarcinoma of the pancreas in a child was reported in 1818 by Todd, as cited by Corner [6]. Less than 50 children have been reported with this lesion. In 1973, Tsukimoto et al. [19] and, in 1976, Taxy [18] reviewed the Japanese and English language literature, respectively; since that time there have been a few further sporadic case reports describing adenocarcinoma of the pancreas in children [2, 12].

These lesions most commonly occur in the head of the pancreas [2, 18, 19]. The age distribution shows a biphasic pattern with most patients presenting in the early teenage years [2]. Many of the children have metastatic disease at the time of diagnosis. The commonest sites for metastases are the liver and lymph nodes [18, 19]. The clinical course is often rapid, with death occurring as the result of metastatic disease or postoperative complications. The prognosis is uncertain [2], but well-localized lesions may be well controlled with radical surgery. Definitive surgery such as pancreaticoduodenectomy would seem to provide the best opportunity for an improved prognosis [2, 10, 12, 13, 19].

Functioning Lesions

The functioning tumors are islet cell adenomas or carcinomas which present with symptoms of hypoglycemia secondary to high levels of insulin production by beta cell lesions or, less frequently, with symptoms of gastrointestinal ulceration secondary to gastric acid hypersecretion resulting from gastrin overproduction by delta cell lesions [1, 10]. In children, it is rare for Cushing's syndrome to be produced by ectopic ACTH production and also rare for islet cell tumors to be the site of such ACTH secretion [11]. Two such cases have been reported [11]. In one, a 9-year-old boy, the lesion was easily detected on CT when all other radiological studies had failed to reveal the lesion [11].

Other Masses

Berger (1983) [3] has used CT to document a case in which there was invasion of the pancreatic head by an adjacent neuroblastoma and a further case of metastatic undifferentiated neuroectodermal tumor to the pancreas. We have recently seen a boy with a pelvic sarcoma of neurogenic origin who presented with metastases in the head and tail of the pancreas (Fig. 9.10). Sarcomas of the pancreas are exceedingly rare. Other mass lesions of the pancreas apart from pseudocysts include abscesses, which may complicate pancreatitis and congenital cysts [1]. The congenital cysts are rare; they are usually multiple, asymptomatic, and may be associated with polycystic involvement of other organs.

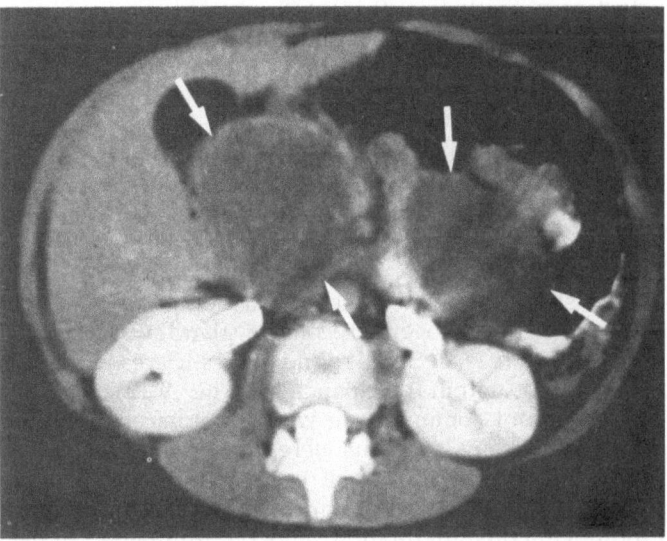

Fig. 9.10. A 9-year-old boy with left pelvic neurogenic sarcoma. At the time of presentation two metastatic masses are noted in the upper abdomen (*arrows*). The right mass is in the pancreatic head and the left in the pancreatic tail. Their position within the pancreas was proven histologically.

Cystic Fibrosis

We have used abdominal sonography extensively to study cases of cystic fibrosis, particularly those in which there is abdominal pain. When the pancreas is visualized, it is usually smaller than normal and has increased echoes, although infrequently it may appear within normal limits. Willi et al. [20] reported one case of cystic fibrosis in which an echogenic pancreas was seen on sonography. At autopsy the exocrine part of the pancreas was replaced entirely by fat, and the endocrine component was altered by fibrosis. The pancreas, however, was within normal limits in size. In only 2 of 24 patients with cystic fibrosis did these authors find enlargement of the pancreatic head. Both patients had clinical and laboratory evidence of pancreatitis, and in both the pancreatic tissue was relatively anechoic because of edema.

Occasionally, the pancreas and other abdominal viscera may not easily be visualized in these patients on sonography. This may be due to the unusual shape of the upper abdomen caused by hyperinflation of the lungs, the small size of the left lobe of the liver, and the large amount of gas in the bowel caused by malabsorption. In these situations, CT is necessary in order to image the viscera of the upper abdomen adequately. In 1983, Daneman et al. reported the appearances of the pancreas on CT in three such patients with cystic fibrosis [8]. All three had severe exocrine pancreatic insufficiency with steatorrhea. In two, abdominal CT was performed to rule out an upper abdominal lesion as the cause for fever and not to evaluate the pancreas specifically.

In two patients (Fig. 9.11), CT revealed complete fatty replacement of the entire pancreas (average −100 HU). The fat maintained the shape of the pancreas, and its site was confirmed by its relationship to the splenic vein and superior mesenteric artery and vein. In one of these an autopsy confirmed the fatty replacement of the entire pancreas. The pancreas was normal in size.

In the third patient, the sonographic and CT studies showed that the pancreas was somewhat enlarged. The echogenicity of the gland was markedly increased. Small round anechoic areas were noted within the pancreas (Fig. 9.12). These did not communicate with the adjacent arteries and veins and thus were interpreted as probably representing small cysts within the pancreas. CT showed the pancreas to have an inhomogeneous attenuation, and CT numbers

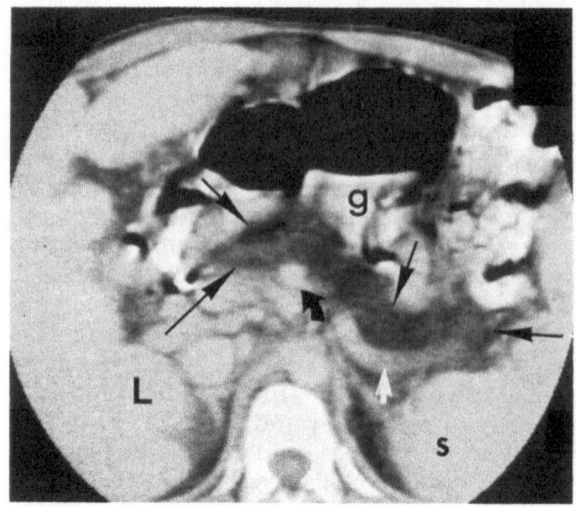

Fig. 9.11. An 18-year-old girl with cystic fibrosis was investigated with abdominal CT to rule out the presence of an upper abdominal abscess. CT scans were performed during the intravenous injection of contrast material. The pancreatic body and tail (*black arrows*) are visualized and are replaced by fat (−90 to −120 HU). *L*, liver; *s*, spleen; *g*, Gastrografin-filled bowel; *white arrow*, splenic vein; *curved black arrow*, superior mesenteric vein. Other retroperitoneal vascular structures represent collaterals because of portal hypertension. (Daneman et al. 1983 [8])

registered positive values of 20–40 HU but no negative values. Tiny areas of high attenuation were thought to represent calcification, and small areas of low attenuation were thought to correspond to the small anechoic structures noted on sonography. These changes noted on sonography and CT were interpreted as being the result of a combination of fatty replacement, fibrosis, calcification, and cyst formation within the pancreas (Fig. 9.12). However, this has not been proven histologically. Macroscopic cysts within the pancreas in patients with cystic fibrosis are indeed rare [4]. There was no clinical or laboratory evidence of pancreatitis in this patient. More recently, we have studied three further cases of cystic fibrosis and found fatty replacement of the pancreas in all. In one, macroscopic cysts replaced the pancreatic head (Fig. 9.13).

The changes on CT and sonography that we have reported reflect the late changes in the pathogenesis of the lesion in cystic fibrosis [14]. These changes have been alluded to in another publication [7].

There is a spectrum of severity of clinical findings and morphological changes in the pancreas of patients with cystic fibrosis at all ages [14, 15].

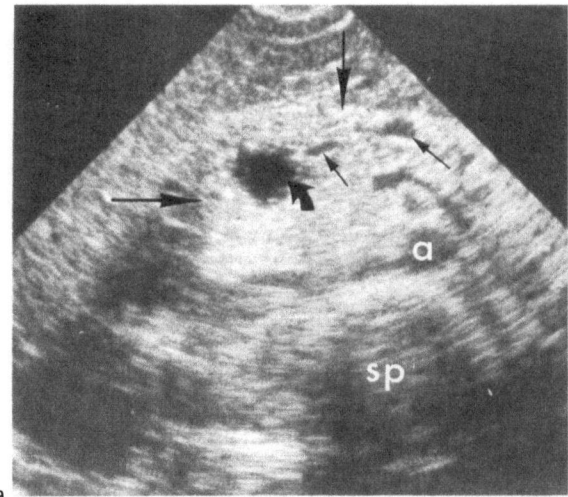

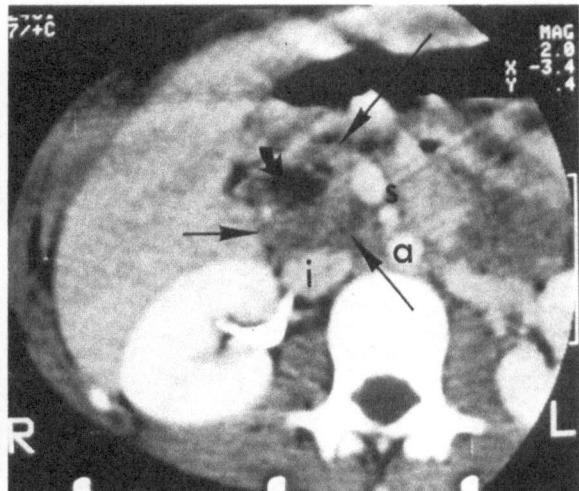

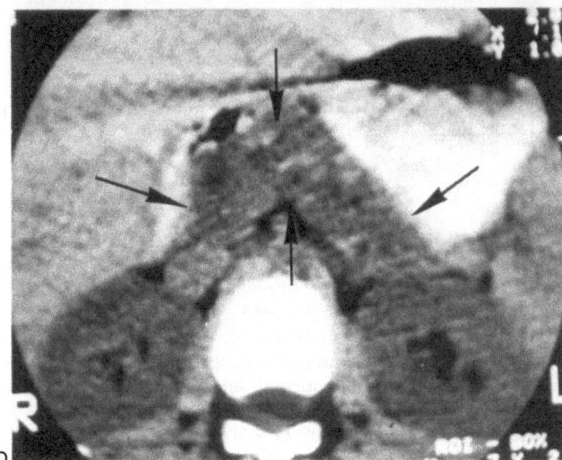

Fig. 9.12a–c. A 12-year-old boy with cystic fibrosis and abdominal pain but no laboratory evidence of pancreatitis. **a** The transverse abdominal sonogram shows the head of the pancreas (*long arrows*) is enlarged and has increased echogenicity. The common bile duct (*curved arrow*) is dilated. Small echopoor areas (*small arrows*), which did not communicate with the common bile duct or the surrounding major vessels, were thought to represent small cysts within the pancreas. **b,c** CT scans before (**b**) and during (**c**) intravenous contrast injection. The pancreas (*arrows*) is enlarged with an inhomogeneous attenuation. Tiny areas of high attenuation are thought to represent pancreatic calcification, and small areas with lower attenuation are thought to represent the small cystic structures noted on the sonogram. (Motion artifact is due to patient's tachypnea.) *sp*, spine; *a*, aorta; *i*, inferior vena cava; *s*, between superior mesenteric artery and vein; *curved arrow*, bile duct. (Daneman et al. 1983 [8])

About 15% of patients have sufficient pancreatic function to prevent steatorrhea. In some of these patients, only minimal pathological lesions are found. Patients with severe, long-standing symptoms of malabsorption may show marked fibrosis, fatty replacement, and cysts in the pancreas. In the most advanced stages of cystic fibrosis, the exocrine tissue of the pancreas is replaced by a mass of fat [14].

We have recently reviewed the autopsy findings in 27 patients with cystic fibrosis who died at the Hospital for Sick Children, Toronto, during the past 5 years (unpublished data). In 15 patients (55%) whose mean age was 17.3 years (range 9–24 years), the pancreas showed diffuse fatty replacement similar to that illustrated in Fig. 9.11. In 12 patients with minimal or no fat replacement, the mean age was lower (10.7 years), but the ages of these patients ranged from 1 month to 22 years. Four of these patients died

in early infancy, whereas five were more than 15 years old at the time of death. These data indicate that diffuse fatty replacement of the exocrine pancreas is relatively common in patients with cystic fibrosis. Although this change tends to occur more frequently in older patients and represents a late phenomenon, it can also be found in younger individuals.

It is of interest to note that the severity of pulmonary disease in patients with cystic fibrosis seems to correlate with the degree of pancreatic insufficiency [9]. Up to the stage where total or mean total fat replacement of the pancreas occurs, there is no correlation between histological findings and pancreatic function as judged by pancreatic function tests. The availability of non-invasive techniques (such as sonography and CT) to monitor the progression of pancreatic disease may thus be useful in assessing the prognosis of patients with cystic fibrosis as well as in

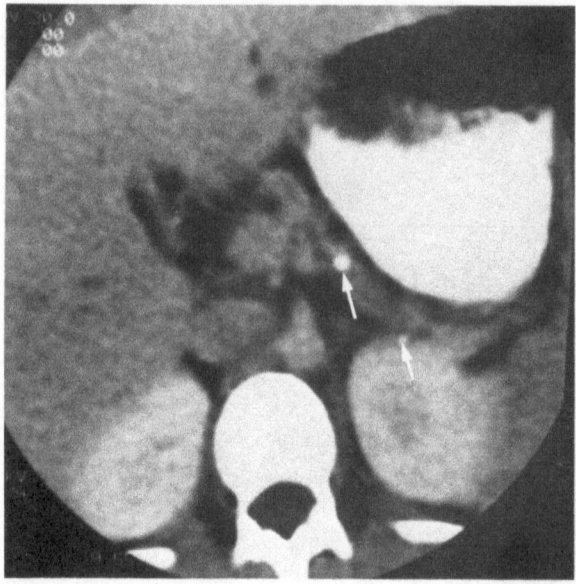
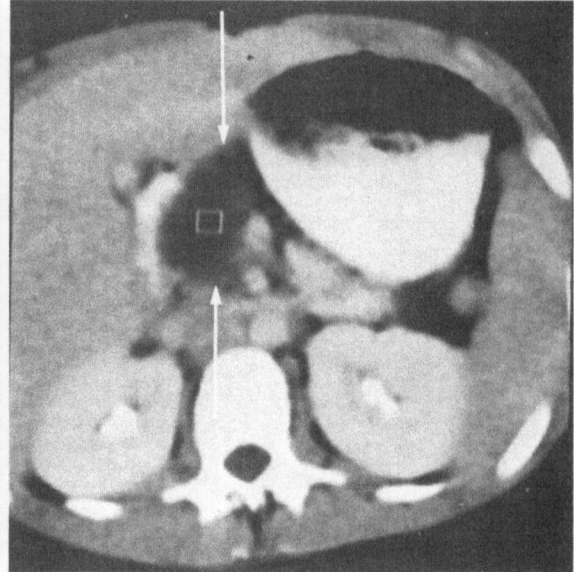

a   b

Fig. 9.13a,b. A 16-year-old girl with cystic fibrosis and abdominal pain. Scan **a** shows calcification in the pancreatic tail (*arrows*) and scan **b** shows macroscopic cyst formation (*arrows*) in the pancreatic head.

the diagnosis and follow-up of other conditions characterized by fatty replacement of the pancreas, such as Schwachman's syndrome of metaphyseal chondrodysplasia with pancreatic insufficiency and neutropenia. The exact clinical significance of these CT findings requires further investigation.

References

1. Altman AJ, Schwartz AD (1983) Tumors of the liver and pancreas. In: Malignant diseases of infancy, childhood and adolescence. Saunders, Philadelphia, pp 524–537
2. Benjamin E, Wright DH (1980) Adenocarcinoma of the pancreas of childhood: a report of two cases. Histopathology 4:87
3. Berger P (1983) Computed tomography of the pancreas in children. In: Siegelman S (ed) Computed tomography of the pancreas. Churchill Livingstone, New York
4. Churchill RJ, Cunningham DG, Henkin RE, Reynes CJ (1981) Macroscopic cysts of the pancreas in cystic fibrosis demonstrated by multiple radiological modalities. JAMA 245:72–74
5. Coleman BG, Arger PH, Rosenberg HK, Mulbern OB, Ortega D, Staugger D (1982) Gray scale sonographic assessment of pancreatitis in children. Paper presented at 25th Annual Meeting of the Society for Pediatric Radiology, New Orleans, May 1982
6. Corner BD (1943) Primary carcinoma of the pancreas in an infant aged seven months. Arch Dis Child 18:106
7. Cunningham RJ, Cunningham DG, Henkin RE, Reynes CJ (1980) Computed tomography in the evaluation of liver disease in cystic fibrosis patients. J Comput Assist Tomogr 4:151–154
8. Daneman A, Gaskin K, Martin DJ, Cutz E (1983) Pancreatic changes in cystic fibrosis: CT and sonographic appearances. AJR 141:653–655
9. Gaskin K, Gurwitz D, Durie P, Corey M, Forstener G (1982) Improved respiratory prognosis in patients with cystic fibrosis with normal fat absorption. J Pediatr 100:857–862
10. Grosfeld JL, Clatworthy HW, Hamoudi AB (1970) Pancreatic malignancy in children. Arch Surg 101:370
11. Hecht ST, Brasch RC, Styne DM (1982) CT localization of occult secretory tumors in children. Pediatr Radiol 12:67–71
12. Horie A, Hoshinobu Y, Yasunori K, Miwa A (1977) Morphogenesis of pancreatoblastoma, infantile carcinoma of the pancreas. Cancer 39:247
13. Moyhan RW, Neerhout RC, Johnson TS (1964) Pancreatic carcinoma in childhood. J Pediatr 65:711
14. Oppenheimer EH, Esterly JR (1975) Pathology of cystic fibrosis: review of the literature and comparison with one hundred and forty-six autopsied cases. Perspect Pediatr Pathol 2:241–278
15. Park RW, Grand RJ (1981) Gastrointestinal manifestations of cystic fibrosis: a review. Gastroenterology 81:1143–1161
16. Robey G, Daneman A, Martin DJ (1983) Pancreatic carcinoma in a neonate. Pediatr Radiol 13:284–286
17. Smith WL (1982) The pancreas. In: Franken EA (ed) Gastrointestinal imaging in pediatrics. Harper and Row, Philadelphia, pp 459–467
18. Taxy JB (1976) Adenocarcinoma of the pancreas in childhood. Report of a case and a review of the English language literature. Cancer 37:1508
19. Tsukimoto I, Wtanabi K, Lin J, Makajima T (1973) Pancreatic carcinoma in children in Japan. Cancer 31:1203
20. Willi UV, Reddish JM, Teele R (1980) Cystic fibrosis: its characteristic appearance on abdominal sonography. AJR 134:1005–1010

Chapter 10

Adrenals

Introduction

Sonography is the modality of choice in investigating neonates suspected of having adrenal disease, as the glands are relatively large in this age group and are easily visualized with this technique.

After the neonatal period the adrenal cortex rapidly involutes and the glands are not as easily detectable on sonography. Small lesions may not be as readily visualized as on CT. We have thus used CT as the initial imaging modality in older patients in whom there is a high clinical index of suspicion for a small adrenal lesion. However, lack of ionizing radiation makes sonography an ideal modality for screening the adrenal area in older patients, in whom there is a lower clinical index of suspicion for an adrenal lesion, and also for assessing the adrenal bed in the postoperative period.

The sensitivity of CT to detect the adrenal glands in any particular child depends on the amount of retroperitoneal fat present and the thickness of the CT slices, as well as on the cooperation of the patient, with particular regard to the ability to suspend respiration. With fast high-resolution scanners, adequate sedation and meticulous attention to technique the adrenal glands can indeed be visualized in the vast majority of children of all ages.

In children, CT plays a major role in the initial investigation and follow-up of patients with known or suspected adrenal neoplasms or adrenal hyperplasia. Neoplasms of the adrenal medulla, such as the ganglioneuroblastoma group and pheochromocytoma, may also occur in the chromaffin tissue of the sympathetic chains anywhere from the base of the skull down into the pelvis. This has an important bearing on the investigation of patients suspected of having these lesions, particularly when no mass is palpable. Although sonography is useful in detecting lesions of the adrenal and sympathetic chain of the upper abdomen and lower pelvis, the presence of gas limits its ability to delineate these lesions in the lower abdomen, upper pelvis, and chest. The exact role of CT and its relationship to other modalities in the investigation of the various adrenal lesions is discussed below.

Technique

Patients undergoing CT examination of the adrenals are given dilute contrast material orally approximately 5 min before a scout radiograph of the abdomen is taken. From this radiograph two to three levels are chosen for scans to be performed prior to intravenous contrast injection so that the area of the adrenals can be roughly gauged. Adjacent slices, each 5 mm thick, are then performed all the way through the region of both adrenals during the rapid bolus injection of intravenous contrast material. Rarely, further scans following the injection of contrast may be required to delineate the adrenal areas more thoroughly. Patients who are being studied for the presence of nonpalpable lesions of chromaffin tissue such as pheochromocytoma and neuroblastoma may require further scans of the rest of the abdomen and pelvis, and occasionally the chest as well.

Anatomy

Shape and Relationships

The adrenal glands are pyramidal or triradiate structures enclosed within Gerotas fascia and surrounded by a variable amount of fat. The shape of the gland results in a variety of cross-sectional appearances depending on the orientation of the gland and the level of the gland included in a particular cross-sectional CT slice. Different shapes may be seen in the same gland on different slices. Scans through the entire gland, are therefore, essential to exclude lesions with certainty, as the gland may appear normal on one image and abnormal on another.

The right adrenal usually has an oblique, linear or inverted "V" configuration and is visualized on a CT slice immediately above the upper pole of the right kidney (Fig. 10.1; see also Fig. 8.1, p. 90). This gland lies immediately behind the inferior vena cava, between the right diaphragmatic crus medially and the right lobe of the liver laterally.

The left adrenal appears as an inverted "V" or "Y" but occasionally may appear triangular or linear (Fig. 10.1; see also Fig. 8.1, p. 90, Fig. 9.5, p. 111, and Fig. 14.3, p. 212). This gland lies more medial, more anterior and usually more caudal than the right adrenal. The superior limit of this gland is visualized anteromedial to the upper pole of the left kidney and more caudal in relationship to the ipsilateral kidney than the right. The splenic vein lies lateral to the left adrenal gland. The adrenal glands enhance after the administration of intravenous contrast material. This is better appreciated in patients with adrenal hyperplasia.

Size

The number of 5-mm thick adjacent scans required to demonstrate both adrenal glands in

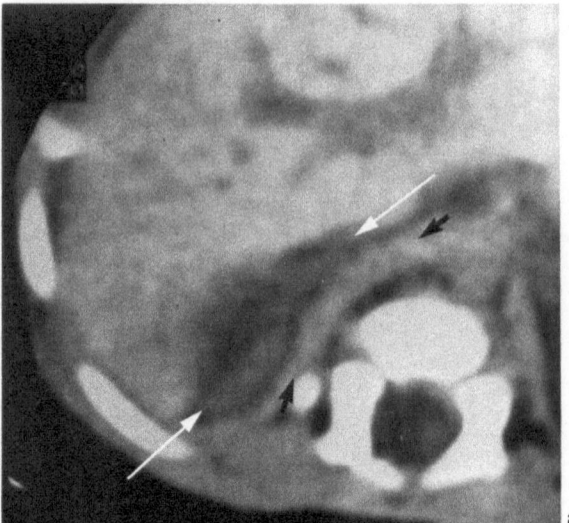

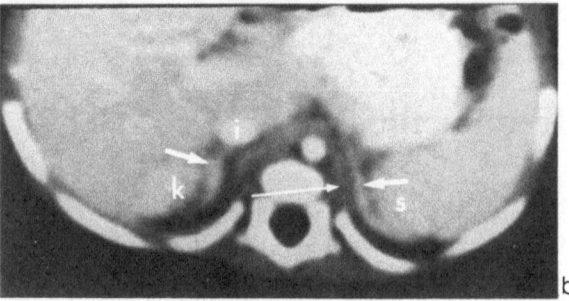

Fig. 10.1a. Normal right adrenal (*white arrows*) in a neonate. The adrenal lies medial to the right lobe of the liver and lateral to the right crus of the diaphragm (*black arrows*). Note the thickness of the adrenal in comparison with the adjacent crus. **b** Normal right and left adrenals (*short arrows*) in a 6-month-old child. Note the relationship of the right adrenal to the upper pole of the right kidney (*k*) and inferior vena cava (*i*) and the left adrenal to the left diaphragmatic crus (*long arrow*) and spleen (*s*).

their entirety varies depending on the age and size of the child. Measurements of the normal variation of the length and thickness of the adrenal limbs have not been documented in children. Except at the apex of the gland, where the limbs converge, the adrenal limbs have a uniform thickness with straight margins. Assessment of adrenal size in the absence of an easily visible mass within the gland is essentially subjective. Comparison of the adrenal limb thickness with the adjacent diaphragmatic crura is helpful as normal adrenal limbs are equal to or less than the thickness of the crura in older children but are equal to or thicker than the crura in normal neonates or older children with adrenal hyperplasia.

In some patients with clinical and laboratory evidence of hyperplasia, the adrenals appear normal on CT, because a large increase in cortical thickness is required before hyperplasia can be recognized. In hypoadrenalism the adrenals usually appear normal on CT because cortex atrophies leaving the medulla intact and cortical atrophy alone cannot be detected on CT. This explains why the opposite gland is normal on CT in patients with functioning adrenal neoplasms. This also applies to the remainder of a gland (if visualized) in the presence of a functioning neoplasm (see Fig. 10.12).

Hyperplasia

"Adrenal hyperplasia" refers to the condition where hyperplasia of the adrenal cortex occurs. In the neonatal period, adrenal hyperplasia may occur because of congenital defects in adrenal enzymes which result in virilization and the adrenogenital syndrome. Although the cortex is normally extremely prominent in the neonatal period and the glands are easily visualized with sonography, there has been no large study reporting the value of sonography in the assessment of adrenal hyperplasia in this age group. The diagnosis can usually be made easily, based on clinical and biochemical findings.

In older children, adrenal hyperplasia may be a primary phenomenon or may occur secondary to overstimulation of the adrenal cortex by a pituitary adenoma. In this age group, the commonest endocrine syndrome resulting from adrenal hyperplasia is Cushing's syndrome, caused by excessive glucocorticoid production. The endocrine syndromes produced by adrenal hyperplasia are more often pure syndromes in contrast to the endocrine abnormalities found with adrenocortical neoplasms, which may produce mixed syndromes [27, 58].

The literature regarding the use of CT in adrenal hyperplasia is virtually limited to the experience in adults. In 50% of adults with clinical and biochemical evidence of hyperplasia the CT appearance of adrenal glands is normal, because a large increase in thickness of the cortex is required before a change will be evident on CT. When changes due to hyperplasia are recognized on CT the limbs of the glands appear thickened but the normal adrenal configuration is maintained. The thickening involves the glands bilaterally and symmetrically. This is in contrast to the vast majority of adrenal mass lesions, which tend to be unilateral, with the opposite gland appearing normal on CT.

Occasionally, hyperplasia may produce focal nodules within the gland. These are usually microscopic but occasionally may be up to 2 cm in diameter. These nodules appear identical to small neoplasms on CT, and, if the remainder of the glands are not thickened, the distinction between a small neoplasm and a hyperplastic nodule cannot be made on the basis of the CT findings alone.

At the Hospital for Sick Children, Toronto, we have used CT to study the adrenals in six children with clinical and biochemical evidence of adrenal hyperplasia and Cushing's syndrome. In three patients the glands appeared to have thickening of the limbs bilaterally and symmetrically on CT (Fig. 10.2). The increased retroperitoneal fat made visualization of the glands extremely easy. In the other three the glands appeared normal. There was no correlation between the degree of enlargement of the glands and the clinical or biochemical severity of the Cushing's syndrome. All six patients had CT of the pituitary fossa after a focal adrenal lesion had been excluded on abdominal CT. In five patients the pituitary appeared normal, but an adenoma of the pituitary gland was found in the sixth. Although pituitary adenomas are a rare cause of adrenal hyperplasia in children, a CT scan of the pituitary gland is mandatory when a focal lesion of the adrenal has been excluded on CT (Fig.10.2c).

We have also examined one 7-year-old boy who presented with precocious puberty. CT showed thickening of the adrenal limbs bilaterally (Fig. 10.2d). On the left a focal nodule was also noted (Fig. 10.2e). This was felt to represent changes caused by congenital adrenal hyperplasia with an associated hyperplastic nodule.

Pseudotumors

Normal splenic and pancreatic variants may simulate adrenal masses on excretory urography and sonography. Even on CT, vascular, visceral, and gastrointestinal structures may simulate adrenal masses. This is a result of the relative

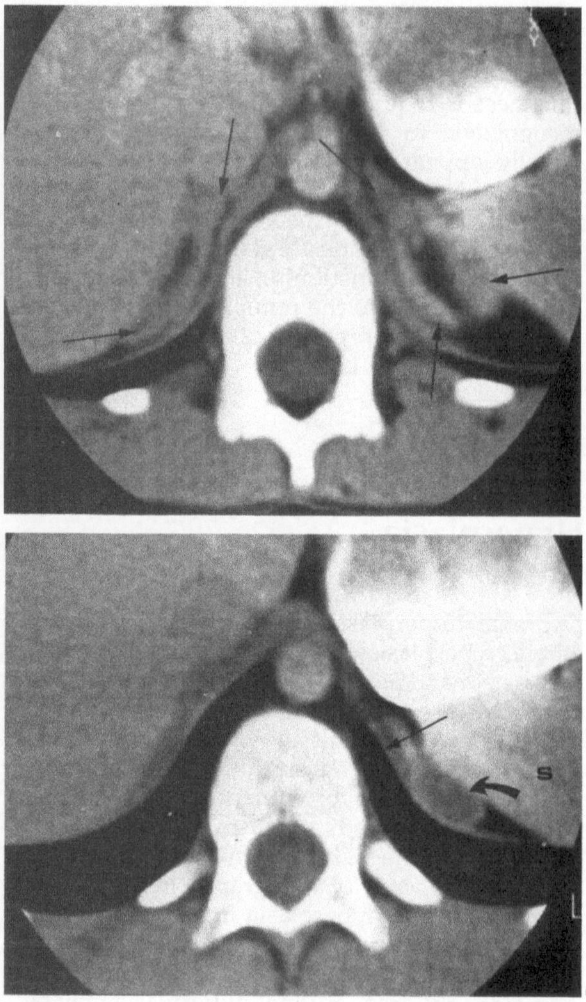

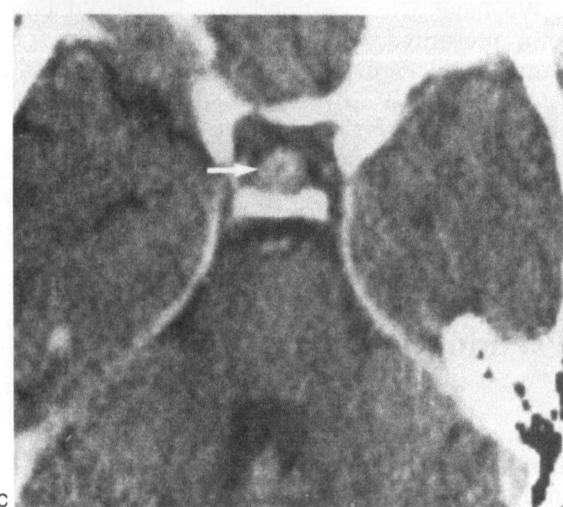

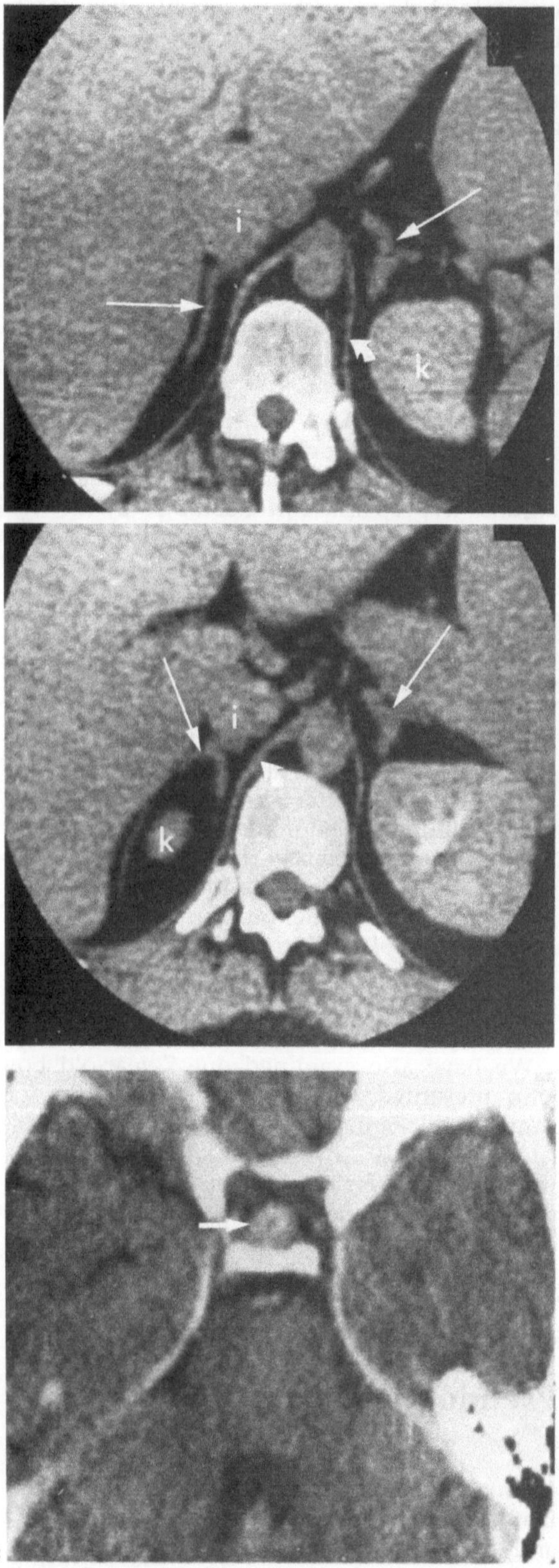

Fig. 10.2a–c. A 15-year-old girl with Cushing's syndrome. **a, b** Scans through the adrenal areas following the intravenous injection of water-soluble contrast material. Note that the adrenals (*arrows*) are uniformly thickened and are much thicker than the adjacent diaphragmatic crura (*curved arrows*). The appearances are that of adrenal hyperplasia, and the left adrenal shows more marked changes than the right. The left adrenal has an inverted "Y" configuration and lies anterior to the upper pole of the left kidney (*k*). The lateral limb of the right adrenal is seen in **a** and lies between the crus and liver and behind the inferior vena cava (*i*). In **b** the two limbs of this adrenal are noted on either side of the upper pole of the right kidney (*k*). Note the increased amount of retroperitoneal fat caused by the Cushing syndrome. (Compare the thickness of these adrenals with the normal adrenals illustrated in Figs. 8.1, 9.5, and 14.3.) **c** CT of the head after intravenous contrast administration shows the presence of a pituitary adenoma (*arrow*), the cause for the adrenal hyperplasia. **d, e** A 7-year-old boy with precocious puberty. Note the large adrenal glands in **d** (*arrows*). In a higher scan (**e**) a nodule (*curved arrow*) is present in the left adrenal lying between the spleen (*s*) and left hemidiaphragm (*long arrow*). It is difficult to differentiate this hyperplastic nodule from the adenoma shown in Fig. 10.12. However, the thickness of the remainder of the glands is a clue to the etiology of the nodule.

paucity of retroperitoneal fat in children and consequent poor delineation of adjacent structures. These pseudomasses will easily be recognized as normal structures on CT if meticulous attention is paid to technique in outlining the gastrointestinal tract with dilute oral contrast material and the vasculature by rapid bolus injection of intravenous contrast.

On the left, prominent, medial, splenic lobulations or accessory spleens may produce rounded structures resembling adrenal masses in cross section (see Fig. 14.3, p. 212). The splenic lobulation can be seen to become continuous with the spleen on adjacent slices and the adrenal can be visualized separately. Such splenic pseudo-tumors enhance to the same degree as the spleen following intravenous contrast injection (see Chap. 14, p. 210). The lateral aspect of the left adrenal lies adjacent to the splenic vein behind the body of the pancreas. Paucity of retroperitoneal fat makes delineation of these structures impossible, and the pancreatic body may simulate an adrenal mass. Rapid bolus injection of intravenous contrast will opacify the splenic vein well and thus delineate the normal adrenal posteromedially and the normal pancreatic body anterolaterally (see Fig. 9.5, p. 111). Poorly opacified duodenum, small bowel, and gastric fundus may also simulate left adrenal masses.

Pseudotumors on the right are less common. Failure to recognize the normal relationship of the right adrenal to the back of the inferior vena cava may lead one to suspect that the cava is an adrenal mass. Intravenous contrast injection will give better delineation of the cava as a vascular structure (Figs. 10.1, 10.2).

In children, vessels such as the renal vessels on the right and the splenic artery on the left seldom simulate adrenal masses as they do in adults, when these vessels are more tortuous.

Neoplasms

Adrenal neoplasms can be classified as those arising from the adrenal medulla and those from the cortex. The incidence of the various types of adrenal neoplasms in childhood differs from that in adults. The adrenocortical neoplasms may be either carcinomas or adenomas. Medullary neoplasms include neuroblastoma, ganglioneuroma, and pheochromocytoma. Neuroblastoma is by far the commonest type of neoplasm; the remainder account for under 10% of all adrenal neoplasms. The medullary lesions arise from chromaffin tissue and therefore may also arise in the sympathetic chain anywhere from the base of the skull down into the pelvis. The CT appearances of these lesions, whether they occur in the adrenal medulla or the sympathetic chain of the abdomen, will be described in one section. Other mass lesions of the adrenals such as cysts, abscesses, myelolipomas, and metastases are extremely rare in childhood.

Children with adrenocortical or medullary neoplasms may present with distant effects of the tumor such as hypertension, endocrine syndromes and metastases [11, 18]. CT has been shown to be the most acurate imaging modality in the localization of clinically nonpalpable, occult masses [11, 18, 19]. The accuracy of CT in the diagnosis of adrenal masses exceeds 90% in adults, and masses as small as 0.5 cm have been detected [1, 13, 14, 15, 40, 47, 49, 53, 64]. The smallest masses cause a focal convexity to the normal straight margin of the involved adrenal limb. This appearance is more important than absolute measurement.

The smallest mass lesion that we have detected in the adrenal in a child was approximately 1 cm in diameter and was easily visualized on CT [11, 18]. The relative lack of retroperitoneal fat in children will make the detection of small lesions that are seen in adults more difficult. Adrenal masses in children are usually over 1 cm in diameter when they present clinically because of their distant effects. To date, we have not failed with CT to detect any adrenal mass lesion in a child suspected of having such a lesion in the absence of a palpable mass. Indeed we have used CT in several children suspected of having adrenal pathology based on clinical and laboratory findings, and in all of them CT was useful in excluding pathology in the adrenals. In none of these patients have we found a mass developing at a later date.

Even in the presence of a palpable mass, CT is the most important modality in the initial delineation of the exact site and size of the mass as well as its relationship to adjacent viscera and vessels [6, 11, 55, 56]. Large adrenal masses replace or compress the remainder of the involved adrenal, which is usually not identifiable. The direction of displacement of surrounding viscera is helpful in localizing the mass to the adrenal, but with very large masses in this region it may be difficult on CT to determine the exact site of origin of such a mass. CT is also the most accurate modality in the documentation of metastatic disease in the abdomen and chest as well as in the post-therapeutic follow-up of these patients.

Medullary and Sympathetic Nervous System Lesions

Neuroblastoma

Neuroblastomas, ganglioneuroblastomas, and ganglioneuromas arise from neural crest cells that give rise to the sympathetic ganglia and adrenal medulla. Therefore abdominal and pelvic neuroblastomas may occur either in the adrenal medulla or in the sympathetic chains as they pass through the diaphragm down into the pelvis. Rarely, these lesions may arise at somewhat ectopic sites where neural crest tissue is found, such as the mesentery. By far the commonest type of these lesions is the malignant neuroblastoma. Ganglioneuromas are far less common. Neuroblastomas may in some cases mature into the more benign form of ganglioneuroma. This maturation may include part or all of the primary tumor or metastases.

Neuroblastoma is the most common extracranial malignancy in childhood and the most common malignant tumor of infancy. The vast majority of neuroblastomas are diagnosed before 5 years of age with a peak incidence at 2 years. The lesions are thought to be congenital in origin and are often diagnosed at birth. Rarely, these lesions may occur in adults, even the elderly.

Surgery is the prime modality for therapy in this tumor. Response to chemotherapy and radiotherapy is poor. Therefore, clinical staging of the disease at the time of diagnosis is the major determinant of whether surgery is possible or not and will ultimately determine the prognosis [17, 37, 55]. The staging of these tumors is summarized in Table 10.1.

Neuroblastomas most commonly present in the abdomen as a palpable mass. However, at times the mass may be small and nonpalpable, and in such cases presentation may well be due to the distant effects of the tumors such as metastases or opsomyoclonus. Whether the primary lesion is palpable or not, CT has proved to be the most useful modality in the delineation of the exact origin and anatomical extent of the primary tumor as well as metastases within the abdomen. This has proved true both at the time of presentation and during follow-up.

Table 10.1. Staging of neuroblastomas

Stage I
Tumor confined to the organ or structure of origin and completely excised

Stage II
Tumor extending beyond the organ of origin but not crossing the midline. Regional homolateral lymph nodes and intraspinal extension are classified as Stage II unless the primary lesion crosses the midline

Stage III
Tumors that cross the midline in continuity or bilateral lymph node involvement

Stage IV
Metastatic disease involving the skeleton, viscera, soft tissues, or distant lymph nodes

Stage IV S
Disease that would otherwise be staged at I or II but has remote metastases confined to one or more of the following sites: liver, skin, or bone marrow (but not bone itself)

The advent of the imaging modalities with cross-sectional anatomy has forced us to reassess the manner in which we stage neuroblastoma. These imaging modalities have shown that many tumors that cross the midline (stage III) may well be pushing blood vessels ahead of them rather than infiltrating around the vessels to cross the midline. Such well-defined lesions are operable despite their crossing of the midline. Other lesions which may not cross the midline may indeed be invading the kidney or surrounding the larger vessels and for this reason may be inoperable. In 1982, Armstrong et al. [4] published a review of 67 children with neuroblastoma seen at the Hospital for Sick Children, Toronto between 1976 and 1980. Stark et al. [56] have published their data regarding an extensive review of the value of CT both at the time of diagnosis and recurrence in 38 and 52 patients respectively. These latter authors have confirmed our findings that CT is the most sensitive single test (100%) for the detection and delineation of the primary tumors. The exact relationship of the mass lesions to the surrounding viscera and vessels is exquisitely displayed in scans that are performed with adequate opacification of bowel and vasculature (see Figs. 10.3–10.8).

Extremely small neuroblastomas may have a somewhat homogeneous attenuation but the vast majority of the larger lesions have an inhomogeneous attenuation appearance with large areas of poorer vascularity centrally. Paraspinal lesions often infiltrate around the larger abdominal vessels. Invasion of the lesion into the liver and kidneys may also be delineated (Figs.

10.3, 10.4, 10.5). However, in many of these instances compression of the adjacent viscera may lead to the appearance of infiltration on CT; indeed this is one of the pitfalls of this modality. Longitudinal sonographic scans may well be more accurate in delineating this.

Stark et al. [55] found calcification in 79% of the cases that they studied, and the type of calcification varies. It may be punctate, globular, or be present as rim calcification. Rim enhancement of the lesions is also occasionally seen. Unfortunately the presence of calcification does not differentiate the benign ganglioneuroma from the malignant neuroblastoma. Stark et al. [55] considered the rim calcification to be the most specific pattern for neuroblastoma.

At CT, lymph node and liver metastases may well be delineated and these vary in size (see Figs. 10.6, 10.7). Stark et al. [55] found that CT alone accurately staged 82% of cases; however, when complemented by bone marrow biopsy, staging accuracy was 97%.

Intraspinal involvement of tumor occurs in approximately 15% of patients. Calcification is rarely seen in the intraspinal component [46]. In the series reported from our institution by Armstrong et al. [4] 11 patients were found to have intraspinal extension and in 6 this was unsuspected clinically. If a neuroblastoma is operated on without the knowledge of intraspinal extension there is a risk of intraspinal hemorrhage and subsequent damage to the cord. It is

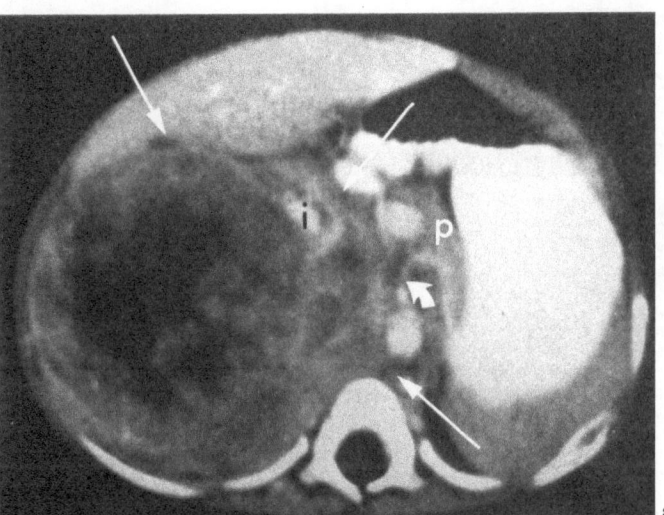

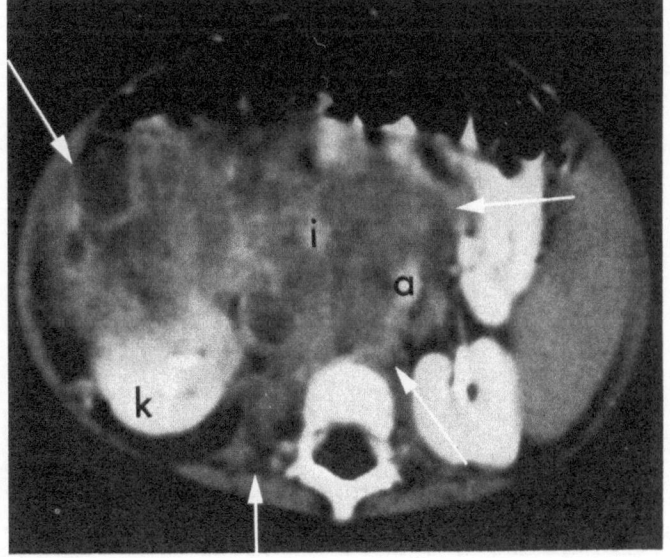

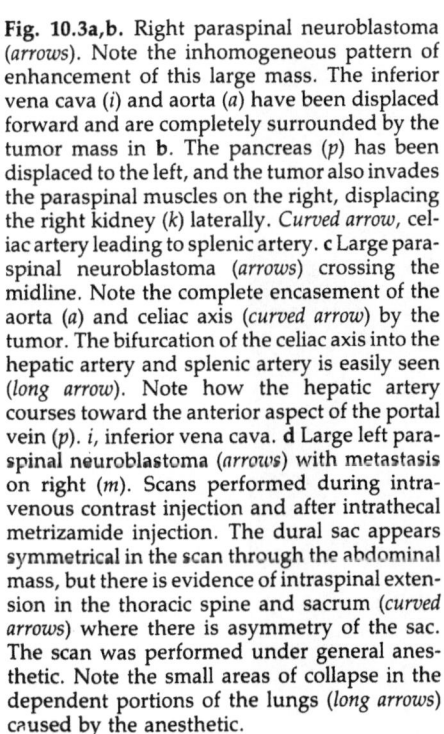

Fig. 10.3a,b. Right paraspinal neuroblastoma (*arrows*). Note the inhomogeneous pattern of enhancement of this large mass. The inferior vena cava (*i*) and aorta (*a*) have been displaced forward and are completely surrounded by the tumor mass in **b**. The pancreas (*p*) has been displaced to the left, and the tumor also invades the paraspinal muscles on the right, displacing the right kidney (*k*) laterally. *Curved arrow*, celiac artery leading to splenic artery. **c** Large paraspinal neuroblastoma (*arrows*) crossing the midline. Note the complete encasement of the aorta (*a*) and celiac axis (*curved arrow*) by the tumor. The bifurcation of the celiac axis into the hepatic artery and splenic artery is easily seen (*long arrow*). Note how the hepatic artery courses toward the anterior aspect of the portal vein (*p*). *i*, inferior vena cava. **d** Large left paraspinal neuroblastoma (*arrows*) with metastasis on right (*m*). Scans performed during intravenous contrast injection and after intrathecal metrizamide injection. The dural sac appears symmetrical in the scan through the abdominal mass, but there is evidence of intraspinal extension in the thoracic spine and sacrum (*curved arrows*) where there is asymmetry of the sac. The scan was performed under general anesthetic. Note the small areas of collapse in the dependent portions of the lungs (*long arrows*) caused by the anesthetic.

Fig. 10.3c,d (*overleaf*)

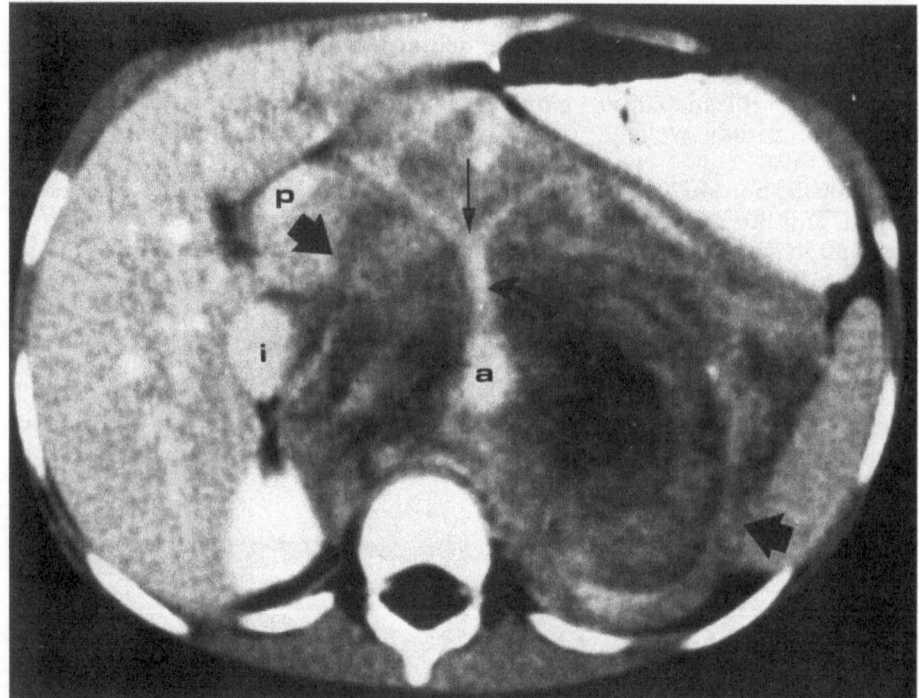

Fig. 10.3c

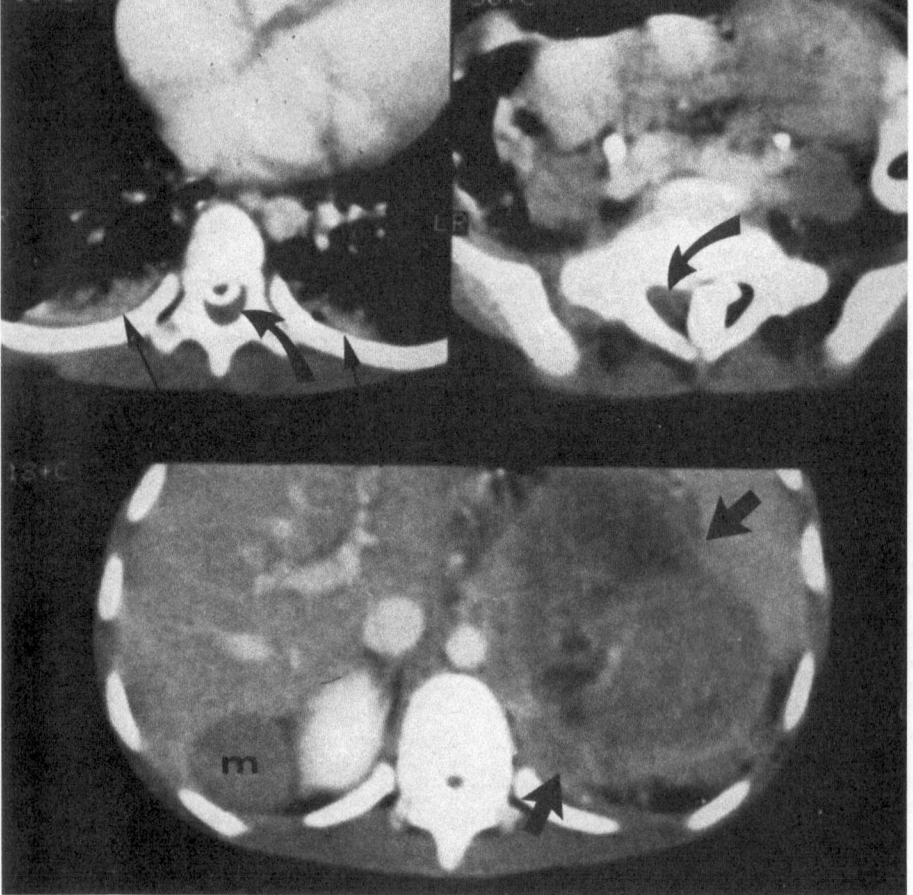

Fig. 10.3d

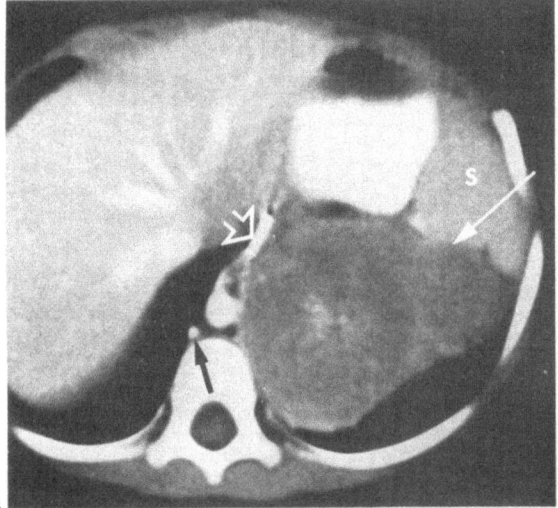

a

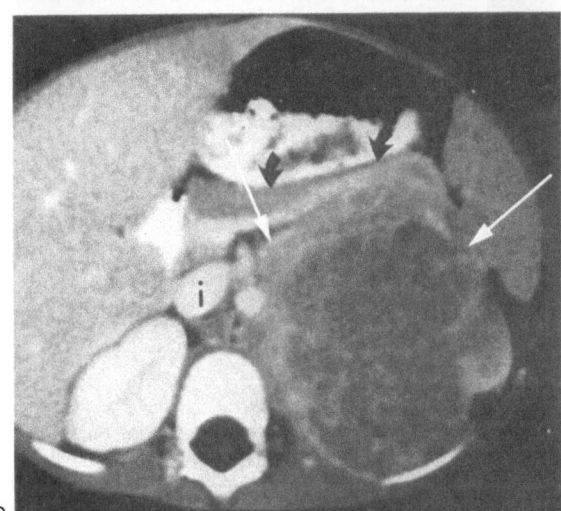

b

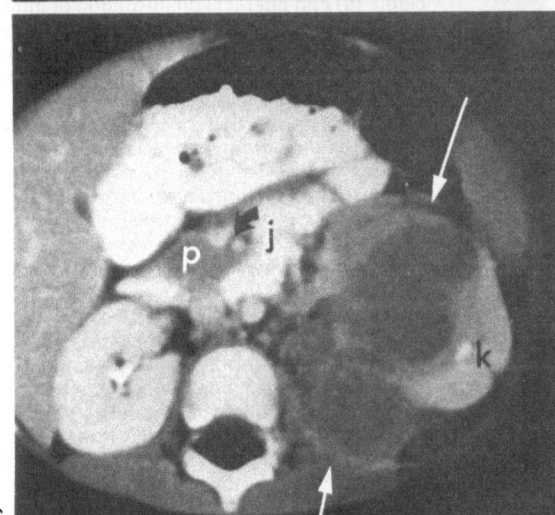

c

Fig. 10.4a–c. Large left adrenal neuroblastoma (*arrows*). The lesion extends from the level of the diaphragm in **a** inferiorly to infiltrate the left kidney (*k*) in **c. a** The spleen (*s*) and esophagus (*open arrow*) are displaced forward. *Black arrow*, azygous vein. **b** The pancreas (*curved arrows*) and splenic vein have been displaced forward and tumor is noted infiltrating behind the aorta and inferior vena cava (*i*). **c** The remaining renal parenchyma (*k*) is displaced laterally and the appearances on this image are indistinguishable from a tumor arising primarily in the kidney. *p*, pancreatic head; *j*, jejunum. *Curved arrow* indicates superior mesenteric artery and vein.

thus important for the surgeon to know pre-operatively whether intraspinal extension exists or not as this will alter the surgical approach and radiotherapy. For this reason any patient with a mass lesion in the abdomen with a propensity to extend into the spinal canal should be studied on CT after the instilation of dilute metrizamide into the intrathecal space. The study should also be performed during rapid bolus injection of intra-venous water-soluble contrast. A careful study performed with this meticulous attention to technique will give more information regarding the site and extent of extraspinal and intraspinal components of the tumor, as well as the presence of metastases to lymph nodes and liver, than all other modalities combined.

Intrathecal metrizamide should be used in those patients with any clinical signs or symp-toms suggesting intraspinal extension, widening of the intervertebral foramina or destruction of adjacent bone on plain radiographs or in those patients in whom sonography shows close prox-imity of the lesion to the spinal canal, particularly with those arising from the sympathetic chain rather than the adrenal.

Tumor growth into the spinal canal may dis-place the spinal cord and dural sac without com-pression of the structures. This displacement may be slight but is sufficient for diagnosis as the epidural space is usually constantly symmetri-cal, particularly in the thoracic spine, provided there is no scoliosis. Larger tumors may flatten or impinge on one side of the dural sac and may even cause a complete block to the flow of con-trast material. The largest mass of the intraspinal component does not always correspond to the same level as the paraspinal primary tumor. This is because the neoplasm may extend up or down the spinal canal as a thin sheet of tumor and may expand into a larger mass at a distance from the primary paraspinal tumor. A metrizamide injection is not used in all patients with neu-

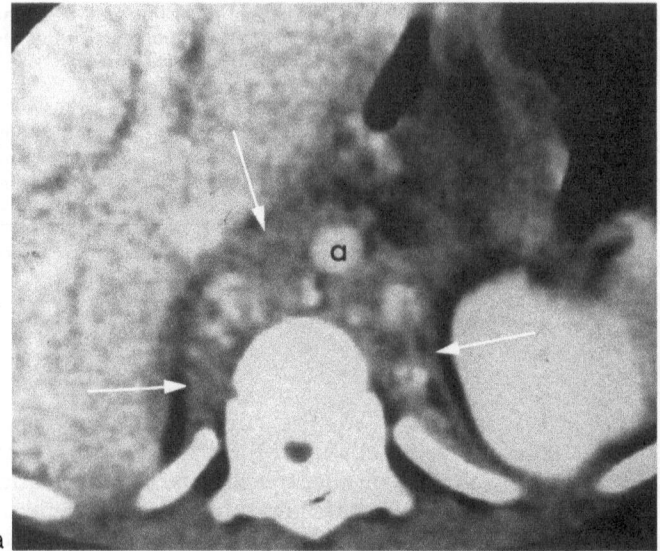

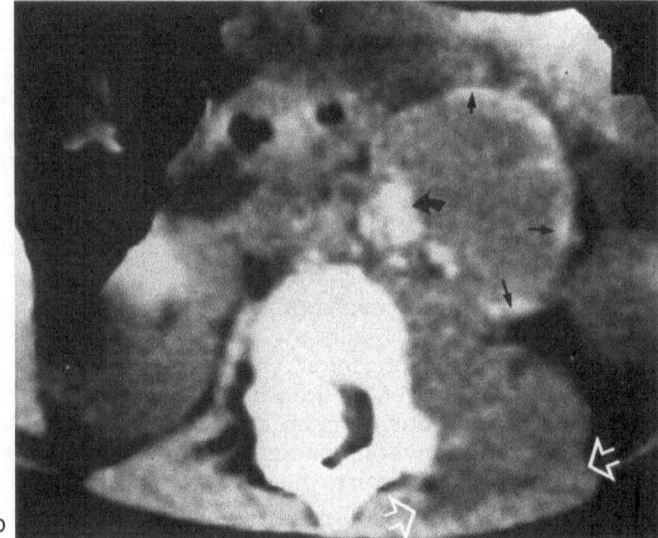

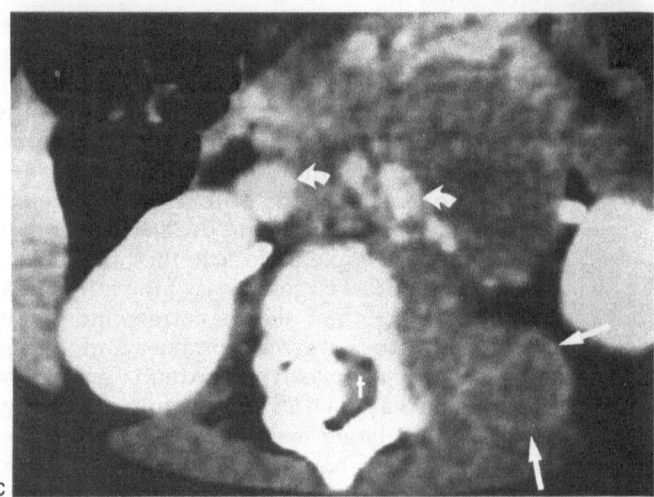

Fig. 10.5a–f. Extensive paraspinal neuroblastoma in a 9-month-old girl. **a** Calcified tumor is noted bilaterally in the retrocrural area (*arrows*) displacing aorta (*a*) forward. Scans before (**b**) and after (**c**) administration of intravenous contrast material are lower in the abdomen through the level of the lower poles of the kidneys. Curvilinear calcification (*short arrows* in **b**) and globular calcification (*curved arrows* in **b** and **c**) are present in the mass. **b** Note infiltration of the tumor into the posterior paraspinal muscles on the left (*open arrows*). After the administration of intravenous contrast (**c**), rim enhancement is noted, particularly in the posterior part of the tumor (*arrows*). **b,c,d** Metrizamide, which was administered to the child prior to the CT study, can be easily seen outlining the dural sac. The sac is asymmetrical, with tumor (*t*) in the extradural space on the left. This is seen to best advantage in image **d** when viewed at a bony window setting. **e** Denser calcification, which includes globules and curvilinear masses, is noted in the tumor (*arrows*) below the level of the kidney. **f** A follow-up CT study after chemotherapy shows that the tumor mass is markedly smaller at the level of the lower pole of the kidney (*k*). The residual mass (*small arrows*) is heavily calcified. *a*, aorta. *Curved arrow*, left ureter.

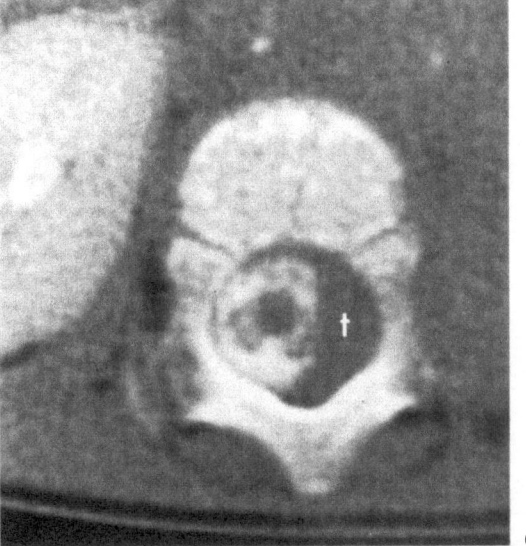

d

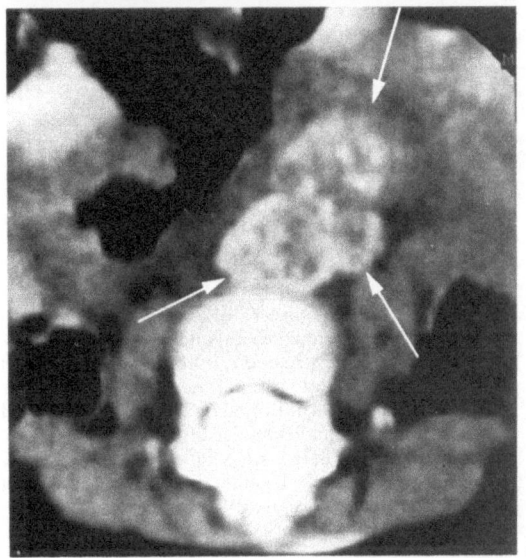

e

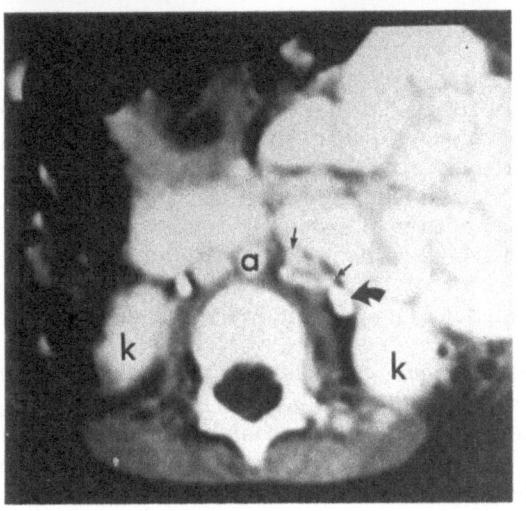

f

roblastoma. It is not used in those lesions arising in the adrenal glands or when the lesion lies anteriorly and is at a distance from the intervertebral foramina. Intraspinal extension occurs more commonly in the thoracic region than in the abdomen. CT metrizamide myelography need not be used in all follow-up studies unless surgery is contemplated.

Sonography remains the modality of choice in children with suspected or palpable neuroblastomas. This study will help delineate the site of origin of such lesions and will allow one to tailor the type of CT examination to be performed. This is particularly important with regard to the decision as to whether metrizamide should be injected into the intrathecal space prior to CT or not. Lesions arising anteriorly or in the adrenal need not have a CT metrizamide myelogram. Other paraspinal lesions should all be studied with CT metrizamide myelography and adequate opacification of bowel and major vasculature by bolus injection of intravenous contrast material. A careful study performed in this way is the most important in the evaluation of the abdominal and pelvic extent of these lesions as well as their intraspinal component and also for the detection of lymph node and liver metastases. The delineation of the exact extent of these lesions is extremely important because surgery is the modality of choice for therapy and because the size of the lesion determines prognosis.

Radionuclide bone scans are mandatory in all patients with neuroblastoma because of the high incidence of bone metastases. These studies should be performed both at the time of diagnosis and during follow-up when decisions have to be made regarding therapy. Plain radiographs of positive areas are useful to confirm the degree of bony involvement. The technetium-99m methylene diphosphonate (^{99m}Tc-MDP) is taken up by many neuroblastomas. This aspect of the radionuclide study is useful when abdominal masses are present and their exact character cannot be determined by other modalities. However, other pediatric malignancies also take up this radionuclide, including adrenal carcinomas, hepatoblastomas, and even Wilms' tumors, although the incidence of uptake in these tumors is very much less than in neuroblastoma. The reason for uptake is not related to the presence or amount of calcification in the tumor but is probably related to the areas of necrosis.

Neuroblastoma metastasizes to lung very much less commonly than other pediatric soft tissue malignancies [62]. For this reason, chest

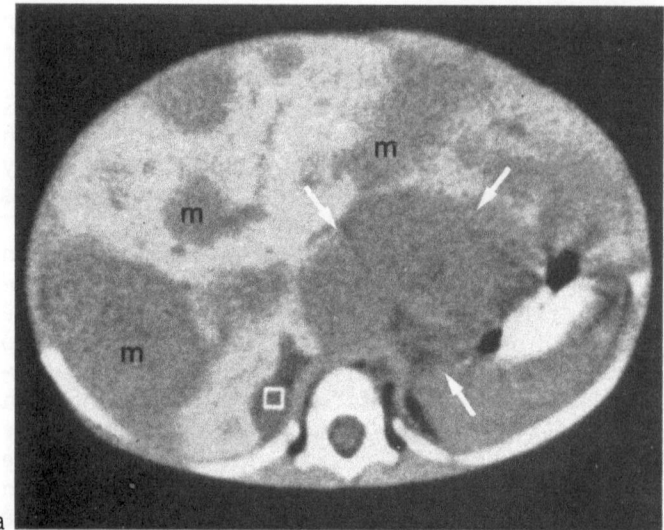

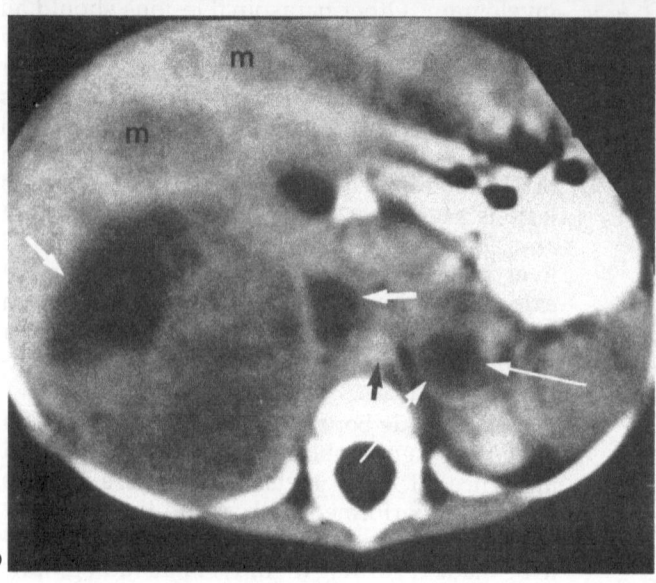

Fig. 10.6a. A 6-week-old boy with left adrenal neuroblastoma (*arrows*) and multiple liver metastases (*m*). (Stage IV S.) **b** A 4-week-old girl with bilateral adrenal neuroblastomas. The right lesion is indicated by *short white arrows* and the much smaller left lesion by *long white arrows*. Notice the large areas of very poor enhancement in both lesions representing areas of diminished vascularity and necrosis. Liver metastases (*m*) are also present. *Black arrow*, aorta.

CT to evaluate the lungs is not performed in the search for pulmonary metastases when these lesions are initially diagnosed or during follow-up unless such lesions are noted on plain radiographs. Involvement of the lungs by direct extension or by metastatic involvement occurs more commonly in the later phases of the disease.

Of the 439 children with neuroblastomas seen at the Hospital for Sick Children, Toronto between 1919 and 1984, 13 had bilateral adrenal lesions (see Fig. 10.6b). These patients presented between 1 day and 34 months of age. Twelve had presented with an abdominal mass; this was thought in each case to be unilateral. All 13 had metastatic disease, and the pattern of involvement suggested that these patients be classified as stage IV S. The survival of this group is extremely poor and suggests that bilaterality of the lesion in the adrenals should exclude patients from the stage IV S type. Documentation of bilaterality is extremely important at diagnosis or during follow-up because it may influence management and survival.

Opsomyoclonus and the Investigation of Occult Neuroblastoma   Opsomyoclonus is a rare presenting feature of neuroblastoma in children and occurs in approximately 2% of patients with neuroblastoma [63]. In 1927, Orzechowski first intro-

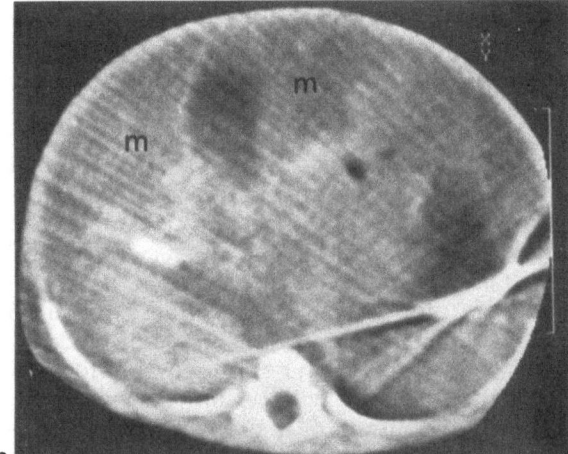

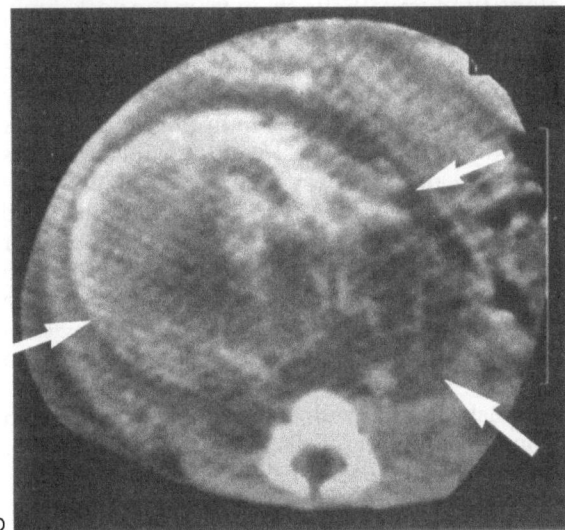

Fig. 10.7a,b. Neonate with a large right paraspinal neuroblastoma and extensive liver metastases. Unfortunately, artifacts caused by the nasogastric tube and blankets are present. **a** Note the extremely low attenuation of the liver (*m*). This was due to extensive necrosis of the liver metastases. **b** The main paraspinal lesion (*arrows*) is heavily calcified.

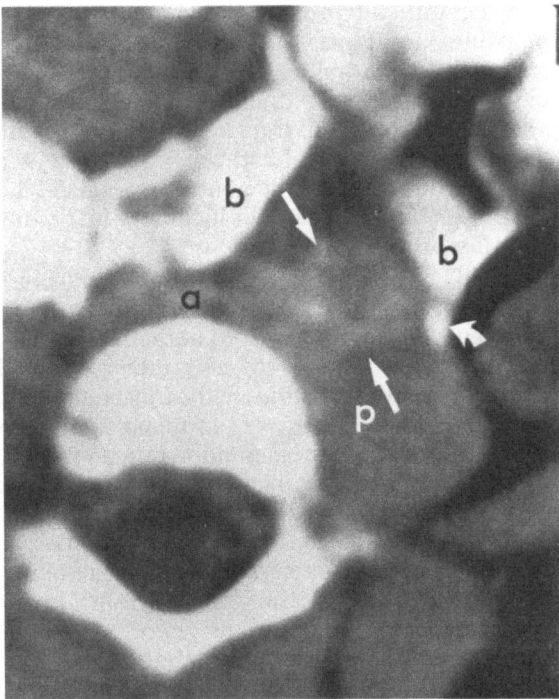

Fig. 10.8. A 1-year-old boy with opsomyoclonus. CT shows a very small left paraspinal neuroblastoma (*arrows*) displacing the left ureter (*curved arrow*) laterally. *b*, opacified bowel; *p*, psoas muscle; *a*, aorta.

duced the term "opsoclonus" to describe intermittent jerky eye movements occurring in all directions [45]. In 1962, Kinsbourne described the association of opsoclonus with myoclonic jerks and cerebellar ataxia [36]. These patients were originally diagnosed as having acute cerebellar pathology of unknown etiology. In 1968, Solomon and Chutorian were the first to draw attention to the association between neuroblastoma and opsomyoclonus [54]. Altman and Baehner, in 1975, reviewed the 28 patients that had been reported in the literature up to that time and established that there was a good prog-

nosis for children with neuroblastoma presenting with opsomyoclonus [2]. Approximately 50% of children with opsomyoclonus have an occult neuroblastoma [31, 42, 51].

The exact nature of the association between opsomyoclonus and neuroblastoma remains to be determined. There is some evidence that the cerebellum is indirectly involved by the disease process [9, 16, 44, 67]. Bray's [9] proposed pathogenesis for this condition included: (1) infection by an unknown virus which simultaneously attacks neural crest tissue and the cerebellum; (2) production by the neuroblastoma of a hormone or metabolite of a hormone which affects the cerebellum; and (3) production of an autoantibody by the patient directed against the neuroblastoma and the cerebellum. None of these theories have been proven or disproven.

Many children with persistent or recurrent opsomyoclonus may be labelled by the clinician as having encephalopathy of unknown etiology after a posterior fossa neoplasm has been ruled out. They constitute a diagnostic problem [5, 28, 33, 43, 51] because the existence of neuroblastoma is often not suspected. Even when occult neuroblastoma is suspected, the diagnosis may be difficult to confirm when there is no palpable tumor mass, when the urinary catecholamines are not increased, and when the plain radiographs of the chest and abdomen are normal. Children presenting with opsomyoclonus should thus be investigated intensively for an occult neuroblastoma [2, 12, 18, 39, 50] and this should include a full radiological workup.

In 1983, Farrelly et al. [18] reviewed our experience with the ten patients with opsomyoclonus and neuroblastoma on record at the Hospital for Sick Children, Toronto, to assess the role of CT relative to other modalities in the investigation of these patients. There were four males and six females. The ages at presentation ranged from 13 months to 3 years (mean age 17.9 months). None of the patients had a palpable mass or symptoms and signs referable to local effects of the mass at the time of original presentation. In two patients, the lesions arose in the adrenals, and in the remaining eight the lesions were paraspinal (three abdominal, one thoracoabdominal, three thoracic, and one thoracocervical). At presentation the urinary catecholamines were increased in only five patients. Histologically, eight of the tumors were neuroblastomas, one was a ganglioneuroblastoma, and one was a ganglioneuroma. All ten children are alive at intervals from 1.5 to 10.25 years after diagnosis (median follow-up 3.25 years). Since that report we have studied one further child with neuroblastoma and opsomyoclonus with CT.

In some series [48], a high diagnostic yield based on plain radiographic findings alone is quoted. In our series, at the time of initial presentation, 60% of the patients had no demonstrable tumor on plain radiographs (chest or abdomen); excretory urography was negative in 50% of the abdominal lesions, and 50% of patients who had ^{99m}Tc-MDP bone scan showed no uptake of the radionuclide in the lesion. In combination, these three modalities did demonstrate the neuroblastoma in five of six patients who had CT. The lesions were diagnosed promptly and accurately in all six patients who had CT (Fig. 10.10). In only one patient did CT detect the tumor when all other modalities were negative. Prompt diagnosis of opsomyoclonus-related neuroblastoma by CT in this way avoids unnecessary investigations of the central nervous system, e.g., brain scan, pneumoencephalogram, and cerebral angiogram.

In addition, CT significantly shortened the time interval between initial presentation and final diagnosis. The average time taken from initial presentation to diagnosis was 4.75 days for four patients who had CT during their first hospital admission and 11.4 months for four who did not have CT. In the two patients who did not have body CT until their second admission, the diagnosis of neuroblastoma was delayed for 14 and 18 months, respectively. The number of hospital admissions for investigation of opsomyoclonus was less in patients who had CT (6 admissions in 6 patients) compared with those who did not have CT (11 admissions in 6 patients). CT is thus the most useful modality available in locating an occult neuroblastoma in children presenting with opsomyoclonus.

The vast majority of neuroblastomas are solitary lesions and the tumor may arise anywhere along the sympathetic chain from the neck down into the pelvis, as well as in the adrenals. Although plain radiographs, excretory urograms, and ^{99m}Tc-MDP bone scans individually failed to locate the lesion in approximately 50% of patients in our series, we do believe that it is useful to perform less expensive, noninvasive studies initially in an attempt to localize the lesion. If the location of the tumor is known prior to CT then this examination can be limited to studying the area in question and can also be tailored to suit the needs of each individual patient. This will also enable the radiologist to use the maximum amount of contrast intravenously to opacify the vasculature in the region being examined and display the relationship of the mass to the surrounding viscera and vessels with greater accuracy. In addition, this makes the most effective use of CT time, which is at a premium. Prior localization of the tumor to the paraspinal regions should encourage the radiologist to arrange the CT examination after the injection of metrizamide into the lumbar subarachnoid space in order to define more accurately the presence or absence of extradural tumor extension.

In children presenting with opsomyoclonus and no palpable tumor, we therefore recommend initial utilization of less expensive, noninvasive localizing studies such as plain radiographs of the chest and abdomen, ultrasound of the abdomen and pelvis, and ^{99m}Tc-MDP bone scans. Body CT can then be tailored to suit the needs of each individual patient [18].

Ganglioneuroma

Ganglioneuroma is the most mature benign type of lesion arising in neural crest tissue. These

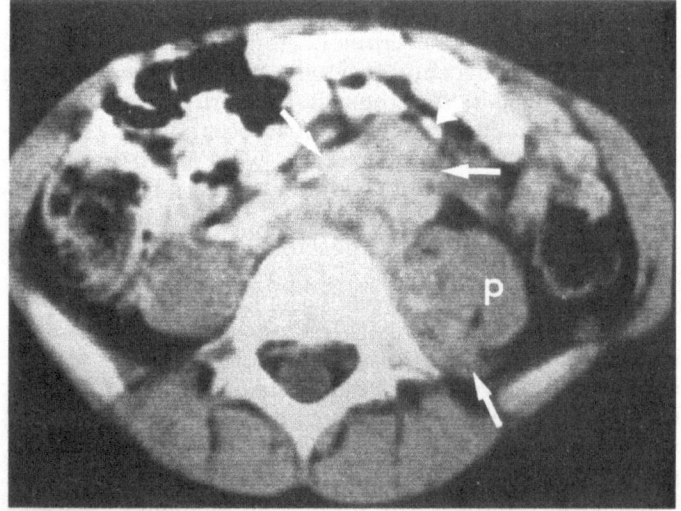

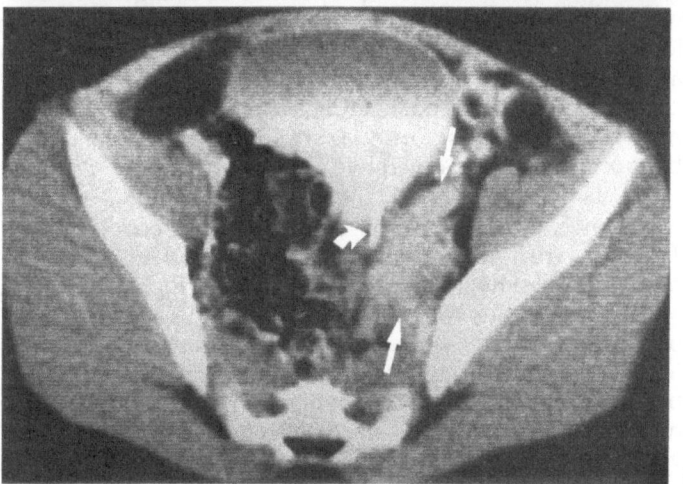

Fig. 10.9a,b. A 7-year-old boy with paraspinal ganglioneuroma (*arrows*). In **a** note the extension of the mass posteriorly on the left, medial to the psoas muscle (*p*). *Curved arrow,* left ureter.

lesions are far less common in the pediatric age group than neuroblastomas. CT used in the same way as described above for neuroblastoma is the modality of choice in the documentation of the site and extent of these lesions (Fig. 10.9). However, the appearances of ganglioneuromas on CT are similar to those of neuroblastomas, and the presence or absence of calcification is not useful in differentiating them. Therefore, differentiation depends on a histological search through these lesions once they have been removed. It should be remembered that neuroblastomas can mature into ganglioneuromas both in the primary lesion or in metastases. Once the lesions have become a ganglioneuroma continued growth does not necessarily represent malignant degeneration. In a few reported patients and in one seen in the Hospital for Sick Children, Toronto, previously irradiated neuroblastomas that have matured into a ganglioneuroma may undergo late malignant degeneration into a malignant Schwannoma.

Pheochromocytoma

Pheochromocytoma is a potentially curable secretory tumor which can arise from adrenal or extra-adrenal sites. Of all pheochromocytomas, 5% occur in children, and these lesions account for 0.2% of all neoplastic disease at the Hospital for Sick Children, Toronto. In children, 30% may be extra-adrenal and most of these occur in the upper abdomen [19, 28]. Multiple lesions have been reported in from 30% to 70% of children and are found mainly in those children with a family history of pheochromocytoma [3, 28]. Children with pheochromocytoma usually present with sustained rather than intermittent hypertension. Pheochromocytomas occur with an increased incidence in patients with neurofibromatosis, Von Hippel–Lindau syndrome, and in the syndrome of multiple endocrine adenomatosis (pheochromocytoma, hyperparathyroidism, and medullary thyroid carcinoma).

Accurate and noninvasive radiological localization of these tumors is an important prerequisite for successful surgical management. Preoperative delineation of local invasion and metastatic disease is important as the malignant potential of these tumors is difficult to assess on histological grounds. The proportion of malignant lesions in adults is 10% [3, 28], but is even less in children. CT compares favorably with angiography in the localization of pheochromocytomas in most adult series and has now replaced angiography as the initial investigation [15, 26, 35, 41, 60, 66].

In 1984, Farrelly et al. [19] documented our experience at the Hospital for Sick Children, Toronto, with the radiological localization of nine pheochromocytomas in five children. Eight of the nine lesions were studied with CT [19]. In our group, there were four males and one female. The initial age at presentation ranged from 8–13 years. The two patients with multiple tumors presented with second lesions 1 and 6 years respectively after their primary tumors were diagnosed. Six of the nine lesions were adrenal in origin (three in right adrenal, three in left adrenal). Of the three extra-adrenal tumors, two were within the upper abdomen and one in the posterior mediastinum. None of the lesions were palpable clinically. The diameters of the tumors ranged from 1.5 cm to 6.5 cm and all except one were 3 cm or greater in diameter. No patient had metastatic disease. We have subsequently seen a boy with a malignant right adrenal lesion who presented with metastatic disease to a thoracic vertebra and lung and with local infiltration into the retroperitoneum.

Plain radiographs of the abdomen in all of our patients revealed no abnormality. A soft tissue mass in the posterior mediastinum was visible in the single patient with a primary intrathoracic pheochromocytoma. Intravenous pyelography with nephrotomography identified tumors in all four patients with adrenal lesions at initial presentation. These lesions were all over 3 cm in diameter. This investigation failed to detect both

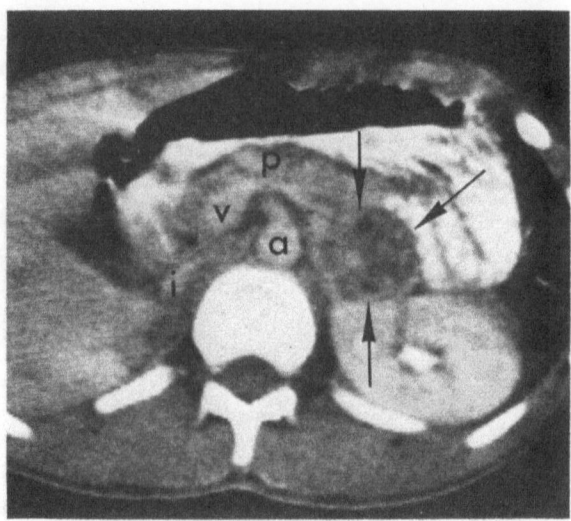

Fig. 10.10. A 17-year-old boy with left adrenal pheochromocytoma. CT shows mass (*arrows*) anterior to upper pole of left kidney. The attenuation of the mass is inhomogeneous, and the anterior surface of the kidney is somewhat flattened. *a*, aorta at origin of superior mesenteric artery; *i*, inferior vena cava; *v*, portal vein; *p*, pancreas. (Farrelly et al. 1984 [19])

extra-adrenal and intra-abdominal lesions and was not performed at the time of the recurrent lesions. The appearances of pheochromocytomas on CT in our patients were similar to those described in the adult literature (Fig. 10.10). Enhancement is not a characteristic feature but was seen in three of our original eight lesions. Rim enhancement was seen in one of our more recent patients and has been reported by other authors. Areas of decreased density within the lesion represent necrosis and hemorrhage. Calcification is rare.

Very few other pediatric patients with pheochromocytoma have been investigated with CT. When we combine the 10 tumors in our experience and the only other 6 tumors examined by CT in the pediatric literature [28, 60, 61], successful localization was achieved in 13 (81%) of these 16 lesions. False negative results appear to be due to examinations on old scanners with long scan time.

Most pheochromocytomas are 2 cm or greater in diameter at the time of presentation [19, 57]. With use of fast scan times and meticulous attention to technique (especially with regard to adequate opacification of the bowel with water-soluble contrast material and opacification of the vasculature by performing scans during the intravenous injection of contrast), detection of these lesions should be relatively easy even in children where there is a paucity of retroperitoneal fat.

Excretory urography with nephrotomography is thus only useful in adrenal lesions. Sonography may be useful in detecting lesions in the adrenals and upper abdomen but is generally limited by bowel gas in the lower abdomen. These modalities are therefore not essential prior to the performance of CT of the whole abdomen and pelvis in the search for multiple lesions. Angiography did detect the small 1.5-cm diameter lesion in our series that was missed on our older 2-min CT machine. It failed, however, to detect two lesions that were diagnosed easily on CT. Therefore, we do not rely on angiography as heavily as we did previously. This avoids an invasive procedure, which also has the added complication of contrast-induced hypertensive episodes in these patients. Arteriography may be useful to define important vascular relationships, particularly with lesions adjacent to the renal arteries [19].

Pheochromocytomas may occur in the sympathetic ganglia from the neck down to the sacrum as well as in the adrenals [8, 19, 28, 59]. Most extra-adrenal lesions occur in the upper abdomen [19]. It is therefore our policy to perform CT of the abdomen and pelvis as the initial investigation in patients suspected of having a pheochromocytoma. Adjacent scans of 1 cm in thickness are performed from the level of the xiphisternum down to the pubic symphysis. If the adrenals are not well visualized, 5-mm scans through the adrenal areas should then be done. The entire abdomen and pelvis should be scanned in the search for multiple lesions. Although lesions in the pelvis are rare [28], we believe that this area should be included in the examination.

Pheochromocytomas of the chest are uncommon (see Fig. 4.27, p. 48), and routine chest CT is not performed unless a lesion is suspected on a chest radiograph or the abdominal and pelvic CT reveals no lesion but there is still strong clinical and biochemical evidence of pheochromocytoma. We feel that it is prudent to perform chest CT in the latter situation, although we are not aware of the diagnosis of pheochromocytoma having been made on CT in the presence of a negative chest radiograph. In the rare instances of malignant abdominal pheochromocytoma, chest CT is of value in determining the presence or absence of metastatic disease in the lungs [60].

Adrenocortical Neoplasms

Adrenocortical neoplasms have been reported at all ages [24, 25, 30]. The mean age of occurrence is 38 years in males and 28 years in females [34]. Adrenocortical lesions are rare in the pediatric age and account for only 0.3% of all neoplasms at the Hospital for Sick Children, Toronto [10]. They are much less common than neuroblastoma but slightly more common than pheochromocytoma.

The clinical and endocrine findings of the 17 patients (13 carcinomas, 4 adenomas) that were reported from our institution by Daneman et al. in 1983 [11] are similar to those reported in previous series [65]. Carcinoma is much more common than adenoma, the ratio being 3:1 [27, 58, 65]. There was an overall female preponderance (10 F, 3 M) in the carcinoma group, and all four patients with adenoma were female [11]. The mean age of presentation for the carcinoma group was approximately 6 years and for the adenoma group 3 years.

Children with adrenocortical neoplasms usually have functioning tumors, the clinical presentation being indistinguishable from isosexual or heterosexual precocious puberty resulting from adrenal hyperplasia or from nonadrenal causes. Even with time-consuming and sophisticated hormonal investigations laboratory data in these patients are often inconclusive. Thus there is often a delay from the onset of symptoms and signs to the time of final diagnosis [27, 58, 65]. Benign and malignant disease cannot be differentiated on the basis of the endocrine status of the child either clinically or by hormonal tests.

Androgenic effects such as virilization in girls and pseudoprecocious puberty in boys constitute by far the commonest type of endocrine syndrome seen in patients with adrenocortical neoplasms and were in fact found in all patients in our series. Cushing's syndrome, feminization, and hyperaldosteronism are much less common [7, 21, 27, 58, 65]. Some of the children in our series had mixed syndromes — a feature of adrenal neoplasms as opposed to hyperplasia, which usually produces pure syndromes [27, 58]. Nonfunctioning adrenocortical tumors are extremely rare in childhood [23, 58]. The presence of local abdominal symptoms and signs such as abdominal mass and pain are more common in patients with carcinoma. Adrenocortical neoplasms have been reported in association with hemihypertrophy, brain tumors, and hamartomatous lesions [20], but none of these features were noted in our group of patients.

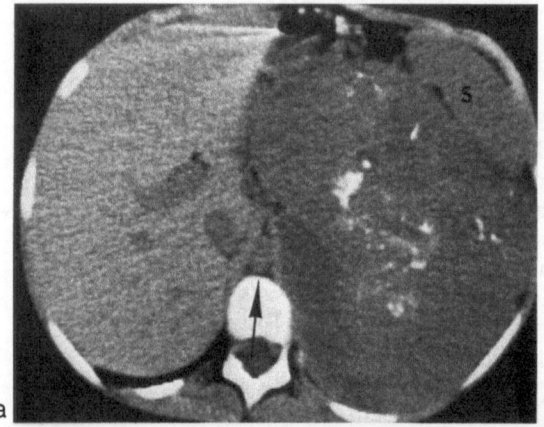

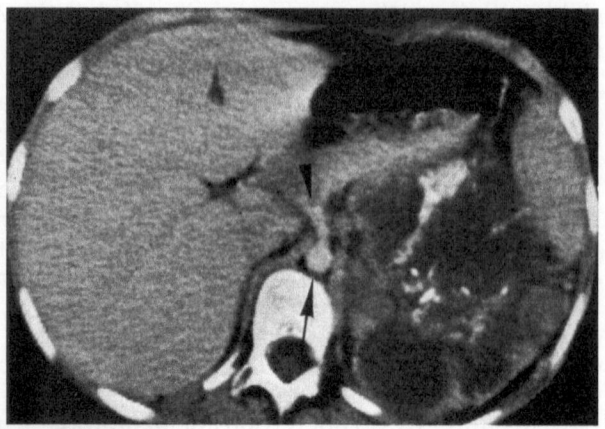

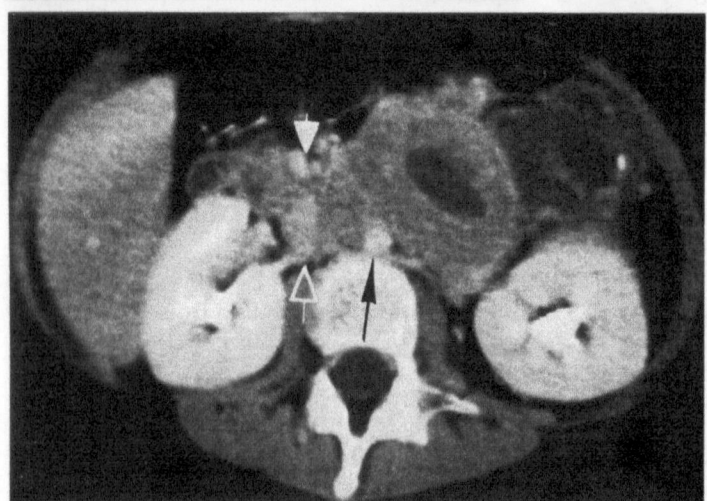

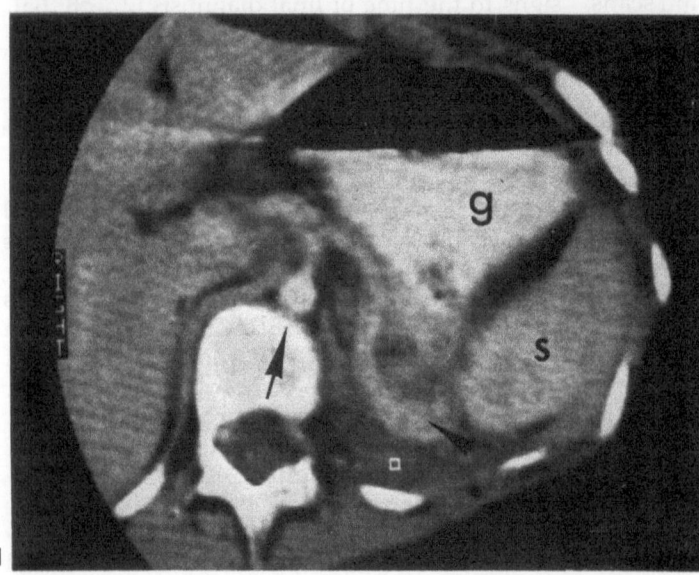

Fig. 10.11a–d. An 11½-year-old girl with a left adrenal carcinoma measuring 16 × 10 cm × 9 cm in diameter. **a** Abdominal CT performed prior to the injection of intravenous contrast. Large left adrenal mass with calcification displacing the aorta to the midline (*arrow*) and the spleen (*s*) anteriorly. **b,c** Abdominal CT performed following chemotherapy and radiotherapy. Scans have been performed during the intravenous injection of contrast material. The mass is much smaller with a more inhomogeneous density because of areas of necrosis, and more calcification is evident. The major vessels of the abdomen are clearly delineated by the scans performed during intravenous contrast enhancement. *Black arrow*, aorta; *closed white arrow*, superior mesenteric artery and vein; *open white arrow*, inferior vena cava; *black arrowhead*, celiac axis. **d** Abdominal CT performed during the injection of intravenous contrast following surgical removal of the carcinoma. The *square cursor* indicates the scar tissue in the adrenal bed. *Arrow*, aorta; *arrowhead*, splenic vein; *s*, spleen; *g*, stomach. (Daneman et al. 1983 [11])

Fig. 10.12a–c. A 2½-year-old girl with a right adrenal adenoma measuring 3 × 1.5 cm in diameter. Abdominal CT scans performed after intravenous contrast enhancement. **a** A well-defined, homogeneous mass in anterior part of right adrenal. Posterior limb of right adrenal mass remains intact (*arrow*). **b,c** Lower scans show relationship of mass to upper part of right kidney. "Claw" (*arrows*) of renal tissue suggests mass may be intrarenal or invading the kidney. Identical appearances have been seen with small adrenal carcinomas. (Daneman et al. 1983 [11].)

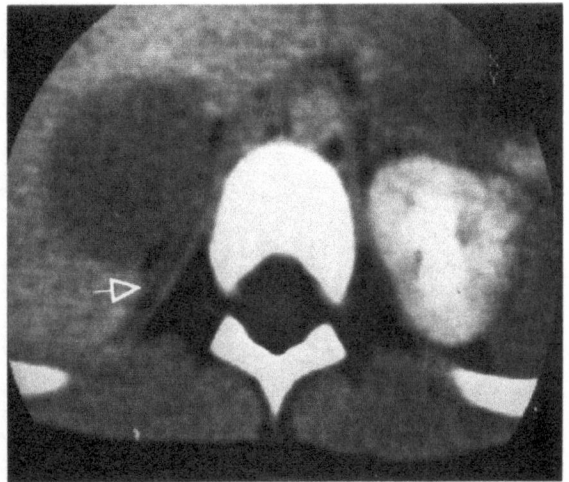
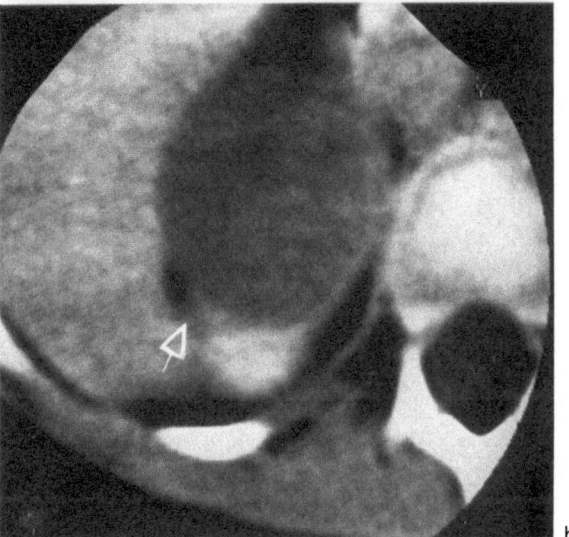
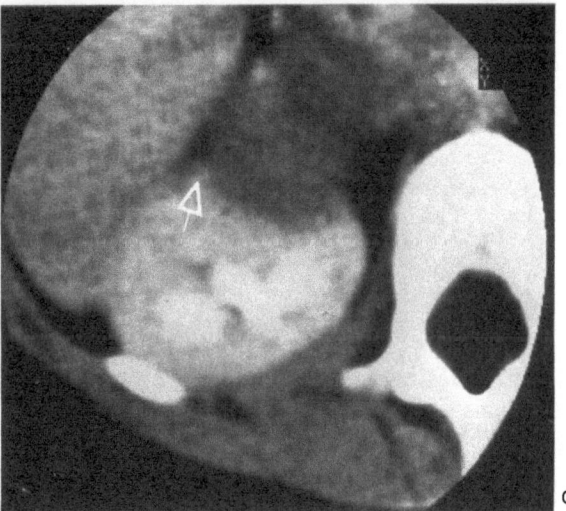

Differentiation of benign from malignant lesions is difficult with all imaging modalities. On plain abdominal radiographs the visualization of a soft tissue mass is much more common with carcinomas. Calcification is seen more commonly in carcinomas [11, 38] and is not related to the size of the tumor.

On excretory urography the ipsilateral kidney may appear normal (five of our patients) or show subtle or gross displacement of the upper pole depending on the size of the adrenal lesion [34, 38, 58]. Nonfunction of the kidney caused by invasion of the kidney by a carcinoma was the only sign suggesting malignancy in our series and was noted in only one of our patients.

Eight of our patients had preoperative abdominal CT, and, of these, three had preoperative sonographic examinations as well. Sonography and CT were equally successful in defining the extent of the primary and excluding metastatic disease in the three patients with large carcinomas (largest diameter 16 cm, smallest 8 cm) who were examined with both modalities. These lesions had an inhomogeneous attenuation on CT and a complex echo pattern on sonography, reflecting the areas of hemorrhage and necrosis seen macroscopically in these large carcinomas (Fig. 10.11; see also Fig. 16.1, p. 250).

In the four patients with smaller lesions (two carcinomas, two adenomas; largest diameter 6 cm, smallest 1.5 cm), CT revealed the presence of smaller adrenal masses with more homogeneous attenuation but could not differentiate benign from malignant disease (Fig. 10.12). On CT the relationship of the lesion to the upper pole of the kidney in one patient with a carcinoma and one patient with an adenoma made it difficult to differentiate whether the lesion was intrarenal or invading the kidney rather than being totally extrarenal. Although none of these smaller lesions were studied with sonography, we believe they would have been detected with this modality, and longitudinal scans might have resolved the problem of questionable renal invasion.

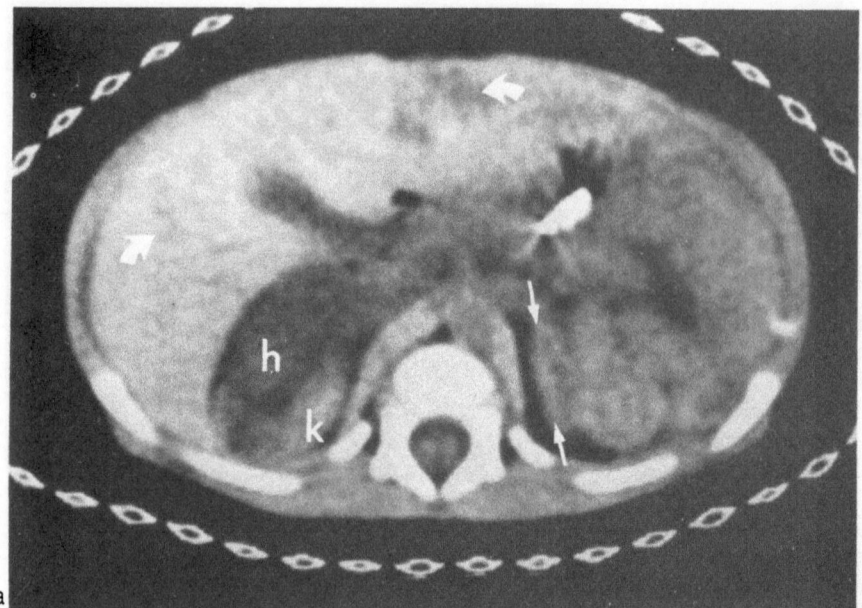

a

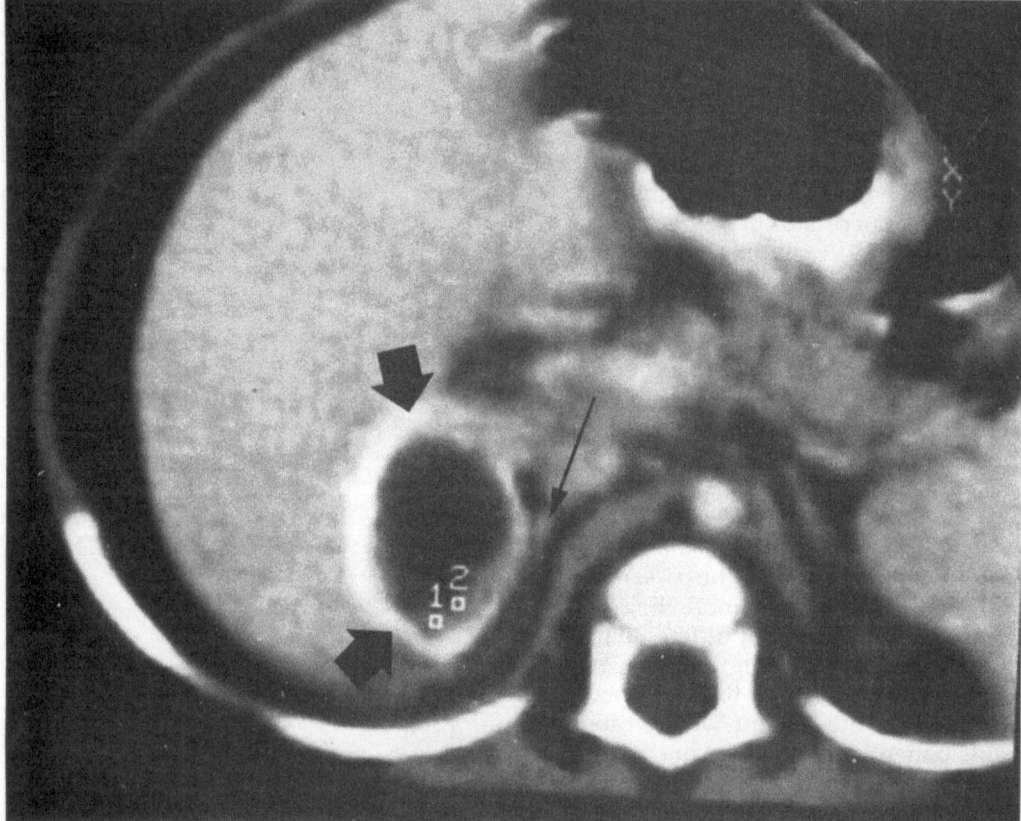

b

Fig. 10.13a. Right adrenal hemorrhage (*h*) in a neonate with history of birth asphyxia. *k,* upper pole of right kidney; *arrows,* normal left adrenal. Note low-attenuation areas in liver (*curved arrows*) caused by ischemic necrosis. **b** Follow-up CT of infant with right adrenal hemorrhage during the neonatal period. The old hemorrhage (*arrows*) has a typical rim of calcification around the periphery. The remaining unaffected medial limb (*long arrow*) of the right adrenal can be faintly seen lying between the hemorrhage in the lateral limb and the crus of the diaphragm. Occasionally adrenal hemorrhage is limited to only a segment of the gland.

The clinical presentation of children with adrenocortical neoplasms is thus nonspecific. Prompt localization of the primary lesion to the adrenal will diminish the delay from the time of presentation to the time of final diagnosis and hopefully ensure a better survival rate [27, 65]. The smallest lesion in our series had an average diameter of approximately 2 cm and was easily seen on CT. The relative lack of retroperitoneal fat in children may make the detection of smaller lesions on CT more difficult than in adults. Adrenal carcinoma is a highly malignant and locally invasive tumor, extensive local invasion being present in just over 50% of the carcinomas in our series. Since the only curative treatment is complete surgical removal, the exact extent of the lesion should be accurately defined preoperatively.

We believe that any child presenting with endocrine symptoms or laboratory findings suggesting an adrenocortical neoplasm should have a CT performed after the oral ingestion of Gastrografin and during intravenous contrast enhancement [11]. This study should accurately define the site and extent of the primary lesion and display the relationship of the mass to the great vessels of the abdomen as well as revealing the presence of metastatic disease in the lymph nodes, liver, or extension into the inferior vena cava. If a lesion is in fact found in an adrenal in this study, a CT scan of the lungs is mandatory. Routine sequential postoperative CT of the adrenal bed and chest are imperative for accurate follow-up.

Angiography, adrenal venography and venous sampling, and radioactive ^{131}I iodocholesterol scans may be reserved for those rare patients in whom the CT has not been helpful [22]. Angiography is also useful in providing a preoperative "road map" for surgeons in children with very large carcinomas.

Miscellaneous

Adrenal Hemorrhage

Adrenal hemorrhage is most commonly seen in asphyxiated neonates. The hematoma, which may be bilateral, is easily visualized on CT (Fig. 10.13). However, sonography is the modality of choice in the initial diagnosis of neonates suspected of having adrenal hemorrhage and in their follow-up. The characteristic progression of sonographic changes in the presence of normal urinary vanillylmandelic acid levels is useful in confirming the diagnosis. Occasionally the hematoma may involve only a segment or one limb of the gland, the remainder of the gland appearing normal on CT in this situation (Fig. 10.13b). On follow-up scans rim calcification may become visible as the hematoma resolves (Fig. 10.13b).

We have also had the opportunity to scan a child who had an adrenal hemorrhage following adrenal venography. The hematoma appeared to have a high attenuation on CT because of the presence of both blood and extravasated contrast material.

Adrenal Calcification

Adrenal calcification is easily detected on CT and the causes for this have been well documented in the past. In 1983, Hill et al. [29] reported the appearances of the adrenals in two young children with acid lipase deficiency. This entity leads to an abnormal accumulation of cholesterol esters and triglycerides in many tissues and is manifested in two forms: Wolman's disease, which is usually fatal in infancy, and cholesterol ester storage disease, which is clinically milder. In a 38-month-old boy with Wolman's disease, CT showed an enlarged liver with diminished attenuation and enlarged adrenals with cortical calcification. In the 13-month-old girl with cholesterol ester storage disease the liver was enlarged but its attenuation appeared normal and the adrenals showed no abnormality.

References

1. Abrams HL, Siegelman SS, Adams DF, Sanders R, Fingerg JH, Hessel SJ, McNeil BJ (1982) Computed tomography versus ultrasound of the adrenal gland: a prospective study. Radiology 143:121–128
2. Altman AJ, Baehner RL (1976) Favourable prognosis for survival in children with coincident opsomyoclonus and neuroblastoma. Cancer 37:846–852
3. Altman AJ, Schwartz AD (1983) Tumors of the sympathetic nervous system. In: Malignant diseases of infancy, childhood and adolescence. Saunders, Philadelphia, pp 368–388
4. Armstrong EA, Harwood-Nash DCF, Fitz CR, Chuang SH, Pettersson H, Martin DJ (1981) CT of neuroblastomas and ganglioneuromas in children. AJR 139:571–576
5. Berg BO, Ablin AR, Wang W, Skoglund R (1976) Encephalopathy associated with occult neuroblastoma. J Neurosurg 41:567–572

6. Berger PE, Kuhn JP, Munschauer RW (1978) Computed tomography and ultrasound in the diagnosis and management of neuroblastoma. Radiology 128:663–667

7. Bhettay E, Connici F (1977) Pure oestrogen-secreting feminizing adrenocortical adenoma. Arch Dis Child 52(3):241–243

8. Brasch RC, Gooding CA (1980) Extracranial computed tomography in children: initial clinical experience and radiation dose considerations. Prog Pediatr Radiol 7:100

9. Bray PF, Ziter FA, Lahey ME, Myers CG (1969) The coincidence of neuroblastoma and acute cerebellar encephalopathy. J Pediatr 75:983–990

10. Chan HSL (1982) Carcinoma of the adrenal gland in children. In: Humphrey GB, Dehner LP (eds) Pediatric oncology, vol II. Martinus Nijhoff, The Hague, p 370

11. Daneman A, Chan HSL, Martin DJ (1983) Adrenal carcinoma and adenoma in children: a review of 17 patients. Pediatr Radiol 13:11–18

12. Davidson M, Tolentino V, Sapir S (1968) Opsoclonus and neuroblastoma (letter). N Engl J Med 279:948

13. Dunnick NR, Schaner EG, Coppman JL, Strott CA, Gill JR, Nassar Javadpour (1979) Computed tomography in adrenal tumors. AJR 131:43–46

14. Dunnick NR, Doppman JL, Gill JR, Strott CA, Keiser HR, Brennan MF (1982) Localization of functional adrenal tumors by computed tomography and venous sampling. Radiology 142:429–433

15. Eghari M, McLoughlin MK, Rosen IE, St. Louis EL, Wilson SR, Wise DJ, Yeung HPH (1980) The role of computed tomography in assessment of tumoral pathology of the adrenal glands. J Comput Assist Tomogr 41(1):71–77

16. Ellenberger C Jr, Campa JF, Netsky MG (1968) Opsoclonus and parenchymatous degeneration of the cerebellum. Neurology (NY) 18:1041–1046

17. Evans AE, D'Angio GJ, Randolph J (1971) A proposed staging for children with neuroblastoma. Cancer 27:374–378

18. Farrelly C, Daneman A, Chan HSL, Martin DJ (1984) Occult neuroblastoma presenting with opsomyoclonus: utility of computed tomography. AJR 142:807–810

19. Farrelly C, Daneman A, Martin DJ, Chan HSL (1984) Pheochromocytoma in childhood: the important role of computed tomography in tumour localization. Pediatr Radiol 14:210–214

20. Fraumeni JF Jr, Miller RW (1967) Adrenocortical neoplasms with hemihypertrophy, brain tumors, and other disorders. J Pediatr 70(1):129–138

21. Ganguly A, Bergstein J, Grim CE, Yum MN, Weinberger MH (1980) Childhood primary aldosteronism due to an adrenal adenoma. Pediatrics 65(3):605–609

22. Gross MD, Freitas JE, Swanson DP, Woodbury MC, Schteingart DE, Bierwaltes WH (1981) Dexamethasone-suppression adrenal scintigraphy in hyperandrogenism: concise communication. J Nucl Med 22(1):12–17

23. Gyepes MT, Lindstrom R, Merten D, Goller D, Lachman R, Lippe B (1976) Hormonally active adrenal adenomas and carcinomas in children. Ann Radiol 20(1):123–131

24. Hajjar RA, Hickey RC, Samaan NA (1975) Adrenal cortical carcinoma: a study of 32 patients. Cancer 35:549–554

25. Harrison JH, Mahoney EM, Bennett AH (1973) Tumors of the adrenal cortex. Cancer 32:1227–1235

26. Hattery RR, Sheedy II PF, Stephens DH, Van Heerden JA (1981) Computed tomography of the adrenal gland. Semin Roentgenol XVI(4):290–300

27. Hayles AB, Hahn HB Jr, Sprague RG, Bahn RC, Priestley JT (1966) Hormone-secreting tumors of the adrenal cortex in children. Pediatrics 37(1):19–25

28. Hecht ST, Brasch RC, Styne DM (1982) CT localization of occult secretory tumours in children. Pediatr Radiol 12:67–71

29. Hill SC, Hoeg JM, Dwyer AJ, Vucich JJ, Doppman JL (1983) CT findings in acid lipase deficiency: Wolman disease and cholesterol ester storage disease. J Comput Assist Tomogr 7(5):815–818

30. Karstaedt N, Sagel SS, Stanley RJ, Melson GL, Levitt RG (1978) Computed tomography of the adrenal gland. Radiology 129:723–730

31. Keating JW, Cromwell LD (1978) Remote effects of neuroblastoma. AJR 131: 299–303

32. Kenney PJ, Siegel MJ, McAlister WH (1982) Congenital intraspinal neuroblastoma: a treatable simulant of myelodysplasia. AJR 138:166–167

33. Kinast M, Levin HS, Rothner DA, Erenberg G, Wacksman J, Judge J (1980) Cerebellar ataxia, opsoclonus and occult neural crest tumour. Am J Dis Child 134:1057–1059

34. King DR, Lack EE (1979) Adrenal cortical carcinoma. Cancer 34:239–244

35. Kinkhabwala MN, Conradi H (1972) Angiography of extra-adrenal pheochromocytomas. J Urol 108:666

36. Kinsbourne M (1962) Myoclonic encephalopathy of infants. J Neurosurg Psychiatry 25:271–276

37. Koop CE, Johnson DG (1971) Neuroblastoma: an assessment of therapy in reference to staging. J Pediatr Surg 6:595–600

38. Korobkin M, White EA, Kressel HY, Moss AA, Montagne JP (1979) Computed tomography in the diagnosis of adrenal disease. AJR 132:231–238

39. Korobkin M, Clark RE, Palubinskas AJ (1972) Occult neuroblastoma and acute cellular ataxia in childhood. Radiology 102:151–152

40. Kuhns LR (1981) Computed tomography of the retroperitoneum in children. Radiol Clin North Am 19(3):495–501

41. Laursen K, Damgaard-Pedersen K (1980) CT for pheochromocytoma diagnosis. AJR 134:277

42. Leonidas JC, Brill CB, Aron AM (1972) Neuroblastoma presenting with myoclonic encephalopathy. Radiology 102:87–88

43. Martin LS, Griffith JR (1971) Myoclonic encephalopathy and neuroblastoma. Am J Dis Child 122:257–258

44. Moe PG, Nellhaus G (1970) Infantile polymyoclonia-opsoclonus syndrome and neural crest tumours. Neurology (NY) 20:756–764

45. Orzechowski C (1927) De l'ataxie dysmetrique des yeux:remarques sur l'ataxie des yeux dite myoclonique (opsoclonie, opsochorie). J Psychol Neurol 35:1–18

46. Pettersson H, Harwood-Nash DCF (1982) Neoplasms. In: CT and myelography of the spine and cord. Springer, Berlin Heidelberg New York, pp 59–72

47. Reynes CJ, Churchill R, Moncada R, Love L (1979) Computed tomography of adrenal glands. Radiol Clin North Am XVII(1):91–104

48. Roberts KB, Freeman JM (1975) Cerebellar ataxia and "occult neuroblastoma" without opsomyoclonus. Pediatrics 56:464–465

49. Sample WF, Sart DA (1978) Computed tomography and gray scale ultrasonography of the adrenal gland: a comparative study. Radiology 128:377–383

50. Sandok BA, Kranz H (1971) Opsoclonus as the initial manifestation of occult neuroblastoma. Arch Ophthalmol 86:235–236

51. Senelik RC, Bray PF, Lahey E, Van Dyk HJL, Johnson DG (1973) Neuroblastoma and myoclonic encephalopathy: two cases and a review of the literature. J Pediatr Surg 8:623–632

52. Siegel MJ, Sagel SS (1982) Computed tomography as a supplement to urography in evaluation of suspected neuroblastoma. Radiology 142:435–438
53. Solomon A, Kreel L (1980) Computed tomographic assessment of adrenal masses. Clin Radiol 31(2):137–141
54. Solomon GE, Chutorian AM (1968) Opsoclonus and occult neuroblastoma. N Engl J Med 279:475–477
55. Stark DD, Moss AA, Brasch RC, de Lorimier AA, Albin AR, London DA, Gooding CA (1983) Neuroblastoma: diagnostic imaging and staging. Radiology 148:101–105
56. Stark DD, Moss AA, Brasch RC, de Lorimier AA, Albin AR, London DA, Gooding CA (1983) Recurrent neuroblastoma: the role of CT and alternative imaging tests. Radiology 148:107–112
57. Stewart BH, Bravo EL, Haaga J, Meaney TF, Tarazi R (1978) Localization of pheochromocytoma by computed tomography. N Engl J Med 299:460–461
58. Stewart DR, Morris Jones PH, Jolleys A (1974) Carcinoma of the adrenal gland in children. J Pediatr Surg (91):59–67
59. Stringel G, Ein SH, Creighton R, Daneman D, Howard N, Filler RM (1980) Pheochromocytoma in children — an update. J Pediatr Surg 4:496–500
60. Thomas JL, Bernardino ME, Samaan NA, Hickey RC (1980) CT of pheochromocytoma. AJR 135:477–482
61. Tisnado J, Amendola MA, Karsten FK, Shirazi KK, Beachley MC (1980) Computed tomography versus angiography in the localization of pheochromocytoma. J Comput Assist Tomogr 6:853–859
62. Towbin R, Gruppo RA (1982) Pulmonary metastases in neuroblastoma. AJR 138:75–78
63. Williams TH, House RF Jr, Burgert EO Jr, Lynn HB (1972) Unusual manifestations of neuroblastoma: chronic diarrhea, polymyoclonia-opsoclonus and erythrocyte abnormalities. Cancer 29:475–480
64. Yeh HC (1980) Sonography of the adrenal glands; normal glands and small masses. AJR 135:1167–1177
65. Zaitoon MM, Mackie GG (1978) Adrenal cortical tumours in children. Urology 12(6):645–649
66. Zelch JV, Meaney TF, Belhobek GH (1974) Radiologic approach to the patient with suspected pheochromocytoma. Radiology 111:279–284
67. Ziter FA, Bray PF, Cancilla PA (1979) Neuropathological findings in a patient with neuroblastoma and myoclonic encephalopathy. Arch Neurol 36:51–53

Chapter 11
Kidneys

Introduction

Radiographic visualization of the urinary tract has been feasible for many years by means of various urographic techniques such as excretory urography, nephrotomography, retrograde and antegrade urography, cystography, and radionuclide scans. Despite this, the introduction of sonography and CT has added a new dimension to the delineation of the detailed, normal anatomy and pathology of the urinary tract. Both of these techniques have enabled the radiologist to visualize all surfaces of the kidney and the renal parenchyma more fully and to delineate the relationship of the kidney to the surrounding peri- and pararenal spaces and retroperitoneal structures with much greater ease. In contrast to excretory urography and radionuclide renal scans, sonography and CT are capable of defining detailed renal anatomy independent of renal function. These two modalities are thus useful in the investigation of patients in renal failure and in those with contrast media sensitivity. The increased spatial and contrast resolution of CT has added greater accuracy to the delineation of small parenchymal lesions and to the detection of small areas of calcification in the renal parenchyma and collecting system. The introduction of sonography and CT has helped the clinician and radiologist to rely less on more invasive techniques such as angiography.

Indications

In many clinical situations in pediatrics, sonography has come to replace excretory urography as an initial imaging modality [1]. Such situations include the investigation of patients with abdominal pain, an abdominal mass, or urinary tract infection. In many children, modalities such as sonography, renal scintigraphy, or excretory urography serve as the definitive procedure; however, in some children, CT is required to delineate the urinary tract in further detail. Renal CT is usually used following these less expensive and less invasive procedures.

We have found that CT is more accurate than sonography and excretory urography in determining whether an abdominal mass is intra- or extrarenal and is the most accurate modality in defining the exact site, size, and extent of renal neoplasia [7, 35]. We have thus used CT to assess the abdomen in all children with renal neoplasia at the time of initial presentation and in follow-up. CT has also proven more accurate than excretory urography and sonography in defining small parenchymal lesions such as multiple, small bilateral Wilms' tumors and cysts in patients suspected of having renal cystic disease. CT is also the most accurate modality in detecting changes in attenuation within the kidney such as nephrocalcinosis and nephrolithiasis. CT has been used extensively to assess patients with abdominal trauma and has been shown to be extremely accurate in defining small traumatic lesions of the kidney. Occasionally, CT is used to confirm the normality of the urinary tract or to clarify suspicious areas of the kidney noted on previous studies such as sonography or excretory urography.

CT is rarely used to delineate the renal anatomy of children with congenital anomalies of the kidneys or in children with urinary tract infection. However, in occasional patients, the CT examination may supply additional diagnostic information not obtained by other techniques. Patients with transplanted kidneys are usually successfully studied by sonography and renal scintigraphy, and rarely is CT of further use.

Technique

When using CT to examine the kidneys, the technique employed in each individual patient varies depending on the type of information that is required. The study should thus be tailored to suit the needs of each individual patient.

In the majority of patients, scans are only performed after the oral administration of dilute water-soluble contrast material to give adequate opacification of the bowel. A scout computed radiograph is first obtained to localize the position of the kidneys. Two sets of cross-sectional scans are then obtained, one before and one during rapid bolus injection of intravenous contrast material. This is the technique of choice, particularly in children with known or suspected renal neoplasia or trauma. Only a limited number of scans prior to the injection of intravenous contrast are obtained to "map out" roughly the renal areas and their relationship to surrounding viscera, and these scans may be 2 cm apart. The main purpose of these scans is to determine where to perform the scans during rapid intravenous bolus injection of contrast in order that the major vessels of the abdomen and their relationship to normal viscera and pathological lesions may be maximally delineated.

A dose of 2–3 ml/kg of Hypaque 60% (maximum dose 120 ml) is used and is injected as a rapid intravenous bolus during the following set of scans. Injection is made into a large vein in one of the upper extremities as this shows better enhancement of the renal vasculature. Injection into a foot vein will often cause such dense

enhancement of the inferior vena cava that disturbing streak artifacts from cardiac and respiratory motion may be present. Adjacent scans 1 cm thick are then performed through the entire region of interest. Thinner scans may be useful occasionally in infants, or if it is felt that the thicker scans do not reveal sufficient detail of the kidneys in a particular area.

This set of scans usually provides the most valuable information as it is at this time that the true nature of soft tissue masses and visceral relationship can be determined. Meticulous attention to technique with regard to vascular delineation in this manner and also with regard to adequate opacification of the bowel with oral contrast material give the maximum amount of information required to aid in making decisions concerning patient management.

Uncommonly, further delayed scans after the intravenous injection of contrast material may be required to delineate the kidneys in further detail, particularly if there is poor renal function, and also to exclude bowel as the cause of soft tissue masses adjacent to the kidney.

Scans of the lower abdomen and pelvis may occasionally be necessary to visualize the ureters and bladder respectively. These scans can also be done after intravenous contrast has been given, as the delineation of vascular structures is not usually as crucial in the pelvis as it is in the upper abdomen. A scout digital radiograph or abdominal radiograph at the end of the study will display the opacified urinary tract in a similar manner to an excretory urogram. Although this does not usually add further information it may prove pleasing to clinicians.

If the renal CT is being performed in the search for renal calcification only, adjacent slices through the entire length of both kidneys are necessary. Oral and intravenous contrast material are not usually necessary. Occasionally, this type of study may provide all the information that is required in a particular patient. If the relationship between a particular area of calcification and the collecting system is to be determined, further scans after the intravenous injection of contrast material may be helpful. In this situation a smaller dose of contrast may be sufficient (e.g., 1 ml/kg of 60% Hypaque).

Anatomy

The kidneys are easily visualized on CT scans in all children and infants. However, the lack of retroperitoneal fat makes delineation of the renal margins less distinct in smaller children than in adults. Despite this, the entire margins of the kidneys are better delineated than with excretory urography, and the size of the kidneys can be accurately gauged.

Renal density is homogeneous (32–60 HU) on precontrast scans. The calyces are usually not visualized. Areas of the normal collecting system may project into the parenchyma and occasionally may be visualized as small irregular areas of water density, giving the kidney a slight inhomogeneous density. The true nature of these low-density areas will be confirmed on postcontrast scans, when they enhance after contrast enters the collecting system.

In the renal hilum, which is usually directed anteromedially, the pelvis and vascular structures are often visualized in older children; however, because of the lack of fat, they may only be visualized after bolus injection of contrast in younger children and infants. The veins are larger than the arteries and lie more anteriorly.

The physiological principles of contrast material excretion apply to CT as they do to excretory urography. There is a linear relationship between iodine concentration and the CT numbers measured in the kidneys. The par-enchymal CT numbers will thus be dependent on the method of contrast delivery, time after injection, and the renal function. Normal kidneys may enhance to 80–120 HU after intravenous contrast administration. CT allows the most optimal visual evidence of contrast material excretion of the kidneys and thus it is of great use in the assessment of very poorly functioning kidneys, when an extremely small amount of contrast excretion by a thinned parenchymal rim can be visualized.

When contrast material is injected as a single, rapid bolus and scans are performed in rapid sequence, there is a regular pattern of enhancement noted in the renal vessels, parenchyma, and collecting system. The first phase is that of an arteriogram, with opacification of the renal arteries and, slightly later, the veins, in parallel with opacification of the aorta. This is followed by the nephrographic phase, which can be divided into two parts. The first part is that of cortical opacification. The cortex enhances as a regular band (4–6 mm thick) along the periphery of the kidney with extensions into the central portions of the kidney at the columns of Bertin (Fig. 11.1a). The medullary pyramids appear less dense at this time and appear as triangular areas around the central portion of the kidney. The second part of the nephrographic phase is that of a diffuse dense nephrogram as the medullary pyramids become enhanced to the same extent as the cortex. The final phase of enhancement is noted when excretion of contrast occurs into the collecting system. At this time, the density of the

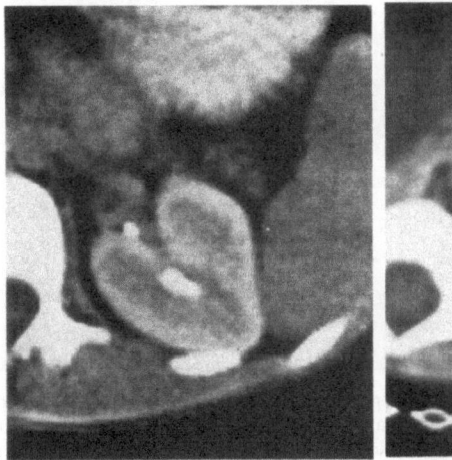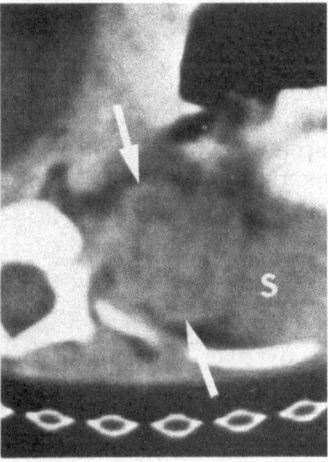

Fig. 11.1. a Normal left kidney in a 10-year-old girl. The cortex has enhanced more markedly than the medulla and appears as a strip of tissue surrounding the medulla. In the anterior aspect of the kidney a column of Bertin crosses the parenchyma. In the central portion of the kidney the area of even higher attenuation is due to concentrated contrast within the collecting system. **b** Normal neonatal kidney (*arrows*). Note the marked fetal lobulation around the periphery of the kidney and the slightly higher attenuation of the cortex. *s*, spleen.

nephrogram may fade and contrast may be noted to be somewhat denser in the medullary rays than in the cortex. When the collecting system is filled with contrast, the detailed anatomy of the calyces is not as well delineated as it is on excretory urography. Often the calyces, pelvis, and ureters appear to be somewhat more distended than they do on an excretory urogram or a scout computed radiograph taken at the end of the examination. Subtle calyceal changes or deformity, or clubbing are better assessed on a urogram than on the cross-sectional CT images.

Normal Variants and Congenital Anomalies

The vast majority of variations of renal shape, rotation, and position can be adequately evaluated with excretory urography and sonography [3, 10, 11, 12, 16, 26, 29, 32, 34, 36]. Occasionally, CT is necessary to confirm the absence of an abnormality when the findings on these other studies are equivocal. Knowledge of the CT appearance of these normal, anatomical variations is essential when attempting to differentiate these appearances from disease processes. However, it is uncommon that CT is the only imaging modality that will provide the necessary information required to make this differentiation.

Occasionally, areas of prominent fetal lobulation (Fig. 11.1b), columns of Bertin, or focal areas of prominent, compensatory, parenchymal hypertrophy (following pyelonephritis or contralateral nephrectomy) may simulate renal mass lesions on sonography or excretory urography. These areas will enhance on CT to the same extent (sometimes greater) as renal parenchyma in contrast to pathological mass lesions. CT may also prove necessary to rule out mass lesions in kidneys that are congenitally of unusual shape and which may be difficult to assess adequately with sonography or excretory urography, for example horseshoe kidney, ectopic pelvic kidneys (Fig. 11.2), crossed-fused ectopia, dysplastic kidneys (Fig. 11.3), and duplex kidneys (Fig. 11.4; see also Fig. 16.2, p.252).

Ectopic kidneys may simulate mass lesions in the abdomen, but their true nature will be recognized after intravenous contrast injection. Enlargement of the liver or spleen may cause displacements of the kidney simulating mass lesions. With renal ectopia or agenesis and fol-

lowing nephrectomy, loops of bowel fill the renal fossa (see Fig. 7.2, p.87, and Fig. 7.3, p.88), together with the pancreatic tail (see Fig. 9.6, p.113) on the left and liver on the right. These structures may simulate renal tissue or recurrent mass lesions if adequate attention is not given to opacification of bowel and vessels. Occasionally, the upper moiety of a duplex kidney may appear as a mass on excretory urography and on precontrast CT scans.

Pathology

Cysts

Sonography is the modality of choice in the investigation of children with known or suspected renal cystic disease [17]. Indeed CT is seldom required in these children. Functional information about the kidneys can be obtained by renal scintigraphy or excretory urography.

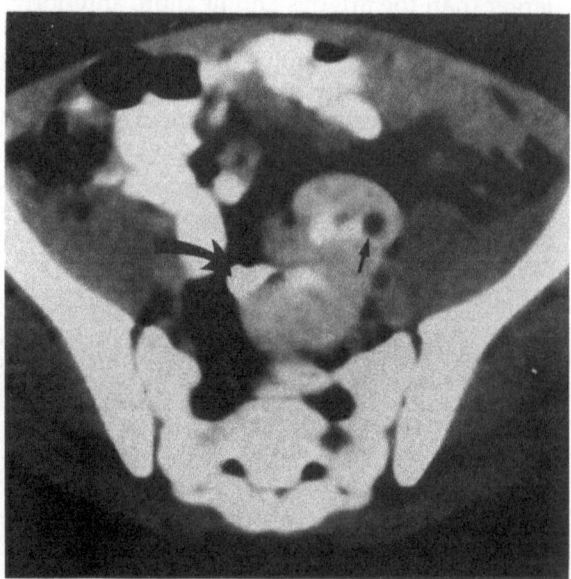

Fig. 11.2. Ectopic pelvic left kidney in an 8-year-old boy with abdominal trauma and hematuria. The kidney lies across the promontory of the sacrum. It has an unusual shape, and the pelvis (*curved arrow*) is minimally distended. A small cyst (*straight arrow*) is noted in the anterior part of the kidney adjacent to one of the calyces. CT was useful in this instance for the exclusion of further underlying renal pathology as sonography could not delineate the detailed anatomy of this kidney because of overlying bowel gas.

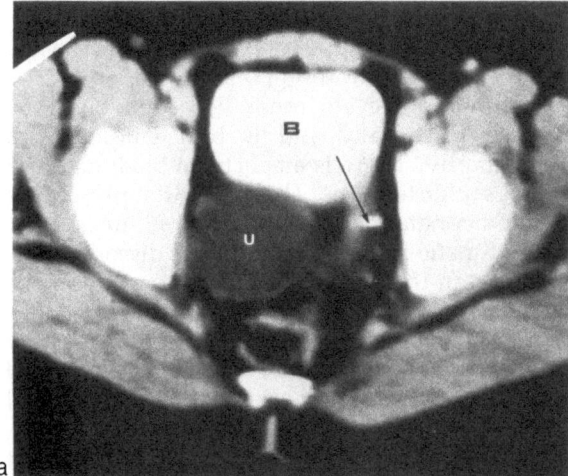

a

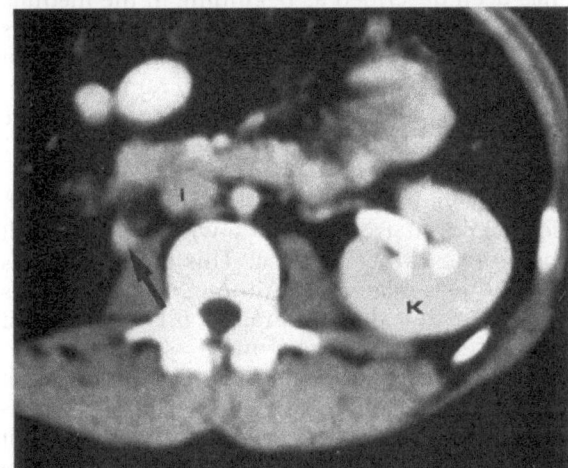

b

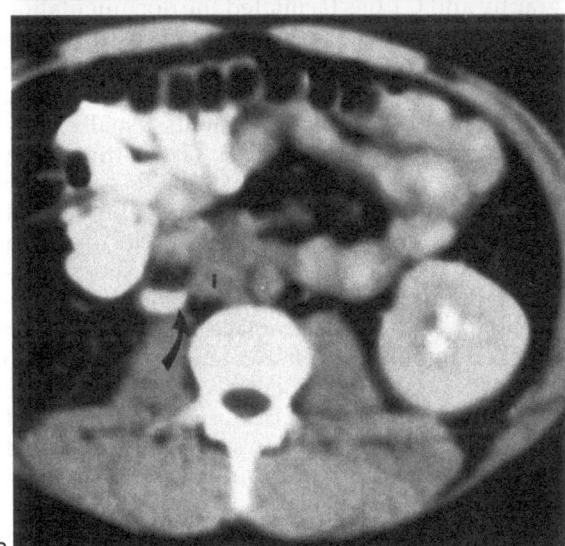

c

Fig. 11.3a–c. A 12-year-old boy with no functioning right kidney noted on renal scan following trauma. CT shows a markedly dilated ureter (*u*) in **a** and an extremely small volume of functioning renal parenchyma (*large arrow*) at the upper end of the ureter in **b**. In scan **c** (between **a** and **b**) contrast which has been excreted by this kidney is noted layering out in the posterior aspect of the dilated ureter (*curved arrow*). Note how sensitive CT is for detecting excretion in a very poorly functioning remnant of renal tissue. The left kidney (*k*) and ureter (*long arrow* in **a**) are normal. *B*, bladder; *i*, inferior vena cava. Diagnosis: atrophic right kidney from chronic obstruction.

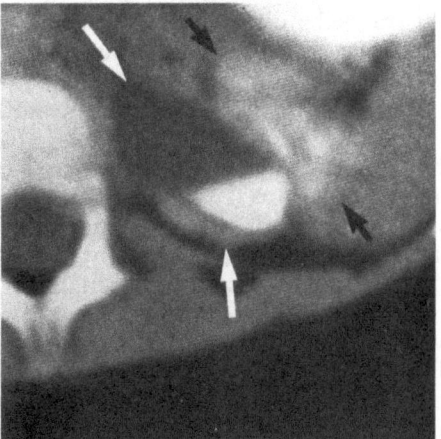

a

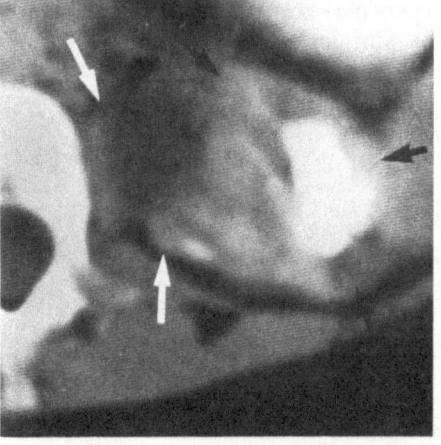

b

Fig. 11.4a,b. A 5-year-old girl with urinary tract infection. Scans **a** and **b** were performed after the injection of intravenous contrast material. A duplex kidney is noted on the left. The upper moiety is marked with the *white arrows* and the lower moiety lying inferolaterally with the *black arrows*. The upper moiety has an extremely thin layer of renal parenchyma, which is seen in scan **a** adjacent to the dilated collecting system draining this moiety. This tissue is functioning, as evidenced by the contrast material which has passed into the ureter and is layering out posteriorly. The lower moiety has a much larger volume of functioning renal parenchyma, although its collecting system is somewhat dilated in scan **b**. This anatomical relationship had been difficult to delineate with sonography and CT offered useful information in this regard.

Simple cysts are extremely uncommon in childhood [20]. These lesions are well marginated, have water attenuation values, and fail to enhance after intravenous contrast administration. We have seen such a renal cyst on CT in a 14-year-old boy with a hepatocellular carcinoma. We have also seen an identical lesion in the cortex of the right kidney of another child with multiple Wilms' tumor in the left kidney. The lesion on the right was associated with an area of nephroblastomatosis. Kuhn and Berger [20] have described a child with a right Wilms' tumor in whom CT showed multiple simple cysts in the left kidney which were confirmed at surgery.

Multicystic dysplastic kidney usually presents in the newborn period as a flank mass and, although it is usually easily evaluated by sonography, it may occasionally be difficult to differentiate from ureteropelvic junction obstruction. CT does not usually add further useful anatomical information, and functional information is readily obtained with renal scintigraphy. On CT, multiple cystic structures are present which replace the renal tissue almost entirely (Fig. 11.5). The cysts vary in size and thin trabeculae separate them. In some areas larger remnants of renal tissue may persist which enhance very poorly. Occasionally, the distribution of the cysts may simulate calyces and a renal pelvis, thus simulating a hydronephrosis, as

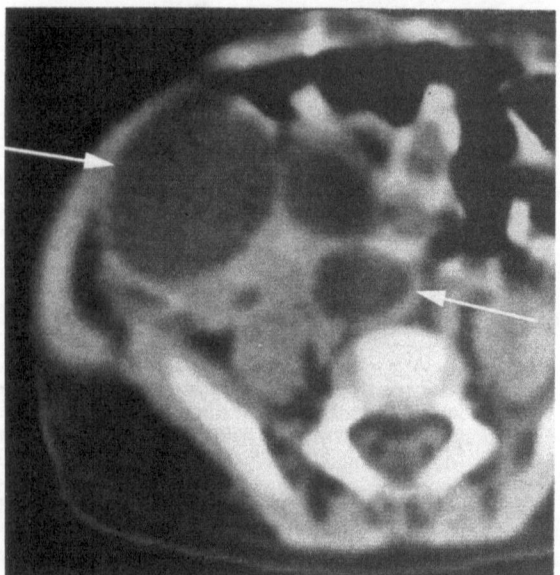

Fig. 11.5. Neonate with right flank mass. CT after intravenous contrast enhancement shows large cysts (*arrows*) replacing the left kidney. This is typical of a multicystic dysplastic kidney. Some solid parenchymal elements are noted in the posterior aspect of this mass.

with sonography. In adults multicystic dysplastic kidney may appear as a shrunken cystic kidney with calcification [27].

Infantile polycystic renal disease involves the kidneys bilaterally and is best studied with sonography. There is a spectrum of clinical and sonographic features. Those children presenting in the neonatal period have large kidneys, poor renal function, and minimal liver disease. Presentation in the later stages of the first decade is associated with less severe renal abnormalities but more prominent hepatic changes caused by fibrosis. In the infant, CT shows marked renal enlargement, prominent fetal lobulation, and prolongation of the cortical phase of enhancement [20]. In the older child, renal involvement has been described as beginning in the medulla and extending to the cortex [20]. Multiple areas of diminished attenuation are noted throughout the kidney. These areas probably represent ectatic tubules. However, the sonographic findings in these children are usually diagnostic, and CT is rarely required.

We have used sonography to screen and follow children from families with known adult polycystic kidney disease. This entity involves the kidneys bilaterally. Although sonography is more sensitive than urography, CT with contrast enhancement is even more sensitive than sonography in documenting the presence of very small cysts. CT shows cysts of varying numbers and sizes depending on the degree of involvement (Fig. 11.6). The advent of sonography and CT has facilitated the documentation and follow-up of this condition in its early phases in the pediatric age group. A similar appearance of multiple cysts may also be seen in tuberous sclerosis, although these patients usually have angiomyolipomas (see p.157). High attenuation values in cysts in adult polycystic disease have been documented [21] and are probably related to cyst hemorrhage. We have not documented this appearance in children. The cysts are distributed randomly throughout the renal parenchyma and may replace almost all the functioning renal parenchyma which is noted to enhance between the cysts. The kidneys are often involved asymmetrically [27]. Involvement of other abdominal organs such as the liver and pancreas may also be present, although rarely in children.

Multilocular cystic nephroma is a localized cystic lesion of the kidney. The lesion contains multiple cystic spaces with thick walls and septations [20, 27]. The lesion is extremely rare in children.

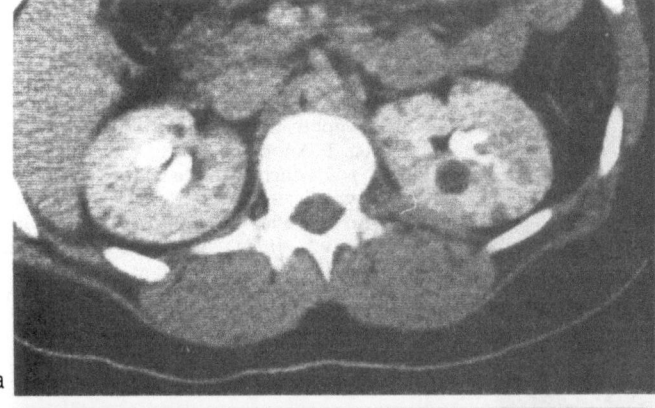

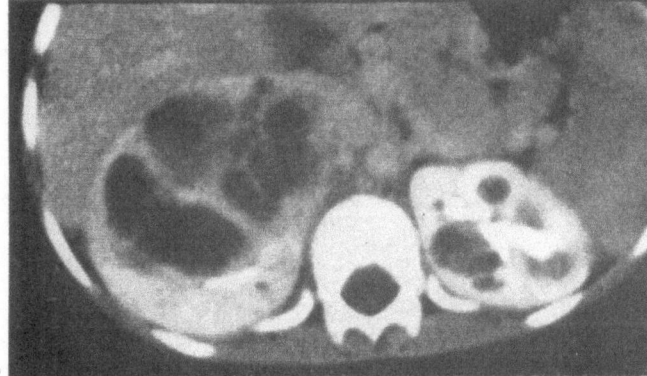

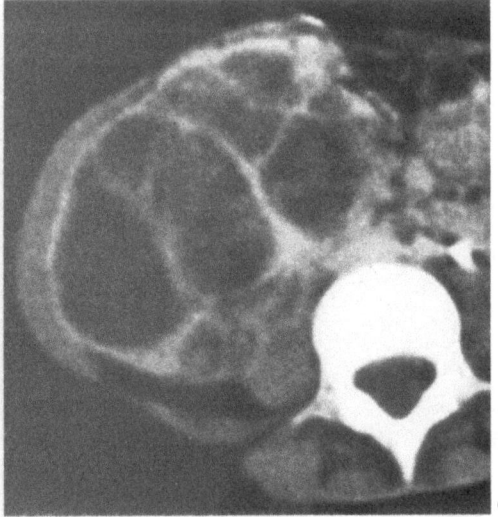

Fig. 11.6a. A 14-year-old boy with adult polycystic disease. The bilateral cysts are represented by round and somewhat irregular areas of low attenuation within the renal parenchyma. **b,c** An 8-year-old girl with more extensive cyst formation in the kidneys caused by adult polycystic disease. Note the replacement and expansion of the lower pole of the right kidney by huge cysts in image **c**.

Renal Vein Thrombosis

Renal vein thrombosis is a condition that typically occurs in the neonatal period in infants who have suffered dehydration or asphyxia. An associated adrenal hemorrhage may also be present. The diagnosis of renal vein thrombosis is best made with sonography. The kidney is enlarged with a disorganized heterogeneous echo pattern.

We have used CT in three neonates with renal vein thrombosis. In all three the kidneys were enlarged and the attenuation pattern was very inhomogeneous in scans without contrast enhancement (Fig. 11.7). Intravenous contrast was not given because of the poor renal function. Diminished renal function, as seen on urography, would be expected. In one patient, calcification of the venous thrombosis was noted on CT in many of the intrarenal veins and extending out into the inferior vena cava. Late changes caused by renal vein thrombosis include renal atrophy. Tumor thrombus in the renal vein and inferior vena cava may be seen with renal tumors such as Wilms' tumor (see Fig. 11.15) and renal cell carcinoma (see Fig. 11.22; see p.167).

Attenuation Changes

Most lesions of the renal parenchyma have a lower attenuation than normal renal parenchyma. Such lesions include cysts (see Figs. 11.5, 11.6), infections (see Figs. 11.9, 11.10), tumors (see Figs. 11.11–11.23), and infarcts.

Nephrocalcinosis and nephrolithiasis are the commonest causes of areas of increased attenuation in the kidney. Renal stones and calcifications are indeed very much less common in children than in adults. We have used sonography as the modality of choice for the detection of small areas of renal calcification (nephrocalcinosis or nephrolithiasis). We have used CT for this purpose when the sonographic findings are equivocal. On CT, stones appear as structures of high attenuation. Scans are best performed without administration of intravenous contrast material, which may obscure small stones. Adjacent scans 0.5 or 1 cm thick should be obtained through the whole length of the kidney. The effects of stones, such as hydronephrosis and urinary extravasation, are easily documented by CT.

We have had the opportunity to study three

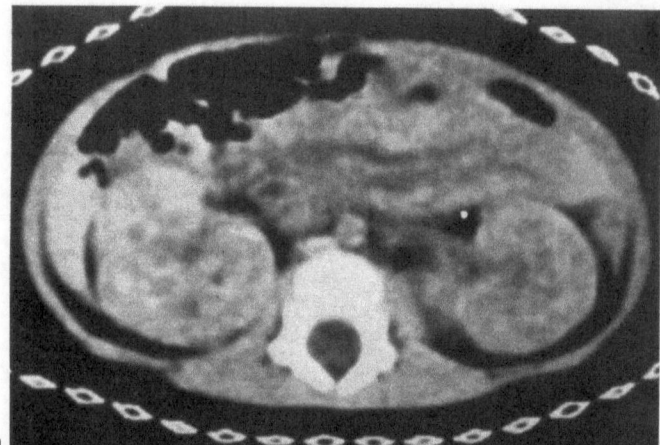

a

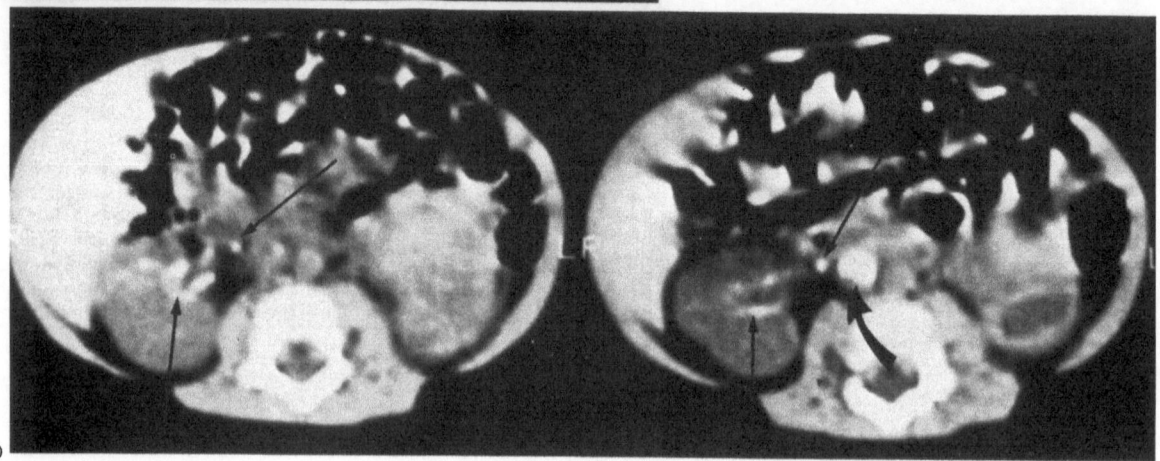

b

Fig. 11.7a. Asphyxiated neonate with hematuria. Scan performed without contrast enhancement shows enlargement of both kidneys. The attenuation of the kidneys is inhomogeneous. The findings were felt to be related to renal venous thrombosis associated with the asphyxia. **b** Another neonate with renal vein thrombosis which extended into the inferior vena cava. Scans without contrast enhancement show calcified thrombosis in inferior vena cava (*curved arrow*). Note the calcification extending into the right kidney caused by calcification in the renal vein and intrarenal veins (*long arrows*).

patients who showed unusual increased attenuation of the kidney. In one, an 11-year-old girl with leukemia, calcifications were noted filling the collecting systems, simulating the appearance seen after intravenous contrast administration (Fig. 11.8a). In two others with thalassemia major, areas of increased attenuation were noted within the renal parenchyma (Fig. 11.8b). Although not proven pathologically, we feel that this represents iron deposition from chronic blood transfusion programs.

Inflammation

In the past, excretory urography and, more recently, sonography have been the modalities of choice in children with known or suspected renal inflammatory disease. The vast majority of children with acute or chronic inflammatory dis-

ease of the kidneys will never come to CT. However, CT is useful when changes on other modalities are equivocal and further information is required for correct management, and also when perirenal disease is suspected. In this latter regard we have found that CT is more sensitive than sonography.

Areas of acute inflammation within the kidney usually have a lower attenuation than the normal renal parenchyma and may simulate a mass with ill-defined margins (Fig. 11.9). Following intravenous contrast injection the affected parenchyma may show patchy or striated inhomogeneous enhancement or may fail to enhance. Perinephric fluid collections (Fig. 11.9) and retroperitoneal inflammatory changes (Fig. 11.10) may also be present. The margin of the kidney may be ill defined adjacent to these retroperitoneal changes, and swelling and increased enhancement caused by inflammation may be present in the adjacent muscles (Fig. 11.10).

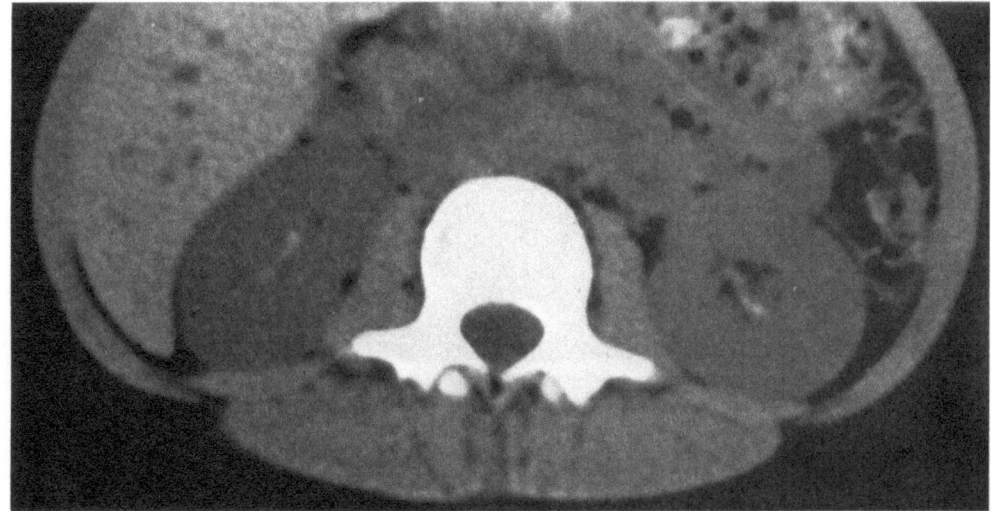

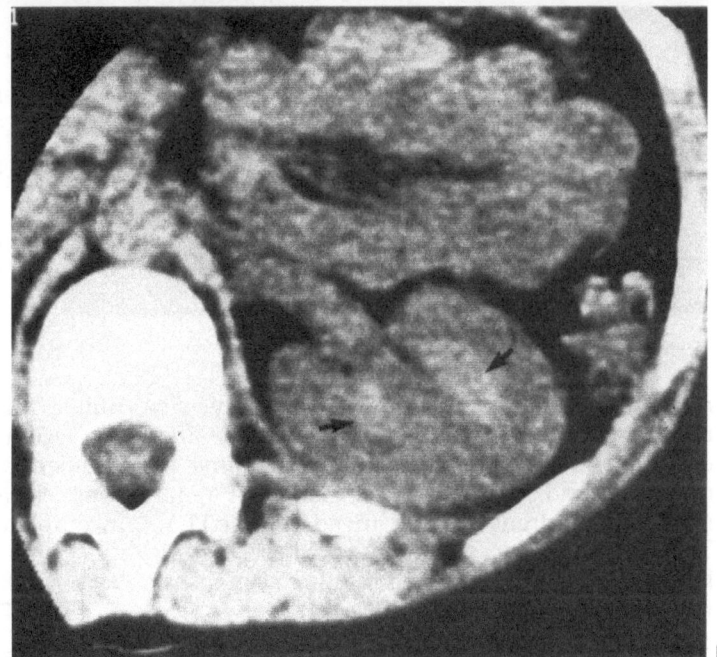

Fig. 11.8a. An 11-year-old girl with acute lymphocytic leukemia and decreased renal function. CT without contrast enhancement shows small areas of calcification within both renal collecting systems. CT is more sensitive than other modalities in the detection of small areas of calcification. **b** An 18-year-old girl with thalassemia and hemochromatosis caused by repeated blood transfusions. Note the two areas within the kidney (*arrows*) with higher attenuation values. Although this finding was not proven pathologically, it was felt to be probably related to iron deposition. This type of change in these patients is unusual and we have only seen it in one other patient.

Abscess formation is extremely rare at our institution. Abscesses appear as well-defined masses of low attenuation that fail to enhance centrally and have an irregular wall of varying thickness and degree of enhancement [27]. Gas within the kidney caused by emphysematous changes is extremely rare in children [20].

In the later phases of inflammatory renal disease CT shows local scarring (Fig. 11.10), atrophy, and cortical thinning, but these features can be documented by sonography. Calyceal deformities are better visualized on excretory urography.

We have not had the opportunity to study xanthogranulomatous pyelonephritis with CT. The kidney is replaced by tissue of low attenuation and there may be complete fatty replacement [27]. Calcification and stones may also be found.

Neoplasia

In pediatric renal disease the greatest impact of CT has been in the initial assessment and follow-up of patients with known or suspected

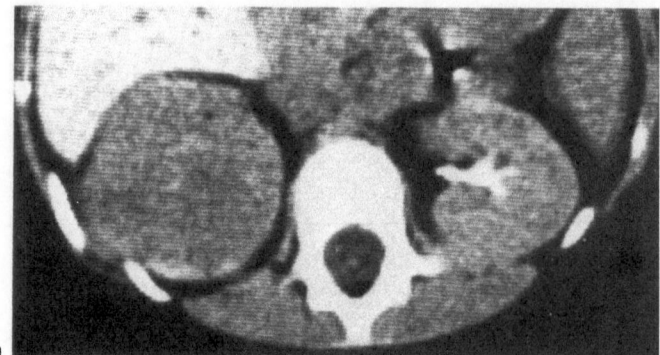

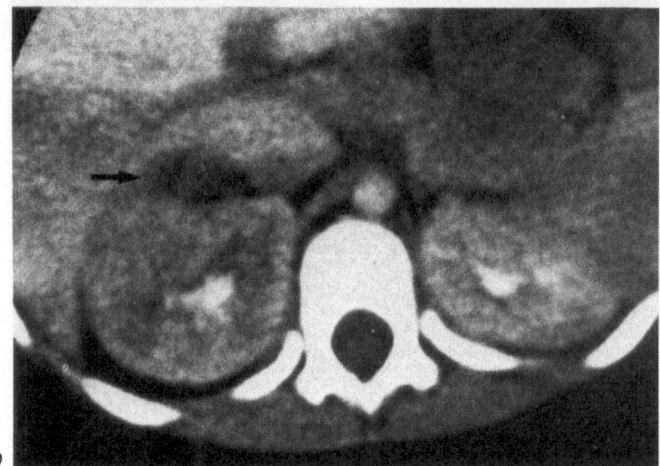

Fig. 11.9a,b. A 6-year-old girl with hematuria. Scans performed after the injection of intravenous contrast. **a** The upper pole of the right kidney is not functioning and has a lower attenuation than the left. **b** Anterior to the mid portion of the right kidney a small perinephric fluid collection is noted (*arrow*). These changes are due to an acute pyelonephritis in the upper pole of the kidney with associated adjacent edema.

renal tumors. In this regard CT has played a major role in the delineation of the site and extent of malignant neoplasms at the time of diagnosis and follow-up. The causes of renal masses in children are summarized in Table 11.1. The CT appearances of many of these benign lesions have been described in other sections of this chapter.

Benign

Mesoblastic nephroma Mesoblastic nephroma is a benign renal tumor that usually presents in the neonatal period as an abdominal mass [2, 15]. Indeed, it is the commonest renal neoplasm to present in the first 3 months of life. The lesion consists primarily of connective tissue, with spindle-shaped cells, that grows between the renal tubules and replaces most of the renal parenchyma. Synonyms for this lesion include fetal renal hamartoma and leiomyomatous hamartoma. For many years mesoblastic nephroma was believed to be part of the spectrum of Wilms'

tumor, but in the late 1960s it was realized that this lesion was indeed a separate entity with an excellent prognosis if completely removed; however, local recurrence may occur if it is incompletely removed.

Table 11.1. Renal mass lesions in children

Benign

1. Compensatory hypertrophy
2. Hydronephrosis — UPJ obstruction
3. Hematomas
4. Inflammatory and abscesses
5. Cysts
    simple
    multilocular
    multicystic dysplastic
    polycystic syndromes
6. Nephroblastomatosis
7. Mesoblastic nephroma
8. Angiomyolipoma

Malignant

1. Wilms' tumor
2. Rhabdoid and clear cell sarcoma
3. Renal cell carcinoma
4. Other sarcomas
5. Lymphoma

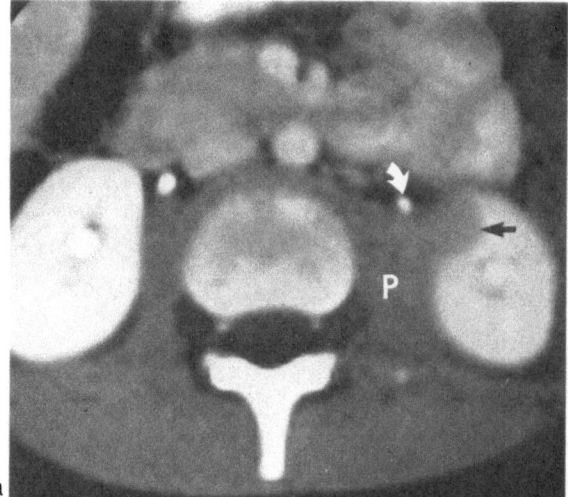

Fig. 11.10a–c. A 10-year-old boy with urinary tract infection. Excretory urography was considered normal apart from a scoliosis concave to the left in the lumbar region. Scans performed during intravenous injection of contrast. **a,b** In **a** the anteromedial aspect of the left kidney (*black arrow*) has not enhanced in the same way as the remainder of this kidney. The margin of this kidney cannot be separated from the adjacent psoas muscle (*P*). *Curved arrow*, left ureter. There is increased enhancement of the anterolateral aspect of the left psoas muscle (*long white arrow* in image **b**). This muscle is also enlarged in comparison with the right psoas. The findings were considered to represent a severe pyelonephritis involving the kidney and extending locally to involve the psoas muscle, which is showing increased enhancement and swelling caused by the inflammatory process. **c** At 6 weeks after antibiotic therapy the lesion in the anteromedial aspect of the left kidney is still evident but is very much smaller than in **a**. The margin of the kidney at this time is more clearly defined and can be separated easily from the psoas muscle, which is no longer showing any enhancement. The muscle at this time is the same size and shows the same enhancement as the right psoas muscle.

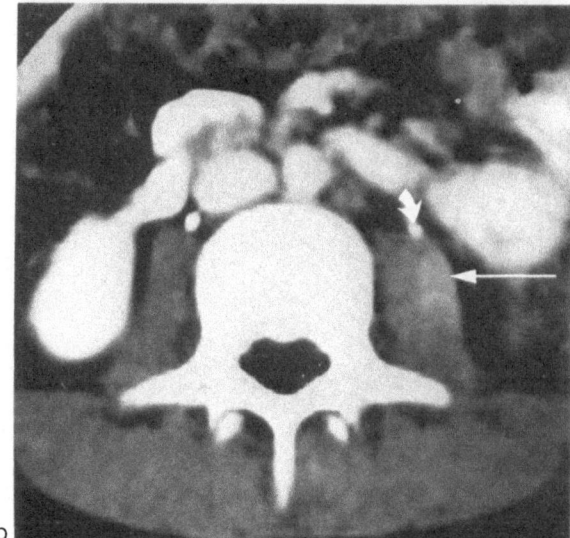

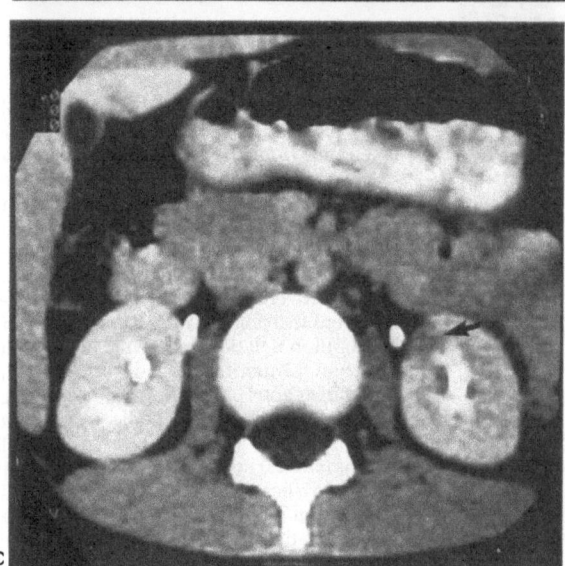

In 1981, Hartman et al. [15] described the radiological/pathological correlation in 20 patients with mesoblastic nephroma. The mass is unencapsulated with a whorled appearance on the cut surface resembling a uterine leiomyoma. The tumor margins blend imperceptibly with the normal kidney. The lesion may penetrate the capsule into perinephric tissue but does not invade the vascular pedicle or metastasize. Hemorrhage and necrosis are uncommon. Two types of cysts may occur: (1) organization of hemorrhage into cystic degeneration and (2) epithelial lined spaces at the junction of the tumor and involved kidney.

In 1985, Kotecha et al. [19] reviewed the 16 cases of mesoblastic nephroma seen at the Hospital for Sick Children, Toronto. Of these children, 8 were studied with sonography and 4 were also studied with CT. Because these lesions usually present in the neonatal period they are quite adequately assessed with sonography and CT has little extra information to add except in larger tumors and with local recurrence. The sonographic appearances reflect the gross pathological appearance, i.e., a solid mass with low-level echoes and anechoic spaces caused by hemorrhage, necrosis, and cyst formation. The CT appearances of this lesion had not received much attention prior to the review by Kotecha et al. [19]. Small lesions have a homogeneous attenuation on CT, and larger lesions have a much more inhomogeneous appearance because of cysts, hemorrhage, and necrosis (Fig. 11.11). In one of

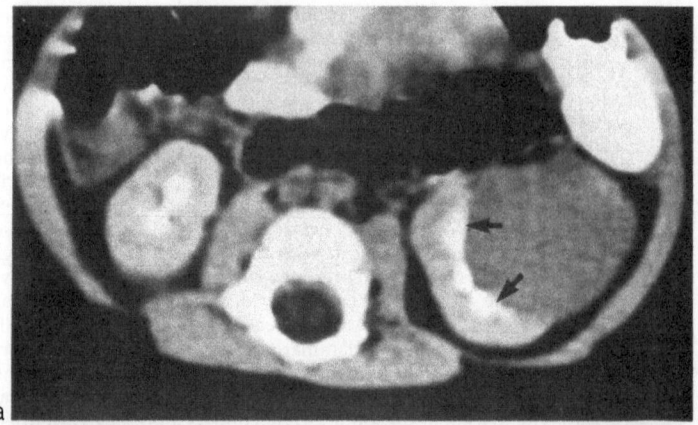

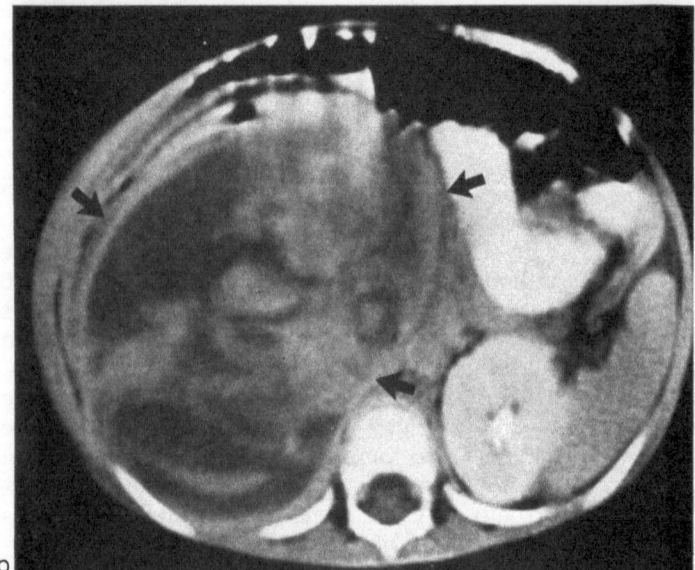

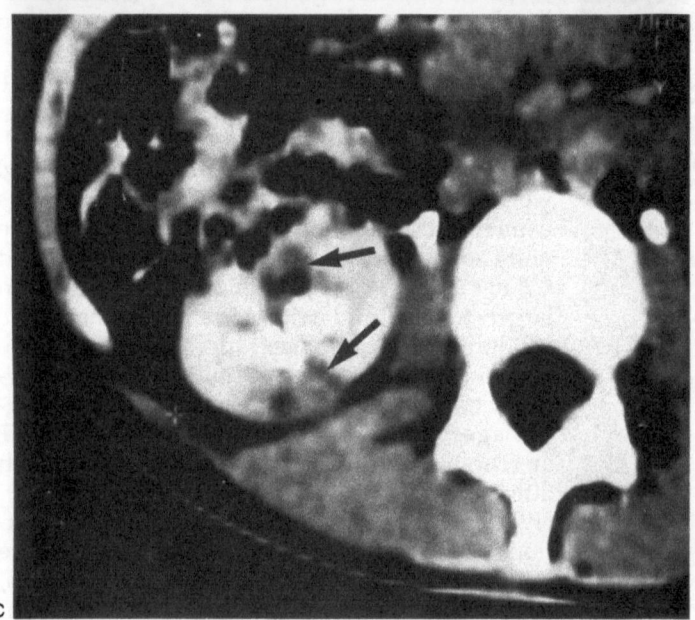

Fig. 11.11. a A 6-week-old boy with left flank mass. CT shows a large soft tissue mass extending from the anterolateral aspect of the left kidney. The lesion has a homogeneous attenuation and enhances less than the adjacent renal parenchyma. The margin between the mass and the remaining kidney is well demarcated (*arrows*). This was a biopsy-proven mesoblastic nephroma. **b** A recurrent mesoblastic nephroma (*arrows*) in the right renal bed following incomplete resection 12 months previously. Note the inhomogeneous enhancement of this lesion. It is indistinguishable from some Wilms' tumors (see Fig. 11.12a). **c** Two small lesions (*arrows*) in the lower pole of the right kidney in a boy with tuberous sclerosis. The attenuation values of parts of these lesions were negative indicating that the lesions represented benign angiolipomas.

the reviewed cases (Fig. 11.11b), CT was extremely valuable in delineating the extent of a large locally recurrent mass. The CT findings are nonspecific, and thus one cannot differentiate this lesion from malignant lesions such as Wilms' tumor on the basis of the CT findings alone.

Angiomyolipoma Angiomyolipoma may occur as an isolated mass lesion of the kidney or may represent one of the renal manifestations of tuberous sclerosis, when it is usually multiple and bilateral [20, 24, 25]. Virtually all children with this lesion have tuberous sclerosis. The lesions consist of varying amounts of fat, large blood vessels, and smooth muscle. We have used sonography primarily to screen children with tuberous sclerosis for any of the renal manifestations. There is a sonographic spectrum of findings with angiomyolipoma [14]. The lesions are usually well defined. Similarly, the CT appearances may vary depending on the quantity of the various components that may be present. Usually there is sufficient fat within these lesions so that the attenuation values of most parts of the mass are negative (Fig. 11.11c). However, if other elements predominate then it may be difficult to recognize the fatty component. Calcification may also be present. Because of the partial volume averaging effect it may be difficult to differentiate very small angiomyolipomas from cysts or other solid renal tumors which may also be seen in tuberous sclerosis. It should also be remembered that occasionally negative values may be observed in Wilms' tumor because of the presence of fat within the tumor [9].

Nephroblastomatosis Nephroblastomatosis is a benign lesion of the kidney characterized by bilateral diffuse proliferation of undifferentiated cells thought to arise from the metanephric blastema [28]. The malignant potential is uncertain and spontaneous regression may occur. This lesion is associated with the development of bilateral or multiple Wilms' tumor [7]. We have found that in children with multiple bilateral Wilms' tumor small areas of nephroblastomatosis may be present pathologically but are usually too small to be recognized even on CT. More massive involvement of the kidney has been described, but we have not had the opportunity to study this type on CT. Nonspecific nephromegaly with distortion of the intrarenal collecting system has also been described [20]. Attenuation values of the tissue are that of normal kidney, but areas may fail to enhance.

Malignant

Wilms' tumor Wilms' tumor or congenital nephroblastoma is the commonest intrarenal neoplasm in children. It has one of the best prognoses for cure of any of the malignant disorders found in childhood. Most children with Wilms' tumor present between the ages of 1 and 5 years, and the peak incidence occurs between 3 and 4 years. The tumor is seldom diagnosed at birth but has been reported occasionally in adults.

The vast majority of children with Wilms' tumor present with an abdominal mass or abdominal pain, which may be discovered by a parent or physician. Hemorrhage into the tumor may be associated with hypertension, anemia, and fever. Occasionally, the child will present with an abdominal mass caused by hemorrhage into the tumor after minor trauma. Bilateral involvement of the kidneys is noted in approximately 10% of children with Wilms' tumor and is usually discovered at the time of the initial diagnosis. Rarely, Wilms' tumor may occur in extrarenal sites — usually in the retroperitoneal area [28].

Gross hematuria is an uncommon presenting symptom, but in 25% of patients microscopic hematuria may be present. Hypertension is uncommonly associated with Wilms' tumor. Rarely, polycythemia may be present and is due to increased production of erythropoietin by the neoplasm. Wilms' tumor has also occasionally been found in association with the nephrotic syndrome.

Approximately 15% of patients with Wilms' tumor have associated congenital abnormalities. These include hamartomas, genitourinary anomalies (such as horseshoe kidney), hemihypertrophy, aniridia, and other eye and heart anomalies. Aniridia is usually of the sporadic congenital type. Approximately 34% of patients with aniridia have Wilms' tumor. Congenital hemihypertrophy associated with Wilms' tumor may involve the entire side of the body or just a segment of a limb, face, or tongue. The tumor is not always on the same side of the body as the hemihypertrophy. Wilms' tumor is also found in relationship to the visceral cytomegaly syndrome described by Beckwith. It is possible that many patients with hemihypertrophy have an incomplete form of Beckwith syndrome. Other tumors associated with the syndrome include hepatoblastoma and adrenocortical carcinomas.

The lesion arises from renal parenchyma and is usually separated from normal kidney tissue by a fibrous pseudocapsule. There are often large areas of necrosis and hemorrhage, and fluid- or blood-filled cysts form as a result of necrosis. The tumor may grow as an exophytic lesion leaving the remainder of the kidney almost normal. On the other hand, growth of the tumor may be within the kidney and a large part of the kidney may be replaced with a rim of parenchyma around part of the tumor or complete disruption of the renal parenchyma. Expansion of the mass may be quite extensive before infiltration of the neoplasm beyond the confines of the kidney is evident. Although metastases are usually via the hematogeneous route, hilar lymph nodes are occasionally involved adjacent to the kidney. Renal vein involvement is not uncommon, and tumor thrombus may be noted to grow or embolize up the inferior vena cava into the heart. Direct extension of tumor into surrounding organs is not common.

The lesion resembles developing embryonic renal tissue with mesenchymal epithelial elements. There is often an abortive attempt at epithelial elements to form tubules and glomeruli. The mesenchymal elements may show differentiation into striated muscle, cartilage, and bone. Anaplastic cells with little differentiation may be present in some tumors.

Factors affecting the prognosis of patients with Wilms' tumor include tumors with unfavorable histology, positive regional lymph nodes, age over 2 years at presentation, and evidence of distant metastases. A good prognosis is indicated histologically by the variety of epithelial differentiation.

Wilms' tumor can be divided into two major histological subgroups: favorable histology (showing no anaplasia and nonsarcomatous) and the unfavorable histology (showing focal or diffuse anaplasia or sarcomatous histology) [28]. The histological findings are obviously important prognostic indicators. The other major factor affecting prognosis and which determines planning of therapeutic regimens is the extent or stage of disease at the time of diagnosis. Therapy has been extremely successful in achieving cures in large numbers of patients with Wilms' tumor. In order to choose the most appropriate regimen and to make fine adjustments in the chemotherapy for a particular patient adequate histological material must be made available and the extent of disease determined as accurately as possible. Imaging techniques are thus extremely important for the accurate estimation of local extent of disease in the abdomen and of metastases at the time of diagnosis. This is also true at the time of follow-up or recurrence.

It has been shown that both false positive and false negative results can occur in the diagnosis of Wilms' tumor with excretory urography [18, 20], and sonography does improve the accuracy somewhat. At the Hospital for Sick Children, Toronto, we have found that CT is the most accurate modality for the delineation of the site and extent of the primary tumor, its relationship to the major abdominal vessels and viscera, the presence of multiple or bilateral lesions, and the presence or absence of spread within the abdomen (e.g., metastases to lymph nodes and liver) and to the lungs.

As outlined in Chapter 16 (see p.245), the modality of choice in the investigation of children with known or suspected abdominal masses is sonography. This modality helps to determine whether the mass is intrarenal or extrarenal and will also display the extent of the lesion and its movement relative to other viscera during real-time examination. In children with Wilms' tumor, sonography has distinct advantages and provides information that complements the subsequent CT study. Sonography is ideally suited for the detection of intravenous extent of tumor into the renal veins and inferior vena cava. Longitudinal real-time images during respiration may determine whether adjacent viscera are involved more easily than transverse CT images (see also Chap. 16, p.247). Information about tumor extent may affect the way in which the CT scan is performed with regard to intravenous contrast enhancement. However, we have found that sonography is not as accurate as CT in the delineation of the exact relationship of the lesion to adjacent vessels, when CT is performed during bolus contrast injection, and is less accurate for delineation of small multiple or bilateral lesions and documentation of lymph node involvement.

The CT appearances of Wilms' tumor have been previously reported by several authors [9, 23, 28]. Examples are illustrated in Figs. 11.12–11.20. Small masses may have a homogeneous attenuation value and, if centrally placed, do not affect the renal outline and, if peripherally placed, do not distort the collecting system. The vast majority of lesions are very large and grow as predominantly exophytic lesions or more centrally, causing gross distortion of the collecting system. On precontrast scans the attenuation of the larger masses is usually inhomogeneous and slightly lower than that of the remaining normal renal parenchyma. However, this inhomogeneity is increased after intravenous contrast administration. Low-attenuation areas are due

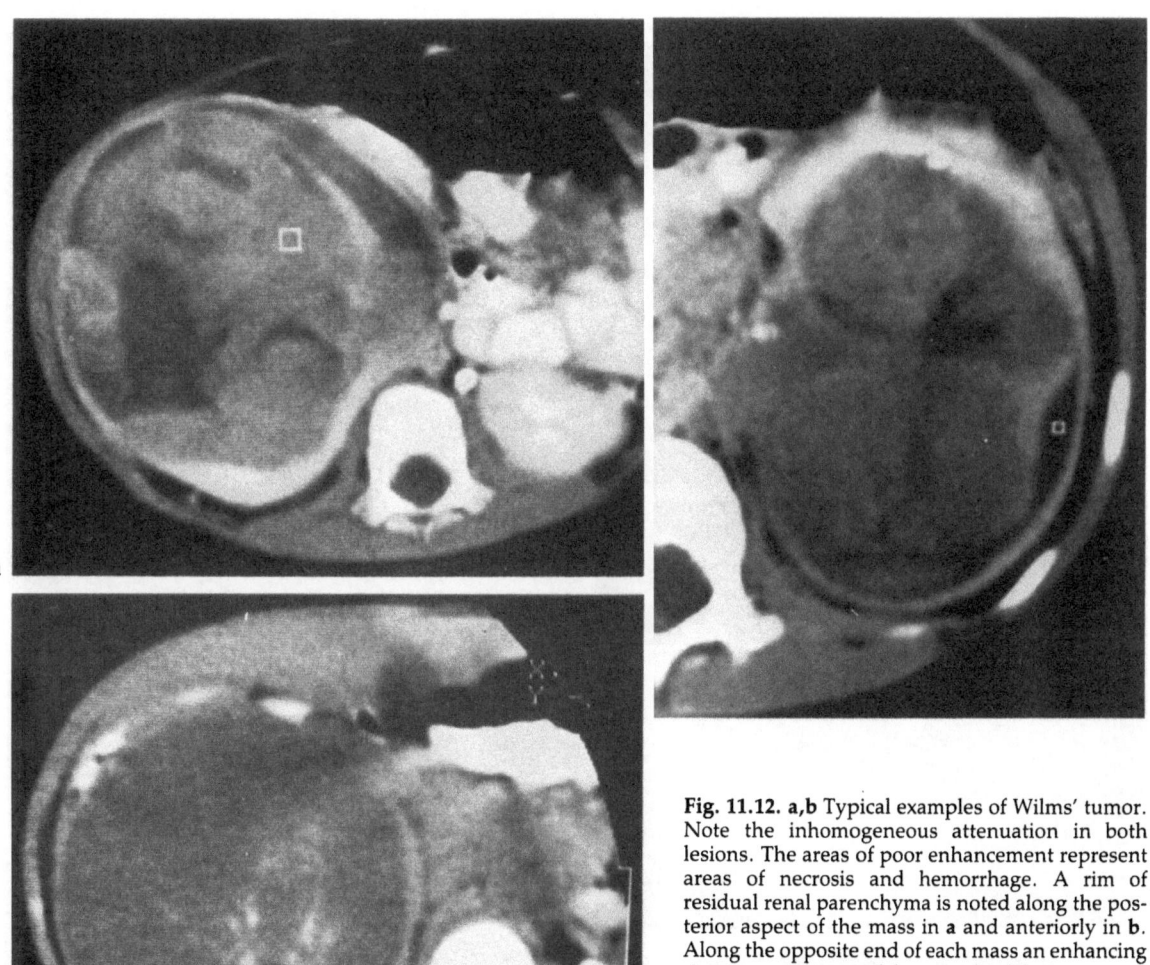

Fig. 11.12. a,b Typical examples of Wilms' tumor. Note the inhomogeneous attenuation in both lesions. The areas of poor enhancement represent areas of necrosis and hemorrhage. A rim of residual renal parenchyma is noted along the posterior aspect of the mass in **a** and anteriorly in **b**. Along the opposite end of each mass an enhancing rim represents part of the capsule of the tumor. **c** A scan performed after injection of contrast material shows poor enhancement of a right Wilms' tumor which has replaced almost the entire kidney. A rim of residual renal parenchyma with some distorted collecting system is noted anteriorly. Some irregular calcification is also noted in the tumor posteriorly.

to poor vascularization and usually relate to areas of necrosis, hemorrhage, or cyst formation. Occasionally, the cystic component may predominate (Fig. 11.14). We have been able to predict from CT findings which tumors are likely to fragment at operation, with tumor spill. These have been large lesions with large areas of necrosis. The remaining functioning renal parenchyma is usually seen as a rim of tissue adjacent to one aspect of the mass. The collecting system may still accumulate contrast in some parts of the residual kidney, and other areas may show marked hydronephrosis caused by obstruction. Calcification, not evident on plain radiographs, may be seen and varies in type from tiny specks and curvilinear calcifications to larger accumulations of varying shapes (see Figs. 11.12, 11.13). Rarely, fat may be seen in the Wilms' tumor [9]. The tumor usually has a pseudocapsule that can often be easily shown surrounding parts of the mass. Children who present with a mass following minor trauma may show areas of hemorrhage in or around the tumor or in the perinephric space (Fig. 11.15). The hemorrhage may have equal or higher attenuation values than the tumor, depending on its age.

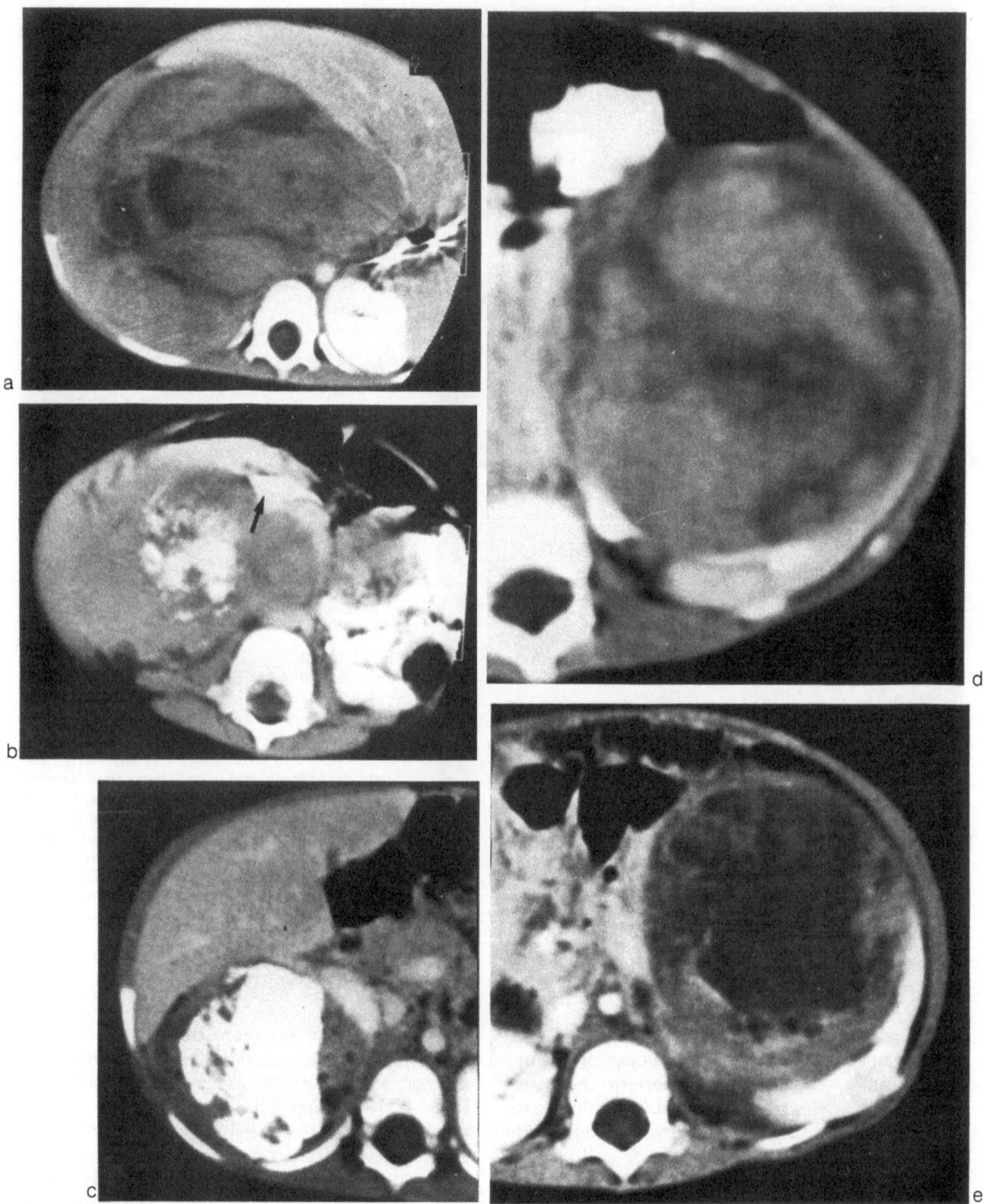

Fig. 11.13. a–c Huge Wilms' tumor crossing the midline from the right flank. **a** Note the inhomogeneous attenuation of the mass. **b** Residual renal parenchyma is noted anteromedially with part of the collecting system (*arrow*). Note the dense calcification in the central part of the tumor in this image. **c** Following intense chemotherapy and radiotherapy the mass has shrunk and is heavily calcified at this time. **d,e** Wilms' tumor at the time of presentation **d** and following chemotherapy **e**. Despite the chemotherapy the mass has only decreased slightly in size in **e**. However, the degree of enhancement has changed dramatically; in **e** there is much less enhancement of the central portion of the mass, indicating tumor necrosis. This change is useful information in assessing response of the lesion to therapy.

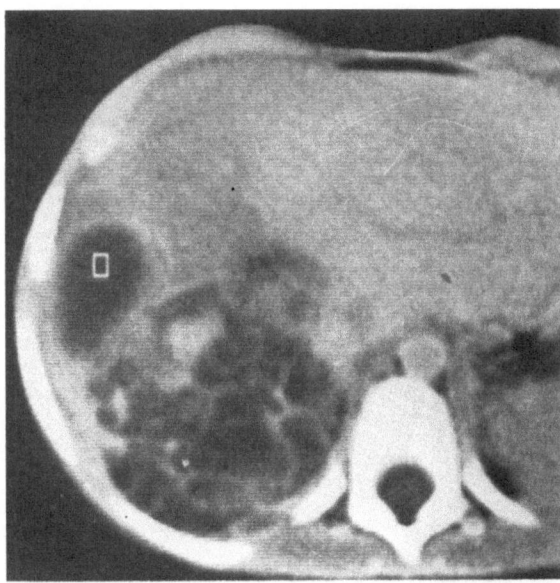

Fig. 11.14. CT scan after intravenous contrast injection shows a poorly enhancing mass in the right upper quadrant. This was a cystic Wilms' tumor. Note the trabeculae between the various cysts. Even though there is a poor line of demarcation between the adjacent liver and tumor no liver invasion was found at operation.

Growth of the lesion into the renal veins and inferior vena cava may be easily documented with CT (Fig. 11.15). This must be differentiated from flow defects in the inferior vena cava when contrast is injected into veins on the dorsum of the foot (see Chap. 8, p.93). Growth of the tumor into the veins may cause occlusion with a persistent nephrogram of the residual renal tissue on the ipsilateral side or on the contralateral side [28].

CT shows small multiple or bilateral lesions exquisitely (Fig. 11.16). Small areas of nephroblastomatosis, which tend to occur in such cases, are not usually evident as they are often only a few millimeters in size. Children with bilateral lesions are often treated with partial nephrectomy, together with adjunctive chemotherapy and radiotherapy, rather than total nephrectomy. CT has proved to be the most valuable modality for the follow-up of such kidneys as they often assume a very unusual shape following such surgery (Fig. 11.17). Small areas of low attenuation within the renal parenchyma following intravenous contrast administration are better appreciated on CT than with sonography. They may represent areas of active tumor, necrotic lesions, or areas of hematoma and scarring. Since CT cannot differentiate their nature, follow-up scans to assess their progress is essential (Fig. 11.17). Enlarged lymph nodes in the retroperitoneum are occasionally seen in patients with Wilms' tumor. Most often these are only slightly enlarged and after removal at laparotomy are usually found to be reactive in nature rather than containing metastatic deposits. It is impossible with CT to determine the histological makeup of these nodes. Larger nodes are usually due to metastases (Fig. 11.18). These usually lie adjacent to the main mass of tumor and may occasionally appear as a lobule off the medial aspect of the lesion. However, the pseudocapsule of the tumor or some residual rim of renal parenchyma may be the clue to the true nature of the apparent lobulation (Fig. 11.18).

The liver is examined thoroughly in all abdominal scans in children with Wilms' tumor. However, the incidence of hepatic metastases at the time of diagnosis in children with Wilms' tumor is very rare (Fig. 11.19). The hepatic metastases are usually focal or multifocal and are nonspecific in appearance, as described in Chapter 12 (see p.89). Hepatic metastases are much more common in the terminal phases of the disease.

Metastatic disease is most commonly found in the lungs. Chest radiographs are mandatory. If no metastases are noted on chest radiographs, then chest CT is imperative as it is much more sensitive. If numerous metastases are noted on chest radiographs, then chest CT is only required during follow-up, if there is a good response to therapy.

Follow-up scans of the abdomen are important in children who have been treated non-operatively or operatively. In those treated non-operatively, sonography is usually sufficient to document the response of the size of the lesion. However, we have occasionally used CT if the lesion does not diminish in size clinically as expected. In some cases a marked change in attenuation values with increased areas of poor enhancement in the tumor will be found, which indicates an increase in tumor necrosis and thus a favorable response to chemotherapy despite a lack of change in size. This has correlated well pathologically [35]. Following chemotherapy and radiation therapy increased calcification may be noted in the tumors (see Fig. 11.13).

Follow-up scans of the renal bed after nephrectomy are useful to rule out early recurrence. Although this can be achieved satisfactorily in many patients by sonography, we have found that CT is somewhat more accurate and appears to delineate the renal bed more clearly when it is

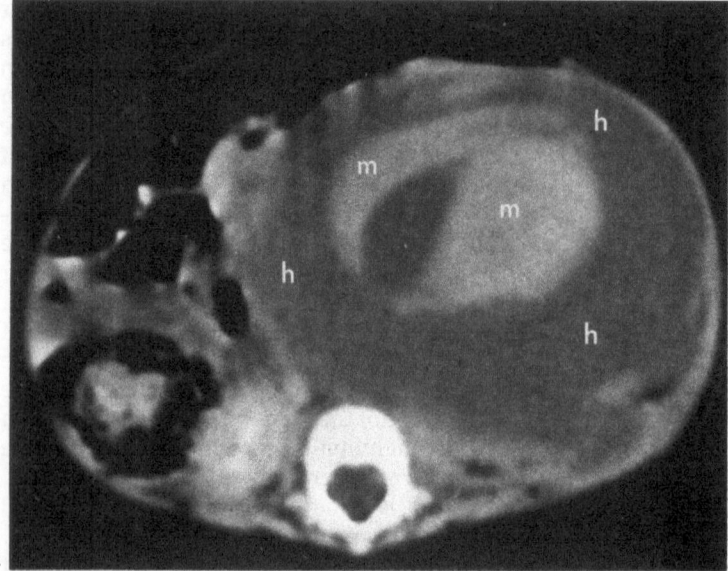

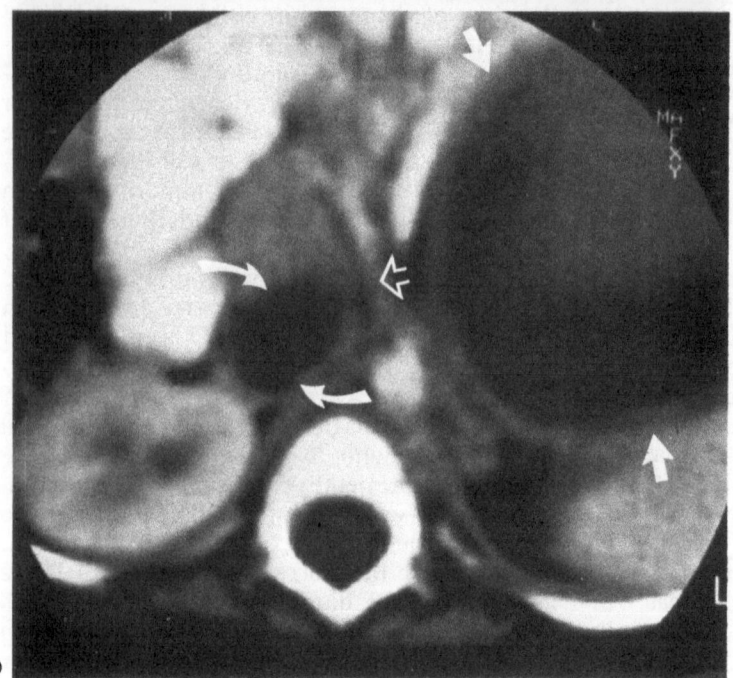

Fig. 11.15a,b. A 15-month-old boy with a large left Wilms' tumor and sudden drop in hemoglobin. **a** CT shows a huge mass in left flank crossing the midline. The enhancing areas centrally (*m*) represent the tumor, and the nonenhancing areas (*h*) represent massive hemorrhage in and around this lesion. **b** Following chemotherapy the mass (*solid arrows*) is much smaller. The *curved arrows* indicate an aneurysmal dilatation of the inferior vena cava, which was filled with necrotic tumor at operation. *Open arrow,* celiac axis.

filled with gas-containing bowel loops. Ideally every child with Wilms' tumor should have a follow-up CT approximately 6–8 weeks after nephrectomy to determine the baseline postoperative CT appearances so that early recurrent disease can be diagnosed with more confidence and not confused with areas of fibrosis or old hematomas. We have used CT in this manner, particularly in those children who have a high possibility of local recurrence. This category has included children with tumors of unfavorable histology, tumor spill at operation, lesions that have invaded the retroperitoneum, lymph node metastases, and those individuals in whom complete removal of tumor is not achieved. Local recurrence usually occurs in the renal bed (Fig. 11.20), and the mass has a nonspecific appearance. Recurrence in other areas such as the pelvis and mesentery may also be seen.

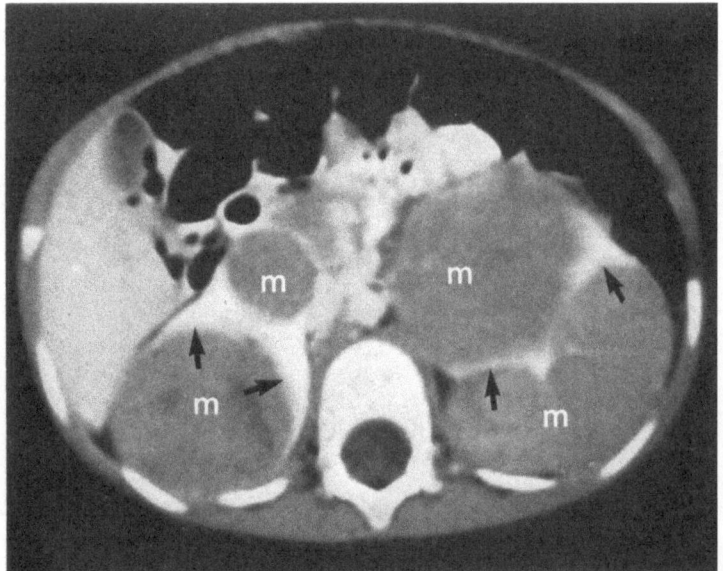

a

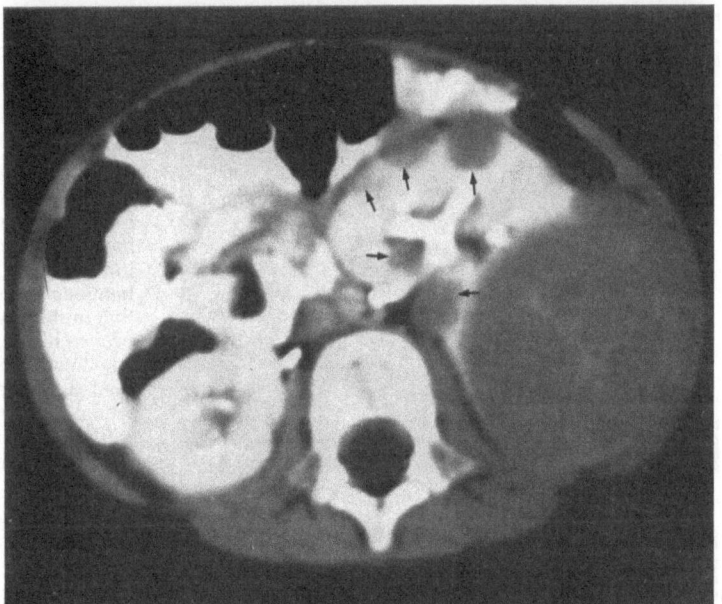

b

Fig. 11.16a,b. A 16-month-old girl with multiple bilateral Wilms' tumors. a Multiple tumor masses (*m*) are noted in both kidneys. Some residual renal parenchyma is noted between these masses (*arrows*). b The lower pole of the right kidney is uninvolved and contains a good volume of normally functioning renal parenchyma. In the left kidney, apart from the large mass in the posterolateral aspect, multiple smaller lesions are noted more anteriorly and medially (*small arrows*).

In order to diagnose early recurrence, meticulous attention to technique is required with regard to gastrointestinal and vascular contrast enhancement. The usual appearances on CT following a nephrectomy should be well understood (see also Fig. 7.2 p.87, Fig. 7.3, p.88, and Fig. 9.6, p.113). Following radiation therapy and chemotherapy, changes may be noted in the liver (as described in Chap. 12, see p.195) and also in the soft tissues and bones.

Some histological groups of renal tumors were formerly classified as part of the spectrum of Wilms' tumor but have recently been recognized as representing other tumor entities. These include the rhabdoid tumor and clear cell sarcoma (Fig. 11.21). These lesions are rare and our experience with the CT appearance in four shows they have a nonspecific pattern which cannot be differentiated from Wilms' tumor. The clear cell sarcomas are characterized by having a high incidence of bone metastases. The rhabdoid lesions have an association with similar lesions in the posterior fossa which may occur at the time of diagnosis of the renal tumor or some years later [28].

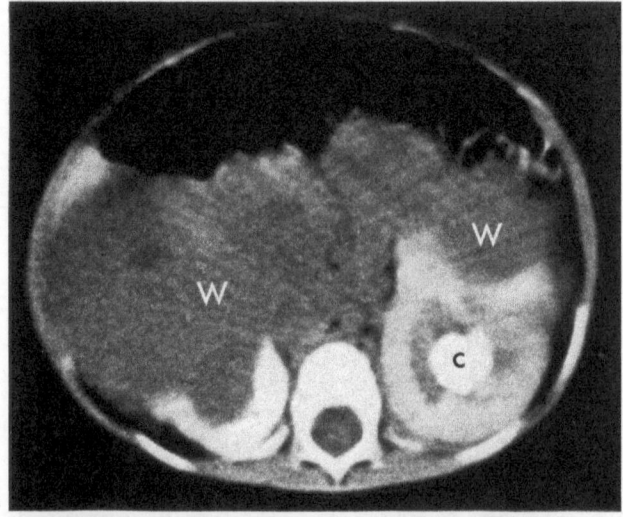

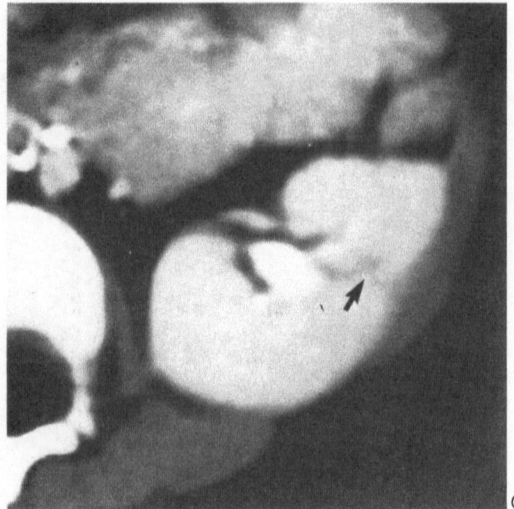

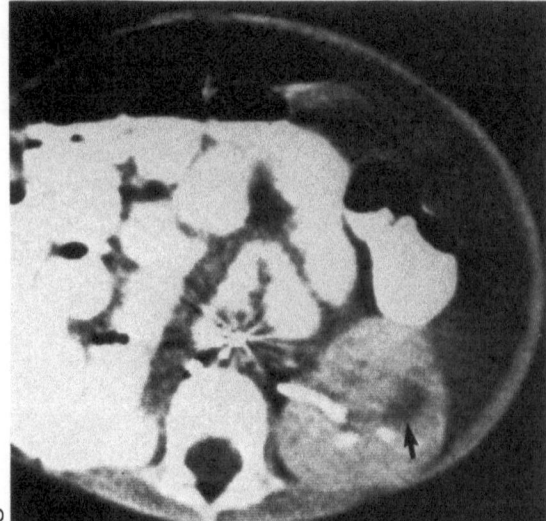

Fig. 11.17a–c. A 15-month-old girl with bilateral Wilms' tumor. **a** Large tumors (*W*) arise from the anterior aspect of both kidneys. There is more remaining normal parenchyma on the left than on the right, although further tumor is noted more centrally on the left, adjacent and medial to the collecting system (*c*). **b** Following right nephrectomy and partial left heminephrectomy CT shows a residual area of low attenuation in the lateral aspect of the left kidney (*arrow*). This was proven histologically to be a recurrent active Wilms' tumor. **c** Following removal of the recurrent lesion CT reveals that the left kidney has an irregular outline and an irregular area laterally that fails to enhance (*arrow*). This probably represents scar tissue but should be followed by CT regularly to diagnose further recurrent disease early.

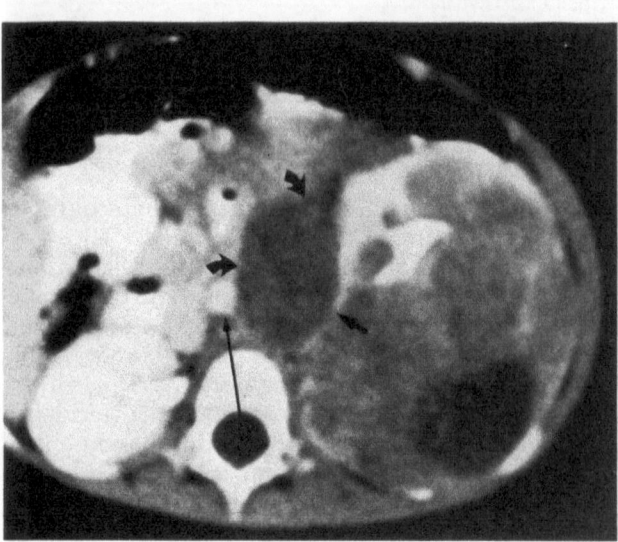

Fig. 11.18. A large Wilms' tumor is noted in the posterolateral aspects of the left kidney with a rim of residual functioning renal parenchyma and collecting system anteriorly. A thin portion of renal parenchyma (*short arrow*) separates the main tumor mass from adjacent metastases in lymph nodes (*curved arrows*). The aorta (*long arrow*) is displaced anteriorly and to the right by the metastases.

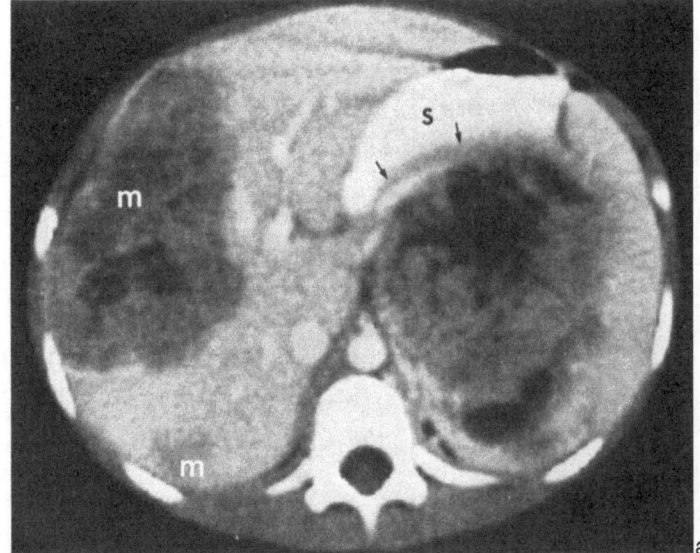

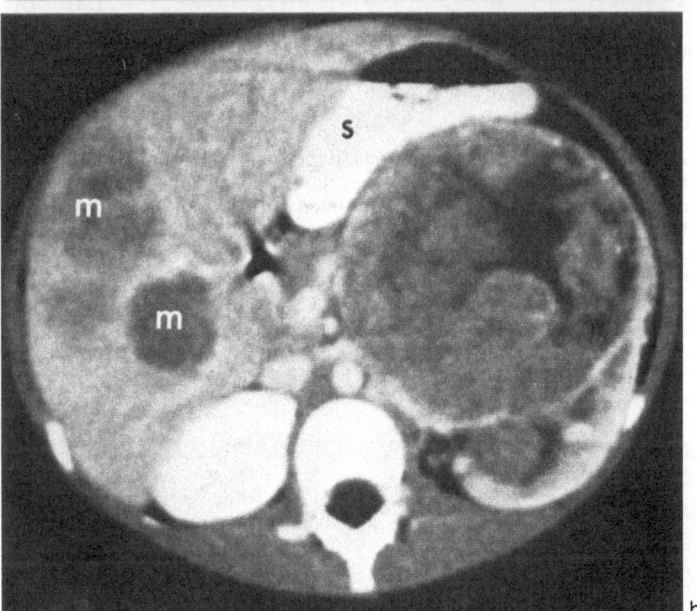

Fig. 11.19a,b. A 10-year-old boy with large left Wilms' tumor displacing the stomach (*s*), pancreatic body and tail (*small arrows*), and splenic vein anteriorly. Multiple liver metastases (*m*) are noted in scans **a** and **b**. Some residual renal parenchyma is noted posteriorly in scan **b**.

Renal cell carcinoma   Renal cell carcinoma rarely presents in the first two decades of life [4, 5, 8, 13, 22, 24, 30, 31]. In an extensive review of more than 1500 patients with renal cell carcinoma, Riches et al. [33] found less than 0.5% of patients presented before 20 years of age. We have reported our experience with 17 such patients (10 F, 7 M; mean age 12 years) seen in a 24-year period at two large institutions in Toronto [6]. The nine patients seen at the Hospital for Sick Children, Toronto, account for 0.2% of all malignant disease in children at this institution and

2% of all intrarenal neoplasms. In the first two decades, the sex incidence of this lesion is almost equal and the peak age of occurrence is approximately 9 years [6]. Children with renal cell carcinoma invariably present with symptoms and signs related to their primary lesion and not caused by metastases. A palpable mass was present in 60%, hematuria in 30%, and pain in 50% of our patients.

One patient in our series had tuberous sclerosis. Renal cell carcinoma is rarely seen in tuberous sclerosis and usually presents in adult-

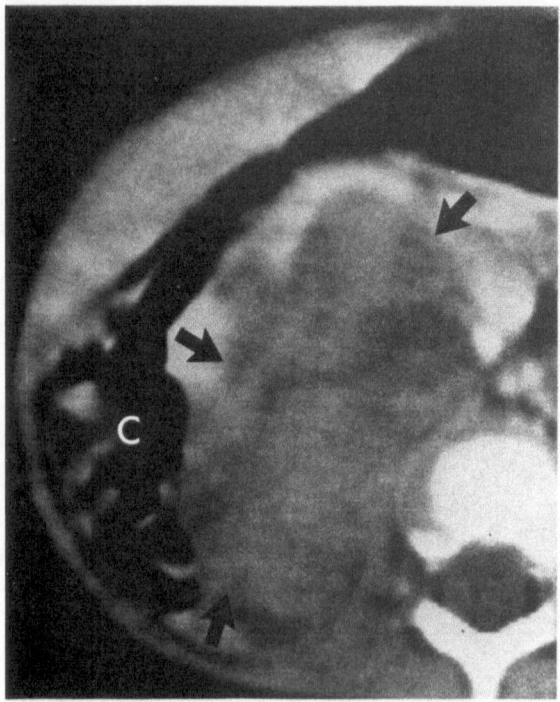

Fig. 11.20. An 8-year-old girl with local recurrence of Wilms' tumor in the right renal bed (*arrows*). The lesion is surrounded anteriorly by Gastrografin-filled small bowel and laterally by gas-filled colon (C).

hood. These lesions may be bilateral and multiple and may occur in association with angiomyolipoma and cysts, which are the more common lesions in patients with tuberous sclerosis [13, 24].

Because the renal mass lesion in children is smaller than that found in Wilms' tumor, plain radiographs may appear normal. A mass was noted in 50% of our patients and calcification in 25% [6]. When present, the calcification tends to be more marked than that found in Wilms' tumor.

Findings on excretory urography, arteriography, ultrasound, and CT are nonspecific [6]. CT was performed in three children in our reported series and in a fourth more recent child. In a 15-month-old boy, a huge mass with homogeneous attenuation was noted with extension around the aorta. In a second patient, the upper part of the involved kidney was diffusely enlarged and the kidney functioned poorly. In the third patient, CT revealed a large solid mass arising from the posterior aspect of the upper pole of the left kidney. In the fourth patient (previously unreported) a huge inhomogeneous mass replaced the entire kidney and extended into the retroperitoneum and into the lumen of the inferior vena cava. Multiple liver metastases were also present (Fig. 11.22).

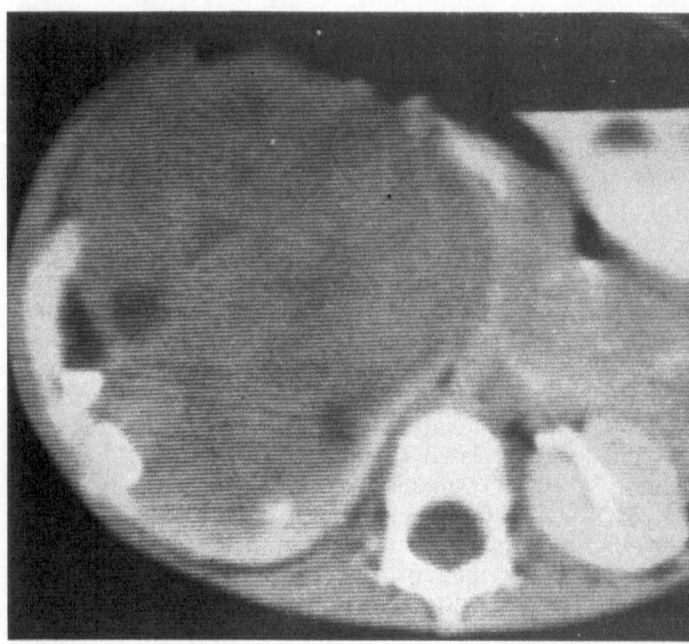

Fig. 11.21. A 6-year-old boy with clear cell sarcoma of the right kidney. A large mass with inhomogeneous attenuation is present, and a rim of renal parenchyma is noted around the posterior aspect of the mass together with some dilated portions of the collecting system. The mass has a nonspecific appearance and resembles a Wilms' tumor on CT.

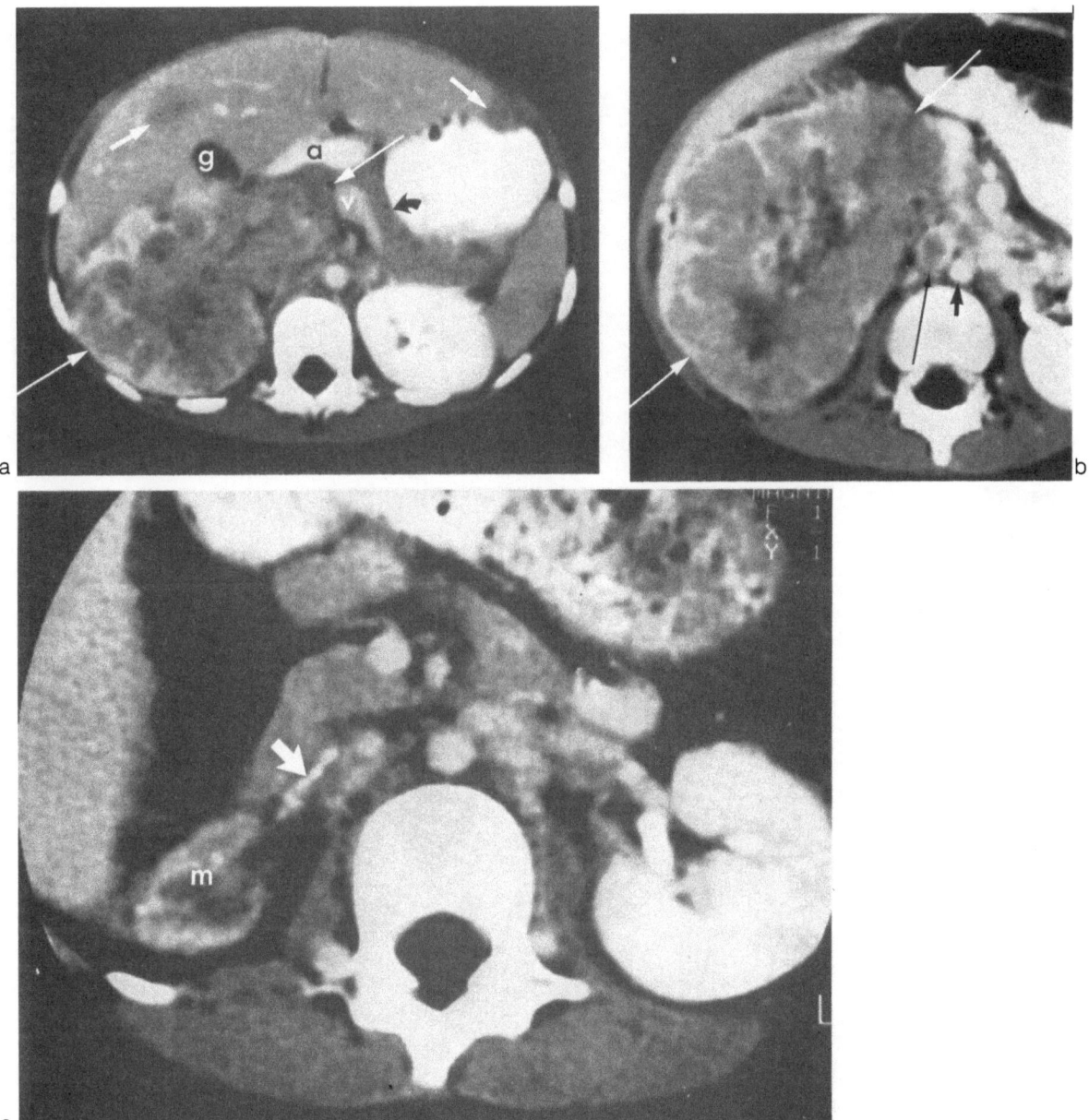

Fig. 11.22a–c. An 8-year-old girl with left renal cell carcinoma (Grawitz tumor). The large left renal mass (*long arrows*) is noted in images **a** and **b**. **a** The portal vein (*v*) and pancreas (*curved arrow*) are displaced toward the left, and the pancreas takes a more anteroposterior course than usual. *Short white arrows*, two liver metastases; *g*, gallbladder; *a*, gastric antrum. The inferior vena cava cannot be visualized. **b** The inferior vena cava (*long black arrow*) shows a large filling defect in the centre representing tumor extension into the vena cava. *Short black arrow*, aorta. **c** Following intensive chemotherapy and radiation therapy the right-sided mass has shrunk to an extremely small size (*m*). Calcification is noted in the residual tumor thrombus in the right renal vein (*arrow*).

Because renal cell carcinoma tends to metastasize locally to retroperitoneal lymph nodes and to the lungs, CT is important in the assessment of the primary lesion and the metastatic disease in the abdomen and lungs at diagnosis and at follow-up. The prognosis depends on the stage of the lesion at diagnosis and is not hopeless as there are a few long-term survivors [6]. Unfortunately, metastatic disease may occur many years after what appears to be an initially

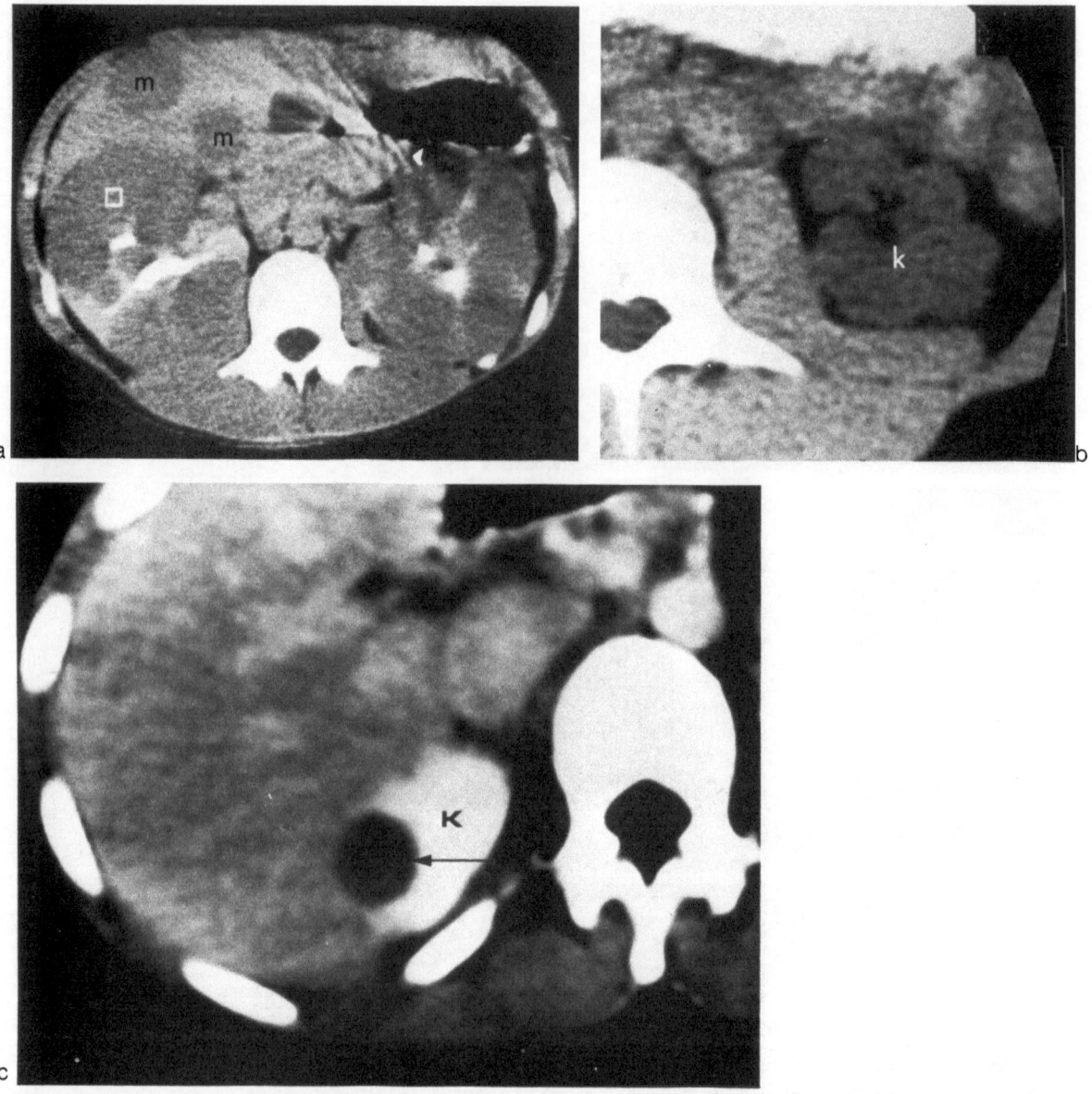

Fig. 11.23a,b. An 11-year-old boy with disseminated metastases from an undifferentiated sarcoma. **a** Liver metastases (*m*) are present as well as huge lesions replacing most of the renal parenchyma. These lesions have a lower attenuation (*square cursor*) than the remaining functioning renal parenchyma. **b** Following intensive chemotherapy the metastases have shrunk in size, and the left kidney (*k*) shows marked scarring with a lobulated appearance. **c** Another boy with lymphoma and focal deposit (*arrow*) in right kidney (*k*).

successful outcome [6]. This rare tumor should thus be included in the differential diagnosis of intrarenal mass lesions, particularly in older children with hematuria and renal calcification on plain radiographs.

Metastases Spread of malignant lesions to the kidney may be either direct or hematogenous. Direct spread may be seen with invasive neuroblastomas adjacent to the kidney. At times it may be difficult to predict from transverse axial scans which cut the tumor – renal interface tangentially whether the kidney is invaded by an adjacent tumor. Often longitudinal sonographic scans with real-time imaging may be more helpful (see also Chap. 16, p.248). Hematogenous spread is very much less common and may occur mainly with sarcomatous lesions (Fig. 11.23). the appearances are nonspecific and may resemble that caused by lymphomatous involvement.

Fig. 11.24a. An 11-year-old boy with hematuria following a motor vehicle accident. Scans following intravenous contrast injection show multiple areas of low attenuation within the renal parenchyma representing intrarenal hematomas. The kidney is surrounded by material of inhomogeneous attenuation related to perirenal hematoma. **b** Right perirenal and intrarenal hematoma (*H*) and urinoma (*U*) following motor vehicle accident. Note the leakage of contrast from the renal pelvis (*P*) into the urinoma. The high-density resolution of CT may enable one to document the exact site of leakage when this may not be apparent on plain films or excretory urography.

──────────────────────────────▶

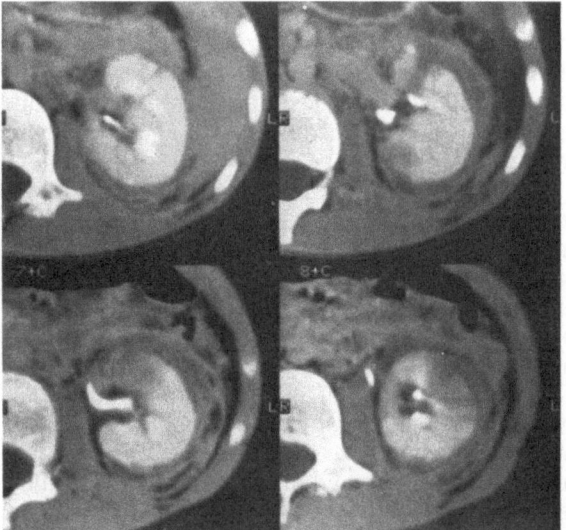

a

Lymphoma Intrarenal lymphoma may be present either as a solitary intrarenal mass, multiple intrarenal masses, or as diffuse bilateral infiltration with nephromegaly. Mass lesions may be well defined or poorly defined (see Fig. 8.5, p.96). In the larger lesions there may be very poor enhancement of the central portion of the mass. Diffuse involvement gives the kidney a lower attenuation than usual, with failure of the lymphomatous tissue to enhance. The intervening normal renal parenchyma shows enhancement but marked distortion, as does the collecting system. The appearance is similar to that seen in Fig. 11.23a. CT may also reveal other evidence of abdominal lymphoma such as para-aortic lymphadenopathy and hepatic or splenic abnormalities. Enlarged retroperitoneal lymph nodes may have secondary effects on the urinary tract such as renal displacement and ureteric obstruction. Primary renal involvement in lymphoma is extremely rare, but renal involvement is not uncommon in patients with far-advanced lymphoma, particularly non-Hodgkin's lymphoma. Leukemia may also infiltrate the kidney in a diffuse manner.

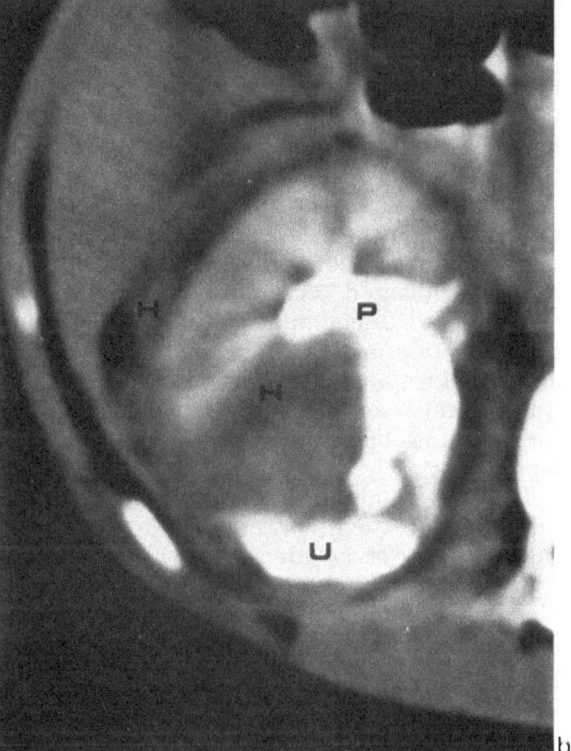

b

Trauma

At the Hospital for Sick Children, Toronto, we have found that CT provides the most accurate anatomical delineation of the kidneys and perirenal tissues in children with blunt abdominal trauma (see also Chap. 16, p.257). The high density and spatial resolution of CT makes this modality highly suited to displaying small parenchymal contusions, perirenal hematomas, and urinomas (Fig. 11.24). Parenchymal injuries range from minor areas or renal contusion to larger areas of parenchymal disruption and fragmentation together with perirenal hematomas. Urinomas occur as the result of disruption of the collecting system and appear as masses of fluid

attenuation. If leakage is still active during the study, contrast-bearing urine will be noted to fill the mass, and the exact site of leakage from the collecting system may well be documented. CT is far more accurate in delineating these types of anatomical renal disruptions than excretory urography and (in our experience) sonography.

Moreover, CT also provides functional information about each kidney, and even small focal areas of devascularization are easily documented (see Fig. 16.8, p.260). Despite this, renal CT is not required in every child suspected of having renal trauma.

It is imperative that both functional and anatomical information be obtained, whichever modality is chosen. Excretory urography and renal scintigraphy provide both functional and anatomical information; either modality may be used alone, particularly in children with hematuria and more minor degrees of injury. The decision whether to use excretory urography or renal scintigraphy may depend on one's familiarity with these modalities; in our department, it depends on what other injuries the child is suspected of having. If liver or spleen injuries are suspected, renal scintigraphy can be combined with liver/spleen scintigraphy (see Chap. 16, p.265), thus reducing the need to move the patient around the hospital. We have found that this combination offers a valuable alternative to CT. If a patient has a head injury and requires a head CT, we also perform an abdominal CT if there is a suspicion of abdominal injury.

Sonography does not provide functional information but may be used to provide complementary anatomical information when lesions have been documented on excretory urography or scintigraphy. Sonography is ideally suited for follow-up of previously documented anatomical abnormalities and may also play a role in the trauma unit as an emergency bedside procedure for the unstable patient prior to emergency laparotomy.

The vast majority of children with renal injuries are treated conservatively. Operative therapy is reserved for those with significant renal vascular injury and those with persistent bleeding, when the hematocrit and blood pressure cannot be kept stable. In children with renal pedicle injuries, as suggested by nonfunction on excretory urography or no flow to the kidney on renal scintigraphy, angiography is necessary prior to surgery.

It should be remembered that renal damage may also occur when the kidney is included in radiation fields in patients treated for malignant disease. Severe changes with renal scarring and loss of renal volume are easily documented on both CT and sonography, although CT will also show the degree of functional damage. Changes in the kidney in children with retroperitoneal neoplasms may also be due to obstruction of the renal vessels and ureters by the mass.

References

1. Alton DJ, Ash J, Daneman A (1984) Pediatric renal imaging. Paper presented at the Annual Meeting of the Canadian Association of Radiologists, Vancouver, June 1984
2. Berdon WE, Wigger HJ, Baker DH (1973) Fetal renal hamartoma — a benign tumor to be distinguished from Wilms' tumor. AJR 118(1):18–27
3. Blank E, Campbell JR (1973) Epidermoid cysts of the spleen. Pediatrics 51:75
4. Cassady JR, Filler R, Jaffe N, Vawter G (1974) Carcinoma of the kidney in children. Radiology 112:691
5. Castellanos RD, Aron BS, Evans AT (1974) Renal adenocarcinoma in children: incidence, therapy and prognosis. J Urol 111:534
6. Chan HSL, Daneman A, Gribbin M, Martin DJ (1983) Renal cell carcinoma in the first two decades of life. Pediatr Radiol 13:1–5
7. Cohen RC, Kelly JH, Chan HSL, Mancer K, Weitzman S, Daneman A, Filler RM (1985) Treatment and prognosis of 32 patients with bilateral Wilms' tumor. Pediatr Surg Int (In press)
8. Dehner LP, Leestma JE, Price EB Jr (1970) Renal cell carcinoma in children: a clinicopathologic study of 15 cases and review of the literature. J Pediatr 76:358
9. Fishman EK, Hartman DS, Goldman SM, Seigelman SS (1983) The CT appearance of Wilms' tumor. J Comput Assist Tomogr 7(4):659–665
10. Forde WJ, Osteolenk DG, Finby N (1960) Renal displacement associated with enlargement of the spleen. AJR 84:889
11. Frimann-Dahl J (1960) Normal variations of the left kidney. Acta Radiol 55:207
12. Gooding GAW (1978) The ultrasonic and computed tomographic appearance of splenic lobulations: a consideration in the ultrasonic differential of masses adjacent to the left kidney. Radiology 126:719
13. Guiterrez OH, Burgener FA, Schwartz S (1979) Coincident renal cell carcinoma and renal angiomyolipoma in tuberous sclerosis. AJR 132:848
14. Hartman DS, Goldman SM, Friedman AC, Davis CJ, Madewell JE, Sherman JL (1981) Angiomyolipoma: ultrasonic-pathologic correlation. Radiology 139:451–458
15. Hartman DS, Lesar MSL, Madewell JE, Lichtenstein JE, Davis CJ (1981) Mesoblastic nephroma: radiologic-pathologic correlation of 20 cases. AJR 136:69–74
16. Karstaedt N, Sagel SS, Stanley RJ, Melson GL, Levitt RG (1978) Computed tomography of the adrenal gland. Radiology 129:723–730
17. Kirks DR, Rosenberg ER, Johnson DG, King LR (1985) Integrated imaging of neonatal renal masses. Pediatr Radiol 147–156
18. Kirks ER (1983) Computed tomography of pediatric urinary tract disease. Urol Radiol 5:199–208
19. Kotecha P, Daneman A, Mancer K, Payton D, Chan HSL, Cheng MY (1985) Sonographic-CT-pathologic correlation of mesoblastic nephroma. Unpublished data
20. Kuhn JP, Berger PE (1981) Computed tomography of the kidney in infancy and childhood. Radiol Clin North Am 19(3):445–460
21. Levine E, Grantham JJ (1985) High-density renal cysts in autosomal dominant polycystic kidney disease demonstrated by CT. Radiology 154:447–482
22. Love L, Neumann HA, Szanto PB, Novak GM (1979) Malignant renal tumor in adolescence. Radiology 92:855

23. Lowe RE, Cohen MD (1984) Computed tomographic evaluation of Wilms' tumor and neuroblastoma. Radio-Graphics 4(6):915–928

24. Lynne CM, Machiz S (1973) Renal cell carcinoma in children: a report of four cases and a review of the literature. J Pediatr Surg 8:925

25. Lynne CM, Nadji M, Carrion HM, Russel E, Bakshandeh K, Politano VA (1979) Renal angiomyolipoma; polycystic kidney and tuberous sclerosis. Urology 14:174

26. Madayag M, Bosniak MA, Beranbaum E, Becker J (1972) Renal and suprarenal pseudotumors caused by variations of the spleen. Radiology 105:43

27. McLennan BL, Lee JKT (1982) Kidney. In: Lee JKT, Sagel SS, Stanley RJ (eds) Computed body tomography. Raven, New York, pp 341–378

28. Miller JH, Laug WE (1985) Urinary tract. In: Miller JH (ed) Imaging in pediatric oncology. Williams and Wilkins, London, pp 252–288

29. Piekarski J, Federle MP, Moss AA, Landon SS (1980) Computed tomography of the spleen. Radiology 135:683

30. Pochedly C, Suwansirikul S, Penzer P (1971) Renal cell carcinoma with extrarenal manifestations in a 10-month-old child. Am J Dis Child 121:528

31. Poole CA, Viamonte M Jr (1970) Unusual renal masses in the pediatric age group. AJR 109:368

32. Rao AKR, Silver TM (1976) Normal pancreas and splenic variants simulating suprarenal and renal tumors. AJR 126:530

33. Riches EW, Griffiths IH, Tackray A (1951) New growths of the kidney and ureter. Br J Urol 23:297

34. Stiris MG (1980) Accessory spleen versus left adrenal tumor: computed tomographic and abdominal angiographic evaluation. J Comput Assist Tomogr 4:543

35. Tiu M, Higa T, Daneman A, Chan HSL (1983) CT-pathologic correlation of Wilms' tumor. Unpublished data

36. Whalen JP, Evans JA, Shanser J (1971) Vector principle in the differential diagnosis of abdominal masses: the left upper quadrant. AJR 113:104

Chapter 12

Liver

Introduction

At the Hospital for Sick Children, Toronto, CT of the liver is most commonly performed to delineate the exact site, size, extent, and character of focal hepatic masses. In this regard CT is particularly helpful in the delineation of primary malignant hepatic neoplasms but it is also valuable when dealing with benign lesions such as cysts and abscesses and also with metastases. CT is also particularly valuable for follow-up of patients with previous surgery for malignant masses. CT is also of benefit for the delineation of hepatic trauma, particularly when trauma to multiple abdominal organs is suspected. Less commonly CT may be performed to delineate the extent and character of diffuse parenchymal diseases more accurately. CT usually has little extra information to offer in the jaundiced infant or child or those patients with portal hypertension, who are usually adequately studied initially with sonography and radionuclide liver studies. Finally, CT of the liver is occasionally performed to delineate equivocal abnormalities noted on hepatic sonography or radionuclide scan.

The vast majority of children who have their liver studied with CT have usually been studied with other modalities such as sonography or hepatic radionuclide scans. All children with suspected hepatic masses are initially studied with sonography. However, in some children CT may well be the initial modality of choice. This is particularly true in children with blunt abdominal trauma when multiple organ involvement is suspected.

Anatomy

The liver is the largest organ in the abdomen and is thus easily visualized in all scans of the upper abdomen. Knowledge of hepatic anatomy is important, especially when attempting to determine whether a focal hepatic lesion is limited to a particular lobe of the liver. This information is vital when planning the surgical approach to such a lesion.

Surfaces

The liver has a smooth parietal surface directed superiorly, anteriorly, and to the right, and this conforms to the shape of the diaphragm and abdominal wall. A more irregular posteroinferior visceral surface is directed toward the left and is related to the viscera of the upper abdomen. It is beyond the scope of this book to detail these relationships further.

Attenuation

The liver has an attenuation value higher than that of other abdominal viscera, and, although absolute values are not useful, the attenuation is relatively homogeneous in individual patients, with values ranging between 50 and 80 HU. This value is usually 1.5 times the attenuation of the spleen [4].

The liver enhances homogeneously following the injection of intravenous contrast material. Experimental work with organ-specific contrast agents has been performed. These agents include a poppy seed oil emulsion and a water-soluble iodinated compound, iosefamate meglumine, but have not been used in children.

Vessels

Contrasted against the liver parenchyma in unenhanced scans are the portal and hepatic veins, which are visualized as branching linear or rounded areas of lower attenuation. The hepatic veins are noted to increase in size as they course superiorly and posteriorly to their junction with the inferior vena cava. The portal veins are recognized as they branch out from the main portal vein as it enters the porta hepatis. The left portal vein courses anteriorly and lies more cranial than the right portal vein, which courses horizontally and to the right, where it divides into anterior and posterior divisions. The veins of the liver show greater enhancement than the liver parenchyma following intravenous contrast administration. The obliterated left umbilical vein courses in the ligamentum teres to the left branch of the portal vein.

In unenhanced scans normal hepatic arteries and intrahepatic bile ducts are not visualized in children. Rapid bolus injection of intravenous contrast material will delineate the hepatic artery as it courses from the celiac artery to enter the porta hepatis anterior to the main portal vein. For a description of the bile ducts see Chapter 13, p. 198.

Lobes

The classic left and right lobes of the liver are demarcated by the falciform ligament and fissure for the ligamentum teres. The falciform ligament is usually not clearly seen because of the apposition of the anterior surface of the liver to the peritoneum lining the inner aspect of the anterior abdominal wall. However, the ligament is visualized when ascitic fluid separates the liver from the abdominal wall. The fissure for the

ligamentum teres contains the obliterated left umbilical vein, which is surrounded by a variable amount of fat. With fast high-resolution scanners the fissure can be visualized in most children, including young infants.

From a surgical standpoint the classic division of the liver is not practical, and a "surgical subdivision" of the liver is necessary. The classic left lobe of the liver (i.e., all the liver to the left of the fissure for the ligamentum teres) is considered to be the lateral segment of the left lobe. The medial segment of the left lobe extends from the ligamentum teres to the right and is demarcated on the right by a major lobe fissure which cannot be seen on the external surface of the liver but can be imagined as a line extending obliquely down from the fossa for the inferior vena cava to the gallbladder. A major hepatic vein courses through this fissure. The porta hepatis divides this medial segment into anterior and posterior portions. Anteriorly the quadrate lobe of the liver lies between the gallbladder to the right and the ligamentum teres to the left. Posterior to the porta hepatis lies the caudate lobe.

This anatomical arrangement is of surgical importance because focal lesions of the right lobe of the liver that extend into the medial segment of the left lobe may still be resectable (i.e., trisegmentectomy). Extension beyond the ligamentum teres into the lateral segment makes the lesion inoperable.

Pathology

Diffuse Parenchymal Disease

The use of CT and sonography in diffuse parenchymal disease of the liver is somewhat limited [13, 20, 24, 32]. CT and sonographic changes in cirrhosis have previously been documented [13, 18, 24]. Cirrhosis may often cause no detectable alteration of the liver on CT [20, 31]. Changes that have been described in cirrhosis include changes in size, shape, and attenuation of the liver [18, 24]. The size of the liver will vary depending on the stage of the disease process and will be small in the end stages of cirrhosis [4, 18]. Occasionally, the right lobe of the liver will decrease in size dramatically, and the caudate lobe will become unduly prominent [13, 31]. Harbin et al. [13] consider the ratio of the measurements of the caudate and right lobes of

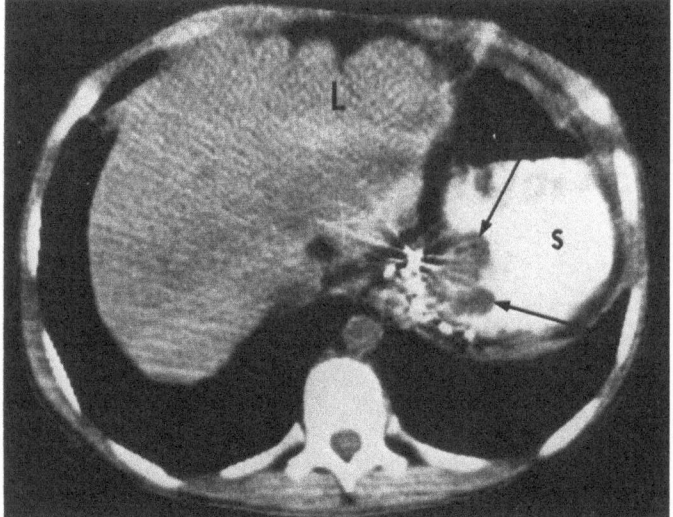

Fig. 12.1. An 18-year-old girl with cystic fibrosis and previous splenectomy and Segura procedure for bleeding esophageal varices. CT performed to exclude an upper abdominal abscess postoperatively reveals cirrhosis with marked lobulation of the anterior aspect of the liver (*L*). *s*, Gastrografin-filled stomach. *Long arrows* indicate residual varices which appear as filling defects at the gastroesophageal junction. The high-attenuation material medial to this is due to surgical clips.

the liver to be the most useful and accurate means that radiologists have available for making the diagnosis of cirrhosis on CT. The value of this ratio has not been established in children.

Regenerating nodules may give a lobulated outline to the liver [4, 18, 20, 31], and CT may be helpful in defining the nature of these nodules in cases showing defects of isotope uptake on technetium sulfur colloid liver/spleen scans. Regenerating nodules have the same attenuation as the surrounding liver (Fig. 12.1).

The attenuation of the liver in cirrhosis is usually normal [18, 31] but may be slightly decreased in a nonspecific uniform manner [4, 24, 31]. Occasionally, the decrease in attenuation may not be uniform and is more circumscribed [24, 30]. This appearance may thus simulate that produced by a focal lesion of the liver (e.g., neoplastic disease or abscesses). These focal changes in cirrhosis, which were first described by Mulhern et al. [24], may vary in response to the administration of intravenous contrast agents, depending on their vascularity; they indicate that fatty metamorphosis and other changes of cirrhosis are not always uniform. The attenuation of the liver will change more dramatically in cases with fatty infiltration and in hemochromatosis related to iron deposition in the liver [4, 20, 24, 31]. Fatty infiltration leads to a lowering of liver attenuation, the degree of lowering depending on the degree of fatty infiltration.

With minimal fat infiltration the attenuation of the liver will decrease but may retain its positive values. With greater deposition of fat the attenuation will be negative (i.e., less than water attenuation). In this situation the venous structures of the liver will have a higher attenuation than the surrounding liver and will appear as if they have been enhanced by intravenous contrast administration (see Fig. 12.3). Iron deposition leads to a marked increase in liver attenuation.

Children with hemolytic anemia on long-term transfusion programs develop increased visceral iron stores known as transfusional hemochromatosis. This is commonly seen in children with β-thalassemia (Fig. 12.2). It has been shown that hepatic CT numbers correlate with hepatic iron content from biopsies [4, 27]. The iron is not only deposited in the liver but also in the spleen, lymph nodes (see Fig. 8.7, p. 97), pancreas (see Fig. 9.4, p. 110), and kidneys (see Fig. 11.8, p. 153).

Desferrioxamine is a chelating agent that has been used at many centers to remove iron from viscera in an attempt to prevent or reverse complications related to increased iron stores. In 1984, Olivieri et al. [27] reported their experience with serial CT scans in 30 transfusion-dependent patients with thalassemia major who were receiving subcutaneous desferrioxamine. The study was designed to measure the efficacy of desferrioxamine and to assess whether the liver attenuation values could be used as a predictor of cardiac dysfunction, which is the major cause for death in these patients. In addition to regular cardiac assessment, serial serum ferritin levels were also measured at 3-month intervals.

The CT scans were performed with the follow-

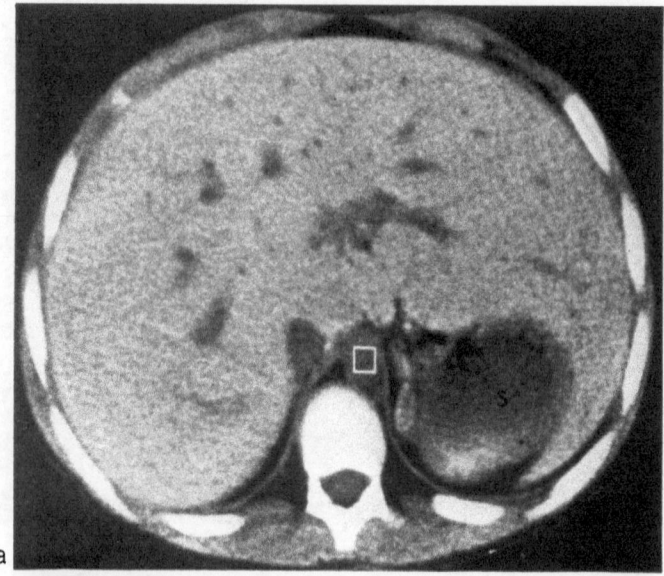

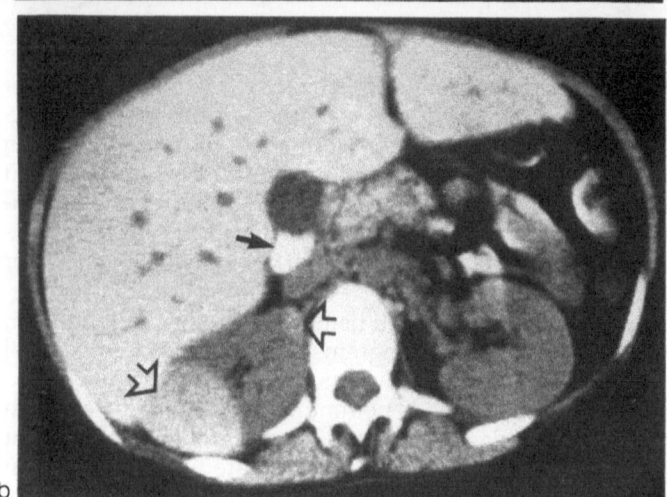

Fig. 12.2a,b. Examples of diffuse increased attenuation of the liver caused by iron deposition (hemachromatosis) as a result of chronic blood transfusions in patients with thalassemia. The increased attenuation of the liver can be appreciated by comparing its attenuation with that of the adjacent abdominal wall muscles. In the patient illustrated in **a** the spleen has been removed and there is marked hepatomegaly with the left lobe passing lateral and posterior to the stomach (*s*). In **b** note also the presence of gallstones (*arrow*) and the areas of high attenuation within the kidney (*open arrows*). The high-attenuation areas in the kidney may be related to iron deposition, but this has not been proven.

ing technique. Four scan levels through the liver were chosen from an initial scout radiograph. These scans were 1 cm thick and 2 cm apart and we ensured that no artifact crossed the liver to interfere with the measurement of the CT numbers. If some artifact was present, one or two further scans would be performed. Hepatic CT numbers were measured with the cursor set at 0.77×0.77 cm in size, and five areas were measured on each scan. The 20 numbers from the 4 scans were averaged, and this number represented the hepatic CT number in Hounsfield units for that patient. Serial examinations were performed 1 year apart. From our findings we divided our patients into two groups. Those in whom the hepatic CT numbers decreased from the first to the second examination and those in whom the hepatic CT numbers remained unchanged.

There were 18 patients in whom the hepatic CT numbers decreased and the mean decrease was from 93 to 76 HU, with a P value of under 0.001. There was a concomitant decline in the mean serum ferritin in all of these patients, with a mean decline from 3800 to 1700 mg/ml, with a P value of under 0.001. All 18 patients have maintained stable cardiac status during the time of observation and in a 12-month follow-up period.

These findings indicate that a decreased hepatic CT number which reflects a decrease in hepatic iron is related to a preservation of cardiac function, suggesting that there is a symmetrical reduction of iron from both the liver and the heart in those patients on desferrioxamine chelation.

There were 12 patients in whom the hepatic CT numbers remained unchanged and in 10 of these this result correlated with no change in the serum ferritin level. Five of these patients have developed cardiac dysfunction.

It is highly significant that in two of these patients with no change in hepatic CT numbers the serum ferritin did decrease significantly, with a P value of under 0.001. Both of these patients have developed cardiac dysfunction over the period of therapy. This suggests that in the majority of patients on desferrioxamine chelation the hepatic CT numbers closely parallel the changes in serum ferritin. However, in a minority of patients when the CT and serum ferritin values are discordant the hepatic CT numbers appear to reflect the effectiveness of chelation more accurately than serum ferritin, that is, the elevated hepatic CT number is associated with the persistence of cardiac iron stores and development of cardiac dysfunction. We therefore cannot observe patients with a declining serum ferritin with complacency if hepatic CT numbers remain high.

Magnetic resonance imaging is capable of showing changes in the liver related to increased iron deposition. It is possible that magnetic resonance imaging may well provide more detailed information regarding iron content within the heart than the indirect methods that we have used with hepatic CT numbers and should be pursued. Direct measurement of attenuation values in the heart is difficult with ungated CT images.

Increased hepatic attenuation has been reported in other conditions. In glycogen storage disease the liver attenuation may be increased, but associated fat deposition makes attenuation values in these patients variable [4]. Berger and Kuhn [4] reported increased size and attenuation of the liver in three children with Crohn's disease following introduction of hyperalimentation. This change was transient. These authors suggested that in such patients there may be a massive deposition of amino acids and protein in the liver, which may not be able to handle the load.

At the Hospital for Sick Children, Toronto, we have occasionally used CT to study the upper abdomen in children and young adults with cystic fibrosis in whom upper abdominal inflammatory processes are suspected, particularly postoperatively. The changes that we have noted in the liver have been quite variable in these patients. This reflects the variable degree of hepatic involvement seen in these patients. However, it tends to be more severe in older patients with cystic fibrosis. Changes in hepatic attenuation may be diffuse as a result of fatty infiltration (Fig. 12.3) or patchy and more focal (Fig. 12.4) reflecting more inhomogeneous involvement. Such changes in the liver on CT are not always associated with clinical manifestations of liver disease. Other changes of cirrhosis such as nodularity of the liver may also be seen (see Fig. 12.1) as well as changes resulting from portal hypertension (e.g., collaterals and varices) (see Fig. 12.1).

Lower attenuation of hepatic parenchyma may also be seen in patients with severe malnutrition, those receiving exogenous steroids, and in association with chemotherapy for malignant disease [1, 4]. We have seen children on treatment for malignant disease who have been noted to have focal areas of lower attenuation within the liver on follow-up scans. These areas usually have an irregular margin. Similar changes have been reported on radionuclide liver/spleen scans [1]. These changes are due to therapy and should not be confused with metastatic disease. Our patients have been well at the time of the scan, and the defects have been noted to resolve spontaneously if they are related to chemotherapy (see Fig. 12.19).

Changes caused by radiotherapy may also be seen if the liver is included in the radiation field. The area involved assumes a lower attenuation than the normal hepatic parenchyma and its margin is usually straight, reflecting the radiation portal (see Fig. 12.21).

Berger and Kuhn [4] have reported the CT findings in two children with congenital hepatic fibrosis. The etiology of this condition is unknown, and children usually present with gastrointestinal bleeding as a result of portal hypertension. Broad bands of fibrous tissue and small cysts are found in the liver. There is associated renal tubular ectasia. On CT, the fibrous bands appear as broad areas of low attenuation, and large areas of poor enhancement in the kidneys probably represent areas of poorly functioning tubules.

In 1983, Daneman et al. [8] reported an unusual appearance of enhancement of the liver on CT in a 7-month-old female with idiopathic

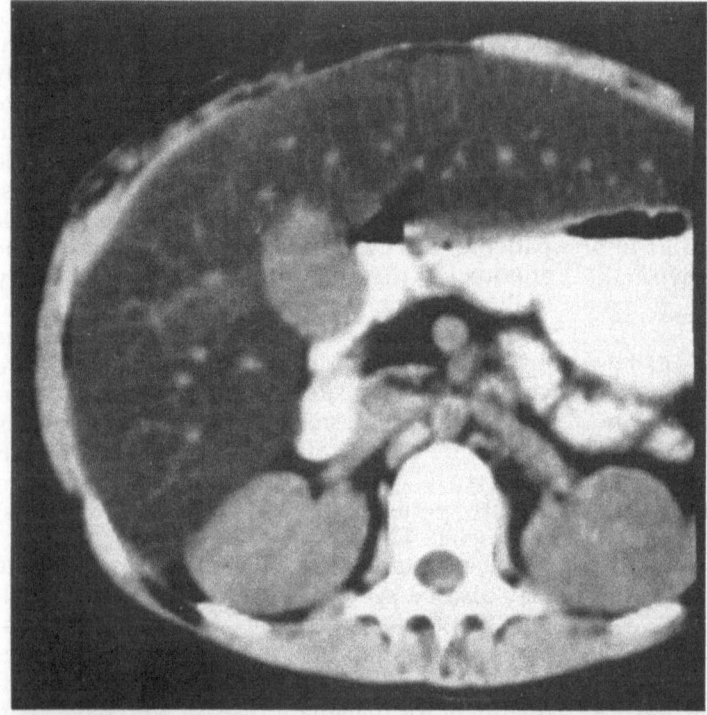

a

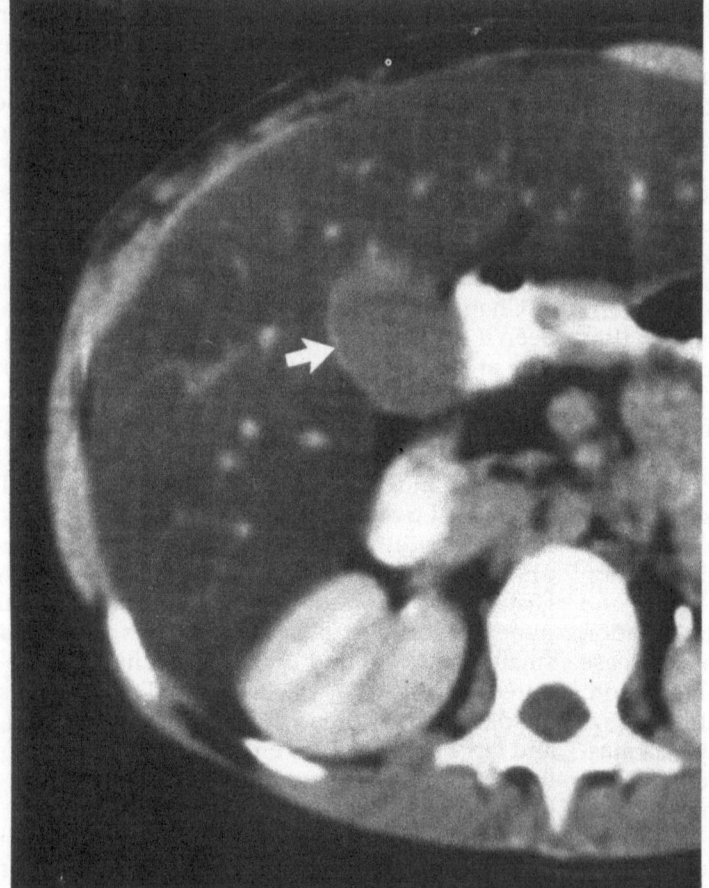

b

Fig. 12.3a,b. A 16-year-old boy with cystic fibrosis and diffuse fatty infiltration of the liver. Scans performed before (**a**) and after (**b**) intravenous injection of contrast material. Note the diffuse low attenuation of the liver. This is easily appreciated when one compares the liver parenchyma with the adjacent musculature. Even without contrast (**a**) the intrahepatic vessels and gallbladder have a higher attenuation than the liver. Under normal circumstances this would be reversed. After the injection of contrast (**b**) the liver has enhanced somewhat and the gallbladder wall (*arrow*) is easily visualized lying between the unenhanced bile within the gallbladder and the low-attenuation liver parenchyma.

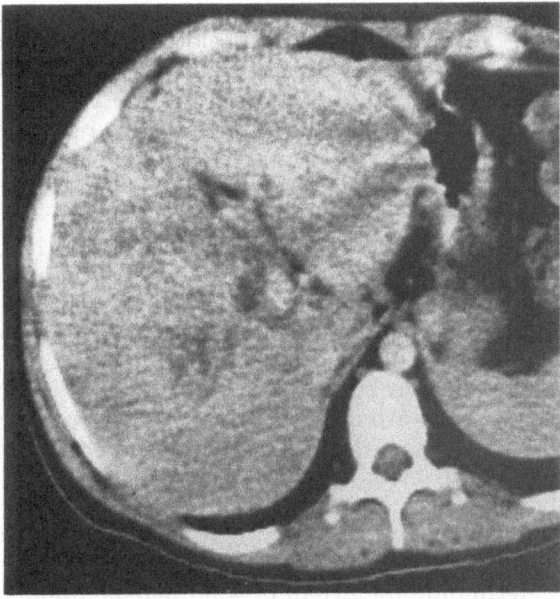

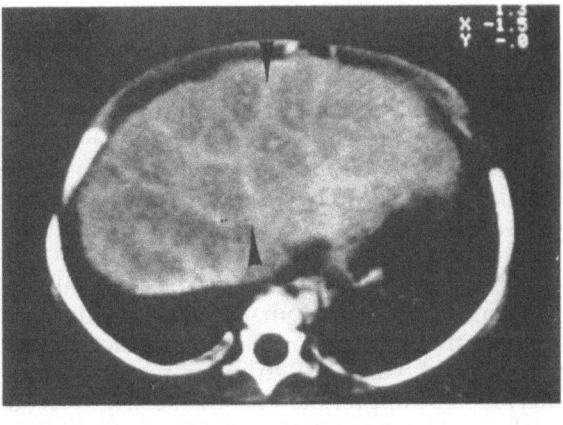

Fig. 12.5. A 7-month-old girl with mixed micro- and macronodular cirrhosis of unknown etiology. CT immediately after rapid bolus intravenous injection of contrast revealed bands of enhancing tissue (105 HU) (*arrows*) surrounding more extensive areas of lower attenuation (95 HU). The bands corresponded to highly vascular bands of fibrous tissue that were shown on liver biopsy. These surrounded areas of more normal liver parenchyma.

Fig. 12.4. A 17-year-old girl with cystic fibrosis. CT shows patchy areas of low attenuation within the right lobe of the liver. This is probably related to cirrhosis, with focal rather than diffuse changes.

cirrhosis. Precontrast scans showed the liver to have a normal homogeneous density throughout. Scans performed immediately after rapid bolus injection of contrast showed an uneven enhancement of the entire liver (Fig. 12.5). Bands of enhancing tissue surrounded more extensive areas that enhanced less markedly. Delayed postinjection scans revealed again an even level of attenuation throughout the liver. The liver biopsy in this patient revealed bands of fibrous tissue surrounding parenchymal nodules. We considered that the areas of greater enhancement on the scans performed immediately after bolus injection of contrast were related to the greater vascularity of these fibrous bands in comparison with the adjacent parenchymal nodules; equilibration of the density in the delayed scans after the injection of contrast was related to an even distribution of contrast material within the extracellular fluid in both the fibrous bands and the parenchymal nodule. This pattern of enhancement had not previously been described. Its diagnostic significance is uncertain and will only become clear if more patients with cirrhosis are scanned immediately after rapid bolus injection of contrast. This technique has been used in adults [21, 25], and similar but not identical changes have been noted in multicentric hepatic lesions [17].

Portal Hypertension

Portal hypertension in children may be due to extrahepatic or intrahepatic causes [3]. Occlusion of the portal vein is the commonest cause of extrahepatic obstruction in children. This is often not associated with sepsis or omphalitis [3]. Cirrhosis is the commonest cause of intrahepatic portal hypertension. This may be due to prenatal hepatic infection, cystic fibrosis, Wilson's disease, cholangitis, and Gaucher's disease [3].

Portal hypertension may produce changes on abdominal CT scans. These signs may be useful signs of underlying disease processes which may aid in the management of such children. However, most of these changes are also visible on sonography and CT is thus not the primary modality for the investigation of such patients. Changes seen on CT include the presence of ascites, splenomegaly, and enlargement of superior mesenteric vein and collateral veins, including esophageal and gastric varices and the umbilical vein.

Ascites is easily documented on CT (see Chap. 17, p. 268). Fluid may accumulate in any of the recesses of the peritoneal cavity. Although minor degrees of splenomegaly are difficult to appreciate on CT, more marked splenomegaly is easily appreciated (see Chap. 14, p. 209).

Measurements of the portal vein and its tributaries on CT have not been done in children. It has been suggested that the diagnosis of portal hypertension can be made when the diameter of the superior mesenteric vein is 2.5 times that of the superior mesenteric artery. Esophageal and gastric varices will be better appreciated when these viscera are distended with dilute contrast material (see Fig. 12.1). The varices appear as rounded soft tissue densities projecting into the contrast material. Barium studies and endoscopy remain the methods of choice for detecting the presence of varices. Retroperitoneal collaterals may also be appreciated on CT (see Fig. 9.11) as well as dilatation of the umbilical vein in the ligamentum teres. We have also used CT to document the presence of cavernous transformation of the portal vein in a boy with portal hypertension in whom bowel gas made delineation of this area impossible on sonography.

Berger and Kuhn [4] have described stretching and distortion of the intrahepatic portal veins in portal hypertension. Hepatic changes caused by underlying cirrhosis may also be noted (see above).

Masses

General Introduction

Hepatic masses are less common than renal and adrenal masses in children. There have thus been few reports describing the CT appearances of hepatic masses in childhood [16, 19, 22, 23]. Benign mass lesions include cysts, mesenchymal hamartomas, abscesses, cavernous hemangiomas/hemangioendotheliomas, adenomas (associated with glycogen storage disease), focal nodular hyperplasia, and hematomas. Malignant lesions include hepatoblastomas, hepatocellular carcinomas, rhabdomyosarcomas, undifferentiated small cell sarcomas, lymphomas/leukemia, and metastases.

Primary malignant hepatic lesions are the third commonest abdominal neoplasms in children, exceeded only by Wilms' tumors and neuroblastomas. Malignant masses are more common than benign hepatic masses. The child with an hepatic mass may be otherwise perfectly well, and a minority appear ill with anemia or weight loss [3]. The treatment of choice with all primary malignant lesions is complete surgical resection. Radiation and chemotherapy can give palliation but are incapable of producing a cure.

The prognosis of these lesions depends on the size and location of the lesion. Radiographic studies are thus extremely important not only for characterization of the lesion but more importantly for the delineation of their site of origin and extent.

The surgical divisions of the liver have been described in the section of hepatic anatomy (see p. 173). The importance of this division is to help one decide preoperatively whether a focal mass is resectable or not.

Hepatic angiography has been used extensively to define the extent of hepatic neoplasms. Failure to reveal the true extent may be due to the presence of arterial and portal vessels crossing the fissure separating the medial segment of the left lobe from the right [4]. Even at surgery it may be difficult to determine whether a tumor of the left lobe extends into the right, or vice versa.

We have found that CT is extremely useful in determining the extent of solid hepatic tumors. The relationship of the mass to the imaginary line joining the inferior vena cava to the gallbladder and the intersegmental fissure of the left lobe containing the obliterated umbilical vein can be easily documented on transverse CT images. We have found that it is far more reliable to ascertain this information on CT than with sonography. Our experience indicates that sagittal and coronal reconstruction images do not add significant information to the transverse images in this regard.

Several previous reports from the Hospital for Sick Children, Toronto, have documented the experience with benign and malignant hepatic mass lesions at our institution [10, 11, 12, 26]. In 1985, Liu et al. [19] reviewed the radiographic findings in 45 children with hepatic masses at our institution. In this study it was found that plain films of the abdomen and excretory urograms were usually nonspecific. Excretory urography may show an intrinsic abnormality in the kidneys, but the renal pathology can usually also be shown with other modalities. Excretory urography thus plays no role in the evaluation of hepatic masses.

Radionuclide sulfur colloid liver/spleen scans are very sensitive and were able to detect all the lesions in our patients. However, the findings are essentially nonspecific. Gallium is taken up by both tumor and inflammatory tissues. The gallium scan provides nonspecific information about the liver lesion itself, although it may show uptake by extrahepatic tumor tissue. This test, however, is somewhat cumbersome, usually requiring delayed scanning at least 24 and 48 h after administration of gallium. Furthermore, the presence of normal gallium activity in the colon can complicate the scan interpretation. In our study the gallium scan missed an abscess in the left lobe. If communication between a liver lesion and the biliary tract is suspected, it may be documented by a ^{99m}Tc-IDA scan.

Sonography has many advantages in pediatrics and should be the initial imaging study used in children with suspected hepatic or upper abdominal masses. It is noninvasive, does not involve radiation, can be quickly performed with real-time equipment, and is relatively inexpensive. This modality can document whether the mass is indeed within the liver and is also useful for documentation of the character and extent of the mass. In some children (e.g., those with hepatic abscesses or cysts) the sonogram may be the definitive investigation as the appearances may be diagnostic in the clinical context. Sonography detected the lesion in 39 of the 40 cases in which it was used and suggested the diagnosis in 16. CT detected all the 38 lesions studied with this modality but gave more information regarding the extent of the lesion than other modalities in 17.

In 1984, Brunelle and Chaumont [6] compared the sonographic and angiographic findings in benign and malignant hepatic lesions (excluding hemangioendothelioma). Although benign and malignant tumors could not be distinguished by their echo pattern, differentiation was possible provided attention was given to the appearance of the intrahepatic vessels on sonography. In all six benign lesions sonography demonstrated a patent portal system despite compression by the tumor. Partial amputation of intrahepatic portal branches was noted in all 16 patients with malignant lesions. These features should also be assessed on CT scans performed during intravenous contrast injection.

It is difficult to assess whether CT is more sensitive than sonography in the detection of small hepatic masses. Meticulous technique is essential to detect such lesions with either modality. In our series, CT detected small hepatic metastases that were missed by sonography in only one patient. However, our impression is that CT performed during rapid bolus infusion of intravenous contrast material will enable one to visualize small lesions more easily than with sonography [19]. Several other children with tiny hepatic lesions (e.g., metastases) missed by both sonography and CT and found only at operation were not included in our series.

At the present time (excluding magnetic resonance imaging) CT gives the best definition of the extent of liver lesions [19]. Hence, if surgical resection of a liver tumor is contemplated, CT should be done, even if sonography is available. With the newer generation scanners the relative lack of body fat in the pediatric age group is not a significant factor in the definition of liver pathology. Optimal CT scan technique is most important [15, 19], including adequate sedation of patients if necessary, performance of both pre- and postenhancement scans, intravenous bolus contrast enhancement, and use of 5- to 10-mm thick cuts with a fast scan time (2 s per slice if possible). With these techniques, CT scanning should be able to define most liver lesions. In addition to giving the best definition of the extent of the mass, CT may show pathology elsewhere in the abdomen or chest, as it is not organ specific. Within the clinical context, the characteristic CT pattern of enhancement is also diagnostic in most hemangiomas [19].

With the advent of the newer modalities, the role of angiography as a diagnostic tool has diminished. Even though it did give additional information in seven of our cases, many of these patients had been examined with the earlier CT and sonographic equipment. In complicated cases, angiography would obviously still play a major role [19]. Its greatest use at the present time is to provide a preoperative "road map" of the abdominal vascular anatomy. Depending on the surgeon's preference, it may be performed in any case when resection is planned but most commonly for malignant lesions. It would also be valuable in cases of vascular pathology such as hepatic artery aneurysm [19] and for embolization techniques, particularly with large hemangiomas not responsive to more conservative therapy. Angiography did not supply any more information about the extent of lesions than the newer generation CT scans. Indeed, our surgeons usually determine operability of a mass based on the CT scan rather than the angiographic findings [19].

In 1985, Miller and Greenspan described their experience with benign and malignant hepatic mass lesions and proposed an integrated imaging approach to the child thought to have a hepatic mass [22]. These authors also proposed sonography as the initial modality. They recommended CT for further investigation of children with malignant lesions and nuclear medicine for those with benign lesions. Indeterminate lesions may be evaluated by either CT or scintigraphy, using the other modality to substantiate the findings [23].

Benign Masses

Cysts   Cysts of the liver are rare and may be solitary or multiple [9, 14, 28, 29]. Multiple small cysts of the liver may be seen in patients with polycystic renal disease as well as in tuberous sclerosis. Sonography is the modality of choice in the assessment of the liver and kidneys in these children, and CT is only worthwhile if sonography is equivocal.

We have recently studied three children with solitary congenital cysts of the liver. In a neonate with the Beckwith–Wiedemann syndrome a cyst projecting from the right lobe of the liver was found on routine abdominal sonography performed primarily to assess the kidneys. This was the only study performed preoperatively. In the other two patients CT was used to delineate the lesions more fully following sonography. Both lesions were well defined with contents of water attenuation. In one patient, a 2-year-old boy, the cyst projected down from the region of the porta hepatis. CT showed the close relationship of the cyst to the main portal vessels exquisitely and thus influenced the type of surgery that was undertaken (Fig. 12.6). In the other patient, an 8-month-old boy, the cyst extended right down into the pelvis (Fig. 12.7). We have only examined one patient, a 12-year-old girl, with a proven hydatid cyst (Fig. 12.8). Hydatid cysts tend to be well demarcated with contents of water attenuation (0–19 HU). In one of the congenital cysts and the hydatid cyst that we have studied, linear septations of higher attenuation were noted crossing the cysts.

Cystic Mesenchymal Hamartoma   Cystic mesenchymal (fibrovascular) hamartoma of the liver usually presents as an enlarging abdominal mass. The child is usually otherwise well. In 1981, Berger and Kuhn [4] reported the CT findings in three children with this lesion. The lesions were large multilocular cystic masses with intervening solid septa and variably sized solid components which enhanced strikingly after intravenous contrast administration. At the Hospital for Sick Children, Toronto, we have relied on sonography for the diagnosis and follow-up of these lesions and have not studied them with CT. The sonographic appearances reflect the multilocular cystic nature of the lesions.

Abscesses   At the Hospital for Sick Children, Toronto, hepatic abscesses are most commonly seen in children with congenital or acquired defects of the immunological mechanism. We have seen liver abscesses most often in patients with chronic granulomatous disease and leukemia. These abscesses may be fungal or pyogenic in origin. Amebic abscesses are exceedingly rare.

Sonography has been used in our department with great success as the initial modality for localization of hepatic abscesses and also as a guide to percutaneous drainage. CT has been used when the response to such therapy is not immediate. However, CT does appear to be somewhat more sensitive than sonography and has delineated small abscesses not seen on sonography. CT is valuable when sonography and radionuclide scans are negative and there is

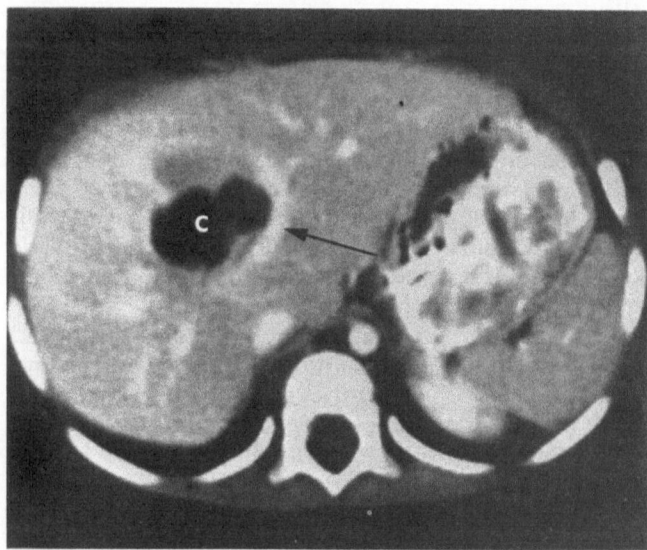

Fig. 12.6. A 12-year-old boy with congenital cyst of liver. CT shows the lobulated cyst (*c*) lying immediately adjacent to the area of the bifurcation of the portal vein. The left branch of the portal vein (*arrow*) lies along the medial aspect of the cyst. This anatomical delineation was important for operative planning.

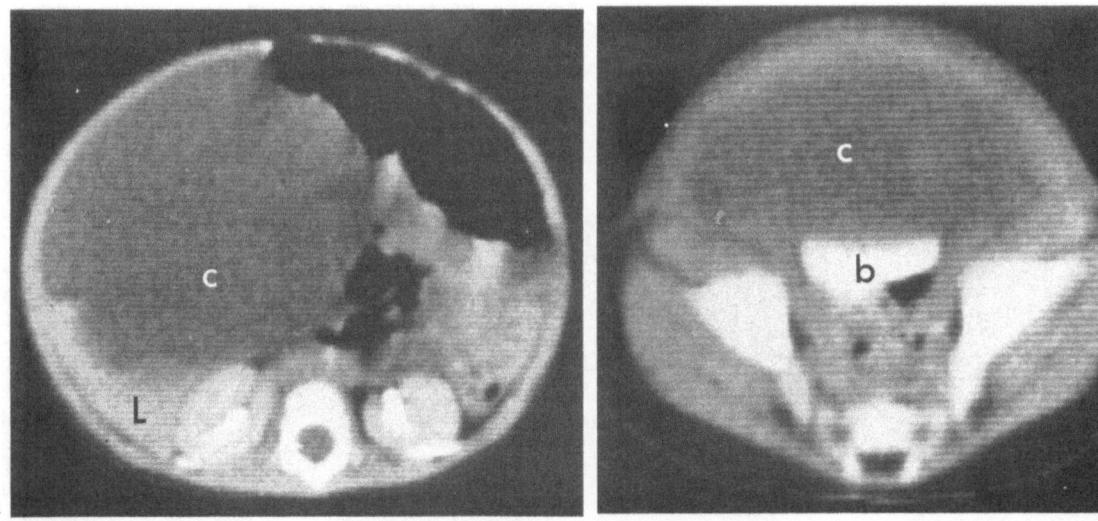

a

b

Fig. 12.7a,b. A 3-month-old boy with abdominal swelling. CT shows a huge cyst (*c*) off the inferior aspect of the right lobe of the liver (*L*). The cyst lies anterior to the bladder (*b*) in the pelvis.

still a strong clinical suspicion of hepatic abscess, and also for the delineation of multiple abscesses.

Abscesses appear as fairly well-defined rounded areas of low attenuation on CT (Fig. 12.9). Rim enhancement may be present along the periphery of the lesion following intravenous contrast administration. Surrounding enhancement of the hepatic parenchyma may be diffuse, indicating adjacent hepatic inflammation (Fig. 12.9). This change is far better appreciated than on sonography. Small bubbles of air not visible on plain radiographs may well be noted. Occasionally, in patients with chronic granulomatous disease areas of calcification within the hepatic parenchyma may be noted; these are due to previous healed abscesses (Fig. 12.10).

Unfortunately, ^{67}Ga scanning is a lengthy procedure but is useful in patients with persistent fever when no hepatic lesions are found on sonography or CT.

Cavernous Hemangioma/Hemangioendothelioma

Hemangioendothelioma (capillary hemangioma) usually presents as multiple discrete masses distributed throughout the liver (Fig. 12.11), whereas cavernous hemangioma presents as a single large mass lesion (Figs. 12.12, 12.13). The diagnosis of these lesions is often suspected clinically as the patient usually presents within the first weeks of life with a hepatic mass often with associated cardiac failure caused by the arteriovenous shunting or thrombocytopenia caused by platelet trapping. Rupture with hemo-

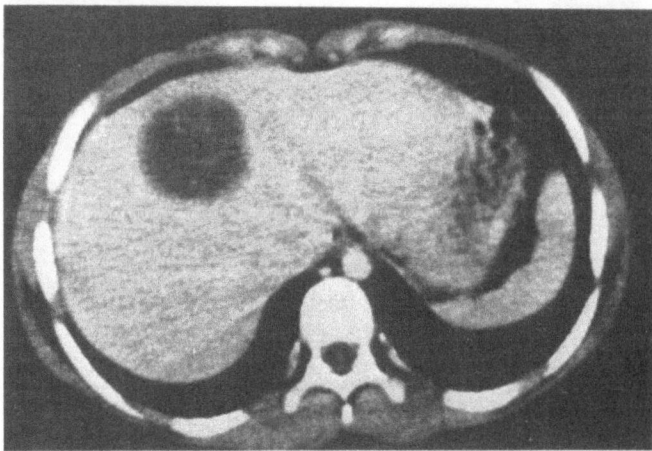

Fig. 12.8. Hydatid cyst of the liver in a 12-year-old girl. Note the higher attenuation linear strands within the cyst.

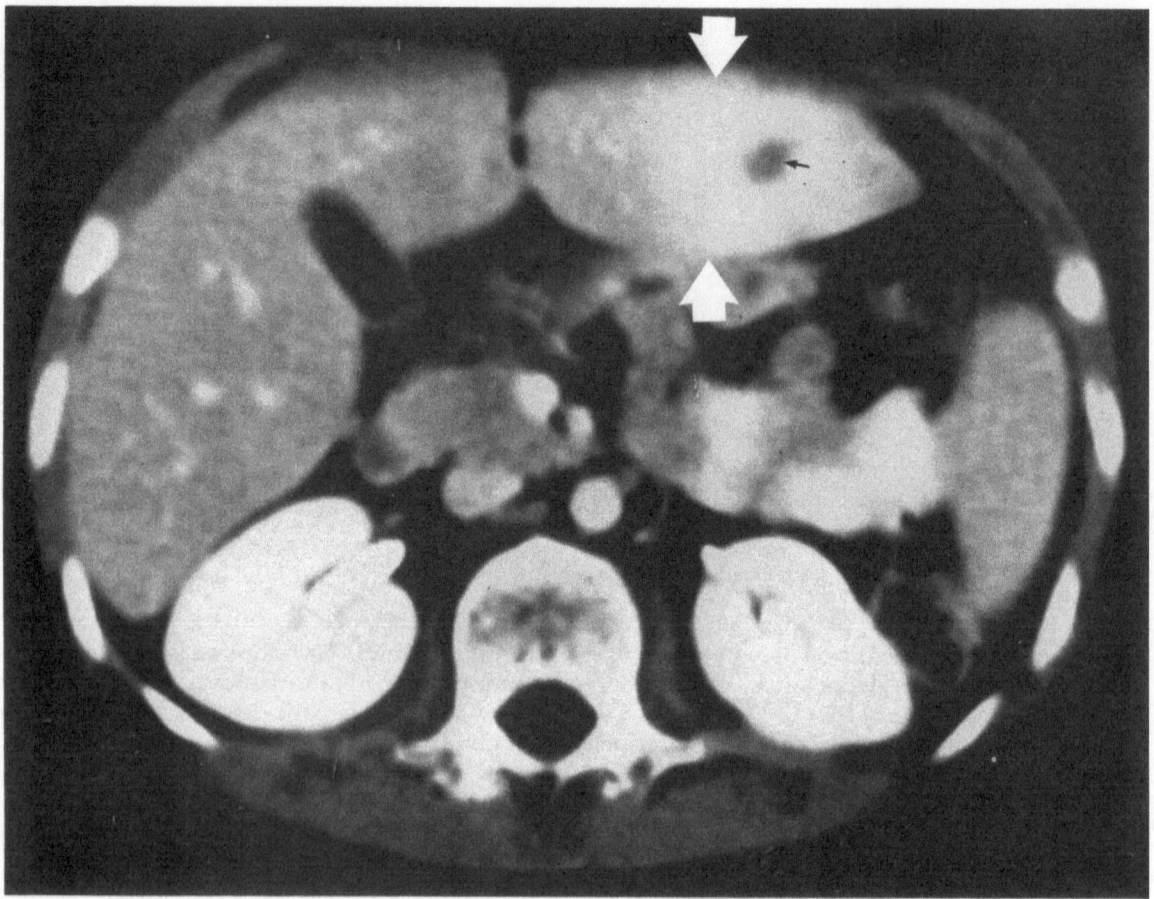

Fig. 12.9. A 6-year-old boy with immune deficiency and fever. CT shows marked swelling of the left lobe of the liver (*arrows*). Note the marked increased enhancement of this lobe compared with the remainder of the liver, which is due to the inflammation in this region. Centrally an area that fails to enhance represents a small abscess which was drained under CT control. The abscess was easily visualized with sonography, but this modality failed to delineate the extensive inflammatory changes in the remainder of the lobe that were so well shown with CT.

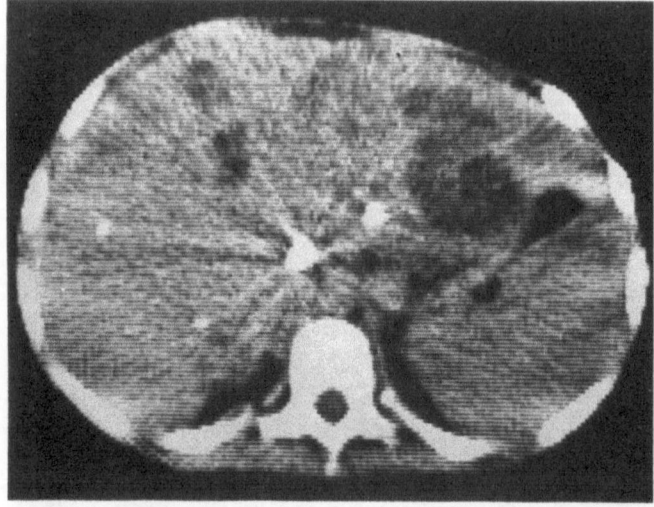

Fig. 12.10. A 12-year-old boy with chronic granulomatous disease. Note the irregular areas of lower attenuation within the liver caused by abscess formation. There are also four areas of much higher attenuation caused by calcification in old healed abscesses.

Fig. 12.11a,b. A neonate with multiple hemangiomas of the liver. The liver is enlarged. Scan **a** (without intravenous contrast enhancement) shows multiple masses within the liver which have lower attenuation values than the intervening parenchyma. Scan **b** (after intravenous contrast enhancement) shows marked enhancement, particularly along the peripheral portions of the masses. This is characteristic for these lesions and is more than that seen with metastatic neuroblastoma. (Courtesy of Dr. Albert Lam, Sydney, Australia)

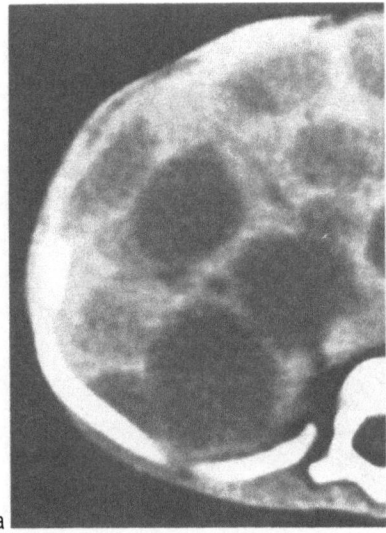 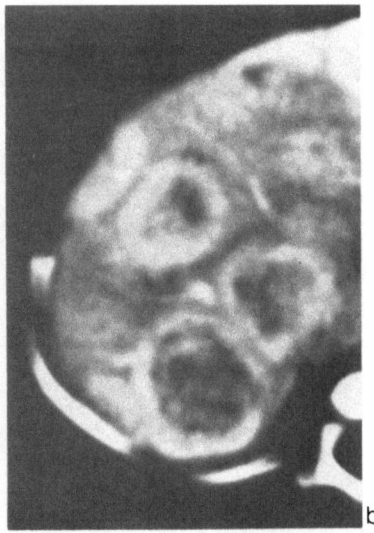

peritoneum may also occur. An abdominal bruit and cutaneous hemangiomas may also be present.

Sonography shows the single or multiple masses within the liver but may also detect enlargement of the aorta above the celiac trunk and enlargement of the hepatic artery and draining veins. The aorta below the celiac artery is usually very much smaller than that above. In the absence of the enlarged vessels radionuclide flow studies may be useful and may show increased perfusion of the lesion with cold defects on the static images. However, occasionally the flow pattern is not specific enough for a diagnosis to be made.

On CT these lesions have a homogeneous or inhomogeneous attenuation lower than that of the surrounding liver parenchyma (Figs. 12.11, 12.12, 12.13). During or immediately after intravenous contrast injection there is striking enhancement, usually of a band of tissue at the periphery of the lesion. However, enhancement may be extremely inhomogeneous throughout (see Fig. 12.12). Large vessels adjacent to the mass may also show striking enhancement (see Fig. 12.13). Delayed scans show rapid washout of the contrast from this peripheral area and increasing enhancement in the more central areas of the mass (see Fig. 12.13). The lesion may indeed become isodense with the liver [2, 15, 23]. However, this appearance is not specific for hemangioma as we have also seen this increase in central enhancement with time occur with hepatoblastoma. Central areas that fail to enhance may be due to hemorrhage. Calcifica-

tion may occasionally be seen at diagnosis but is more commonly encountered in follow-up sonographic studies.

Angiography is only necessary if the diagnosis cannot be made with the previously mentioned modalities and for embolization techniques if complications such as cardiac failure occur and the lesion is unresponsive to more conservative measures such as steroids. These lesions usually regress in 1–2 years. Sonography is the modality of choice for following this regression.

Adenoma   Adenomas of the liver in children are usually associated with type I glycogen storage disease. They have the potential for malignant degeneration. Occasionally, some adenomas may have increased attenuation [23] relative to the liver. This may in part be due to the fatty change in the liver parenchyma with concomitant lower attenuation. Other lesions have a lower central attenuation, often with variable contrast enhancement [23]. Adenomas of the liver are usually well defined and may be multiple. We have not had the opportunity to study these lesions with CT.

Focal Nodular Hyperplasia   Focal nodular hyperplasia most frequently occurs in young women and rarely in children. These lesions are similar to regenerating nodules. The attenuation varies, and the lesions may show enhancement which may be similar to that of the liver or may have areas of low attenuation [22]. They are usually well defined. We have not had the opportunity to study this type of lesion with CT.

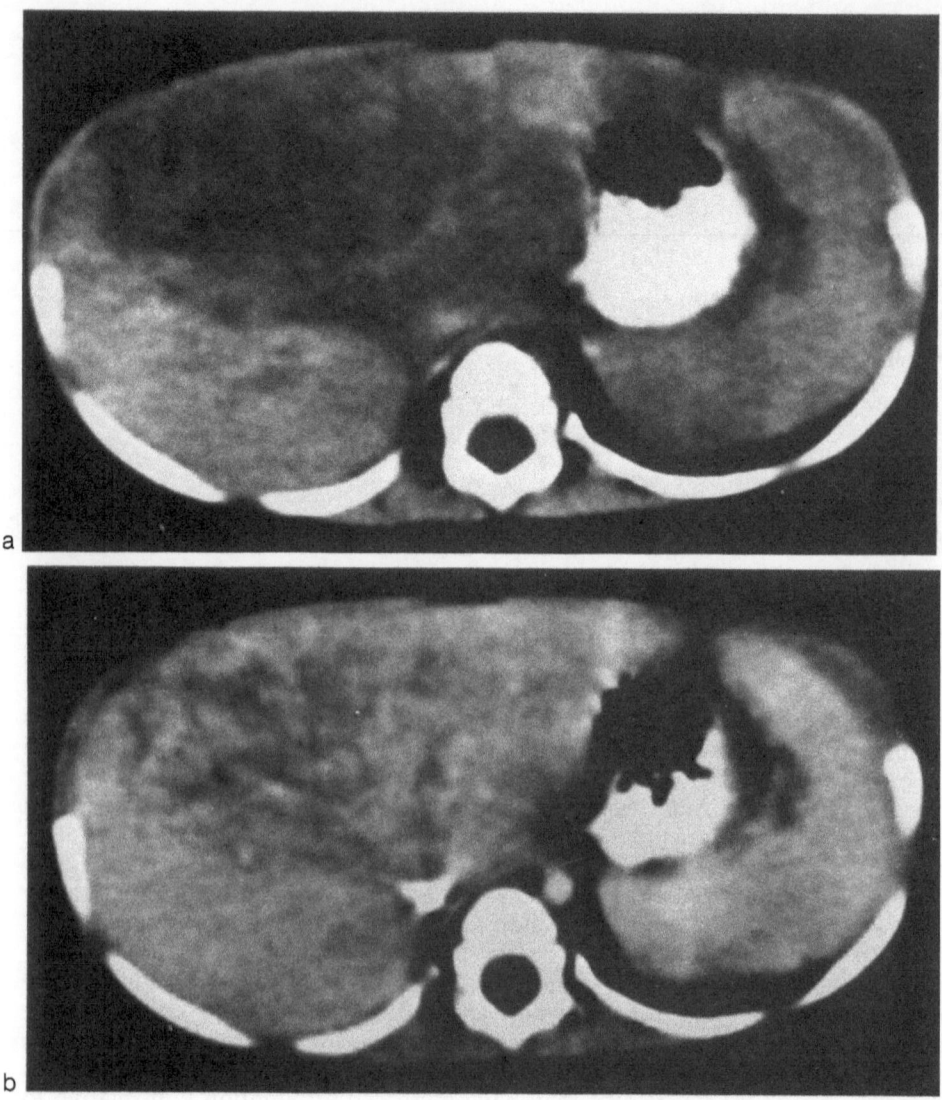

Fig. 12.12a,b. A 3-month-old girl with hepatomegaly. CT shows an irregular area of lower attenuation prior to contrast administration (**a**). Following contrast injection (**b**) the area has enhanced markedly but in an irregular manner. Biopsy proved this lesion to be a hemangioma of the liver.

Malignant Masses

The two commonest primary malignant lesions of the liver in children are hepatoblastoma and hepatocellular carcinoma.

Hepatoblastoma Hepatoblastoma is a poorly differentiated tumor which occurs in children under 3 years of age. The patients most commonly present with an abdominal mass and rarely have associated precocious puberty caused by HCG secretion by the tumor. These lesions are found with increased incidence in patients with Beckwith–Wiedemann syndrome or hemihypertrophy. One of our patients also had biliary atresia.

We have studied nine children with hepatoblastoma with CT. The features are relatively nonspecific. In all the cases the lesion was very easily visualized as an intrahepatic mass of lower attenuation than normal hepatic parenchyma and which enhanced slightly in an inhomogeneous manner (Figs. 12.14, 12.15b).

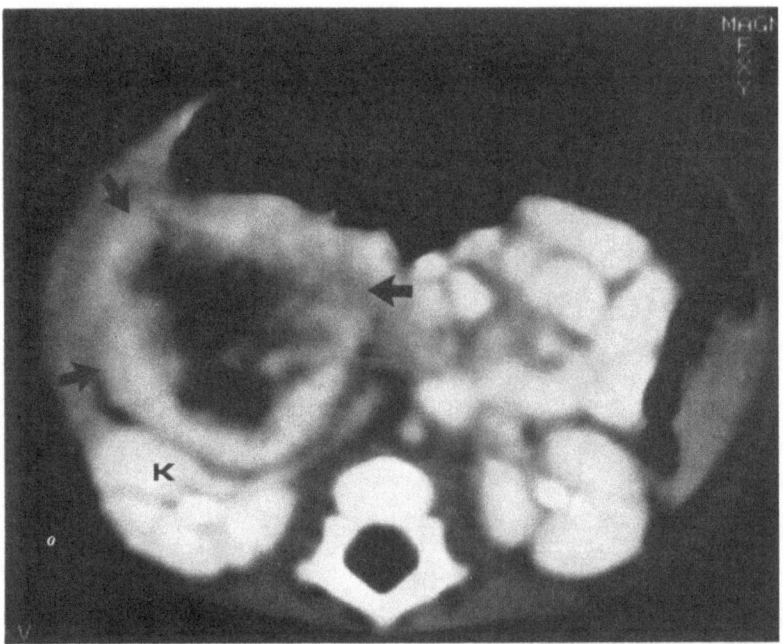

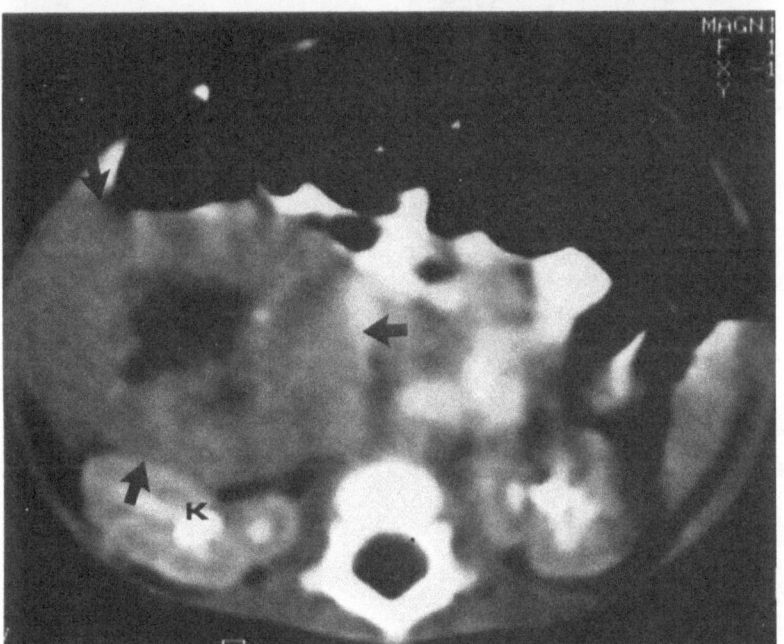

Fig. 12.13a,b. An 8-week-old girl with a right upper quadrant mass (*arrows*). Scan immediately after intravenous contrast injection (**a**) shows intense enhancement of periphery of mass. Delayed scan (**b**) shows decrease in intensity of the peripheral enhancement but progressive slight increased enhancement toward the centre of the mass. This mass was a hemangioma. *K*, kidney.

We have seen two patients in whom central enhancement increased with time similar to that described with hemangiomas. The margins of the lesion are often irregular and poorly defined. Occasionally, cystic lesions have been reported [22]. All of the lesions that we have studied have been solitary. Calcification was seen in two patients. This represents ossifying osteoid which is part of the lesion. Disruption of the adjacent vessels was seen in all patients.

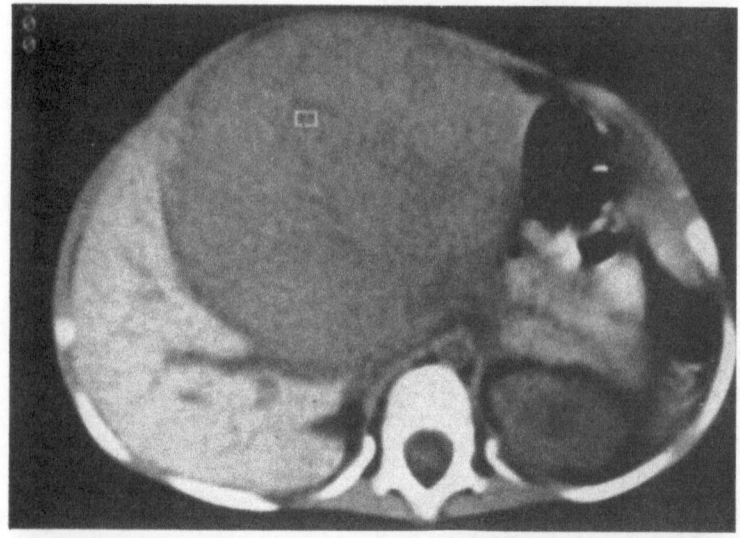

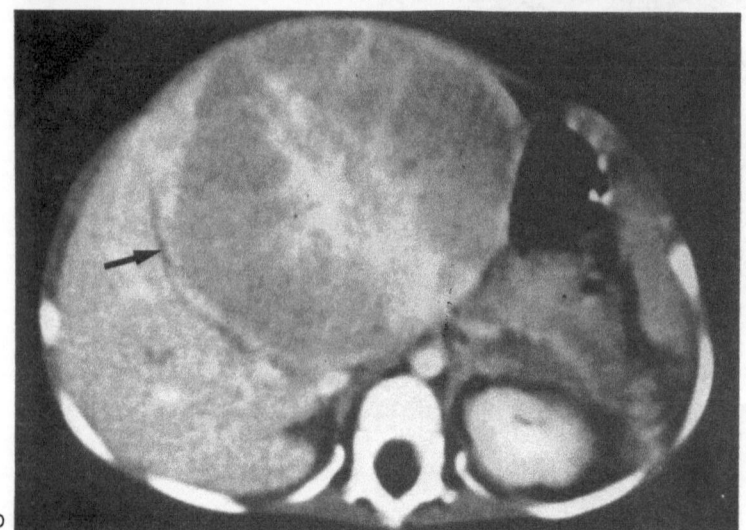

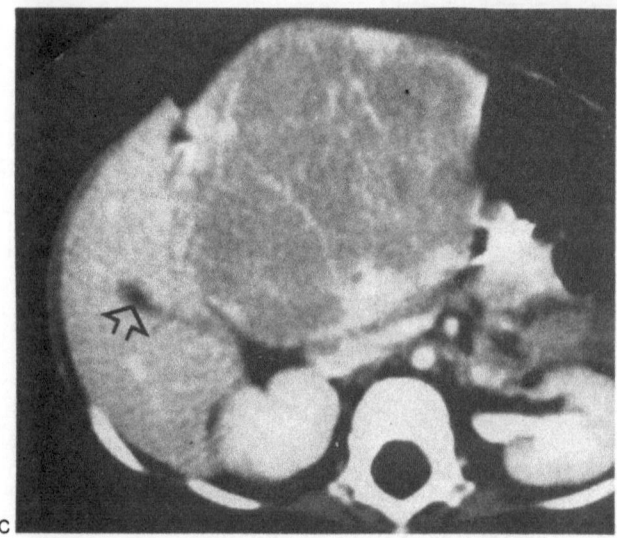

Fig. 12.14a–c. A 6-month-old boy with hepatoblastoma of the left lobe of the liver. The lesion is well defined and has an inhomogeneous attenuation which is lower than that of the adjacent liver before contrast injection (**a**). After contrast injection (**b** and **c**) the lesion has enhanced in an irregular manner, but the attenuation is still, for the most part, less than that of the liver. The ligamentum teres (*arrow* in **b**) demonstrates that this lesion is limited to the left lobe of the liver and is thus resectable. *Open arrow* (in **c**), gallbladder.

The extent of the lesion and its relationship to the major surgical boundaries in the liver must be established. Extrahepatic extension and biliary and portal obstruction may occasionally occur. CT may reveal extension of the tumor into the larger hepatic and portal veins and inferior vena cava. This vascular extension is better assessed with real-time sonography.

The extent of these lesions has been exquisitely defined by our newer 4-s and 2-s CT scanners, and surgical planning of these patients has been based primarily on the CT information. In this regard, CT has proved to be the single most useful modality for the delineation of the extent of these lesions at the time of diagnosis. However, invasion of the diaphragm may be difficult to predict with CT as the transverse axial images at the upper end of the mass cross the mass tangentially. Sagittal and coronal reconstruction images may not be helpful in this regard, and sonography may well provide more information regarding diaphragmatic infiltration with scans performed in the parasagittal plane.

Two of our patients have had preoperative chemotherapy to shrink a massive inoperable tumor. Following such chemotherapy CT may show not only a reduction in the size of the mass but also a change in the attenuation values if there is a good response to chemotherapy. Chemotherapy-induced necrosis causes more areas within the tumor to assume a lower attenuation. If the chest radiograph is normal, CT of the chest is mandatory at the time of diagnosis and also during follow-up as these lesions have a propensity to metastasize to the lung. Osseous and brain metastases are much less common.

Because of the possibility of local recurrence, CT has proved invaluable in the follow-up of children with previously resected hepatoblastoma. Following surgery the liver regenerates rapidly and often assumes a somewhat globular configuration. Following resections of the right lobe the hepatic flexure comes to lie high under the diaphragm behind the remaining liver. Following left lobe resection the stomach and transverse colon lie high in the midline. During large liver resections for any tumor the bile ducts may be damaged; this may necessitate choledochoenterostomy or lead to a postoperative bile leak. Postoperative scans may reveal gas in the biliary tree following choledochoenterostomy or a biloma caused by bile leaks (see Fig. 2.5, p. 16).

Hepatocellular Carcinoma Hepatocellular car-cinoma is a more mature lesion histologically and is less common in childhood than hepatoblastoma. These lesions usually occur in children over the age of 5 years. The incidence of carcinoma and adenoma is increased in children with glycogen storage disease and chronic liver disease. Three of our six recent patients with hepatocellular carcinoma were found to have the fibrolamellar variant, which has a somewhat better prognosis [5, 7].

We have performed CT in six children with hepatocellular carcinoma. The appearances of this neoplasm on CT were similar to those on hepatoblastoma. Hepatocellular carcinoma is seen as a lesion of low attenuation with variable enhancement (usually lower than that of the surrounding hepatic parenchyma) and margination. Ring enhancement has been described [23]. Calcification may occasionally be present. Extension into extrahepatic tissue tends to occur more commonly with hepatocellular carcinoma (Fig. 12.16). The CT appearances are thus nonspecific (Figs. 12.15a, 12.16, 12.17), and it may thus be impossible to differentiate hepatoblastoma from hepatocellular carcinoma based on the CT appearances alone. However, hepatocellular carcinoma tends to be multicentric in origin more commonly than hepatoblastoma. This was a distinguishing feature described by Miller and Greenspan [22]. The masses may indeed be confluent.

The commonest site for metastases is the chest. Chest CT is thus imperative at the time of diagnosis, if no lesions are noted on a plain chest radiograph, and also during follow-up. CT has proved important for the documentation of local extent and spread in the abdomen and chest at the time of diagnosis and during follow-up (Fig. 12.17) and for the documentation of postoperative changes (see Fig. 2.5, p. 16). Therefore, the value of CT for the management of patients with hepatocellular carcinoma is obvious.

Other Primary Neoplasms Other primary neoplasms of the liver are rare and may include small cell sarcomas and, rarely, rhabdomyosarcomas [22]. Their appearance on CT is nonspecific, and it is often impossible to differentiate them from the common primary neoplasms.

Metastases Metastases to the liver may occur with many childhood neoplasms [19, 23]. Neuroblastoma is the commonest neoplasm in childhood to have metastasized to the liver at the time of diagnosis (i.e., stage IV S neuroblastoma in neonates). We have found liver metastases on

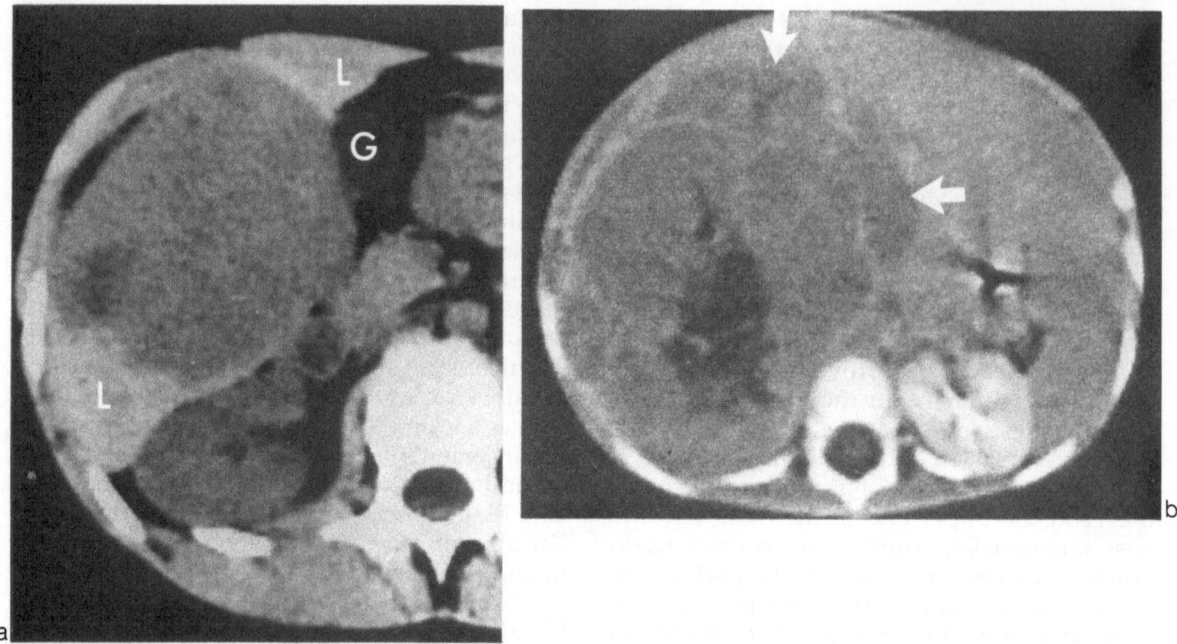

Fig. 12.15a,b. Examples of malignant lesions in right lobe of the liver. **a** Hepatocellular carcinoma of the right lobe of the liver with normal liver noted anteriorly and posteriorly. *G*, gallbladder; *L*, normal liver parenchyma. **b** Hepatoblastoma of right lobe of liver. The scan has been performed after intravenous contrast enhancement and shows inhomogeneous attenuation in the lesion. The margins between the lesion and the remainder of the liver are ill defined (*arrows*). On this single image it is impossible to know whether the lesion arises in the liver or infiltrates the liver from the right flank.

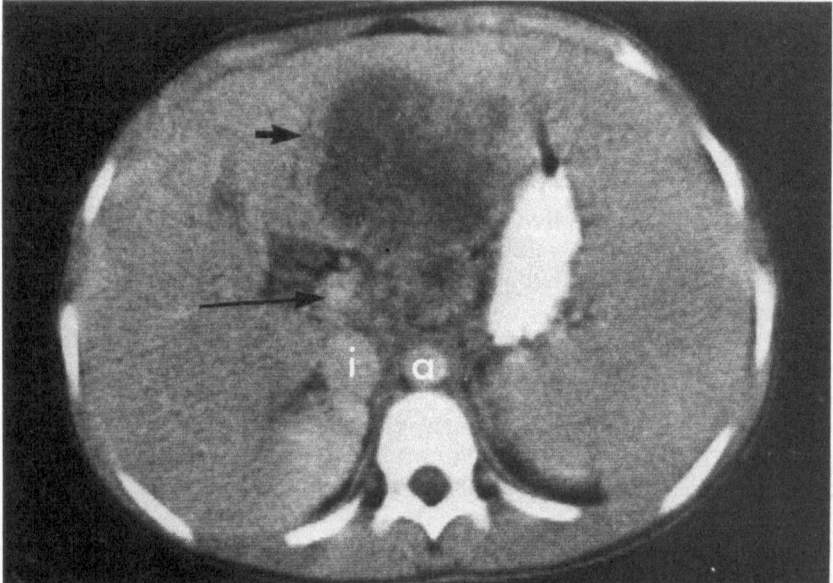

Fig. 12.16. A 12-year-old boy with hepatocellular carcinoma of the lateral segment of the left lobe of the liver. The lesion has a lower attenuation than the adjacent liver and does not cross to the right of the ligamentum teres (*short arrow*). However, the lesion infiltrates posteriorly toward the retroperitoneum. This was an important consideration preoperatively. *Long arrow*, portal vein; *i*, inferior vena cava; *a*, aorta.

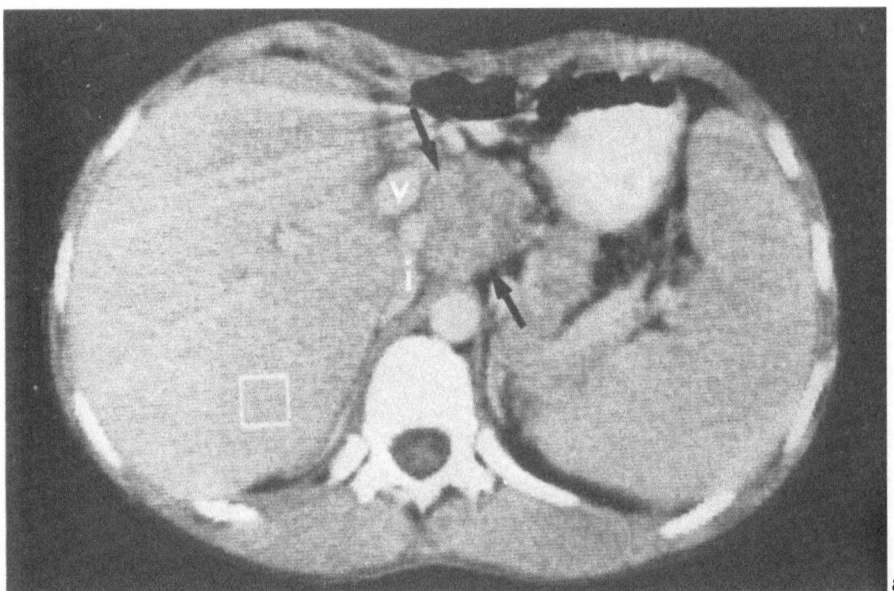

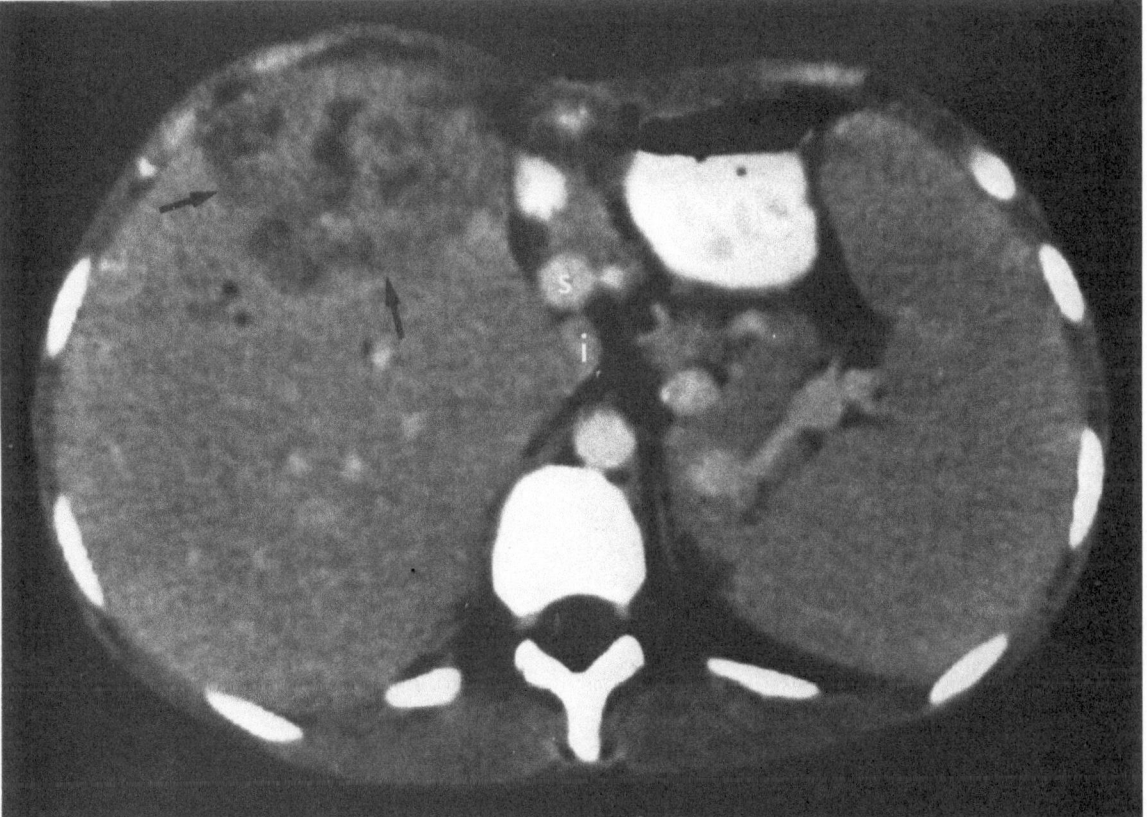

Fig. 12.17a–c. A 12-year-old boy with previously resected hepatocellular carcinoma of the left lobe of the liver together with metastases in lymph nodes above the diaphragm. **a** Follow-up CT shows a recurrent mass (*arrows*) in lymph nodes just to the right of the portal vein (*v*) and inferior vena cava (*i*). Note the distortion of the inferior vena cava and liver postoperatively. **b** Following resection of the recurrent mass this follow-up study shows a recurrence in the anterior aspect of the right lobe of the liver (*arrows*). Small rounded nonenhancing areas within the liver represent slightly dilated bile ducts resulting from early obstruction. *s*, superior mesenteric vein; *i*, inferior vena cava. **c** Chest CT at the same time reveals recurrent metastases in enlarged node (*N*) anterior to the heart (*H*). (**Fig. 12.17c** *overleaf*)

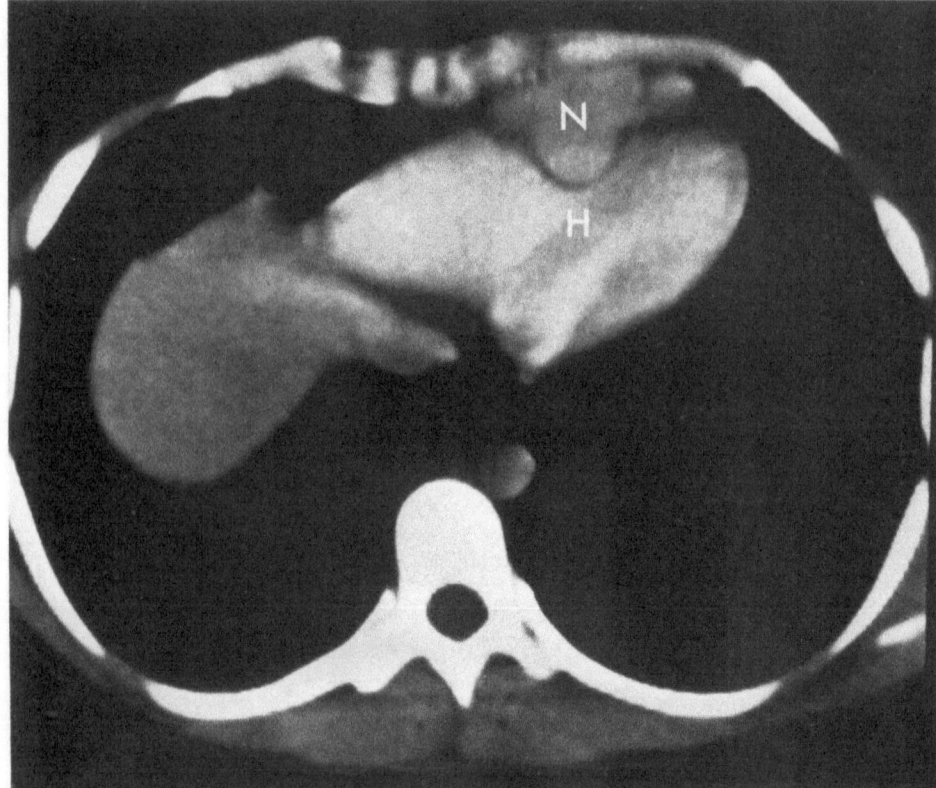

Fig. 12.17c

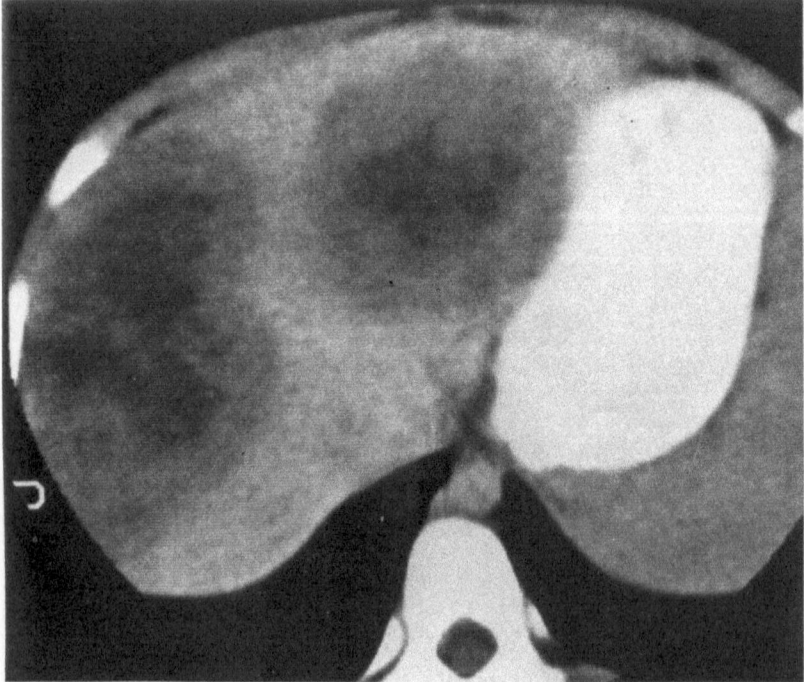

Fig. 12.18. A 10-year-old boy with left Wilms' tumor. CT shows two large metastatic lesions within the liver.

CT at the time of diagnosis in only one patient with Wilms' tumor, a child with renal cell carcinoma, and a boy with undifferentiated sarcoma. Liver metastases are more commonly found later in the disease process with a wider variety of childhood neoplasms.

Liver metastases have a lower attenuation and enhance less than normal liver (Fig. 12.18). They are therefore best visualized after the intravenous injection of contrast material. The contrast between liver and hepatic metastases is best viewed with narrow window settings, but varying settings should be used. Areas of even lower attenuation in the central portion of the metastases represent areas of necrosis (see also Fig. 11.19, p. 165, and Fig. 11.22, p. 167). This may give the lesion a bull's-eye appearance. The enhancing tissue at the periphery has a thick rind. With bolus dynamic scanning techniques lesions as small as a few millimeters have been detected. Calcification may be present in metastases from neuroblastoma or from carcinoma of the gastrointestinal tract [23]. Neuroblastoma may produce extensive replacement of hepatic parenchyma (see Fig. 10.6, p. 132, and Fig. 10.7, p. 133). Ring enhancement may be seen [23].

It has been our experience that CT is more sensitive and diagnoses more and smaller metastases than both radionuclide liver/spleen scanning and sonography. It is this author's view that a radionuclide liver/spleen scan is redundant if an abdominal CT scan is being performed with contrast enhancement to assess a patient with known malignancy at diagnosis or during follow-up. However, no large study has yet been performed to determine the relative accuracy of radionuclide liver/spleen scans, CT, and sonography in the detection of hepatic metastases in children.

Neuroblastoma and Wilms' tumor may both spread directly into the liver. It may be difficult with CT to determine whether spread has occurred or whether this tumor is just in apposition to the liver (see Chap 16, p. 251). The transverse axial CT images cut the tumor tangentially at the tumor–liver interface and may give a false impression of invasion (see Fig. 16.3, p. 253). Sonography is often very useful in determining spread: Longitudinal scans may show a clear line of demarcation between the lesion and the liver, and images viewed in real time will reveal whether the liver moves independently of the mass or not.

The liver should always be thoroughly assessed in children with lymphoma undergoing abdominal CT. Detection of lymphoma in the liver is difficult with any imaging modality. On CT, lymphomatous deposits appear as focal areas of low attenuation with varying shapes and margination (Fig. 12.19). The lesions may be solitary or multiple. Leukemic involvement of the liver frequently causes a nonspecific hepatomegaly together with splenomegaly. It may be difficult to document focal leukemia involvement with CT when this is shown sonographically and with scintigraphy [23].

Trauma

CT and hepatic scintigraphy are reliable methods of detecting traumatic lesions of the liver in children (see also Chap. 16, p. 264). Despite the fact that scintigraphy is somewhat limited as it is organ specific, we have used this modality with great success in many children when only a liver injury is suspected. However, in severe blunt abdominal trauma, particularly when trauma to multiple organ systems is suspected, CT is a better modality as all structures in the abdomen can be exquisitely displayed. In order to achieve this, however, it should be remembered that CT is a much more difficult procedure to perform. Meticulous attention to technique is necessary.

Sonography may be difficult to use in the acutely traumatized child because of abdominal tenderness and bowel gas caused by an associated ileus. Although sonography may be able to detect small amounts of free intraperitoneal fluid, we have found that it often underestimates the size of intrahepatic hematomas in comparison with CT and scintigraphy. However, sonography is extremely useful in the follow-up phase when a liver lesion has already been documented by another modality and the abdominal tenderness has settled.

Plain radiographs are very limited as they only reveal gross changes in liver size and larger quantities of free abdominal fluid.

On CT, the site, size, and exact extent of the hematoma is easily seen and its relationship to the other major vessels and intra-abdominal structures well depicted. Simultaneous evaluation of other abdominal viscera is also achieved. CT shows whether the hematoma is entirely intraparenchymal (Fig. 12.20) or whether there is an associated subcapsular component (see Fig. 16.9, p. 261) and free intraperitoneal blood. Intrahepatic hematomas vary in shape and margination. The more minor lesions may be linear or stellate, and larger lesions may be rounded. Subcapsular hematomas parallel the surface of

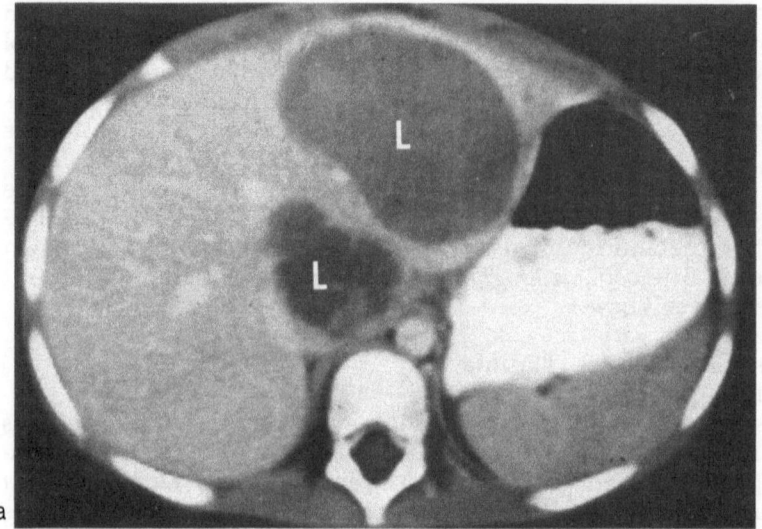

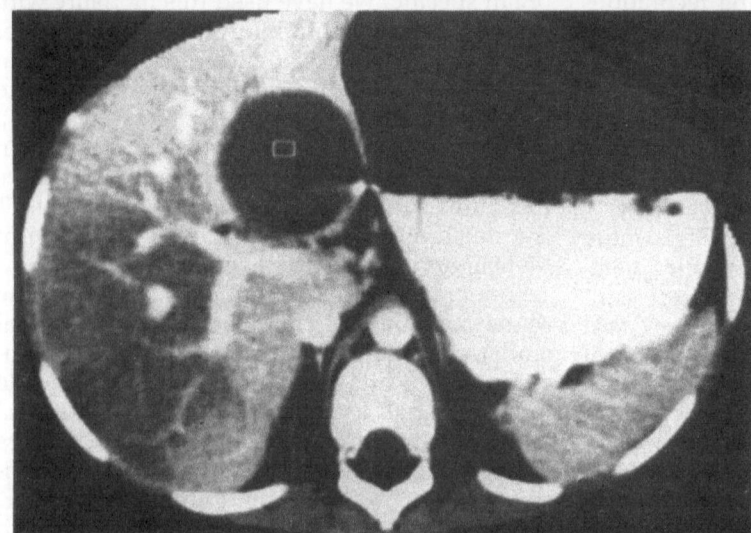

Fig. 12.19a,b. A 4-year-old boy with non-Hodgkin's lymphoma in the liver. **a** CT shows two large focal masses (*L*) within the liver. **b** Follow-up CT shows marked decrease in the size of one of these masses. A large triangular area of low attenuation in the right lobe of the liver was thought to represent parenchymal changes related to chemotherapy. This was noted to have resolved on a later scan.

the liver and may cause a concavity to the liver edge. The attenuation values of hematomas vary depending on the time lapsed from the injury till scanning. The vast majority of hematomas have a lower attenuation than hepatic parenchyma (Fig. 12.20) and the contrast between the two is increased after injection of intravenous contrast material. Higher attenuation values of the hematoma may be seen if the patient is scanned when active bleeding is occurring and contrast leaks from the vessels directly into the hematoma (see Fig. 16.9, p. 261).

The vast majority of liver lacerations and hematomas in children are treated conservatively. Follow-up studies are useful to confirm resolution of the hematoma. For this purpose we have used sonography primarily, but also scintigraphy. Sonography will show a change in size of the lesion and is useful to exclude bile leaks and associated infection. On CT, follow-up studies show that the injured area initially coalesces into a larger defect and then diminishes in size as the density increases until the lesion is invisible. Calcification may occur in the healing lesion.

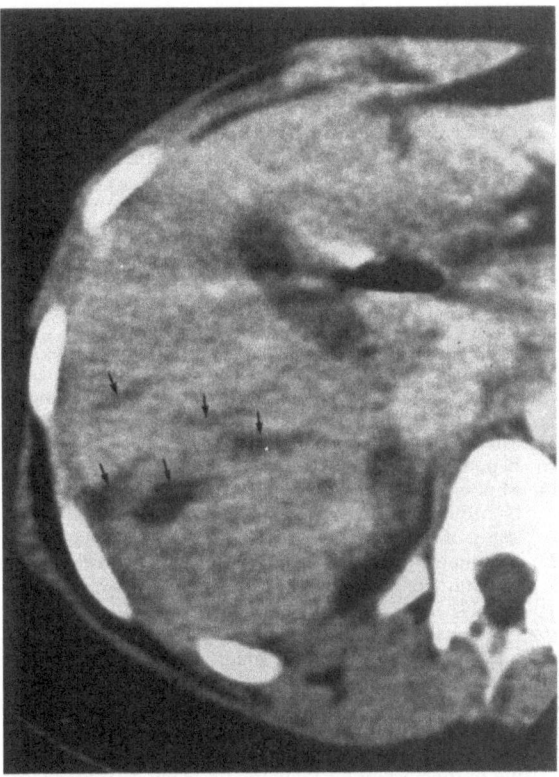

Fig. 12.20. A 12-year-old boy following a motor vehicle accident. CT shows lacerations in the right lobe of the liver. These areas are represented by irregular linear areas of lower attenuation (*small arrows*).

Hepatic injury may also be seen following radiation therapy in children treated for malignant disease. The portion of the liver irradiated assumes a lower attenuation than that of the adjacent normal hepatic parenchyma. These areas must be differentiated from metastases. The margins of radiation-induced liver lesions are usually sharp and straight reflecting the edges of the radiation therapy portals (Fig. 12.21). Changes in echogenicity on sonography and reduction of accumulation of radionuclide on scintigraphy may also be noted in these areas. Radiation-induced changes in the liver appear to be related to veno-occlusive disease and tend to be dose related. Late changes following radiation therapy include shrinkage of the irradiated portion of the liver with resultant deformity of the outline of the liver.

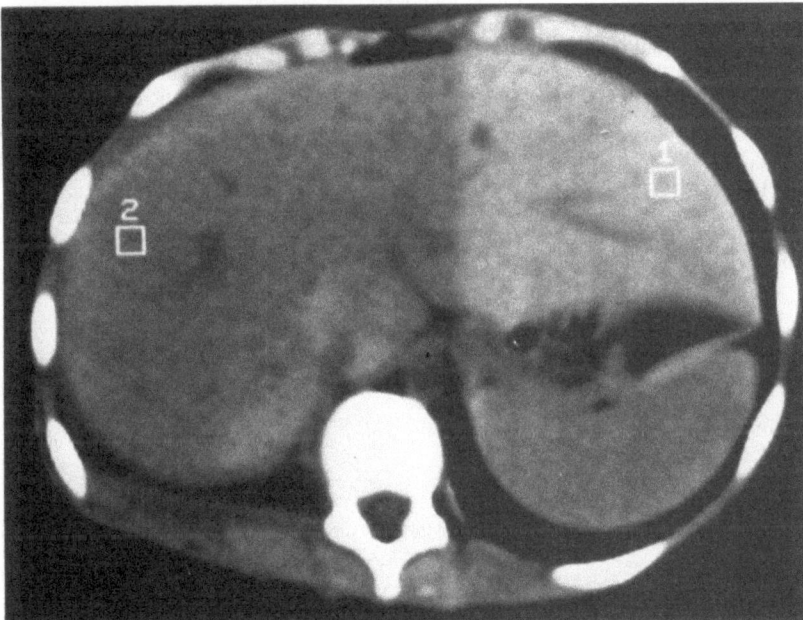

Fig. 12.21. A 12-year-old boy with previous resection of Ewing's sarcoma of the right 11th rib. CT scan following postoperative radiation shows diminution in the size of the upper abdomen on the right compared with the left. There is a linear demarcation between normal liver parenchyma on the left and radiation-damaged parenchyma on the right. The attenuation values measured at 2 were markedly lower than at 1. The linear demarcation is just to the left of the vertebral column, indicating that the radiation has included entire vertebrae in its field.

References

1. Abramson SJ, Barash FS, Seldin DW, Berdon WE (1984) Transient focal liver scan defects in children receiving chemotherapy (pseudometastases). Radiology 150:701–702

2. Barnett PH, Serhouni EA, White RI, Seigelman SS (1980) Computed tomography in the diagnosis of cavernous hemangioma of the liver. AJR 134:439–447

3. Berdon WE, Baker DH, Casarella W (1975) Liver disease in children: portal hypertension, hepatic masses. Semin Roentgenol X(3):207–214

4. Berger PE, Kuhn JP (1981) Computed tomography of the hepatobiliary system in infancy and childhood. Radiol Clin North Am 19:431–444

5. Berman MM, Libbey NP, Foster JH (1980) Hepatocellular carcinoma. Polygonal cell type with fibrous stroma — an atypical variant with a favourable prognosis. Cancer 46:1448–1455

6. Brunelle F, Chaumont P (1984) Hepatic tumors in children: ultrasonic differentiation of malignant from benign lesions. Radiology 150:695–699

7. Craig JR, Peters RL, Edmondson HA, Omata M (1980) Fibrolamellar carcinoma of the liver: a tumor of adolescents and young adults with distinctive clinicopathologic features. Cancer 46:372–379

8. Daneman A, Matzinger MA, Martin DJ (1983) Cirrhosis: an unusual pattern of enhancement on CT. Pediatr Radiol 13:162–164

9. Desser PL, Smith S (1956) Nonparasitic liver cysts in children. J Pediatr 49:297–305

10. Ein SH, Stephens CA (1974) Benign liver tumors and cysts in childhood. J Pediatr Surg 9(6):847–851

11. Ein SH, Stephens CA (1974) Malignant liver tumors in children. J Pediatr Surg 9(4):491–494

12. Giacomantonio M, Ein SH, Mancer K, Stephens CA (1984) Thirty years of pediatric primary malignant liver tumors. J Pediatr Surg 19:523–526

13. Harbin WP, Robert NJ, Ferrucci JT (1980) Diagnosis of cirrhosis based on regional changes in hepatic morphology. Radiology 135:273–283

14. Johnston PW (1968) Congenital cysts of the liver in infancy and childhood. Am J Surg 116:184–191

15. Kaufman RA (1983) Liver-spleen computed tomography. A method tailored for infants and children. CT 7:45–57

16. Korobkin MK, Kirks DR, Sullivan DC, Mills SR, Bowie JD (1981) Computed tomography of primary liver tumors in children. Radiology 139:431–435

17. Kunstlinger F, Federle MP, Moss AA, Marks W (1980) Computed tomography of hepatocellular carcinoma. AJR 134:431–437

18. Levitt RG, Sagel SS, Stanley RJ, Jost RG (1977) Accuracy of computed tomography of the liver and biliary tract. Radiology 124:123–128

19. Liu P, Daneman A, Stringer DA (1985) Diagnostic imaging of liver masses in children. J Can Assoc Radiol (In press)

20. MacCarty RL, Stephens DH, Hattery RR, Sheedy PR (1979) Hepatic imaging by computed tomography. Radiol Clin North Am 17:137–155

21. Marchal GJ, Baert AL, Wilms GE (1980) CT of noncystic liver lesions: bolus enhancement. AJR 135:57–65

22. Miller JH, Greenspan BS (1985) Integrated imaging of hepatic tumors in childhood. Radiology 154: 83–90

23. Miller JH, Greenspan BS (1985) Integrated imaging of hepatic tumors in childhood. Radiology 154:91–100

24. Mulhern CG, Arger PH, Coleman BG, Stein GH (1979) Nonuniform attenuation in computed tomography study of the cirrhotic liver. Radiology 132:399–402

25. Nishikawa J, Itai Y, Tasaka A (1981) Lobar attenuation difference of the liver on computed tomography. Radiology 141:725–728

26. Nguyen L, Shandling B, Ein S, Stephens C (1982) Hepatic hemangioma in childhood: medical management or surgical management? J Pediatr Surg 17(5):576–579

27. Olivieri N, Daneman A, Freedman M (1984) CT scanning of liver iron density in thalassemia major: valuable predictor of cardiac dysfunction. Paper presented at Meeting of the Society for Pediatric Research. San Francisco, June 1984

28. Rosch J, Mayer BS, Campbell JR, Campbell TJ (1978) 'Vascular' benign liver cyst in children: Report of two cases. Radiology 126:747–750

29. Sanfelippo PM, Beahrs OH, Weiland LH (1973) Cystic disease of the liver. Ann Surg 179(6):922–925

30. Scott WW, Sanders RC, Siegelman SS (1980) Irregular fatty infiltration of the liver: diagnostic dilemmas. AJR 136:67–71

31. Stanley RJ, Sagel SS, Levitt RG (1977) Computed tomography of the liver. Radiol Clin North Am 15:331–348

32. Stephens DH, Sheedy PF, Hattery RR, MacCarty RL (1977) Computed tomography of the liver. AJR 128:579–590

Chapter 13

Biliary Tract

Introduction

The normal and pathological gallbladder and biliary tract are usually exquisitely imaged with sonograhy. Radionuclide studies using ^{99m}Tc-labeled N-substituted iminodiacetic acids such as HIDA are valuable in defining the patency and anatomy of the biliary tract in those children in whom it is felt that the anatomical information obtained from the sonographic study is inadequate. These scans are also useful in determining biliary function, particularly in neonates with jaundice and in those children suspected of having cholecystitis. Percutaneous transhepatic cholangiography and endoscopic retrograde cholangiopancreatography may be used to define the detailed anatomy of the biliary tract in selected patients in whom less invasive procedures are equivocal or nondiagnostic.

It is extremely rare to use CT to image the biliary tract specifically in children, as diagnostic information obtained from CT is similar to that obtained with sonography. CT of the gallbladder and biliary tract should thus be reserved for those rare difficult cases in which these structures cannot be adequately examined with sonography either because of excessive bowel gas or rib shadows in patients with an unusual shape to the lower chest and upper abdomen and in obese patients. CT may rarely be of value in delineating abnormalities suggested on radionuclide scans or sonography, or when other studies do not provide a definitive diagnosis.

Occasionally, biliary abnormalities, such as stones, may be diagnosed as incidental findings in patients having CT of the upper abdomen for the investigation of other organs. Intravenous Cholegrafin (meglumine iodipamide) may be used during CT to outline the ducts and may give both anatomical and physiological information [10]. The dose of intravenous Cholegrafin required to outline the ducts on CT is much lower than that necessary for routine cholangiography. The need to use this hazardous contrast material is indeed very limited.

Anatomy

Gallbladder

The gallbladder is easily visualized as a fluid-filled cystic structure lying under the posteroinferior surface of the liver demarcating the right lobe from the quadrate lobe of the left lobe of the liver (Fig. 13.1; see also Fig. 8.1, p. 90). Its position is an extremely important landmark when determining whether a mass lesion of the liver is confined to the right or left lobes. The gallbladder extends inferiorly and to the right for a variable length from the level of the porta hepatis. The gallbladder may lie completely external to the liver or may be partly imbedded within hepatic tissue. That portion of the gallbladder wall which

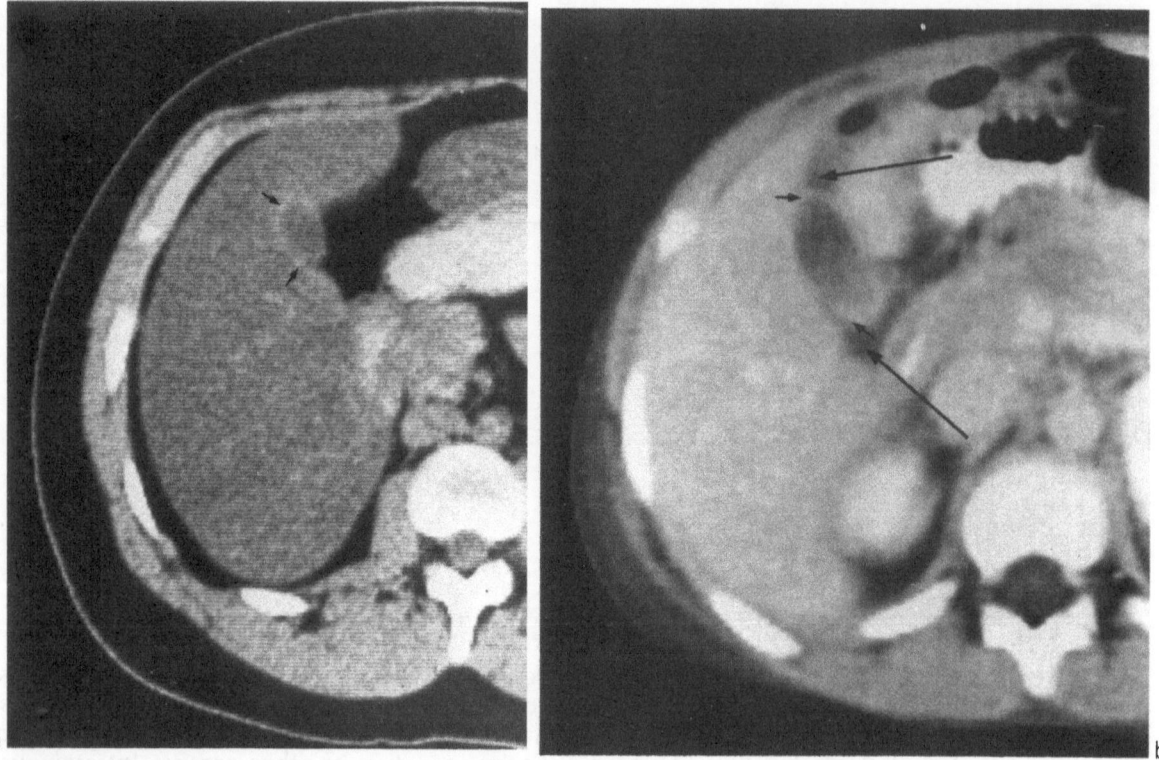

Fig. 13.1a,b. CT scans showing normal gallbladder wall. **a** The gallbladder wall (*small arrows*) can be seen without contrast administration as it is contrasted against a fatty liver which has a lower attenuation than the muscles. **b** The gallbladder wall (*small arrows*) is noted as it is partially surrounded by a very small amount of ascitic fluid (*long arrows*).

is not adjacent to the liver is occasionally distinguished as a rim of soft tissue attenuation surrounding the bile within the lumen and may be better visualized following intravenous contrast enhancement (see Fig. 8.1, p. 90, and Fig. 8.3, p. 93). The gallbladder wall may also be well visualized contrasted against a fatty liver (see Fig. 12.3, p. 178) and in ascites (Fig. 13.1).

Bile in the gallbladder has an attenuation of 0–20 HU. Increased attenuation of bile in the gallbladder may be due to hemobilia (see Fig. 13.7) [5, 15], contrast material from cholecystographic agents (see Fig. 13.4), or from vicarious excretion of water-soluble contrast agents (see Fig. 13.5). Increased attenuation of gallbladder contents 15–48 h following high-dose angiography was reported by Strax et al. in 1982 [22]. This is presumably due to hepatic excretion of small amounts of urographic agents in the presence of normal renal function. We have seen this in only two children, both with Wilms' tumor, in whom CT was performed 24 h after abdominal angiography (see Fig. 13.5). In

adults, other causes of increased attenuation described within the gallbladder include cholelithiasis, milk of calcium bile, tumor, and empyema [22, 23]. The gall bladder contents may appear to have an abnormally high attenuation when contrasted against a fatty liver (see Fig. 12.3, p. 178).

Bile Ducts

The normal intra- and extrahepatic bile ducts are rarely visualized in children who have not received cholegraphic contrast agents. Measurements for normal duct caliber in children have thus not been made. The normal common bile duct can occasionally be seen as it courses through the posterior aspect of the pancreatic head toward the duodenum (see Fig. 13.4; see also Fig. 9.2, p. 109). Slightly dilated intra- and extrahepatic ducts may be easily visualized without the administration of biliary contrast agents (see Fig. 13.8).

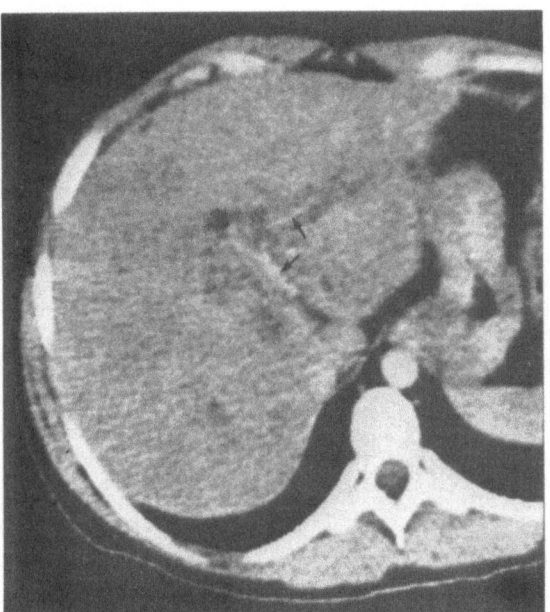

Fig. 13.2. A 16-year-old girl with cystic fibrosis and previously documented biliary duct stones. CT scan following intravenous cholegraphic contrast administration shows delineation of normal-caliber intrahepatic ducts (*small arrows*). Note patchy attenuation of liver caused by cirrhosis.

The intrahepatic ducts lie just anterior to the corresponding portal veins as they course through the liver in the portal tracts. Normal-caliber intrahepatic ducts may be visualized after cholecystographic contrast material administration (Fig. 13.2) or if air is present in the ducts (see Fig. 13.9). Dilated ducts within the liver appear as linear branching or circular areas of low attenuation and become larger as they approach the porta hepatis (see Fig. 13.8). They are differentiated from veins by their failure to opacify following injection of intravenous urographic contrast agents (see Figs. 13.8, 13.10, 13.11) and minimal dilatation is best appreciated after the injection of these contrast agents. Occasionally, connective tissue and fat in the porta hepatis may be visualized as tissue of low attenuation lying adjacent to the main portal veins and should not be confused with dilatation of hepatic ducts. When visualized, this tissue often lies anterior as well as posterior to the veins (Fig. 13.3).

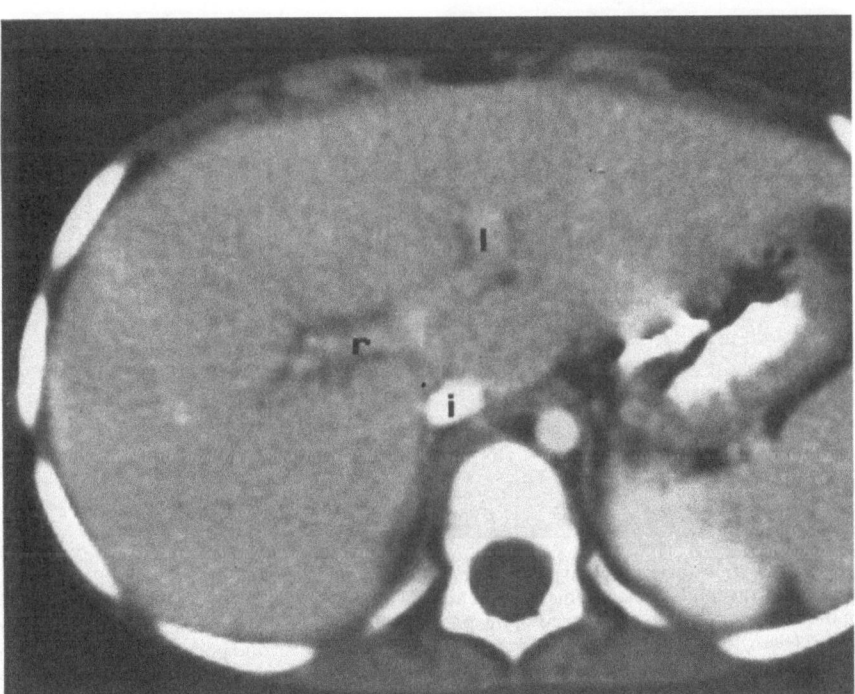

Fig. 13.3. CT scan in a 3-year-old boy through the bifurcation of the portal vein after intravenous contrast administration. Scan shows normal low-attenuation connective tissue on either side of the left branch (*l*) and in front of and behind the right branch (*r*) of the portal vein. *i*, inferior vena cava.

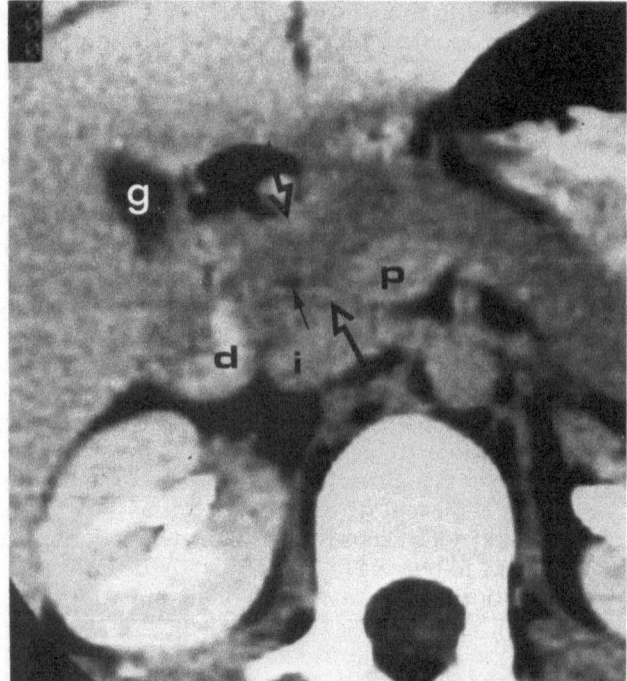

a

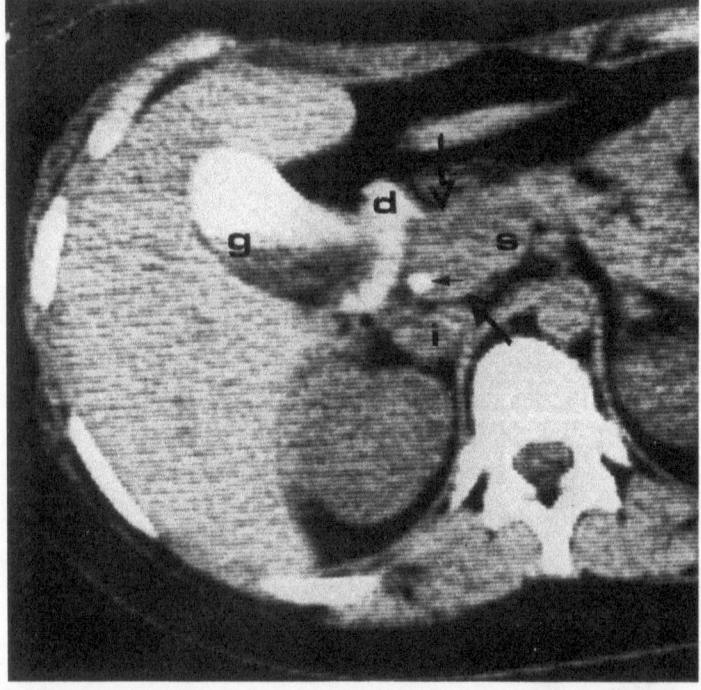

b

Fig. 13.4a,b. CT scans through the head of the pancreas in two patients. **a** After intravenous urographic contrast administration and oral contrast ingestion; **b** after intravenous cholegraphic contrast administration. **a** The unopacified normal common bile duct (*small arrow*) is noted in the posterior portion of the head of the pancreas. **b** Cholegraphic contrast has opacified the gallbladder (*g*) and common bile duct (*small arrow*) in pancreatic head and has passed into the second portion of the duodenum (*d*). This image was obtained with the patient prone but has been inverted to allow easier comparison with **a** — hence the reversed fluid-fluid level of opacified and unopacified bile in the gallbladder. The opacified bile normally lies in the dependent portion of the gallbladder. *s*, superior mesenteric vein; *d*, duodenum (second portion); *p*, portal vein; *i*, inferior vena cava; *g*, gallbladder; *open arrows*, head of pancreas

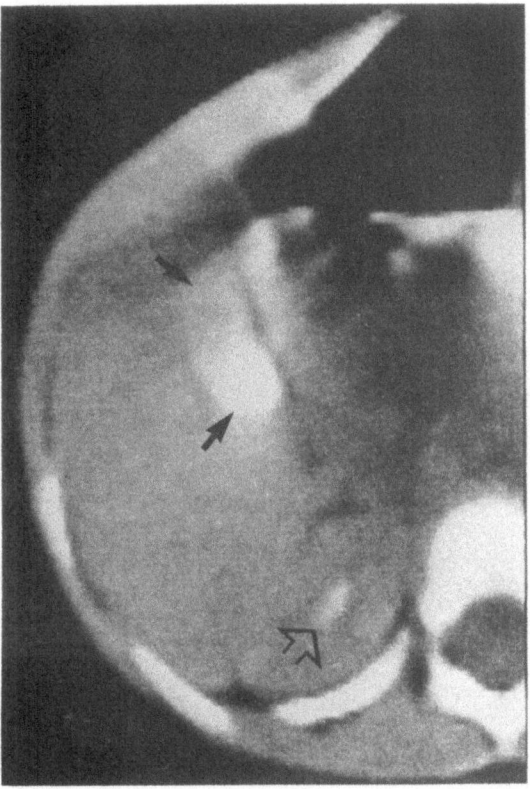

Fig. 13.5. A 3-year-old girl with left Wilms' tumor. CT scan performed 18 h after abdominal arteriography shows opacification of the gallbladder (*arrows*) by the urographic contrast material and also faint persistent opacification of the right renal collecting system (*open arrow*) indicating normal function of the right kidney.

Pathology

Gallbladder

Stones

In children, gallstones are found most commonly in the gallbladder. In many children the cause of the gallstones is idiopathic [9, 17]. There is an increased incidence of gallstones in children with hemolytic anemias and in those who have interruption of the enterohepatic circulation of bile salts, such as in terminal ileal disease [9, 17].

In children being examined in the supine position, gallstones are usually found to lie in the neck of the gallbladder and appear as rounded structures with a high attenuation (Fig. 13.6). When multiple stones are present, it may be extremely difficult to discriminate individual stones on CT.

Trauma

Gallbladder injuries resulting from blunt abdominal trauma are infrequent [21]. A review of 31 patients with blunt gallbladder trauma by Soderstrom et al. in 1981 revealed gallbladder contusion in 20 patients, avulsion in 10, and laceration in 1 [21]. In only one of these 31 patients was the gallbladder the only site of intra-abdominal injury; 83% of the patients had liver lacerations as well. Including these 31 patients, these authors found 101 patients reported in the English language literature with gallbladder injury secondary to blunt trauma. The commonest type of injury was perforation.

Hemorrhage, when present, usually occurs into the peritoneum. Bleeding into the gallbladder has been infrequently described and, apart from trauma, may rarely be related to gallstones, cholecystitis, tumors and vascular disease [11, 13, 18, 20]. Blood may remain within the gallbladder (hemocholecyst) or may enter the intestine via the bile duct causing hematemesis and melena [19].

In 1983, Daneman et al. reported the CT and sonographic findings of a 14-year-old girl in whom hemorrhage into the gallbladder occurred following nonpenetrating abdominal trauma [5]. The material within the gallbladder was noted to have an extremely high homogeneous attenuation on CT performed 5 days following the trauma (Fig. 13.7). This was consistent with fresh blood within the lumen. Sonography revealed the material to have low-level echoes distributed evenly throughout the lumen. A CT scan repeated 11 days following trauma showed no change, but sonography at this time showed that the echogenicity of the material was less than at the previous study.

The source of the bleeding may have been related to a small hepatic laceration with tearing of adjacent veins and gallbladder wall allowing the gallbladder to fill with blood. The frequent association of hepatic laceration [21] with blunt gallbladder trauma favours this hypothesis. A primary cystic duct injury may have been the cause, as a ^{99m}Tc-HIDA scan showed cystic duct obstruction. The patient was treated conservatively and her condition remained stable. She was discharged with no further symptoms or signs related to the biliary tract. She had no previous history of gallbladder disease.

The diagnosis of blunt gallbladder injury is difficult to make preoperatively [8, 21], and radiological studies are generally considered to be unhelpful [7, 21]. The above-mentioned

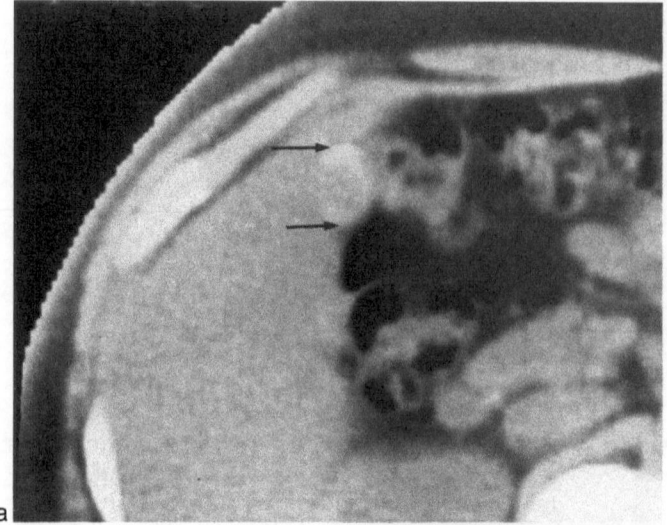

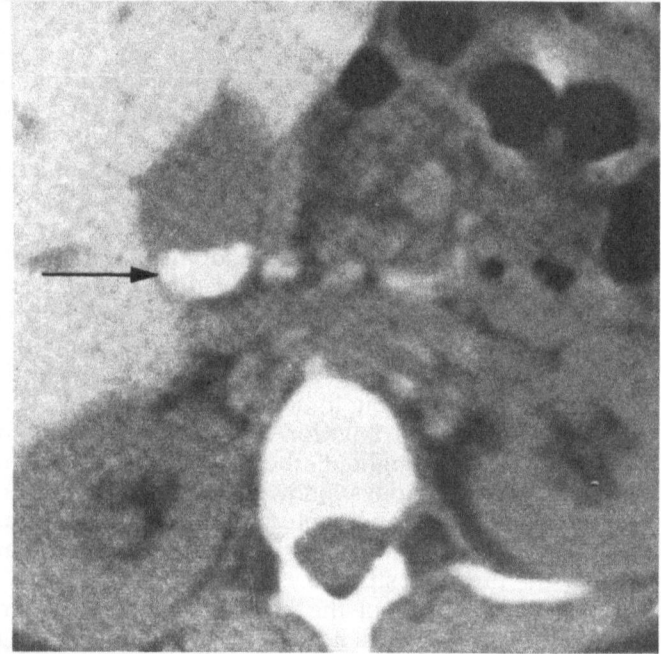

Fig. 13.6. A 17-year-old boy with recurrent right upper quadrant pain. CT shows contracted gallbladder (*arrows*) filled with poorly calcified stone. **b** A 16-year-old boy with thalassemia and multiple stones lying in dependent portion of gallbladder (*arrow*). Note the high attenuation of the liver and retroperitoneal nodes caused by iron deposition.

patient illustrates the value of CT in delineating unexpected injuries in patients with blunt abdominal trauma and serves as a reminder of this rare type of injury. Since then we have seen two further children with blunt abdominal trauma in whom CT showed blood in the gallbladder (see Fig. 16.8, p. 260).

The CT appearance of blood within the gallbladder was initially described by Berland et al. in 1980 [3]. In 1983, Krudy et al. [15] reported an inhomogeneous increase in attenuation of the gallbladder contents caused by hemobilia in an

adult patient following a liver biopsy. These authors found similar CT appearances in two monkeys in whom blood was injected into the gallbladder. In their patient and in the two monkeys, the attenuation of the visualized clot initially became denser, probably as the result of clot retraction and resorption of water by the gallbladder. Small amounts of blood within the gallbladder may lead to a nonhomogeneous increased attenuation of the bile, but more concentrated blood may lead to a homogeneous appearance because of clot formation. The

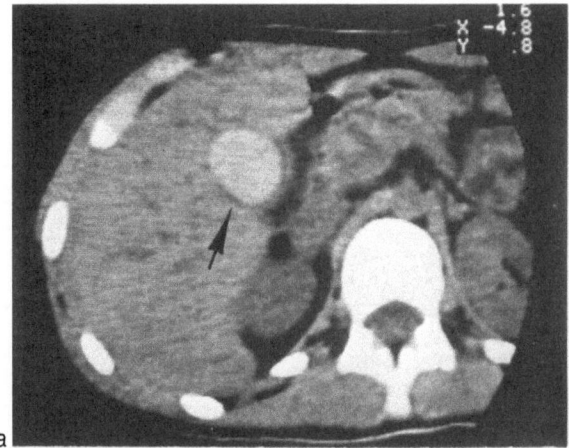

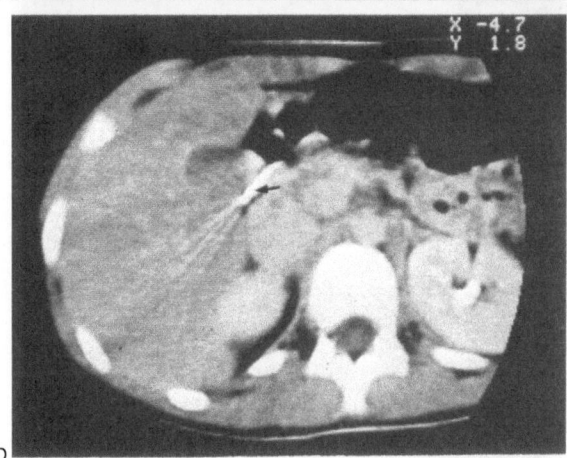

Fig. 13.7a,b. A 14-year-old girl with abdominal pain and a drop in hemoglobin level following a motor vehicle accident. **a** CT scan without intravenous contrast 5 days after trauma shows the gallbladder (*arrow*) filled with material of high attenuation (80 HU). This was thought to be due to blood within the lumen (Daneman et al. 1983 [5]). **b** Scan performed after the injection of intravenous contrast material shows that the attenuation of the contents of the gallbladder are lower than the enhancing liver. Artifact from feeding tube (*arrow*).

increased attenuation of gallbladder bile may persist for weeks, even in the presence of a patent cystic duct [15].

Bile Ducts

Sonography and CT are extremely accurate in detecting dilatation of intra- and extrahepatic ducts in children. Obstructing lesions usually cause dilatation of both the intrahepatic and extrahepatic segments of the biliary tract (Fig. 13.8). Occasionally, however, dilatation of the extrahepatic ducts may occur in the absence of intrahepatic duct dilatation.

In children, dilatation of the biliary tract may occur with choledochal cysts and occasionally in biliary atresia. It may also be secondary to pancreatitis but is rarely due to choledocholithiasis. Obstructing mass lesions in the region of the head of the pancreas and duodenum are extremely uncommon in the pediatric age group. Indeed, in children, the biliary tract usually remains within normal limits even in the presence of adjacent huge mass lesions of the upper abdomen. Trauma to the bile ducts is rare but may be due to surgical procedures such as partial hepatectomy for liver tumors (Figs. 13.9, 13.10).

In 1981, Berger and Kuhn [2] suggested that CT may in fact be more accurate than sonography in detecting slight dilatation of the bile ducts. These authors described two children with biliary cirrhosis without obstruction in whom CT showed minimal dilatation of the intrahepatic ducts but sonography was interpreted as being normal. Furthermore, they reported slight extrahepatic duct dilatation in children following trauma and suggested that this may be secondary to edema at the ampulla of Vater, or a "reflex ileus" of the ducts in response to the trauma.

The two relatively common conditions of the bile ducts in the pediatric age group that require imaging are biliary atresia and choledochal cysts.

Biliary Atresia

Biliary atresia is thought to result from a perinatal insult to both the liver parenchyma and biliary tract [16]. The inflammatory process that affects the ducts leads to irregular sclerosis and eventual obliteration of the duct lumen. The exact pattern of obliteration varies from patient to patient.

Landing has postulated that neonatal hepatitis and biliary atresia represent two ends of the spectrum of a disease entity termed "infantile obstructive cholangiopathy" [16]. The distinction between neonates with neonatal hepatitis from those with biliary atresia is important [12], as treatment of the former is conservative and the latter surgical. However, this distinction is difficult, not only clinically and radiologically, but often also histologically. Occasionally, the correct diagnosis can only be made after an operative cholangiogram.

The preoperative radiological problem in the differentiation of biliary atresia from neonatal hepatitis is to determine whether the biliary tract is patent or not. A radionuclide scan using [99m]Tc-

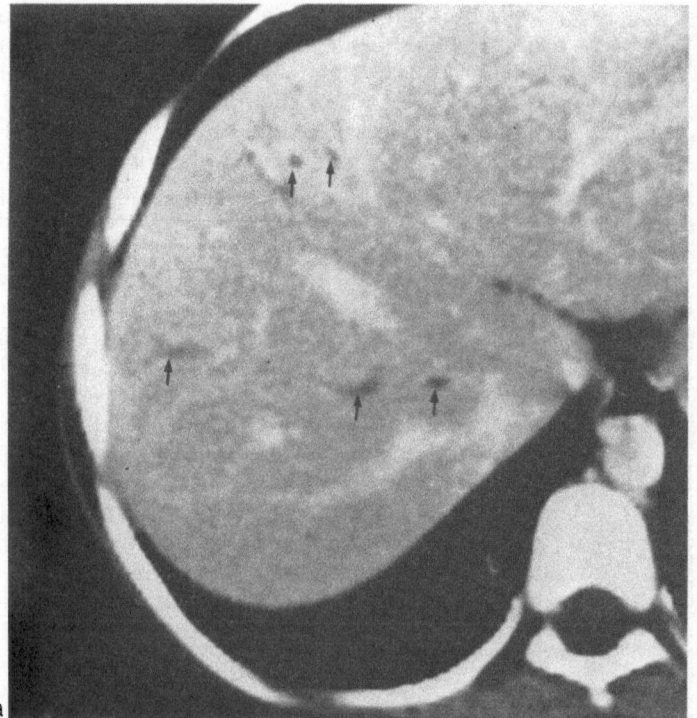

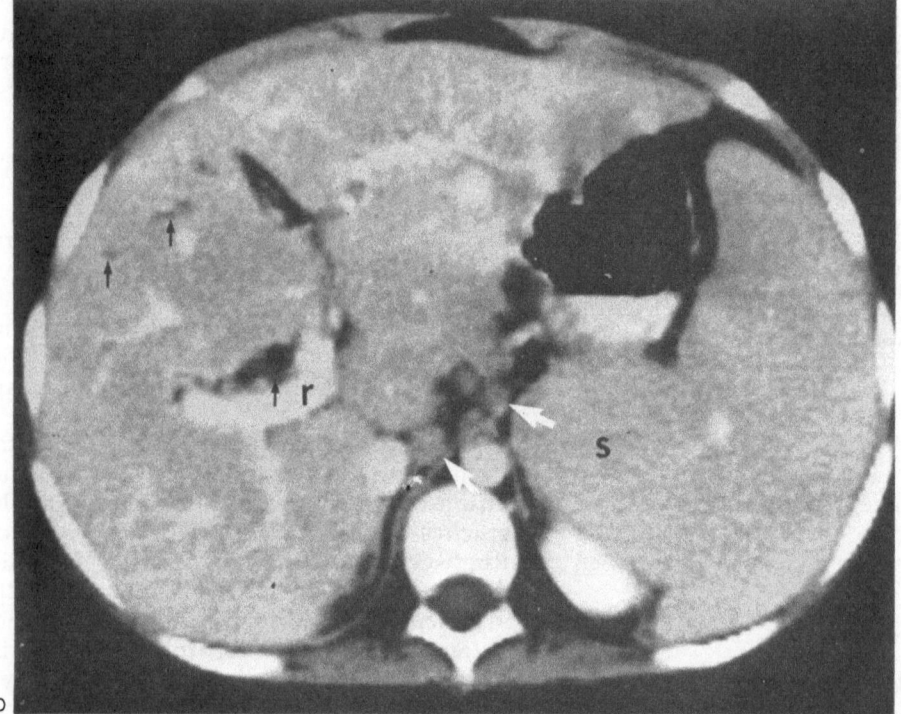

Fig. 13.8c (next page)

Fig. 13.8a–c. A 12-year-old boy with hypogammaglobulinemia. **a,b** CT scans during intravenous contrast administration show intrahepatic linear and rounded areas that fail to enhance (*small arrows*). These represent mildly dilated intrahepatic bile ducts. Note the relationship of the larger ducts anterior to the right portal vein (*r*). Splenomegaly and retroperitoneal lymphadenopathy (*white arrows*) are also present. Note the large medial splenic lobulation (*s*). **c** Scan shows dilated common bile duct (*arrow*) in pancreatic head (*open arrows*). The duct dilatation was thought to be related to obstruction by lymphoid tissue in the duodenum. *v*, superior mesenteric vein. This is the same patient illustrated in Fig. 8.6 and 9.3.

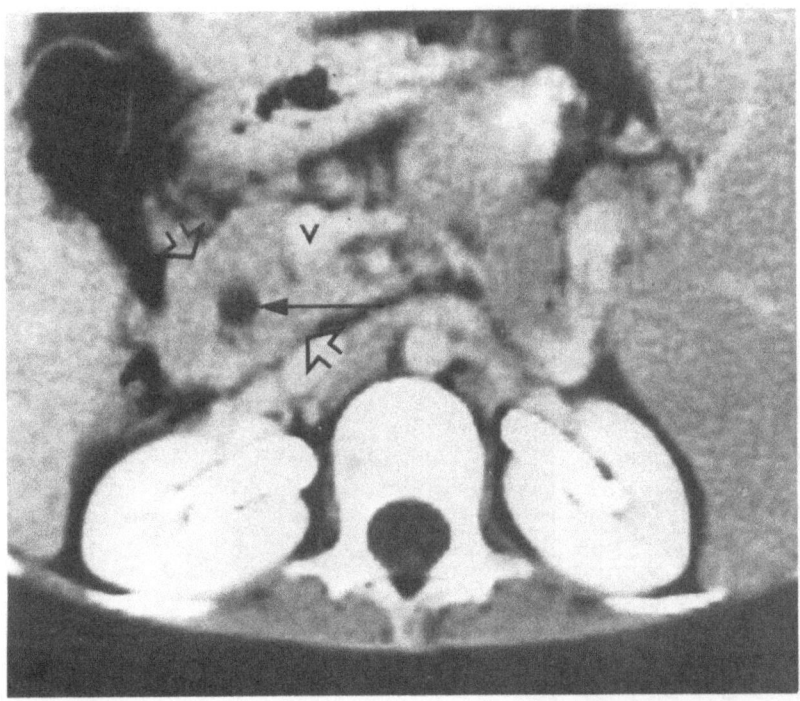

Fig. 13.8c

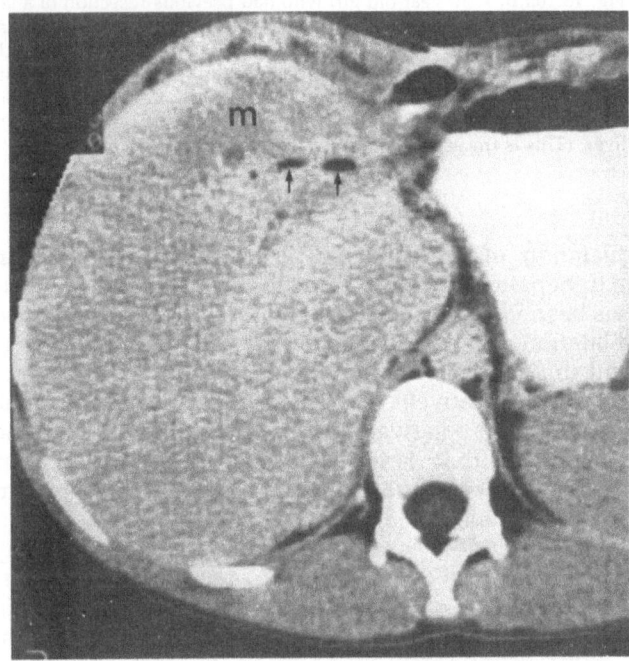

Fig. 13.9. A 12-year-old boy who had a previous resection of a left-lobe hepatocellular carcinoma. Follow-up CT scan shows low-attenuation area (*m*) in anterior aspect of the liver caused by recurrent neoplasm. At the original resection the bile ducts were injured and a choledochojejunostomy was performed — hence the gas in nondilated intrahepatic bile duct radicles (*small arrows*).

labeled N-substituted iminodiacetic acids is the study of choice in attempting to determine whether the biliary tract is patent. Activity will be seen in the gastrointestinal tract in patients with neonatal hepatitis and not extrahepatic atresia.

Previous reports have stated that biliary atresia does not usually cause dilatation of the ducts proximal to or between the sites of complete obstruction [1, 4, 14]. However, 25% of the neonates with biliary atresia that we have studied with sonography have been shown to have

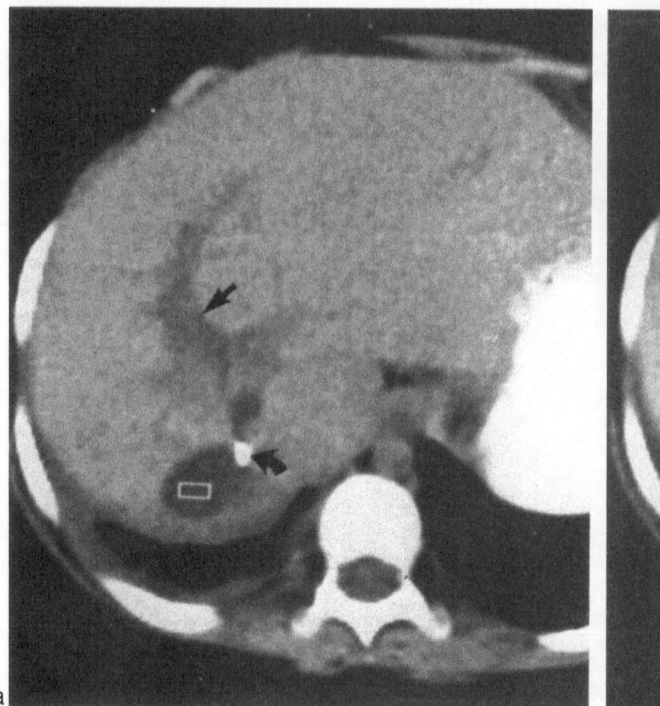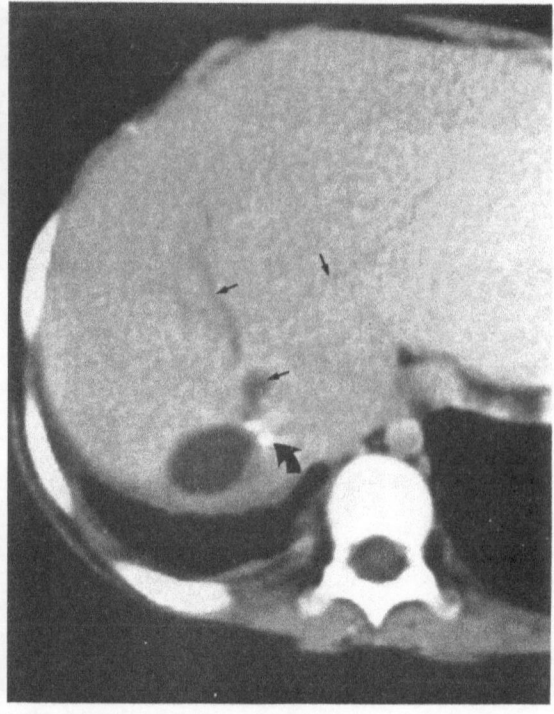

Fig. 13.10a,b. A 10-year-old girl who had previous resection of a large right fibrolamellar hepatic carcinoma. Follow-up CT scans before (**a**) and after (**b**) intravenous contrast administration. **a** Curvilinear low-attenuation areas (*arrow*) represent left portal vascular structures and bile ducts leading posteriorly to a fluid collection marked by the *rectangular cursor*. *Curved arrow*, surgical clips. **b** Scan shows enhancement of the portal vessels equal to that of liver. The curvilinear unenhanced structures (*small arrows*) represent slightly dilated intrahepatic bile ducts. The ducts had been injured at the previous resection. The surgical clips (*curved arrow*) mark the site of this injury where the ducts drain into the "biloma" in the bed of the right lobe of the liver. (This is the same patient illustrated in Fig. 2.5).

dilatation of segments of the intrahepatic or extrahepatic biliary tract; indeed, the gallbladder has been visualized in several [6]. These areas of dilatation are well delineated with sonography, and this information may be useful to the surgeon preoperatively. We have used CT in two patients with biliary atresia. In one we used CT to confirm that large echo-free intrahepatic spaces that were noted on sonography were indeed ducts (Fig. 13.11). In the other, CT was used to exclude the presence of an intra-abdominal abscess.

Choledochal Cyst

Choledochal cysts usually present in later childhood or in adults. Rarely, they may be seen in the neonatal age group. The presenting features may include jaundice, pain, fever, and an abdominal mass. Occasionally pancreatitis or common duct stones may be present [2].

In many of the patients with choledochal cysts, the common bile duct has an anomalous insertion into the pancreatic duct. It is thought that the ventral pancreas fuses with the dorsal pancreas more laterally and cephalad than normal, and the common bile duct thus does not reach the duodenum. It joins the pancreatic duct more proximally leading to elongation of the common pancreatobiliary channel and exclusion of the bile duct from the lower sphincter. This may result in reflux of pancreatic secretions into the biliary tract causing a cholangitis with weakening of the duct wall and partial distal duct obstruction leading to choledochal cyst formation.

Sonography is the modality of choice in the diagnosis and follow-up of patients with suspected or known choledochal cyst. This modality accurately defines the cystic dilatation of the extrahepatic ducts and shows the accompanying intrahepatic duct dilatation as well. CT supplies similar information to sonography and should be reserved for those patients in whom sonography

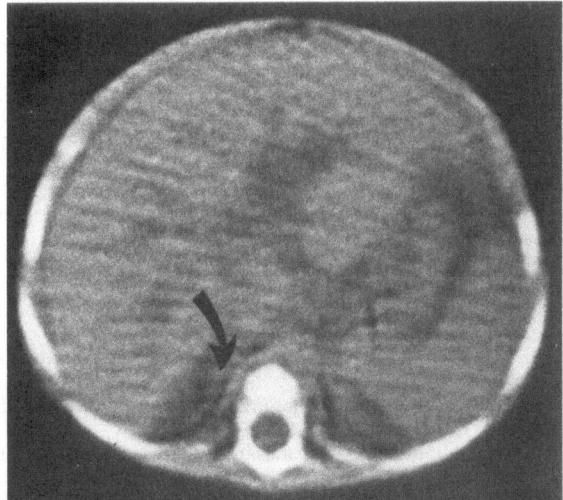

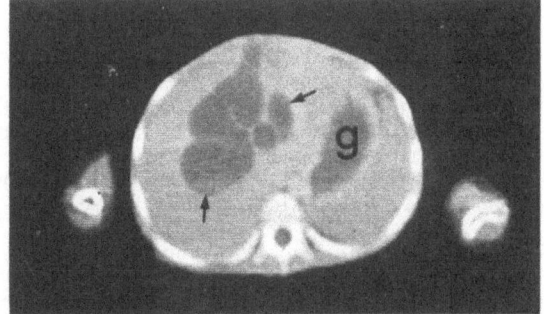

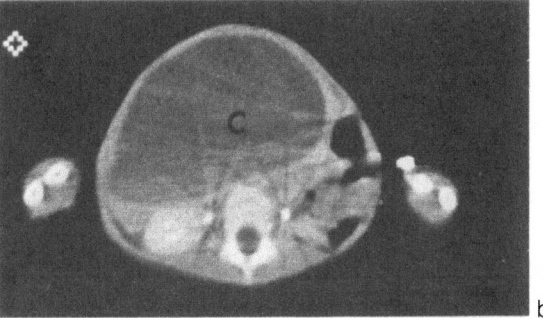

Fig. 13.12a,b. A 4-year-old boy with large choledochal cyst. **a** Scan shows dilated intrahepatic ducts (*arrows*). *g*, stomach. **b** Scan shows the large extrahepatic choledochal cyst (*c*). These images are from an old 2-min scanner, as more recent patients with choledochal cysts have been adequately evaluated with sonography.

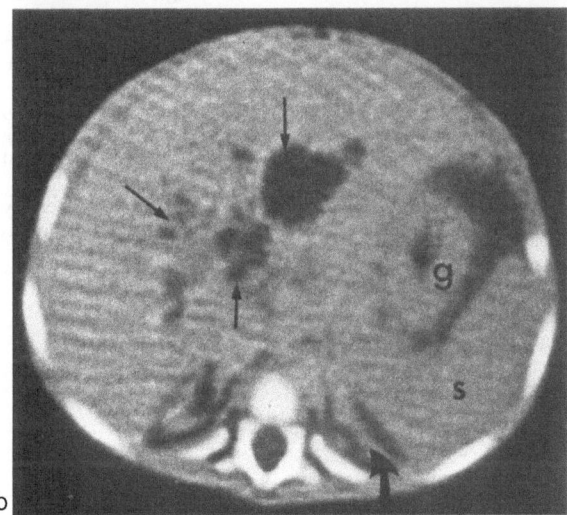

Fig. 13.11a,b. A 4-month-old boy with biliary atresia. CT scans before (**a**) and after (**b**) intravenous contrast enhancement. Large low-attenuation areas in scan **a** are due to the portal venous system and dilated intrahepatic ducts. In **b** the liver and portal veins have enhanced equally, revealing the true size of the dilated duct system (*arrows*). This study was performed in order to confirm that the large intrahepatic fluid-filled structures seen on sonography were indeed dilated ducts and not large tortuous veins. Dilatation of ducts to this degree is very uncommon in biliary atresia but these findings were confirmed at autopsy. *Curved arrows*, adrenals, *g*, stomach; *s*, spleen.

is hampered by bowel gas. On CT the cysts appear as rounded fluid-filled spaces and occasionally may contain some debris or stones (Fig. 13.12). The intrahepatic duct dilatation is also visualized and is usually limited to the more central main hepatic ducts, in contrast to acquired obstruction when dilatation often extends to the periphery [2]. If only extrahepatic

dilatation is present, there is usually an abrupt transition to the normal ducts. In rare cases when one is not certain that the cystic mass is in communication with the biliary tract, intravenous Cholegrafin may be administered. Enhancement of the fluid in the cyst 30 min after infusion will confirm the communication.

If the diagnosis is still in doubt, radionuclide scans using iminodiacetic acid derivatives are helpful. The need to perform endoscopic retrograde pancreatocholangiography or percutaneous transhepatic cholangiography to define the anatomy better preoperatively is not always necessary as the detailed anatomy can usually be obtained at operative cholangiography.

References

1. Abramson SJ, Treves S, Teele RL (1982) The infant with possible biliary atresia: evaluation by ultrasound and nuclear medicine. Pediatr Radiol 12:1–5

2. Berger PE, Kuhn JP (1981) Computed tomography of the hepatobiliary system in infancy and childhood. Radiol Clin North Am 19(3):431–444

3. Berland LL, Doust BD, Foley WD (1980) Acute hemorrhage into the gallbladder diagnosed by computed tomography and ultrasonography, J Comput Assist Tomogr 4:260–262

4. Blane CE, Jongeward RH Jr, Silver TM (1983) Sonographic features of hepatocellular disease in neonates and infants. AJR 141:1313–1316

5. Daneman A, Matzinger MA, Martin DJ (1983) Posttraumatic hemorrhage into the gallbladder. CT 7:59–61

6. Daneman A, Stringer DA, Martin DJ (1984) The value of sonography in children with biliary atresia. Paper presented at the 21st Annual Congress of the European Society for Pediatric Radiology, Florence, Italy, April 1984

7. Evans JP (1976) Traumatic rupture of the gallbladder in a three year old boy. J Pediatr Surg 11:1011–1034

8. Fletcher WS (1972) Nonpenetrating trauma to the gallbladder and extrahepatic bile ducts. Surg Clin North Am 52:711–717

9. Garel L, Lallemand D, Montagne JP, Forel F, Sauvegrain J (1981) The changing aspects of cholelithiasis in children through a sonographic study. Pediatr Radiol 11:75–79

10. Greenberg M, Rubin JM, Greenberg BM (1983) Appearance of the gallbladder and biliary tree by CT cholangiography. J Comput Assist Tomogr 7(5):788–794

11. Hakami M, Beheshti G, Amirkhan A (1976) Hematobilia caused by rupture of cystic artery aneurysm. Am J Proctol 27:56–59

12. Hatfield PM, Scholz FJ, Wise RE (1976) Congenital diseases of the gallbladder and bile ducts. Semin Roentgenol 11(4):235–243

13. Helmlund D, Lundstrom B (1977) Extrahepatic obstruction of the portal vein with bleeding from the gallbladder. Report of a case. Acta Radiol [Diagn] (Stockh) 18:680–682

14. Kirks DR, Coleman RE, Filston HC, Rosenberg ER, Merten DF (1984) An imaging approach to persistent neonatal jaundice. AJR 142:461–465

15. Krudy AG, Doppman JL, Dissonette MB, Girton M (1983) Hemobilia: computed tomographic diagnosis. Radiology 148:785–789

16. Landing BH (1974) Considerations of the pathogenesis of neonatal hepatitis, biliary atresia and choledochal cyst: the concept of infantile obstructive cholangiopathy. Pediatr Surg 6:113–139

17. Newman DE (1973) Gallstones in children. Pediatr Radiol 1:100–104

18. Pilling DW (1979) Haematoma of the wall of the gallbladder. Br J Radiol 52:840–841

19. Saad AS, Rush BF, Devanesan ID, Lazaro EJ (1979) Traumatic hematocele of the gallbladder with hemobilia. J Trauma 19:56–59

20. Sandblom P (1973) Hemobilia. Surg Clin North Am 53:1191–1201

21. Soderstrom CA, Maekawa K, DuPriest RW, Cowley RA (1981) Gallbladder injuries resulting from blunt abdominal trauma. Ann Surg 193:60–66

22. Strax R, Toombs BD, Kam J, Rauschkolb EN, Patel S, Sandler CM (1982) Gallbladder enhancement following angiography: a normal CT finding. J Comput Assist Tomogr 6:766–768

23. Ueda J, Hara K, Ohishi H, Uchida H (1983) High density bile in the gallbladder observed by computed tomography. J Comput Assist Tomogr 7(5):801–804

CHAPTER 14

Spleen

Introduction

Although the spleen is easily demonstrated on CT scans of the abdomen, this modality is seldom used specifically and solely for the purpose of delineating splenic anatomy and pathology in children. Indeed, very little has been written with specific reference to CT scanning of the spleen in the pediatric age group. The appearance of the spleen on CT is always assessed in children having scans to delineate problems involving other areas of the abdomen (e.g., patients with lymphoma or trauma). CT of the spleen is occasionally performed when clarification of an abnormality suspected on the basis of radionuclide or sonographic examination is necessary. We have used sonography successfully as the initial imaging modality to study children with a left upper quadrant mass when the clinician is unsure whether this represents splenomegaly or a separate mass lesion. It is unusual that CT is required to delineate the anatomy of the left upper quadrant in greater detail because of an inadequate sonographic examination.

Anatomy

The superolateral border of the spleen is usually smooth and convex and conforms to the shape of the adjacent abdominal wall and left hemidiaphragm (see Fig. 8.1, p. 90). The anteromedial surface shows a varying degree of lobulation (see Fig. 14.3; see also Fig. 13.8, p. 204). The hilum divides this surface into two areas: The posteromedial area lies above and lateral to the upper pole of the left kidney; the anteromedial surface is related to the greater curvature of the stomach (Fig. 14.1; see also Fig. 8.1, p. 90). These areas have a varying degree of concavity. The tail of the pancreas lies adjacent to the splenic hilum.

Size

Measurements of the normal splenic size on CT in children have not been established. The absolute criteria for the diagnosis of splenomegaly on CT are thus not available. Splenic enlargement is usually based on findings from physical examination and from radionuclide and sonographic studies. The size of the spleen on CT is usually based on subjective findings and an assessment as to the size of the spleen related to adjacent structures. When diffuse splenic enlargement occurs, the general concavity of the visceral surface is often lost as the spleen assumes a more globular shape (Fig. 14.1).

Splenomegaly most often causes inferior displacement of the kidney without local flattening of the upper pole [11, 12, 34]. Occasionally, the kidney may be pushed inferomedially or, rarely, medially or upward [3, 4]. Upward displacement

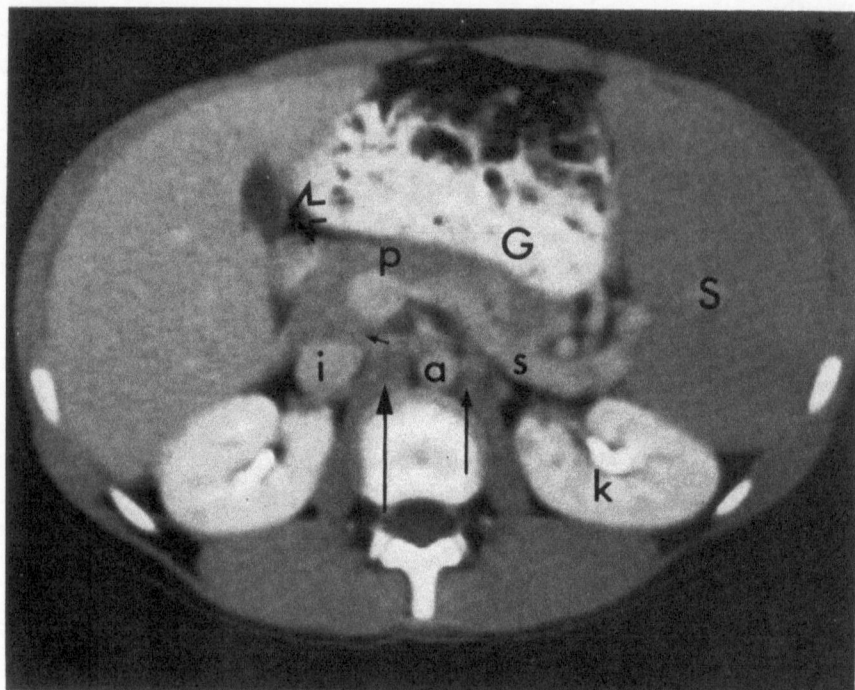

Fig. 14.1. A 12-year-old boy with hypogammaglobulinemia. There is splenomegaly (*S*). Note that the spleen is a little more rounded in shape than that noted in Fig. 8.1. *G*, stomach; *k*, left kidney; *s*, splenic vein; *p*, pancreas; *a*, aorta; *i*, inferior vena cava; *Open arrow* indicates normal gallbladder wall; *arrows* on either side of the aorta indicate the diaphragmatic crura. Although they are asymmetrically thickened they are within normal limits. *Small arrow*, uncinate process of the pancreatic head.

probably occurs when the bulk of splenic tissue lies lateral rather than superior to the left kidney. With splenic enlargement, the left kidney is thus squashed against the psoas muscle and is pushed upward [25] (Fig. 14.2).

Normal Variations and Congenital Anomalies

The size, shape, lobulation, and position of the spleen may vary from patient to patient.

Shape

Variations of splenic shape may appear as suprarenal, pararenal, renal, or pancreatic lesions on excretory urography or sonographic examinations [15, 18, 23, 28]. These splenic variations include prominent splenic lobulation extending medially from the visceral surface of the spleen, accessory spleens, ptotic and rotated spleens, depressed spleens, and splenosis [23, 28, 31].

We have reported our experience with two children in whom flattening of the upper pole of the left kidney was noted on excretory urography [25]. The appearances suggested the presence of an adrenal mass. In both patients, CT revealed the presence of a lobulated spleen, which was the cause for the flattening of the upper pole (Fig. 14.3). Abdominal sonography in both cases revealed no abnormality in the left upper quadrant but did not define the splenic lobulation as the cause for the upper pole flattening as clearly as CT. CT is the most sensitive method of defining the detailed anatomy of the spleen and the remainder of the viscera of the left upper quadrant and readily explains the cause for these pseudomasses more accurately than sonography [4, 25].

Splenic lobules and accessory spleens have the same CT numbers as the remainder of the spleen both before and after intravenous contrast

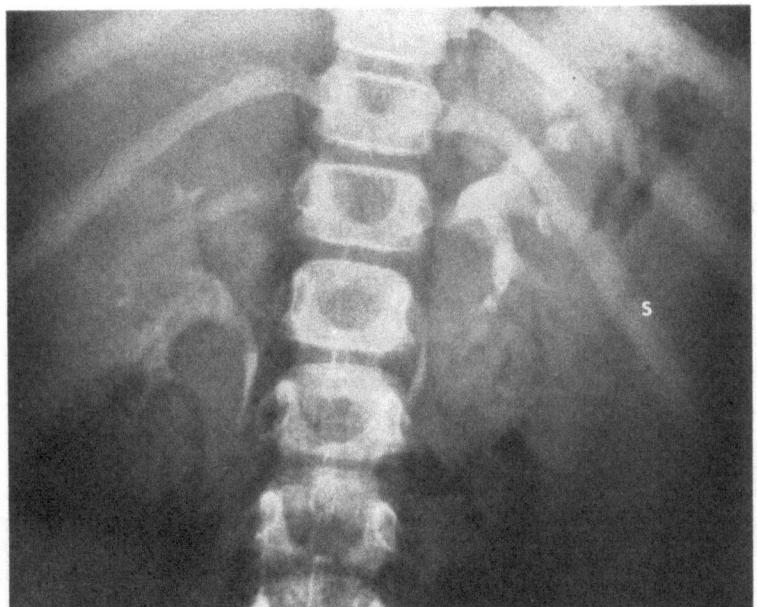

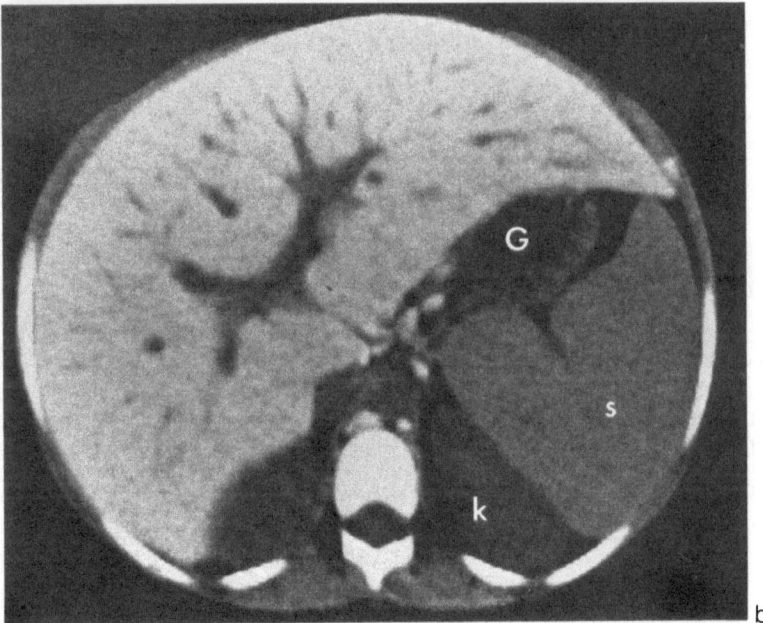

Fig. 14.2a,b. A 10-year-old girl with red cell aplastic anemia and hemochromatosis resulting from repeated blood transfusions. **a** Excretory urogram shows upward displacement of the left kidney. The enlarged spleen (*s*) lies laterally. **b** Abdominal CT scan without contrast enhancement shows hepatosplenomegaly and increased attenuation of the liver, spleen, and lymph nodes. The left kidney is squashed by the spleen lying anterolaterally. Note the prominent splenic lobulation anterior to the kidney (*k*). *G*, stomach (Olutola et al. 1982 [25])

enhancement. Medial splenic lobulations usually lie above or anterior (see Fig. 14.2; see also Fig. 13.8, p. 204) to the upper pole of the left kidney but may lie posteriorly. Clefts between these lobules may pass deeply into the splenic tissue (see Figs. 14.4, 14.6). Accessory spleens are an incidental finding and are seen in 10%–30% of adults but are very rarely visualized on CT in children. They usually lie close to the splenic hilum but occasionally may occur at a distance from the spleen. It is important to recognize the presence of accessory splenic tissue, particularly in patients who have had a splenectomy because of hypersplenism caused by hematological disorders (Fig. 14.5). In this situation accessory spleens may hypertrophy, leading to a recurrence of hypersplenism, and can be detected with CT [1, 21].

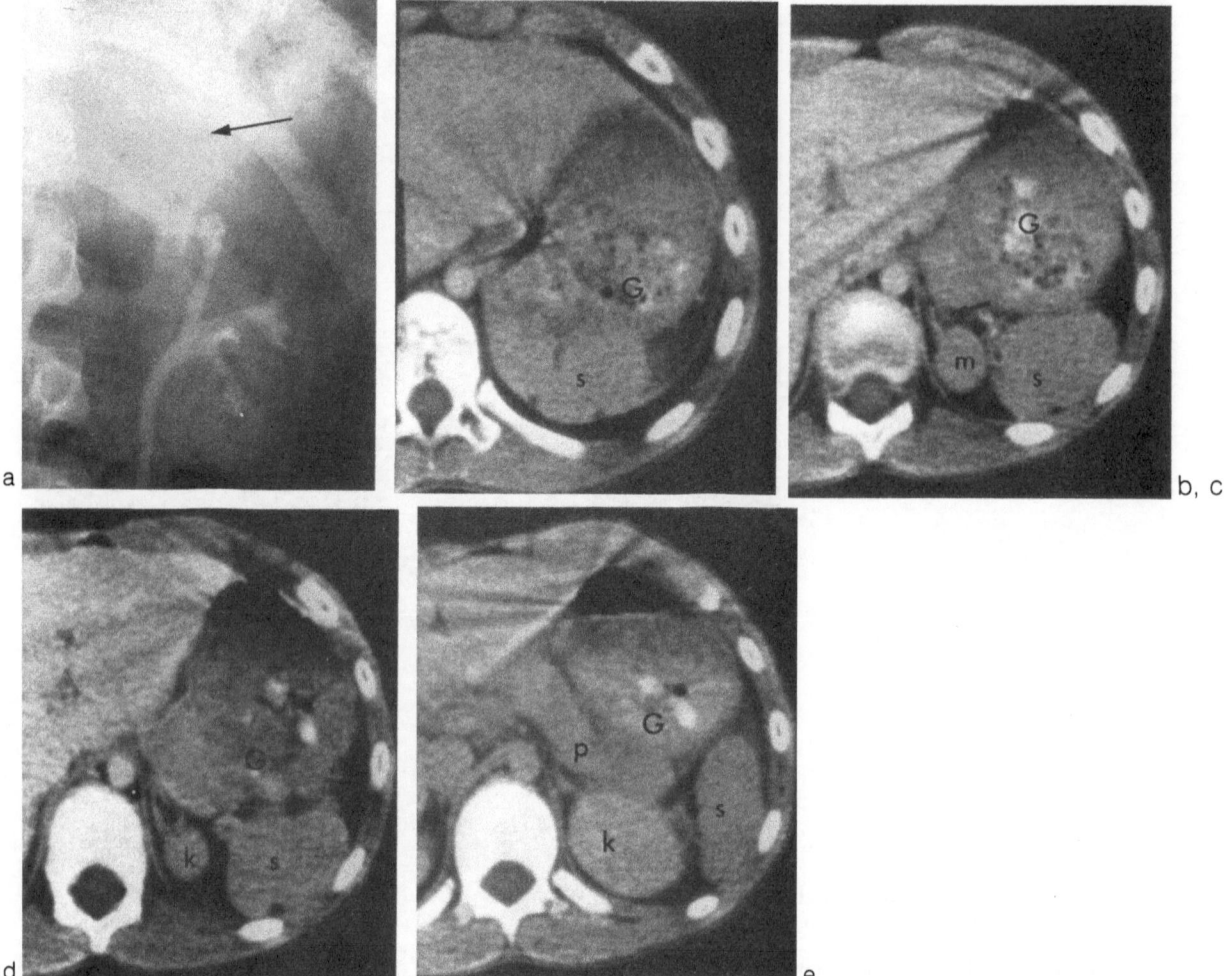

Fig. 14.3a–d. A 10-year-old boy with daytime urinary incontinence. **a** Excretory urogram shows flattening of the upper pole of the left kidney (*arrow*). **b** CT scan of the abdomen reveals a lobulated spleen (*s*). **c** CT scan 10 mm below **b** shows the anterior part of the adrenal to be normal (*arrow*), but a "mass" is noted posteriorly (*m*). This is a prominent lobule of the spleen, the remainder of which lies laterally (*s*). **d** CT scan 15 mm below **c** shows the upper pole of the left kidney (*k*) immediately below the "mass." **e** CT scan 5 mm below **d** shows the pancreas (*p*) anterior to the kidney (*k*). *G*, stomach. (Olutola et al. 1982 [25])

Position

Laxity of the ligamentous attachments of the spleen may allow the spleen to lie in an unusual position in the absence of an abdominal mass or previous operation. More marked laxity of the ligaments allows the spleen to move about the abdomen ("wandering spleen") and to simulate the presence of an abdominal mass. The shape of the "mass" and absence of the spleen from the left upper quadrant should lead one to recognize the true nature of the "mass". This situation is usually of little clinical significance once the nature of the "mass" is recognized, but occasionally such a "wandering spleen" may undergo torsion with compromise of its vascular supply [4, 16, 21, 29, 36].

We have seen one such patient who presented with left upper quadrant pain. Laxity of the suspensory splenic ligaments allowed the spleen to rotate, causing vascular compromise [22]. The unusual rotation was easily recognized on CT (Fig. 14.6).

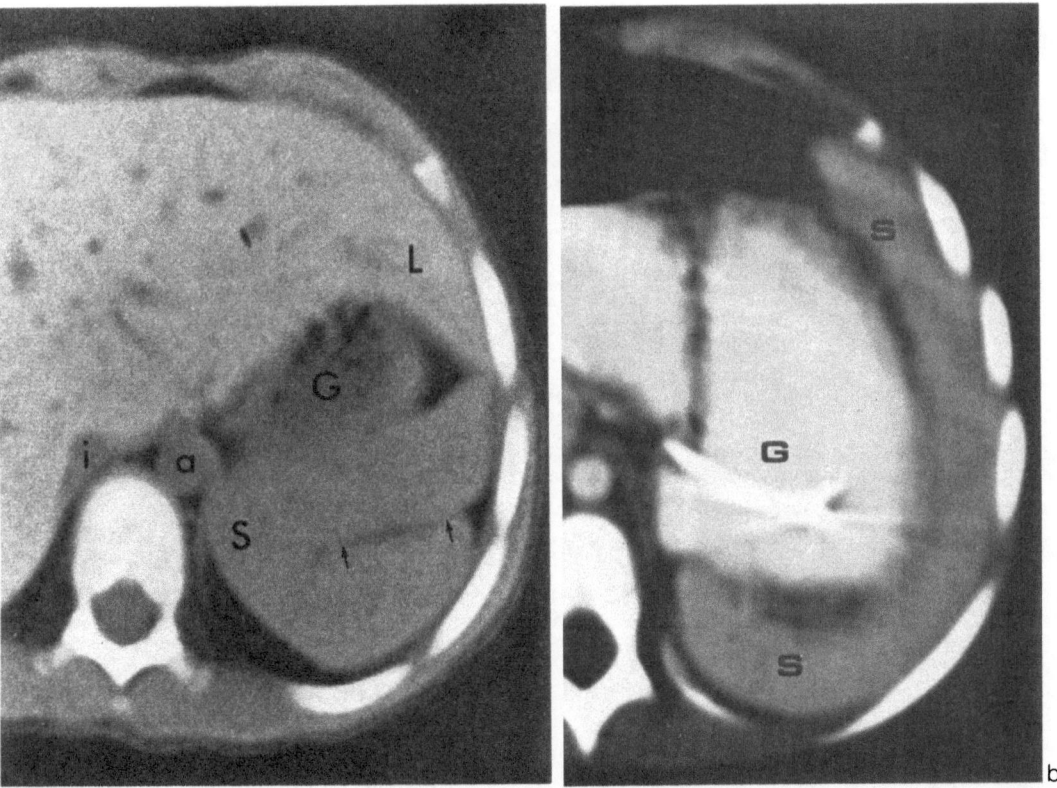

Fig. 14.4a. A 16-year-old boy with thalassemia and hemochromatosis. There is hepatosplenomegaly. The spleen (S) is bilobed and has a large cleft (*small arrows*) from the lateral aspect. L, liver; G, stomach; a, aorta; i, inferior vena cava, **b** Another example of an unusual splenic shape. The spleen (S) has a crescentic shape lying adjacent to the stomach (G).

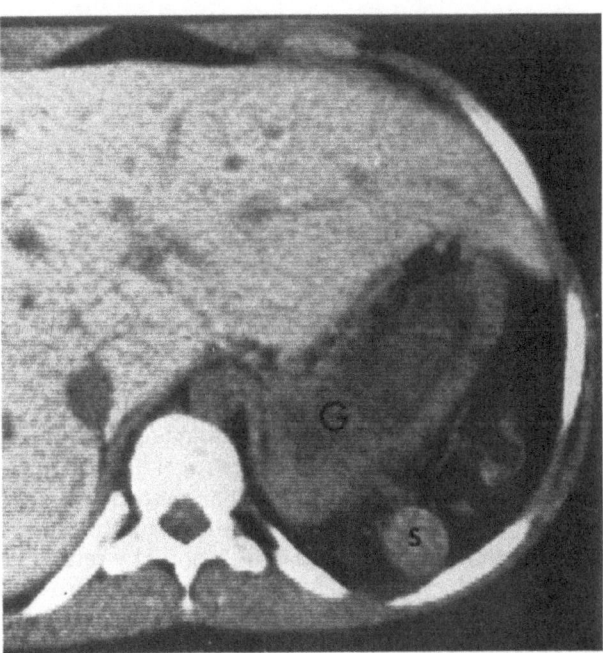

Fig. 14.5. A 10-year-old boy with thalassemia and hemochromatosis who had a previous splenectomy. A small splenunculus (s) is noted on the left in the splenic bed. G, stomach. The liver is enlarged and has an increased attenuation caused by iron deposition.

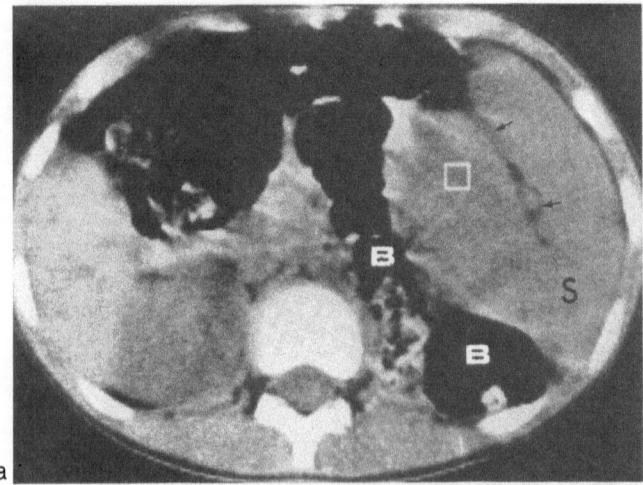

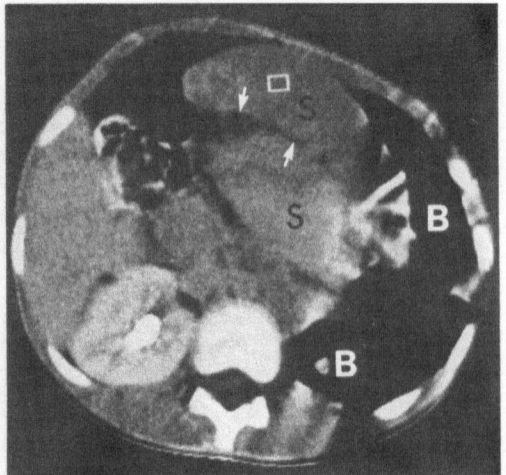

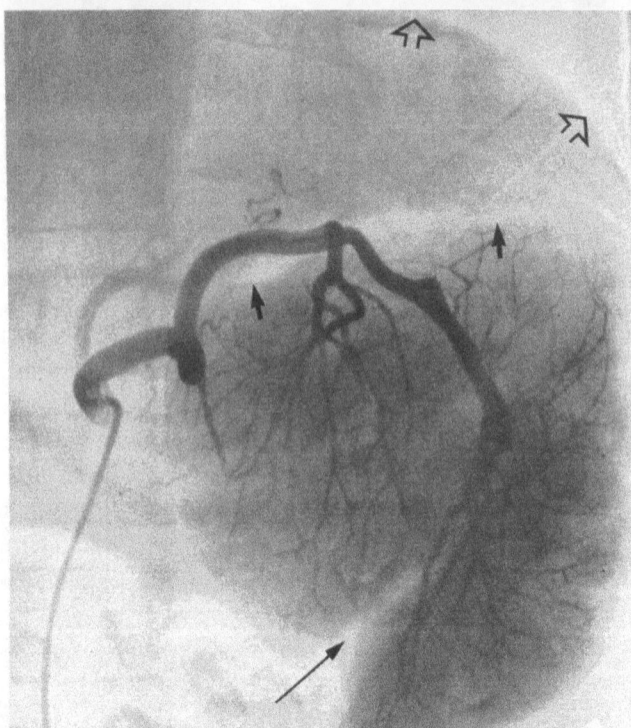

Fig. 14.6a–c. A 13-year-old boy with left upper quadrant pain. **a** CT scan in supine position shows the spleen (*S*) lying more lateral and more anterior than normal. The spleen is bilobed and contains a large cleft (*small arrows*). Small and large bowel (*B*) separate the spleen from the vertebrae. **b** CT scan taken with the patient in a right lateral decubitus position. The image has been reorientated to make comparison with scan **a** easier. Note that the spleen has moved markedly anteriorly and medially compared with its position in **a**. Bowel (*B*) now lies lateral and posterior to the spleen. Note the artifact from the bowel gas obscuring the posterolateral aspect of the spleen. **c** Splenic arteriogram shows that the upper border (*arrows*) of the bilobed spleen is markedly separated from the diaphragm (*open arrows*). *Long arrow* shows the splenic cleft. Laparatomy confirmed the abnormal position of the spleen and revealed areas of ischemia in the isthmus between the two splenic lobes. It was felt that the patient's left upper quadrant pain was related to a "wandering spleen" with intermittent torsion. (Liu and Daneman 1985 [22])

Displacements

The presence of left upper quadrant masses or visceromegaly may cause considerable displacement of the spleen, and, because it is a soft organ, the shape of the spleen changes to accommodate the adjacent mass. The spleen is often pushed markedly upward or anteriorly by retroperitoneal masses such as Wilms' tumor, neuroblastoma, and adrenal carcinoma (see Fig. 10.4, p. 129, and Fig. 10.11, p. 138).

When adjacent organs such as the kidney are removed, the spleen then shifts position to occupy the space that has been vacated. Knowledge of the usual changes in visceral position and the accurate delineation of these viscera in postoperative follow-up scans is important in order to rule out early recurrent tumor. Occasionally, these changes may be somewhat unexpected. In one such patient that we have seen [22], the spleen dropped to an unusually low position following the removal of an adrenal carcinoma and left nephrectomy (Fig. 14.7).

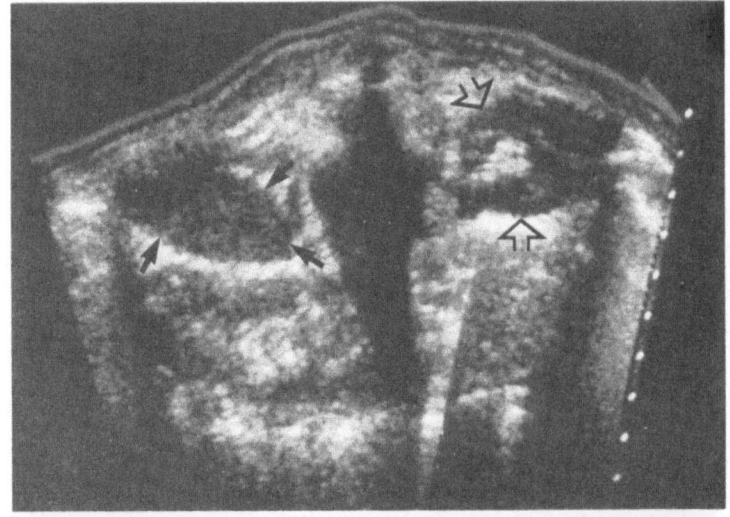

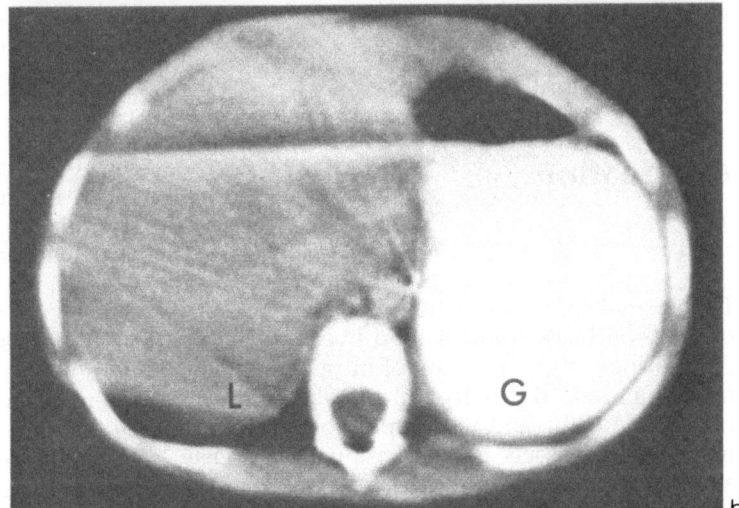

Fig. 14.7a–d. A 4-year-old boy with previous left adrenalectomy and nephrectomy for a large adrenal carcinoma. a Transverse abdominal sonogram in prone position shows the right kidney (*open arrows*). An echogenic "mass" (*arrows*) occupies the left renal fossa. b CT reveals absence of the spleen behind the upper portion of the stomach (*G*). This is the appearance seen in asplenia. However, in images c and d it is noted that the spleen (*arrows*) has descended to occupy the left renal fossa and lies lateral to the psoas muscle (*p*). *k*, right kidney; *small white arrows*, surgical clips. (Liu and Daneman 1985 [22])

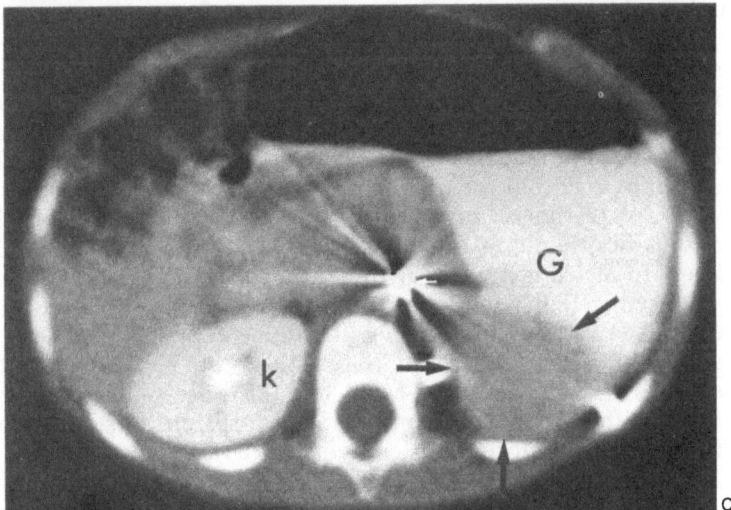

Fig. 14.7d *overleaf* ▶

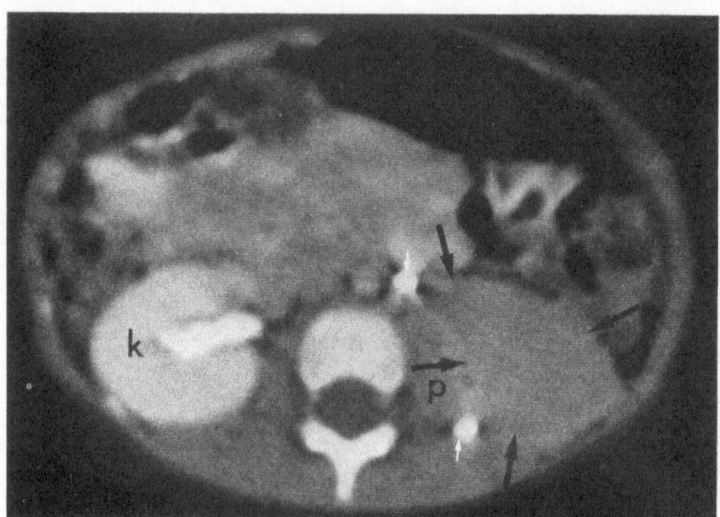

Fig. 14.7d

Attenuation

The normal spleen has a homogeneous attenuation (35–55 HU) — lower than liver but higher than kidney. With injection of intravenous contrast material, the spleen normally enhances homogeneously, and with rapid bolus injection intrasplenic vessels may occasionally be visualized. With diffuse lymphomatous involvement and in storage diseases, the spleen may be enlarged but the attenuation remains normal.

Small areas of increased attenuation within the spleen may represent punctate calcification related to granulomatous disease such as tuberculosis and histoplasmosis [21]. Diffuse, increased attenuation of the spleen is noted in children on chronic blood transfusion programs such as β thalassemia, but the increase in attenuation is not as great as that noted in the liver. In sickle cell anemia, the spleen may be small with a high attenuation caused by repeated episodes of splenic infarction with diffuse deposition of calcium and iron (Fig. 14.8a). Such spleens may take up [99mTC-MDP], and CT is useful in differentiating this uptake in the spleen from uptake in a focus of osteomyelitis in a rib [1, 21].

Focal splenic lesions such as neoplasms (Fig. 14.8), abscesses, infarcts (see Fig. 9.7, p. 114), old hematomas (see Fig. 14.10) and cysts (see Fig. 14.9) have attenuation values less than that of the normal spleen [21]. Neoplasms may have irregular shapes and margins. Splenic abscesses, which are rare in children, may have a spherical outline, may contain air, and have an enhancing rim. Acute infarcts may appear wedge-shaped, with the base of the wedge directed to the splenic margin (see Fig. 9.7, p.114). Cysts have a fluid attenuation with a thin enhancing wall (see Fig. 14.9).

When examining the spleen for such focal lesions, we recommend scanning both before and after intravenous contrast injection. Intravenous contrast enhancement of the splenic tissue may improve the detectability of small focal lesions. Experimental studies using intravenous injection of emulsified liposoluble contrast materials which are taken up by reticuloendothelial cells have shown that the attenuation number of the spleen can be elevated by 80 HU [21]. With this technique, nodules only a few millimeters in diameter can be demonstrated. However, this technique has not been used in children.

Artifacts may give the spleen an inhomogeneous attenuation and may simulate the presence of focal lesions. These streak artifacts are usually related to densities originating from the surfaces of the adjacent ribs or adjacent bowel gas (see Fig. 14.6). The artifacts are more troublesome in patients who cannot suspend respiration adequately but are also occasionally seen in more cooperative patients.

Pathology

Neoplasms

The commonest reason for splenic assessment on CT in children is in patients with lymphoma. The sensitivity for detecting splenic involvement with CT in adults with lymphoma has been reported to be between 50% and 90% [21].

The spleen may appear normal or be enlarged with a normal homogeneous attenuation when there is diffuse, homogeneous, splenic infiltration. The incidence of finding focal abnormalities in such involved spleens varies from series to series (see Fig. 14.8). They are found rarely in Hodgkin's disease and more commonly in diffuse histiocytic lymphoma. Focal lesions are thus the exception rather than the rule. They have a lower attenuation relative to the remainder of the spleen and vary in size, shape, and margination. One-third of patients with

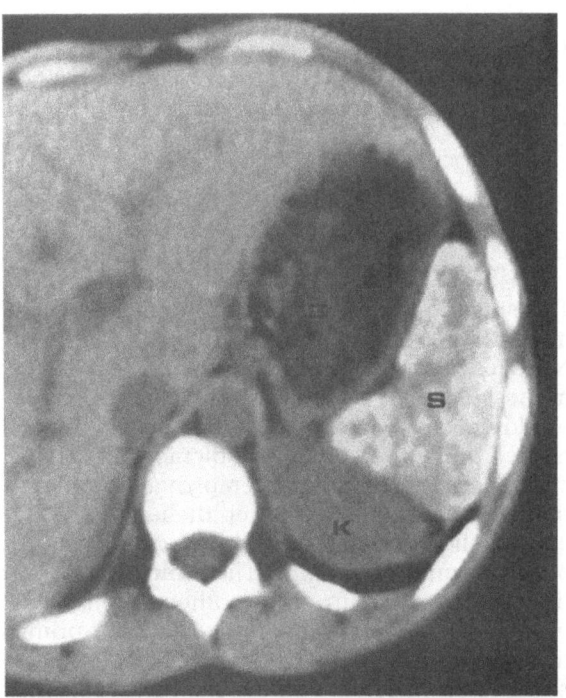

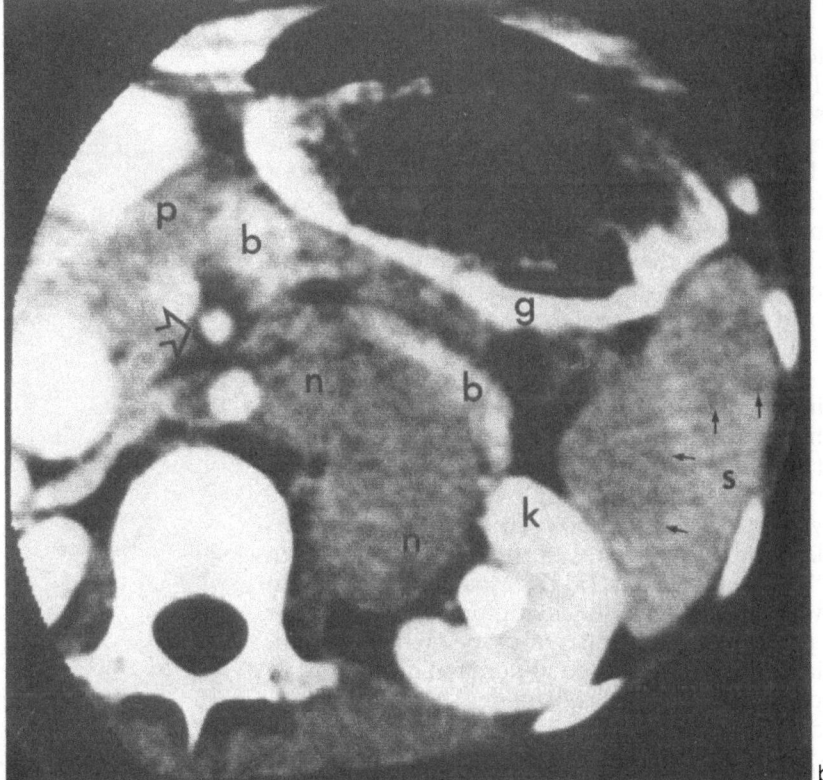

Fig. 14.8a. Example of increased attenuation of the spleen (s) in a boy with sickle cell anemia. This is related to splenic infarctions with deposition of calcium and iron. *G.*, stomach; *K*, left kidney. **b** A 12-year-old boy with Hodgkin's disease. Low-attenuation areas (*small arrows*) in the spleen (s) represent malignant infiltration. These areas are irregular in outline with poorly defined margins. Large retroperitoneal lymph nodes (*n*) displace the left kidney (*k*) laterally and jejunum (*b*) anteriorly. *Open arrow*, superior mesenteric artery and vein; *g*, stomach; *p*, pancreatic head.

Hodgkin's disease and splenomegaly are found to have no splenic involvement at the time of splenectomy. Other primary and secondary neoplasms of the spleen are extremely rare in children.

Cysts

The spleen undergoes cystic changes less commonly than other abdominal viscera [2, 3, 27]. In North America, epithelial cysts are the commonest type of splenic cyst. However, on a worldwide basis hydatid cysts are said to be commoner [3]. Other types of splenic cysts (false cysts) occur secondary to hemorrhage or infarction and are not lined with epithelium [2, 3, 7].

Epithelial cysts of the spleen are considered to be congenital in origin. The lining cells are thought to arise from mesothelial cells that migrate during embryogenesis from the primitive celomic cavity into the splenic anlage. These cells then undergo squamous metaplasia [8, 17]. No skin appendages are present.

Epithelial cysts are usually solitary and unilocular and seldom contain calcification [7, 8, 17]. The lining consists of squamous or stratified squamous epithelium, often with interspersed areas of mesothelial cells, but large areas may be devoid of epithelium [3]. The wall consists of fibrous tissue. The internal surface of the cyst may be smooth or appear trabeculated [2]. The fluid within the cyst may be clear or turbid and has been reported to contain bilirubin, protein, iron, cholesterol crystals, and fat [3, 8, 14, 17, 32, 37].

Epithelial cysts occur rather more commonly in females, and almost half of the reported cases have presented in patients under 15 years of age [3]. The age range of presentation varies from the neonatal period [17, single case report] up to 50 years of age [3]. These cysts produce symptoms late and therefore are often extremely large when they are discovered [3, 17]. Most patients present with an otherwise asymptomatic left upper quadrant mass [3, 8]. Symptoms, when present, include mild left-sided abdominal discomfort or pain and postprandial fullness [17]. Occasionally, mild symptoms may precede the presence of a palpable mass. The physical examination is usually unremarkable except for the presence of the left upper quadrant mass, which is usually nontender. Acute symptoms and signs may be related to trauma, hemorrhage, and infection, to which these large cysts are predisposed [3].

We have recently seen eight patients with epithelial cysts. Four of these were previously reported by Daneman and Martin in 1982 [5]. In all eight, a rim of normal splenic tissue was easily visualized around part of the cyst on sonography. This confirmed the intrasplenic location of the cyst. In three of the cysts, the fluid was completely echo free. Echoes within the fluid were due to fat globules in three cases, infective debris in one, and blood clot in one. All eight cases were well evaluated with sonography and CT was only performed in special circumstances. Only two of our patients had CT. In one patient, known to have tuberculosis and left upper quadrant trauma, the CT study was performed following sonography merely to confirm the absence of granuloma or hematoma in the spleen in addition to the splenic cyst (Fig. 14.9). In the second patient, CT was used to localize the cyst prior to drainage. The cyst was partially drained easily, but the fluid promptly reaccumulated.

In both patients, the cysts appeared well defined with a smooth margin and contained fluid of water attenuation (Fig. 14.9). No rim enhancement or calcification was present. Most

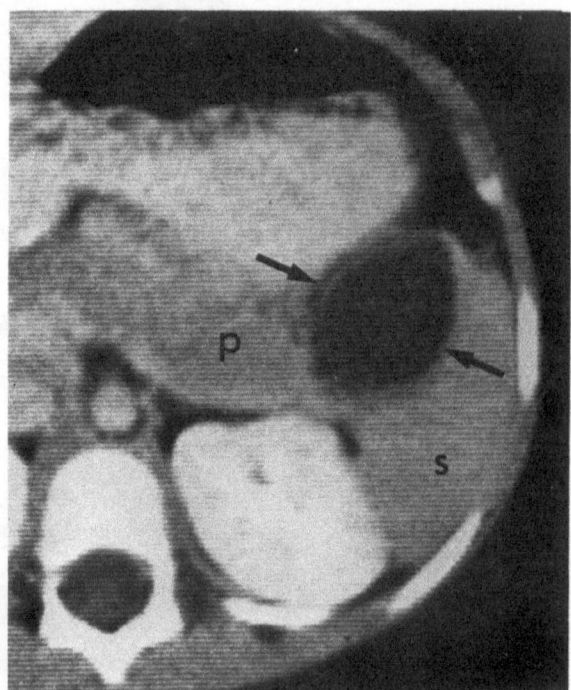

Fig. 14.9. A 10-year-old boy with epithelial cyst (*arrows*) in the anteromedial aspect of the spleen (*s*). The contents of the cyst are of water attenuation. Note the thin enhancing wall along the anteromedial side of the cyst. *p*, pancreas.

of the various types of splenic cysts have this appearance, and it is difficult to differentiate them except on histological grounds [2].

Sonography is thus the modality of choice for evaluation of splenic cysts, and scintigraphy and CT are only required in special circumstances [6, 9, 10, 13, 24, 26, 30, 35].

Trauma

At the Hospital for Sick Children, Toronto, we have used radionuclide liver/spleen scans successfully as the initial imaging modality in the assessment of patients with suspected splenic trauma as well as in follow-up. However, CT is extremely useful in assessing the abdomen in patients with blunt trauma. The sensitivity of CT in detecting splenic injury has been reported to be as high as 100% in recent series [21]. Furthermore, other viscera can be examined simultaneously, and occasionally otherwise unsuspected lesions of other organs are diagnosed in this way. This is a distinct advantage over radionuclide scans. The sensitivity of sonography in evaluating splenic trauma is probably not as high as that of CT.

On CT, subcapsular hematomas appear as crescentic fluid collections along the surface of the spleen and flatten or indent the splenic margin. Hematomas which are 1–2 days old may be iso- or hyperdense relative to the spleen, and intravenous contrast may be necessary to deline-

ate these lesions adequately. After this period, the hematoma gradually loses density and becomes hypodense relative to the spleen [21] (Fig. 14.10). Splenic lacerations are visualized as a cleft or defect in the splenic border and are often accompanied by free intraperitoneal blood. More rarely, intrasplenic hematomas may occur [19, 20, 21].

With the aid of radionuclide spleen scans and CT, the accuracy of the initial assessment and follow-up of patients with splenic trauma has increased. This has led to a more conservative therapeutic approach. Splenectomy for trauma is rarely performed at most institutions. This avoids the complication of severe infection following splenectomy [1].

CT can be useful in detecting the foci of splenosis. This occurs following trauma or operation where there is seeding of the peritoneal cavity with viable splenic tissue [21].

Asplenia/Polysplenia Syndrome

Sonography and CT may be used together with chest radiographs to diagnose visceroatrial situs [33]. Asplenia is characterized by absence of the spleen and abnormal position of the liver (100%). The inferior vena cava and aorta course together on the same side of the spine with inferior vena cava/atrial communication (100%). Polysplenia is characterized by multiple splenules, abnormal position of the liver (80%), and interruption of the hepatic segment of the inferior vena cava with azygous (hemiazygous) continuation (100%) [33] (see Fig. 8.14, p. 104). The associated vascular anomalies are important features for diagnosis.

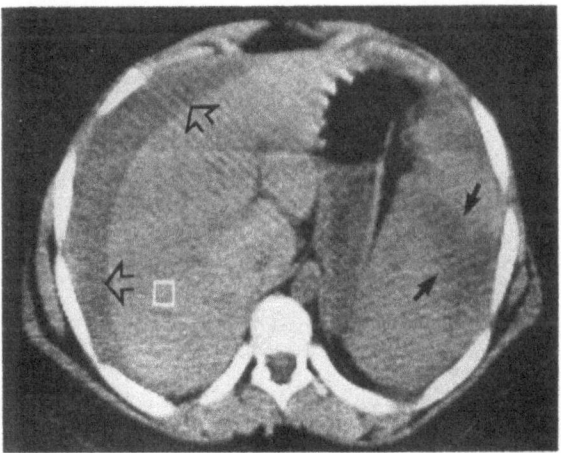

Fig. 14.10. A 12-year-old boy with hemophilia and abdominal trauma. A hematoma (*arrows*) is present in the mid portion of the spleen. A subcapsular hematoma is also noted along the anterolateral aspect of the liver (*open arrows*).

References

1. Berger PE (1982) Computerized tomography. In: Franken EA (ed) Gastrointestinal imaging in pediatrics. Harper and Row, Philiadelphia, pp. 490–529
2. Bhimji SD, Cooperberg PL, Naiman S, Morrison RT, Shergill P (1977) Ultrasound diagnosis of splenic cysts. Radiology 122:787
3. Blank E, Campbell JR (1973) Epidermoid cysts of the spleen. Pediatrics 51:75
4. Carswell JW (1974) Wandering spleen: 11 cases from Uganda. Br J Surg 61: 495–497
5. Daneman A, Martin DJ (1982) Congenital epithelial splenic cysts in children. Emphasis on sonographic appearances and some unusual features. Pediatr Radiol 12:119–125

220

6. Davis PL, Filly RA, Goerke J (1981) In vitro demonstration of an echogenic emulsion: relationship of lipid particle size to echo detection. J Clin Ultrasound 9:263
7. Dembner AG, Taylor K (1978) Gray scale sonographic diagnosis: multiple congenital splenic cysts. J Clin Ultrasound 6:143
8. Faer M, Lynch RD, Lichenstein JE, Madewell JE, Feigin DS (1980) Traumatic splenic cyst. Radiology 134:371
9. Filly RA, Sommer FG, Minton MJ (1980) Characterization of biological fluids by ultrasound and computed tomography. Radiology 134:167
10. Fitzer PM (1976) 99mTC-Pertechnetate angiography and sulphur colloid scans in epidermoid cyst of spleen. Clin Nucl Med 1:60
11. Forde WJ, Ostrolenk DG, Finby N (1960) Renal displacement associated with enlargement of the spleen. AJR 84:889
12. Frimann-Dahl J (1960) Normal variations of the left kidney. Acta Radiol 55:207
13. Glancy JJ (1979) Fluid-filled echogenic epidermoid cyst of the spleen. J Clin Ultrasound 7:301
14. Glancy JJ, Goddard J, Pearson DE (1980) In vitro demonstration of cholesterol crystals' high echogenicity relative to protein particles. J Clin Ultrasound 8:27
15. Gooding GAW (1978) The ultrasonic and computed tomographic appearance of splenic lobulations: a consideration in the ultrasonic differential of masses adjacent to the left kidney. Radiology 126:719
16. Gordon DH, Burrell MI, Levin DC, Mueller CF, Becker JA (1977) Wandering spleen — the radiological and clinical spectrum. Radiology 125:39–46
17. Griscom NT, Hargreaves HK, Schwartz MZ, Reddish JM, Colodny AH (1977) Huge splenic cyst in a newborn: comparison with 10 cases in later childhood and adolescence. Am J Roentgenol Radium Ther Nucl Med 129:889
18. Karstaedt N, Sagel SS, Stanley RJ, Melson GL, Levitt RG (1978) Computed tomography of the adrenal gland. Radiology 129:723–730
19. Kaufman RA (1983) Liver spleen computed tomography. A method tailored for infants and children. CT 7:45–57
20. Kaufman RA, Towbin R, Babcock DS, Gelfand MJ, Guice KS, Oldham KT, Noseworthy J (1984) Upper abdominal trauma in children: imaging evaluation. AJR 142:449–460
21. Koehler RE (1983) Spleen. In: Lee JK, Sagel SS, Stanley RJ (eds) Computed body tomography. Raven, New York, pp 243–256.
22. Liu P, Daneman A (1985) Unusual positions of the spleen: a report of two cases. J Can Assoc Radiol 36:163–165
23. Madayag M, Mosniak MA, Beranbaum E, Becker J (1972) Renal and suprarenal pseudotumors caused by variations of the spleen. Radiology 105:43
24. Mittelstaedt CA, Partain CL (1980) Ultrasonic-pathologic classification of splenic abnormalities: gray-scale patterns. Radiology 134:697
25. Olutola PO, Daneman A, Martin DJ, Alton DJ (1982) Unusual renal distortion and displacement due to the spleen. Pediatr Radiology 12:185–189
26. Piekarski J, Federle MP, Moss AA, Landon SS (1980) Computed tomography of the spleen. Radiology 135:683
27. Propper RA, Weinstein BJ, Skolnick ML, Kisloff B (1979) Ultrasonography of hemorrhagic splenic cysts. J Clin Ultrasound 7:18
28. Rao AKR, Silver TM (1976) Normal pancreas and splenic variants simulating suprarenal and renal tumors. AJR 126:530
29. Sheflin JR, Lee CM, Kretchmar KA (1984) Torsion of wandering spleen and distal pancreas. AJR 142:100–101
30. Shirkhoda A, McCartney WH, Staab EV, Mittelstaedt CA (1980) Imaging of the spleen: a proposed algorithm. Am J Roentgenol Radium Ther Nucl Med 135:195
31. Stiris MG (1980) Accessory spleen versus left adrenal tumor: computed tomographic and abdominal angiographic evaluation. J Comput Assist Tomogr 4:543
32. Thurber LA, Cooperberg PL, Clement JG, Lyons EA, Gramiak R, Cunningham J (1979) Echogenic fluid: a pitfall in the ultrasonographic diagnosis of cystic lesions. J. Clin Ultrasound 7:273
33. Tonkin ILD, Tonkin AK (1981) Abdominal ultrasound and computed tomography in the diagnosis of visceroatrial situs. Paper presented at 24th Annual Meeting of Society for Pediatric Radiology, San Francisco, March 1981
34. Whalen JP, Evans JA, Shanser J (1971) Vector principle in the differential diagnosis of abdominal masses: the left upper quadrant. Am J Roentgenol Radium Ther Nucl Med 113:104
35. Wicks JD, Silver TM, Bree RL (1978) Giant cystic abdominal masses in children and adolescents: ultrasonic differential diagnosis. Am J Roentgenol Radium Ther Nucl Med 130:853
36. Woodward DAKL (1967) Torsion of the spleen. J Surg 114:953–955
37. Zimmerman O, Scheuken JR, Schultz L, Paustian FF (1972) Epidermoid cyst of the spleen: an unusual cause of splenomegaly. J Pediatr Surg 7:374

Chapter 15

Pelvic Viscera and Soft Tissues

Introduction

For purposes of description, pelvic structures can be divided into two components: bony and soft tissue. Details of the anatomy and pathological entities involving the musculoskeletal part of the pelvis are discussed in Chapters 21, 22 and 23. The purpose of this chapter is to describe the anatomy and pathological processes affecting the pelvic soft tissues and viscera and to outline our radiological approach to children with known or suspected abnormalities involving these structures.

In many instances, sonography is the initial modality of choice in the investigation of certain pelvic viscera. In the investigation of disease entities of the uterus, Fallopian tubes, and ovaries in girls, and in children with suspected pelvic abscesses, sonography is usually definitive. The commonest reason for performing CT of the soft tissues of the pelvis in children is to delineate malignant soft tissue masses. The delineation of other soft tissue masses and the search for clinically nonpalpable testes are less common indications. The appearances of benign cystic or fluid-filled lesions on CT is often nonspecific, and these are usually just as easily delineated by sonography. CT, however, may rarely add extra information about such lesions, including urinomas, lymphoceles, seromas, congenital genital malformations, and even abscesses and hematomas. Excretory urography, cystography, and barium studies have been used in the past to define pelvic disease, but their use is limited as small masses may not be detected with these modalities; and indeed, normal structures may simulate masses. Rarely, urographic or barium studies may be necessary to further define abnormalities found on sonography or CT. The relationship of CT to other modalities in the investigation of pelvic diseases will be discussed under the various disease entities.

Anatomy

The soft tissue structures of the pelvis are either bilaterally symmetrical or midline. This anatomical arrangement usually enables one to recognize abnormalities readily. If the patient has been placed in the gantry at a slight angle, suspicious areas on one side of the body should be compared with similar structures in adjacent superior or inferior scans in order to make an accurate assessment of these structures. In order to appreciate these structures optimally, strict attention must be paid to technique.

In the midline anteriorly the bladder is usually filled with sufficient fluid to be visualized easily even without contrast administration. As urographic contrast fills the bladder a fluid-fluid level forms as the opacified urine sinks to the dependent portion of the bladder (see Figs. 15.1, 15.3). Occasionally, turbulence caused by the "jet effect" may be visualized on scans per-

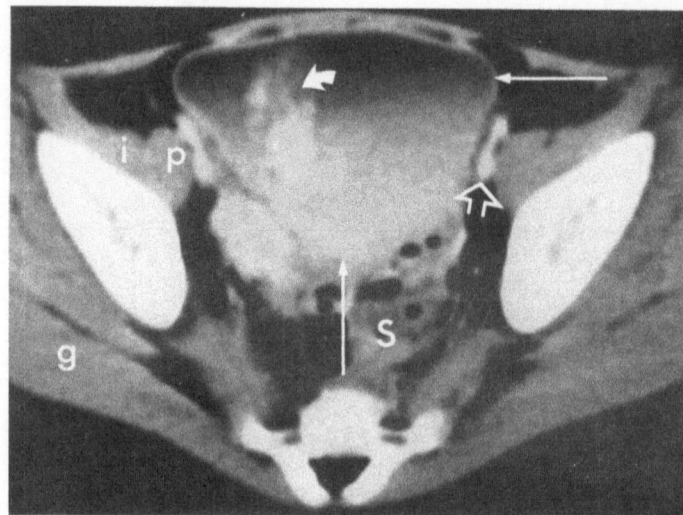

Fig. 15.1. CT through the lower parts of the iliac bones shows the bladder (*long arrows*) with more opacified urine in the more dependent portion of the bladder. Turbulence caused by opacified urine squirting into the bladder is noted on the right (*curved arrow*). *s*, sigmoid colon; *p*, psoas muscle; *i*, iliacus muscles; *g*, glutei; *open arrow*, external iliac artery (anterior) and vein (posterior) between the bladder and the psoas muscle.

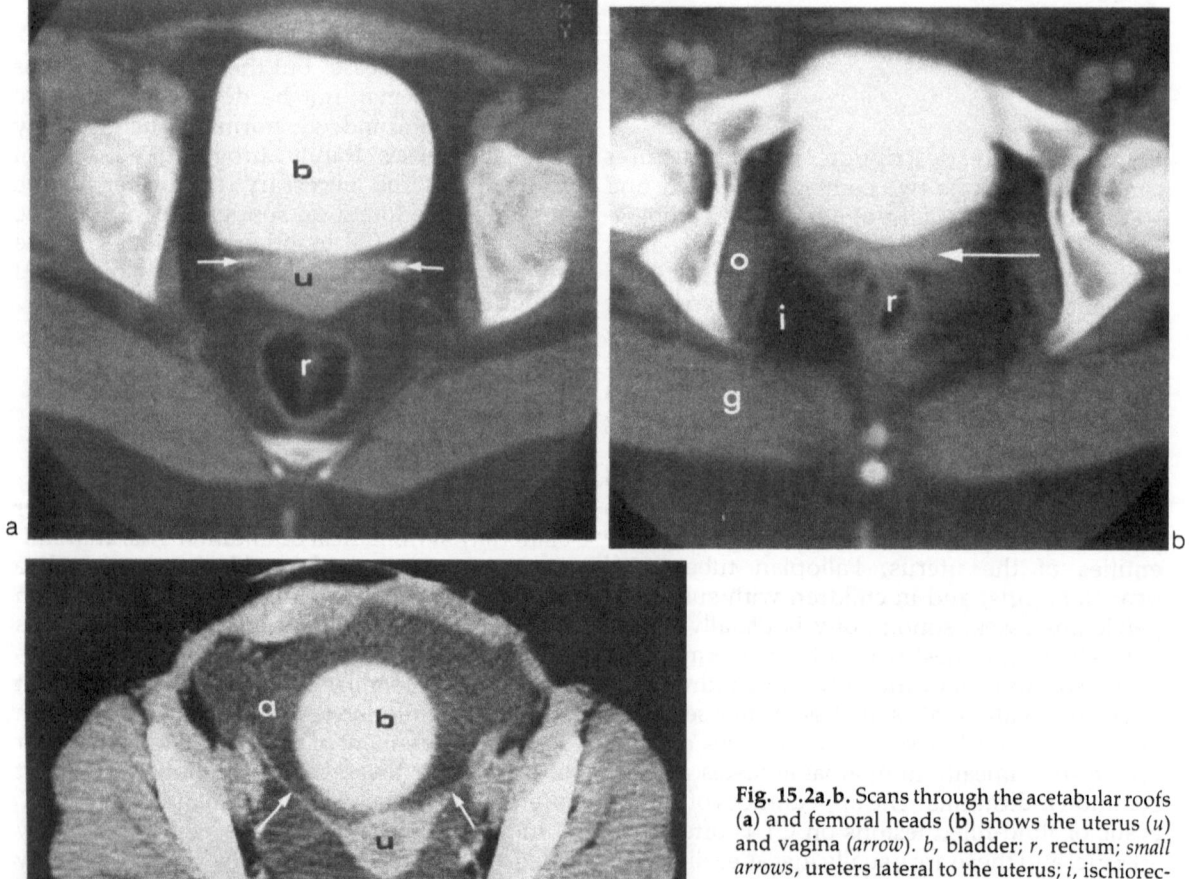

Fig. 15.2a,b. Scans through the acetabular roofs (**a**) and femoral heads (**b**) shows the uterus (*u*) and vagina (*arrow*). *b*, bladder; *r*, rectum; *small arrows*, ureters lateral to the uterus; *i*, ischiorectal fossa; *o*, obturator internus muscle; *g*, glutei. **c** A 15-year-old girl with thickening of the anterior abdominal wall on the right caused by previous surgery who presented with ascites. The ascitic fluid (*a*) is seen surrounding the bladder (*b*) and is also posterior to the uterus (*u*). The fluid outlines the broad ligaments (*arrows*) well.

formed as a bolus of opacified urine squirts into the bladder from a ureter (Fig. 15. 1). As more contrast fills the bladder the urine becomes more homogeneously opacified (see Fig. 15.3).

In young children the reproductive organs are not well visualized. However, in older children the uterus is usually well seen in girls (Fig. 15.2), as are the prostate and seminal vesicles in boys (Fig. 15.3). Distinct planes surrounding these structures are not always present. In the presence of pelvic ascites the uterus can often be easily seen surrounded by fluid posterior to the bladder (see Fig. 15.2). The ovaries are not usually seen well unless enlarged.

The sigmoid colon and rectum are easily recognized posteriorly and usually contain formed stool and air (see Figs. 15.1–15.3). Small bowel fills the remainder of the central portion of the pelvis, and occasionally a redundant sigmoid loop may also be found in this site.

The ureters, if not dilated, will only be visualized after intravenous contrast administration as they course from the lateral pelvic wall (around the lower portion of the uterus in girls) toward the bladder base (see Fig. 15.2). If dilated, they will appear as rounded fluid-filled structures on consecutive scans.

The iliacus muscle lies on the inner aspect of the iliac wing, and the psoas muscle is separated from it in the upper pelvis. Low in the pelvis these two muscles fuse to form iliopsoas as they course toward the lesser trochanter (see Figs. 15.1, 15.2, 15.4). Lying medial to the psoas muscle are the ureter and common iliac and external iliac artery and vein as they course toward the groin (see Figs. 15.1, 15.4). The artery lies anterior and slightly lateral to the vein, and there is often marked asymmetry between the iliac veins on each side of the body. Other vessels and lymph nodes may be difficult to discern, but the vasculature is better appreciated after intravenous contrast administration.

The aorta and inferior vena cava are easily visualized in the lower abdomen, as are the iliac vessels in the pelvis. However, in younger children lack of adjacent fat makes separation of these vessels from neighboring structures difficult. These structures are better seen after injection of intravenous contrast material. Their anatomical relationships are illustrated in Fig. 15.4.

In boys the spermatic cords can be seen anteriorly in the inguinal canals as they course inferiorly toward the testes which appear as oval or rounded soft tissue masses within the scrotum (see Fig. 15.24).

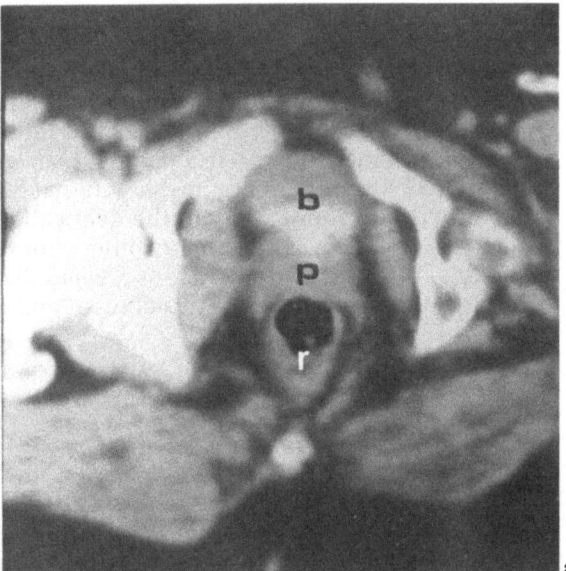

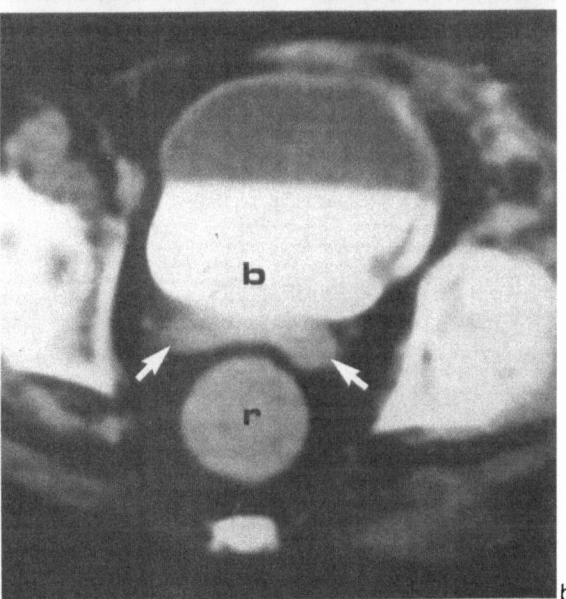

Fig. 15.3a,b. CT scans through the pelvis in a 17-year-old boy show the prostate (*p*) slightly behind the lowermost limit of the bladder (*b*) and the seminal vesicles (*arrows*) behind the bladder in a higher cut. *r*, rectum. The bones and musculature on the left are atrophied compared with those on the right because the patient has a left proximal focal femoral deficiency.

Pelvic Masses

CT plays a vital role in the characterization and delineation of the extent of many soft tissue masses in the pelvis. Based on clinical findings and the site of the mass, CT may well be the initial modality chosen and will often provide definitive information necessary for adequate therapy. This is particularly true of lesions adjacent to bone, such as those in the presacral space or along the lateral pelvic wall, as well as those with clinical evidence of extension into the sacrosciatic notch. Our experience has shown that CT is far superior to sonography in the delineation of such lesions. However, in many other clinical situations, particularly if the lesions are situated centrally in the pelvis and are of a nonmalignant or congenital etiology, sonography should be utilized initially. This may well provide definitive information thus obviating the necessity to proceed to CT in many. CT is occasionally useful in these instances if sonography is nondiagnostic, either because of excessive intestinal gas or because the bladder cannot be adequately distended. For purposes of description, pelvic masses can be grouped according to their sites of origin: presacral, rectal, bladder and genital, and lateral.

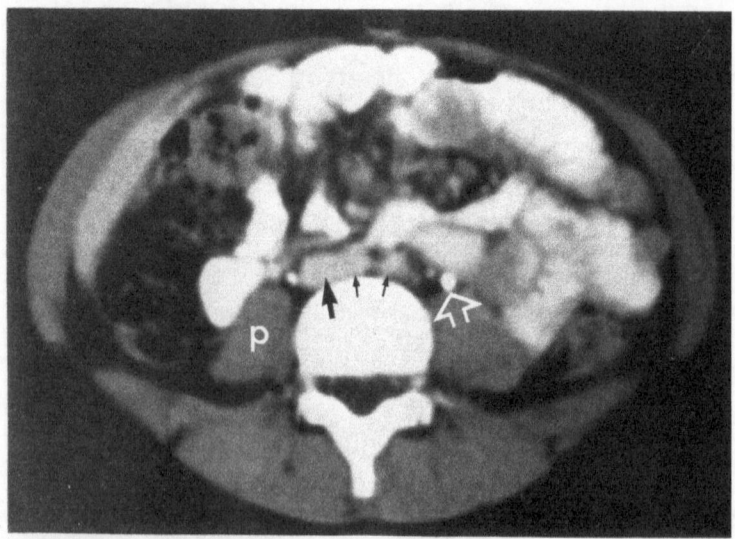

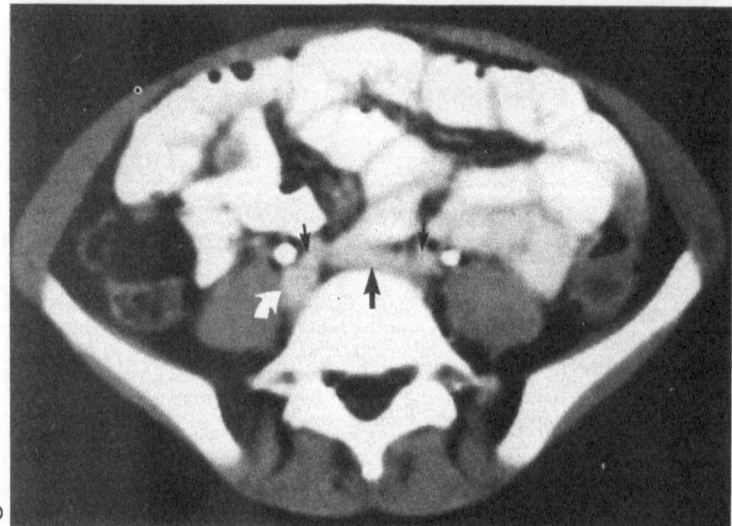

Fig. 15.4c (next page)

Fig. 15.4a–c. CT scans through the lower abdomen and upper pelvis in a 12-year-old boy. **a** The aorta has bifurcated at this site into the common iliac arteries (*small black arrows*), and the inferior vena cava (*large black arrow*) is noted to the right. The ureters (*open arrow*) are easily seen anterior to the psoas muscles (*p*). **b** The common iliac arteries (*small black arrows*) are noted medial to the well-opacified ureters. The left common iliac vein (*large black arrow*) is seen as an enhancing linear structure anterior to the vertebral body, passing from behind the left common iliac artery to the right to meet the right common iliac vein (*curved arrow*). **c** Common iliac arteries (*small black arrows*) are noted as lying slightly anterior to the common iliac veins (*small white arrows*). Both sets of vessels lie anteromedial to the psoas muscles and a little posterior to the ureters at this site.

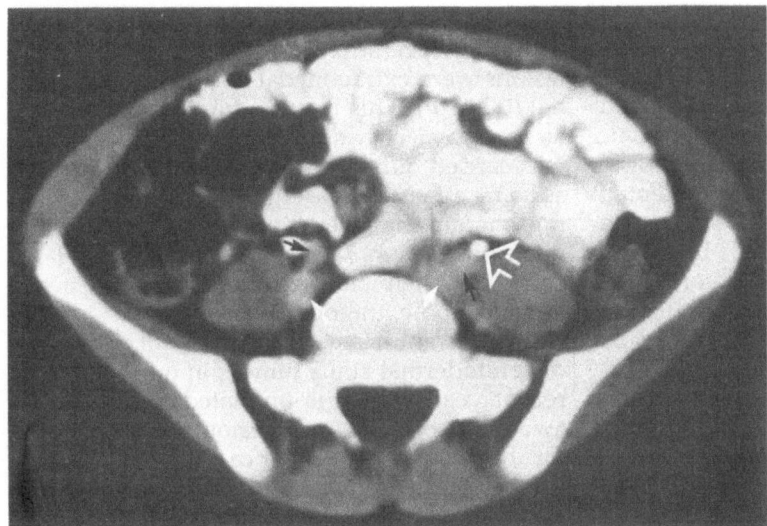

Fig. 15.4c

Presacral Lesions

Lesions that occur in the retrorectal or presacral space include:

1. Extragonadal germ cell lesions including teratomas, endodermal sinus tumors, and embryonal carcinomas
2. Neuroblastomas
3. Anterior meningomyeloceles
4. Lipomas
5. Duplication cysts

CT is the single most important modality in the characterization and delineation of the extent of lesions arising in this site. Extension of these lesions into the buttock is common and is excel-lently displayed with CT, as is the upward extension into the retroperitoneum, which occurs less commonly. Bony destruction and extension of the tumor into the spinal canal is exquisitely demonstrated with CT. CT also defines the effect of these masses on the ureters, bladder, and rectum. CT is the most accurate modality in assessing response of the tumor to therapy and diagnosis of recurrent tumor.

Extragonadal Germ Cell Tumors

The commonest group of lesions that we have seen occurring in the presacral space are the extragonadal germ cell lesions. Indeed, this is the commonest extragonadal site for such lesions to occur.

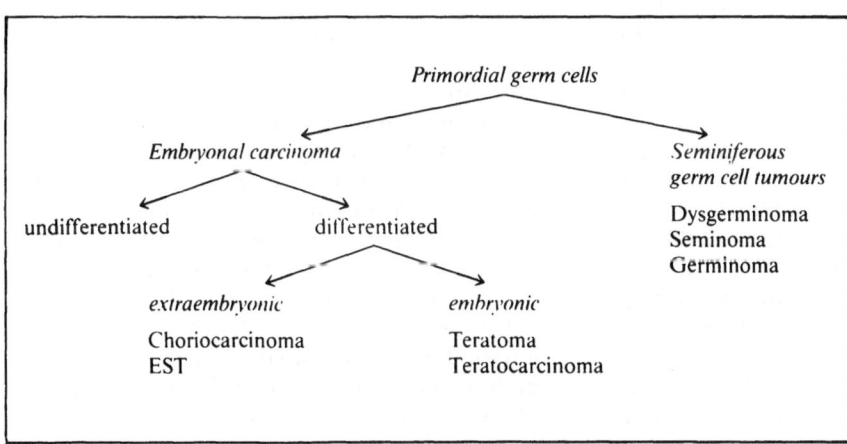

Fig. 15.5. Relationship of germ cell tumors. (O'Sullivan et al. 1983 [18])

Endodermal sinus tumors Endodermal sinus tumors or yolk sac tumors were first described as a distinct entity in 1959 by Teilum [29]. These tumors are derived from totipotential cells that differentiate primarily into extraembryonic structures that resemble the endodermal sinus of the rat placenta [8, 29]. The generally accepted hypothesis regarding endodermal sinus and related tumors is outlined in Fig. 15.5 [18]. According to this theory, primordial germ cells may develop into seminiferous germ cell tumors (dysgerminoma and seminoma) or into tumors that resemble either embryonic structures (teratoma and teratocarcinoma) or extra-embryonic structures (choriocarcinoma and endodermal sinus tumors). The embryonal carcinoma represents the undifferentiated form of the latter groups of tumors.

Supporting this theory is the fact that these tumors may occur either in a pure form or in a mixed form with elements of more than one cell type in the same tumor [3, 8, 12, 28, 29, 30, 32, 34]. Of all endodermal sinus tumors in the pediatric age group, 90% are pure lesions [26]. The prognosis of children with mixed lesions is related to the presence of the most malignant elements, which in the pediatric age group are either endodermal sinus tumors or embryonal carcinomas [5, 8, 34]. Metastatic lesions from these mixed tumors are usually pure endodermal sinus tumors or embryonal carcinomas [8, 34].

Further support for this theory of pathogenesis is the fact that endodermal sinus tumors may develop at the site of previous benign teratomas [5, 11, 12]. This was found in two of our patients (one sacrococcygeal lesion and a nasopharyngeal lesion).

Alpha-fetoprotein, which is formed by the epithelial cells of the endoderm of the fetal yolk sac, is also produced by the tumor, thus lending further support to the hypothesis that endodermal sinus tumor is related to extraembryonic structures [8, 27, 30, 32, 33].

Like other tumors in this group, primary endodermal sinus tumors may either occur in the gonads or in specific extragonadal sites [8, 12]. The extragonadal lesions are thought to develop from totipotential cells that undergo aberrant migration from the yolk sac during embryogenesis and usually occur in the midline [8, 12, 13].

Since the acceptance of endodermal sinus tumors as a distinct pathological entity, reports in the literature have shown that gonadal lesions are much more common than extragonadal lesions [11, 12, 13, 22, 32, 34]. However, in our series, the reverse situation was true: 54% of the lesions were extragonadal and 46% were gonadal (6 M:1 F). This may be due to the fact that a large retrospective study of pathological material was carried out and lesions, initially diagnosed as being other tumors (e.g., adenocarcinoma and mesonephroma) were reclassified as endodermal sinus tumors [26]. Figures from future large series may help clarify the relative incidence of gonadal and extragonadal lesions.

There is an increased incidence of extragonadal endodermal sinus tumors in our hospital in recent years which is unrelated to the greater awareness of this type of lesion. The exact cause for this increase in incidence is uncertain.

In 1983, O'Sullivan et al. [18] reviewed our experience with 24 extragonadal endodermal sinus tumors at the Hospital for Sick Children, Toronto. The clinical and radiological features of these lesions depend on the sites of the primary lesion and the presence or absence of metastatic disease. In our group the age of presentation ranged from the first day of life to 5 years of age (mean = 21 months). There is an overall female preponderance (3 F:1 M), mainly the result of the large number of females presenting with sacrococcygeal lesions (13 F:3 M). Patients with lesions at other sites have an equal sex incidence.

Radiologically the findings are nonspecific, and the primary lesion is characterized by a soft tissue mass, usually with no calcification (Fig. 15.6). Calcification was visible on plain radiographs in only one patient — a recurrent sacrococcygeal lesion following chemotherapy and radiotherapy. In one sacrococcygeal lesion CT revealed calcification not visible on plain films at the time of diagnosis (Fig. 15.7).

By far the commonest site for extragonadal lesions is the sacrococcygeal region [5, 9, 12, 13, 20, 21, 31, 32], and this site accounted for 64% of patients in our series. CT of the pelvis was performed in seven of the patients with sacrococcygeal lesions and revealed a well-circumscribed mass of soft tissue attenuation which was usually homogeneous before and after intravenous contrast enhancement (see Fig. 15.6). In only one case was calcification, not evident on plain films, noted on CT. Enhancement in two patients was extremely inhomogeneous (see Fig. 15.7). CT was the most accurate modality in defining the extent of the mass within the pelvis and its extension into the buttock or abdomen. Following therapy (surgical or nonsurgical) in six patients, CT accurately delineated the presence or absence of recurrence or postoperative changes. Inguinal

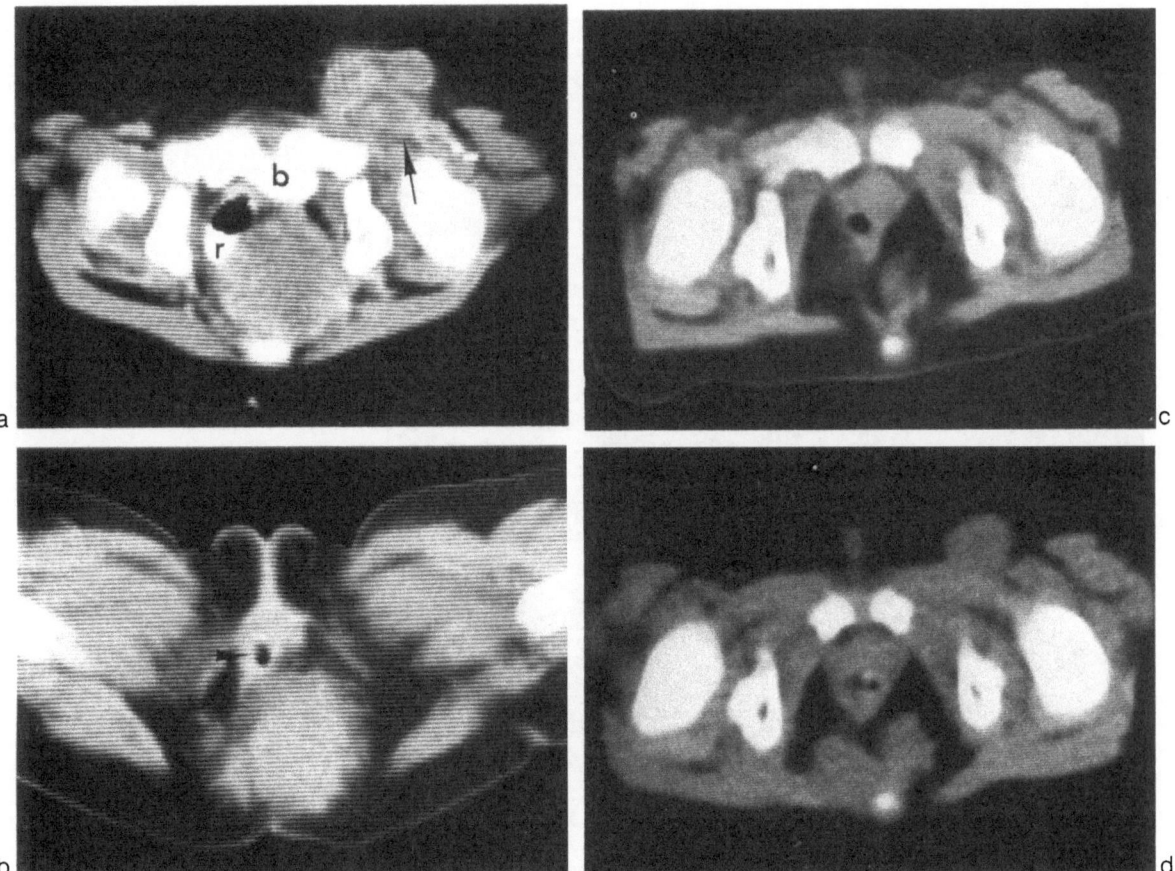

Fig. 15.6a–d. An 11-month-old girl with large sacrococcygeal endodermal sinus tumor. **a** CT of the pelvis at the time of presentation shows a well-defined rounded mass with a homogeneous density anterior to the lower sacrum, pushing the bladder (*b*) forward and the Gastrografin-filled rectum (*r*) forward and to the right. The left inguinal lymph nodes are enlarged because of metastatic spread (*arrow*). **b** Lower scan through perineum shows extension of mass into the left side of the perineum. Anus displaced to the right (*arrow*). **c** Baseline post-therapeutic scan taken 6 months later shows scar tissue anterior to the coccyx. Following chemotherapy the left inguinal lymph nodes are no longer enlarged. **d** A scan taken 7 months later reveals a soft tissue mass in the sacrococcygeal region, larger than the tissue noted in the site on the previous scan, and also enlargement of the left inguinal lymph nodes. These masses represent recurrent tumor at both sites. (O'Sullivan et al. 1983 [18])

lymphadenopathy was noted in two patients at the time of diagnosis (see Fig. 15.6).

Three further patients in our series had lesions in the pelvis, two within the vagina and one in the bladder (see Fig. 15.15). Other sites included anterior mediastinum, retroperitoneum, liver, nasopharynx (see Fig. 20.15, p. 307), and posterior cranial fossa [18]. Other authors have also reported endodermal sinus tumors occurring at these rare sites [3, 6, 10, 16, 17, 19]. Endodermal sinus tumors may also occur in other sites that have not been included in our experience, and these include the face [35], pineal and third ventricle [4, 28, 32], vulva [34], broad ligament [12], prostate [2], and cervix [37].

Endodermal sinus tumors tend to recur locally and also have a high incidence of metastatic disease at the time of presentation [5]. In our series, local recurrence occurred in 20% of patients, and metastatic disease was present at the time of diagnosis or soon thereafter in 50% of patients. The commonest site for metastases was the lungs, and this was found in 33% of patients at the time of diagnosis.

Because of this, it is essential to have an accurate knowledge of the site and extent of the primary lesion and the presence or absence of metastatic disease at the time of diagnosis, in order that the correct mode of therapy may be chosen. In this regard, CT is the most important

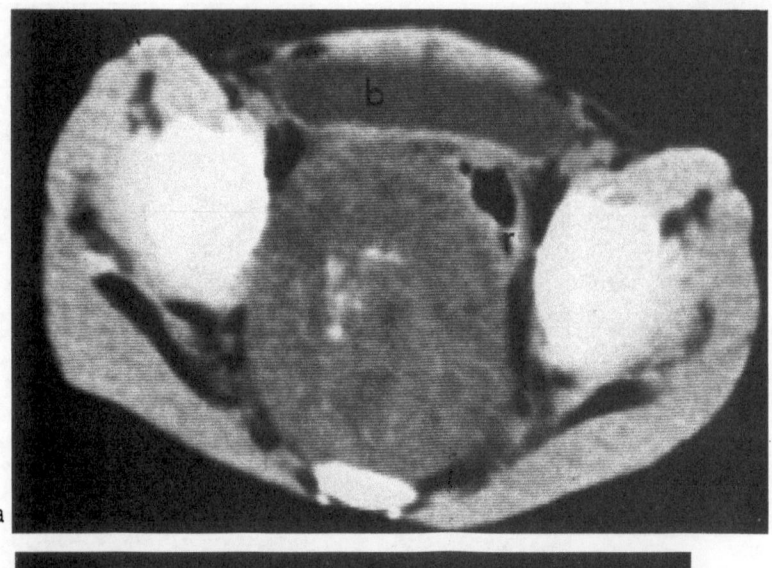

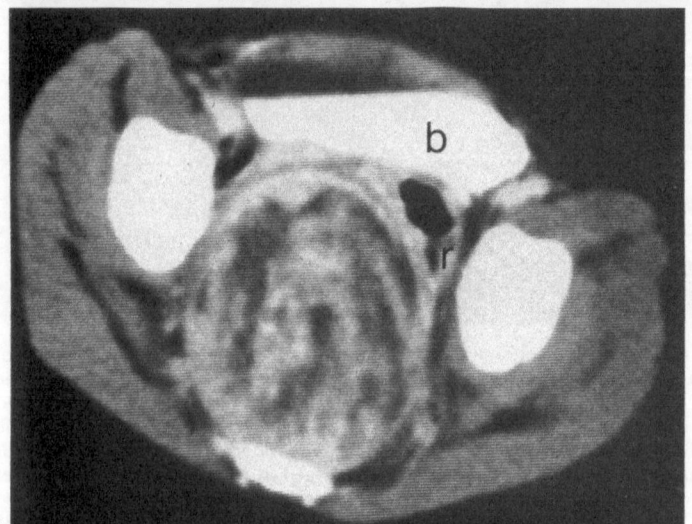

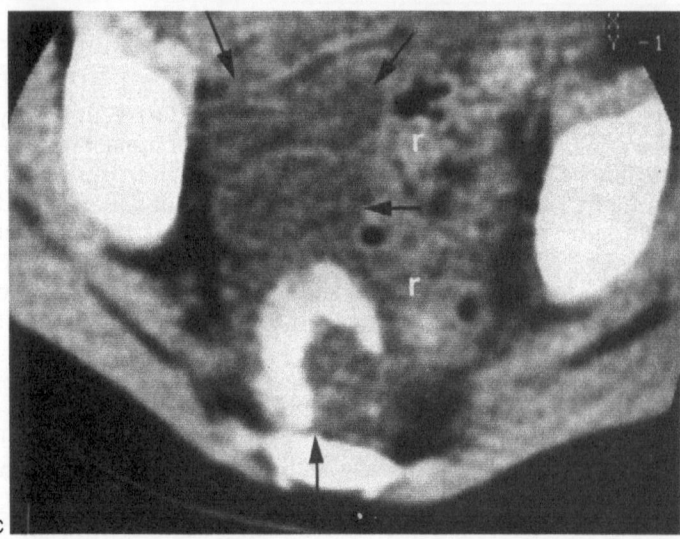

Fig. 15.7a–c. A 2½-year-old boy with a large sacrococcygeal endodermal sinus tumor. **a** Precontrast scan; **b** scan performed during intravenous contrast injection. The oval mass is well defined, and calcification (not seen on plain radiographs) is evident in the precontrast scan. The lesion has an inhomogeneous attenuation better seen on the scan performed during the injection of intravenous contrast. This lesion was considered inoperable. *b*, bladder; *r*, rectum displaced to left. **c** Following chemotherapy the mass (*arrows*) has shrunken considerably and the amount of calcification has increased. This mass was removed surgically, and the patient has no evidence of disease 1 year later. (O'Sullivan et al. 1983 [18])

modality. Because of the high incidence of pulmonary metastases, CT of the chest is mandatory in all patients prior to embarking on any therapy.

During and after therapy, CT examination of the primary site and of the chest are mandatory. Scans of the tumor bed should be performed approximately 6 weeks postoperatively to establish a baseline of the appearances of the postoperative changes and will enable the subsequent early diagnosis of local recurrence to be made with more certainty. These areas can be followed at 3- to 6-monthly intervals, and, if the response is favorable, the length between examinations can be lengthened.

An increase in serum alpha-fetoprotein is diagnostic of recurrence, and levels can be followed during and after therapy as an accurate marker of response, recurrence, or metastatic disease [12, 13, 22, 27, 30, 32, 33]. Our experience has shown that alpha-fetoprotein levels may again become elevated when recurrent lesions are too small to be detected on CT. Repeated follow-up studies are required to monitor the site of the original primary lesion as well as the lungs in order to document the site where the alpha-fetoprotein is being produced, so that correct treatment can be instituted.

Teratomas Teratomas are congenital tumors containing derivatives of all three germ layers. Extragonadal teratomas most commonly occur in the sacrococcygeal region but may also appear in other areas of the midline such as the retroperitoneum, mediastinum, and pineal [7, 23]. Sacrococcygeal teratomas may be divided into four groups depending on their location:

Type 1 — most of the mass is external, presenting as a buttock or perineal mass

Type 2 — most of the mass is external, but there is a significant intrapelvic component

Type 3 — mass has a greater proportion of intrapelvic than extrapelvic component

Type 4 — mass is presacral and sometimes retroperitoneal with no external component

Any of these types may have an intraspinal component. These lesions may present as a buttock or perineal mass or as a result of the pressure effects of the mass on adjacent structures such as urinary tract, bowel, veins, and spinal cord.

Sacrococcygeal teratomas are usually evident at birth, are benign, and occur more frequently in females, in a ratio of 4 to 1 [23]. Malignancy is more commonly seen in males if the lesion is noted at birth or in those that present beyond the neonatal period. Teratomas may be cystic, solid, or mixed. The vast majority of cystic lesions are benign. Malignant degeneration has been estimated to occur in well under 1% of cystic lesions [23] and occurs in the solid components associated with the cysts.

On plain radiographs these lesions appear as soft tissue masses that extend to a variable degree into the buttock and perineum, or pelvis and abdomen, depending on their exact location. Calcification in the mass is frequent, and occasionally well-developed bony elements may be present representing whole body parts. The calcification may be amorphous, punctate, or spiculated. Calcification or bony elements usually indicate a benign lesion and have rarely been reported in malignant lesions [23]. Areas of increased transradiancy may be seen caused by the presence of fat in the lesion. When all these features are present the diagnosis may be made easily from plain radiographs.

Associated bony abnormalities of the spine are infrequent. Large lesions cause growth disturbances of the pelvic bones with widening of the distance between the ischial tuberosities caused by pressure.

The various tissue components of teratomas are well visualized on CT (see Figs. 15.8, 15.9, 15.24c). The lesions may appear cystic or solid, or contain elements of both. In many the cystic component may involve almost the whole lesion and may be extremely large. The contents have attenuation values slightly above that of water and are surrounded for the most part by a thin rim of soft tissue. The solid component (dermoid plug) of these lesions varies in size and may exist as a solid mass projecting into the cyst, a bridge across the cyst, or only a thickened segment of the cyst wall [7]. Calcification, which may be curvilinear or globular, and bone formation occur in the solid components [7]. Fat may also be a component of these lesions. The more dependent elements may contain material of attenuation higher than that of fat because of a mixture of fat, hair, debris, and fluid.

Abscence of a fat plane between a lesion and an adjacent structure can be either normal or due to adherence or invasion [7, 25]. Cystic lesions may well be adherent to adjacent structures and still be benign. Obvious invasion, however, suggests malignancy. This is not commonly seen with sacrococcygeal teratomas in young children.

Most sacrococcygeal teratomas present as large masses, but their size does not correlate with their malignant potential. CT is the most valuable modality in delineating the exact extent of these lesions as well as in defining their tissue character. This information is vital pre-operatively as large lesions are more difficult to remove surgically and hence are associated with a higher morbidity and mortality. Both benign and malignant lesions can be adequately treated surgically if diagnosed early and completely removed. Recurrence may be due to inadequate removal or malignancy.

Sonography is limited in its ability to define the exact extent of these lesions, which are intimately related to bone on many sides and which

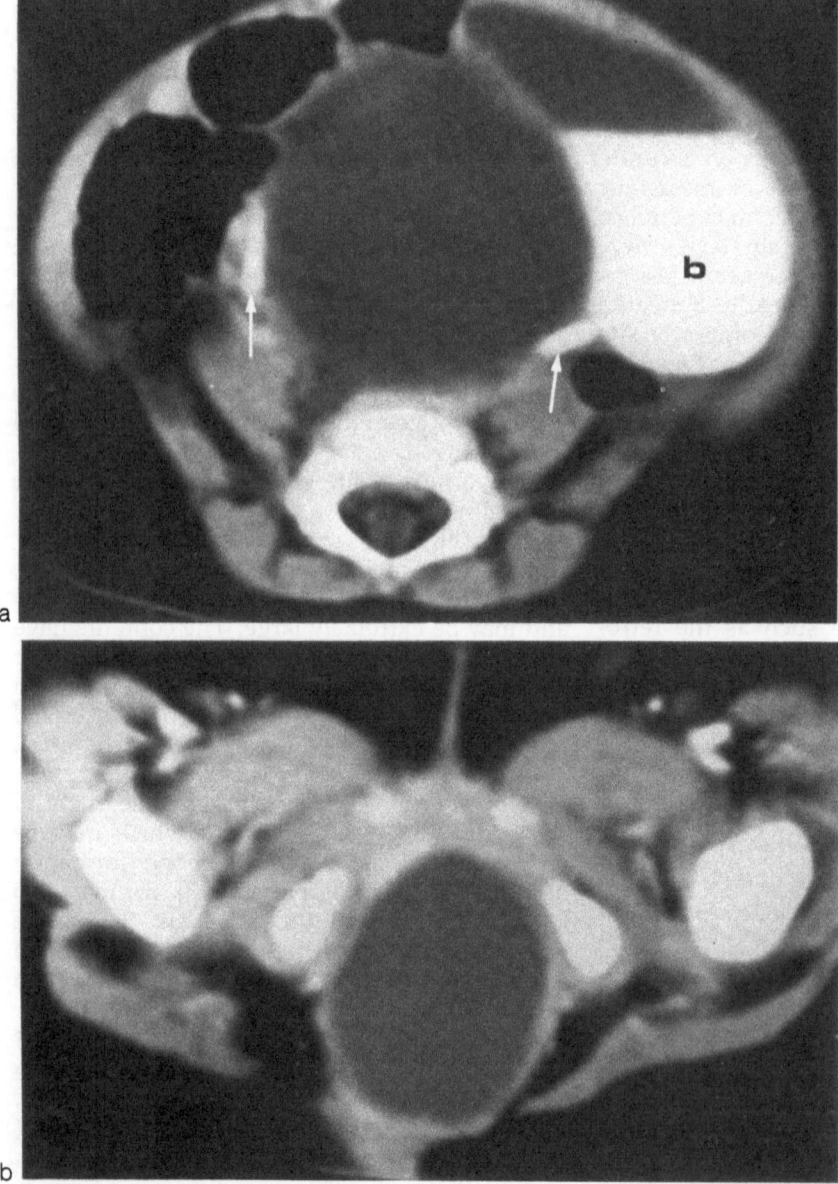

Fig. 15.8c (*next page*)

Fig. 15.8a–c. Large benign teratoma in a neonate. The CT examination has exquisitely demonstrated the exact character and extension of the mass and its effect on adjacent viscera. In scan **a** the mass is seen extending high in the retroperitoneum, with displacement of the ureters (*arrows*) and bladder (*b*). In scan **b** the mass fills the pelvic cavity, and in scan **c** it is seen to extend into the perineum and right buttock. The mass is mainly cystic with an attenuation equal to that of fluid. A small solid component is noted in the lower scans on the right.

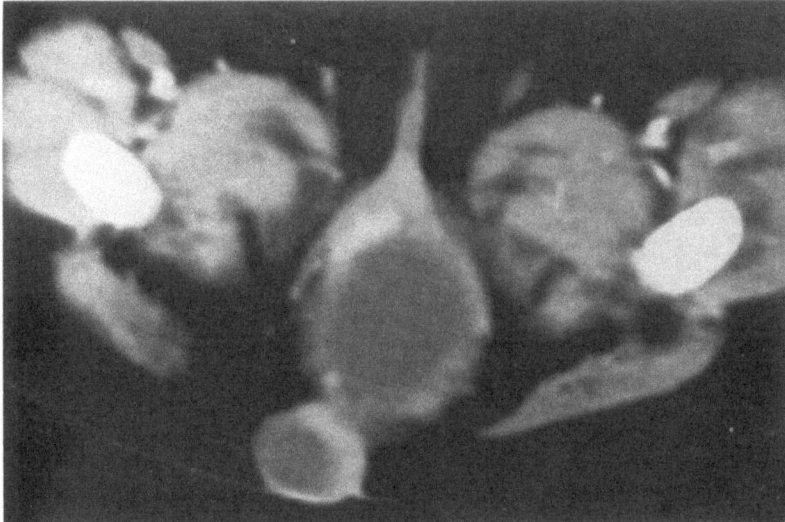

Fig. 15.8c

project into the buttock and perineum. Sonography is also not as sensitive as CT in the delineation of fat or calcium within the lesion.

Neuroblastomas

Neuroblastomas occur far less commonly in the pelvis than in the chest and abdomen [14]. On CT they appear as masses of soft tissue attenuation prior to injection of intravenous contrast. Enhancement may be quite dramatic, and occasionally low-attenuation necrotic areas are noted centrally. Calcification may also be evident in these lesions. Intraspinal extension into the extradural space in the sacrum and lumbar region is often easily visualized on CT even with-

out the injection of metrizamide into the subarachnoid space (Fig. 15.10).

Anterior Meningomyeloceles

Anterior meningomyeloceles are rare lesions and are diagnosed by their associated sacral abnormalities on plain radiographs. CT shows these lesions as fluid-filled structures anterior to the sacrum and also delineates the bony abnormalities. The CT study is best performed after intrathecal injection of metrizamide in order to delineate the communication of these structures to the intraspinal subarachnoid space (Fig. 15.11).

Other Tumors

Other retrorectal masses of soft tissue origin (nerve, fat, connective tissue, duplications) are uncommon, and examples are shown in Figs. 15.12 and 15.13. CT accurately delineates the extension of these lesions as well as giving important information regarding their tissue character.

Rectal Lesions

Rectal lesions are best evaluated with barium enema and endoscopy. In one patient with hypogammaglobulinemia that we have studied, CT showed marked thickening of the rectal wall

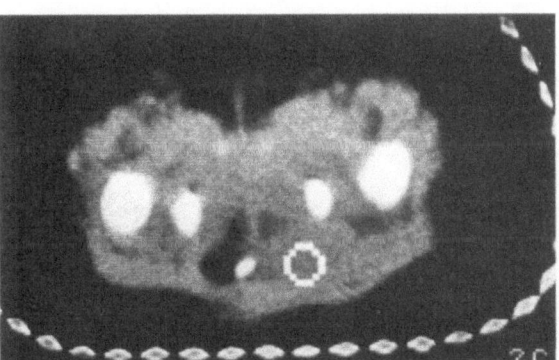

Fig. 15.9. A benign sacrococcygeal teratoma in a neonate. The scan shows the lesion has mainly a solid component, indicated by the *cursor*, with a small area of calcification on the right extremity of the mass.

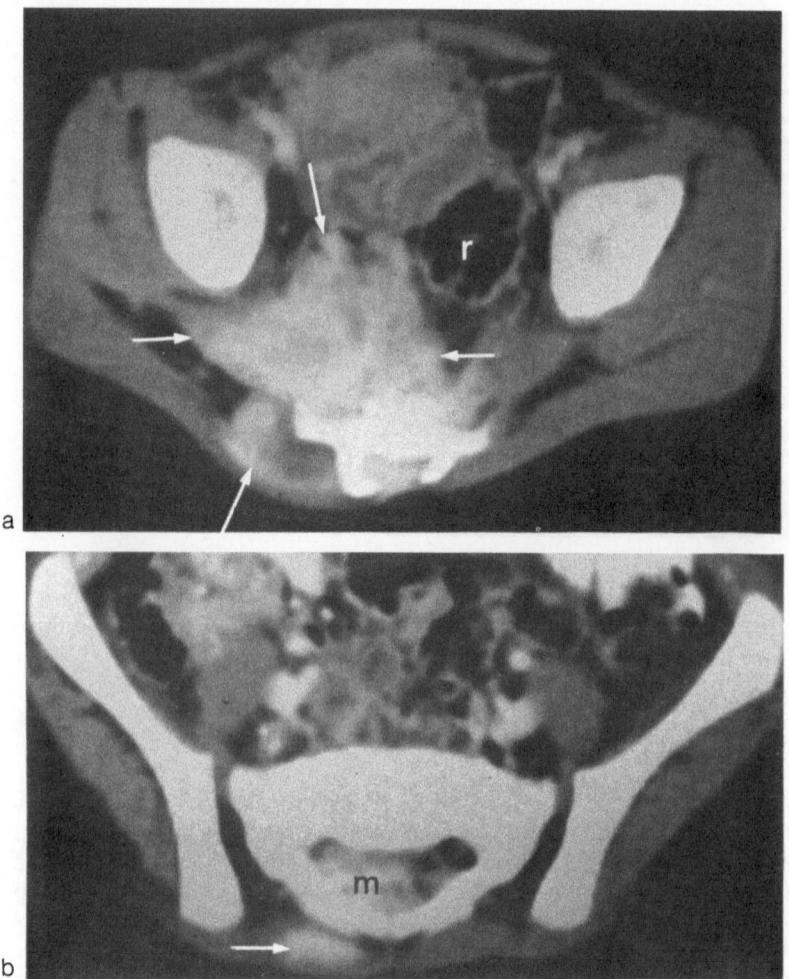

Fig. 15.10a,b. A 2-year-old girl with a retrorectal neuroblastoma. The mass (*arrows*) enhances much more dramatically than the surrounding musculature. In scan **a** extension of the mass through the greater sciatic notch is well visualized, and there is also a component of the mass extending lateral to the sacrum and into the spinal canal. The intraspinal component (*m*) is noted to enhance equal to the remainder of the mass, as noted in both scans **a** and **b**. In **b** a small component is noted posterior to the vertebral body (*arrow*). Note the normal thin rim of enhancement in the wall of the fluid-filled small bowel anterior to the mass and rectum (*r*).

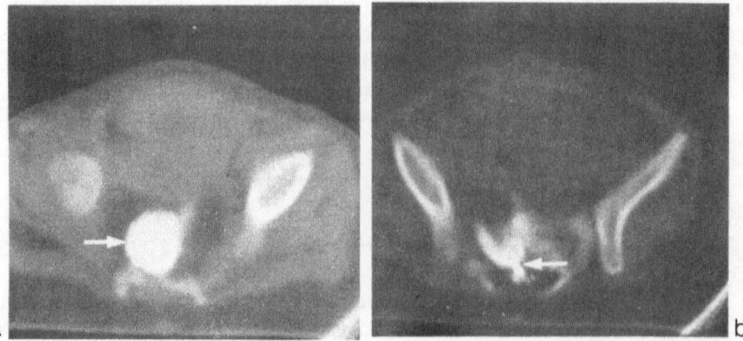

Fig. 15.11a,b. A 1-year-old girl with anterior sacral meningocele. Scans show metrizamide filling the sac (*arrow*) anterior to the sacrum in **a** and the communication (*arrow*) between the sac and subarachnoid space in **b**. Note the sacral defect in scan **a**.

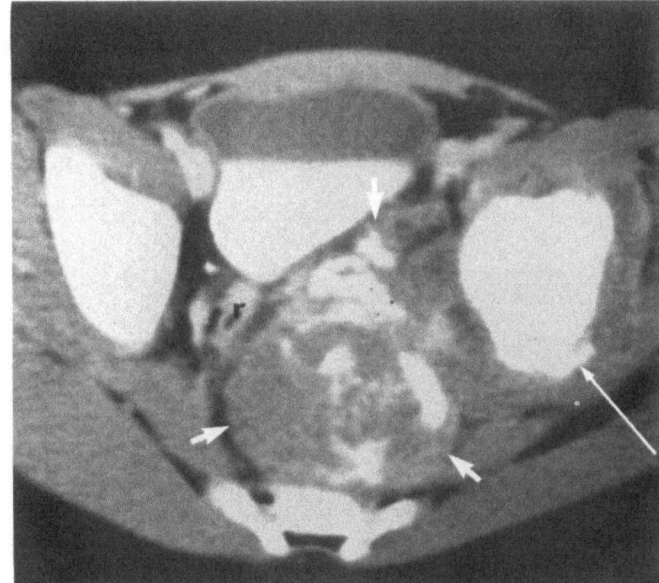

Fig. 15.12. A 9-year-old boy with a malignant Schwannoma of the pelvis shows a large calcified mass (*short arrows*) with reactive bony involvement on the left (*long arrow*). The rectum (*r*) is displaced to the right. This is the same patient as illustrated in Fig. 9.10.

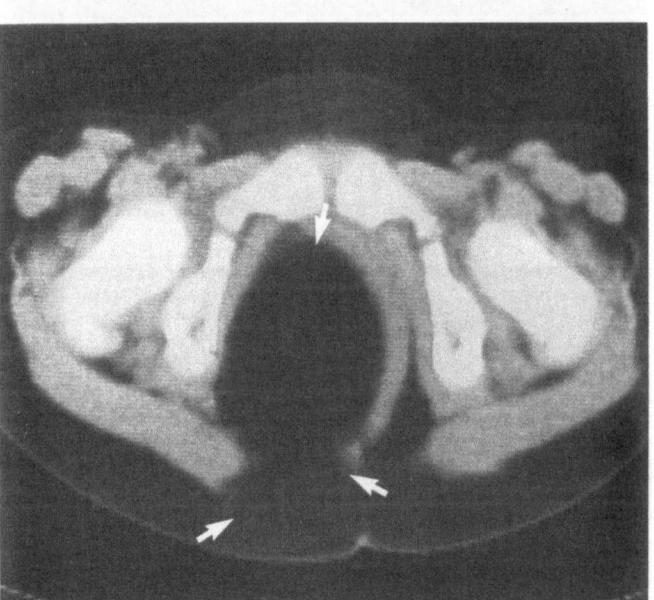

Fig. 15.13. A young girl with a large pelvic lipoma (*arrows*). The attenuation of the lipoma can be seen to be equal to that of the adjacent fat. The lipoma displaces the midline structures to the left.

caused by massive lymphoid hyperplasia. This study was performed after a barium study in order to rule out an associated perirectal mass (Fig. 15.14). CT was also useful to another child with aplastic anemia and severe neutropenia who presented with fever. Rectal examinations and barium enemas were contraindicated in this child, and CT, performed to rule out the presence of a pelvic abscess, showed the presence of rectal wall thickening caused by proctitis.

Bladder and Genital Lesions

Sonography and cystography are the modalities of choice in the evaluation of bladder disease. We have only used CT once specifically to assess a lesion that was localized to the bladder in a child. The patient was a 1-year-old boy with a vesical endodermal sinus tumor. This case is unique in that there are no previous reports of endodermal sinus tumors developing at this site [18]. The lesion was equally well demonstrated by CT and sonography (Fig. 15.15). Rhabdomyosarcomas of the bladder tend to be more extensive and often are extensions from lesions arising in the prostate. CT is very useful for delineating the extent of such lesions (see below).

Sonography is also the initial modality of choice in the evaluation of congenital lesions involving the uterus, such as hydrocolpos, or in patients with ambiguous genitalia. Appropriate genitographic and urographic studies are often necessary following sonography.

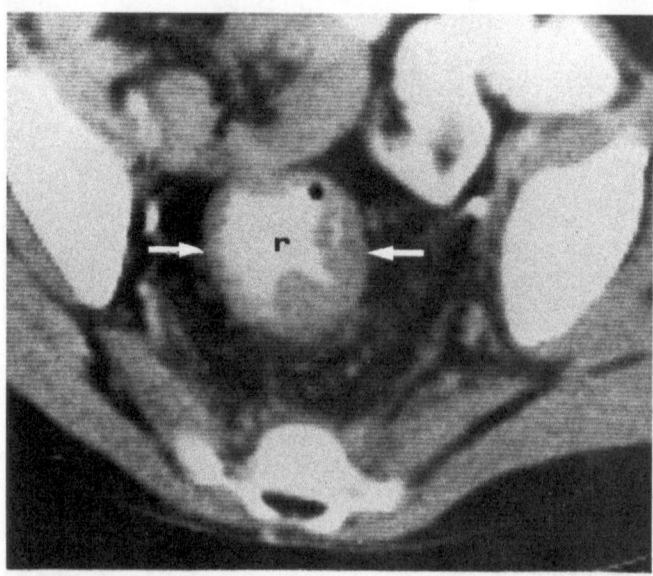

Fig. 15.14. A 12-year-old boy with hypogammaglobulinemia and marked lymphoid hyperplasia of the bowel wall. A scan through the rectum (*r*) shows marked thickening of the bowel wall (*arrows*) in this region as well as nodularity projecting into the lumen and deforming the outline of the dilute water-soluble contrast filling the rectum.

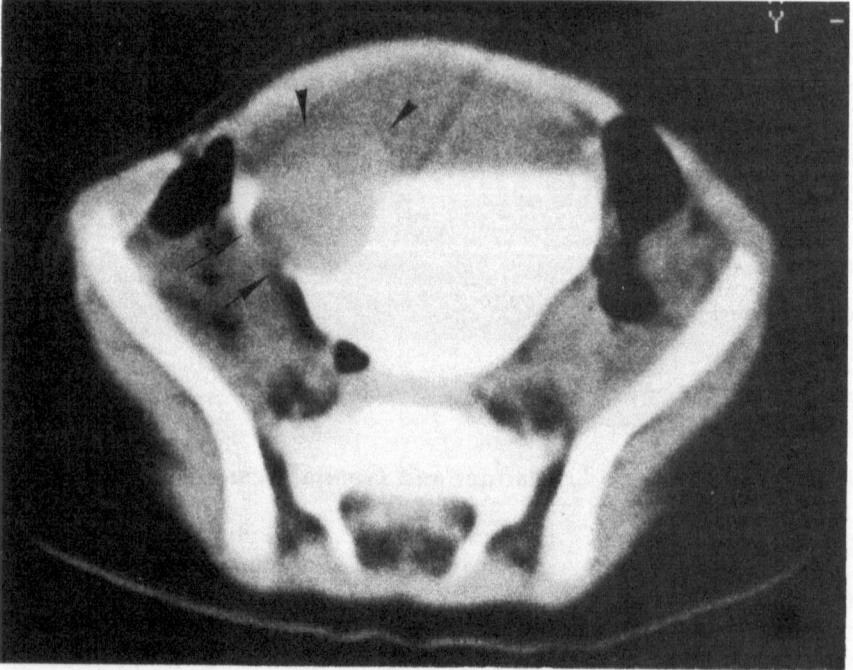

Fig. 15.15. A 1-year-old boy with an endodermal sinus tumor of the bladder. CT scan after intravenous contrast enhancement shows the mass (*arrowheads*) in the right side of the bladder projecting up above the fluid-fluid level caused by the contrast in the urine. The attachment of the mass to the bladder wall is seen laterally (*arrows*).

Lesions of the ovaries are also initially best assessed with sonography. Small follicular cysts are the commonest "mass" lesions of the ovary and are easily visualized on sonography. Larger cysts, including teratomas, are also usually adequately assessed with this modality. These ovarian cysts may well be huge and may be multiloculated. Fat and calcific areas are more accurately delineated with CT and confirm the presence of a teratoma. It has been our experience that CT is almost never necessary to delineate these type of ovarian lesions in greater detail. On CT, ovarian cysts (Fig. 15.16) may resemble hydrocolpos in appearance as the contents are of water density in both lesions, but hydrocolpos is seen to have a thicker wall, which enhances to a greater extent [25].

Ovarian neoplasms account for 1% of childhood neoplasms and may present at any time in the pediatric age group but most frequently occur at puberty. Solid mass lesions of the ovary occur in older teenage girls and most commonly are germ cell tumors and granulosa tumors [1]. In these children sonography is usually adequate

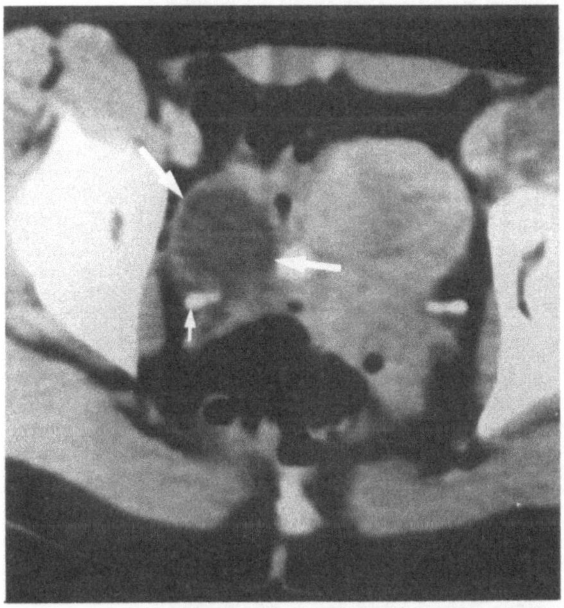

Fig. 15.16. A 15-year-old girl found to have a right ovarian cyst (*long arrows*) on a pelvic study being performed to assess a possible soft tissue mass anterior to the left hip. The right ureter (*small arrow*) is seen behind the ovarian cyst. The cyst has an enhancing rim. Unopacified bowel loops are on the left.

to assess the primary lesion, but it has been our experience that CT is more accurate in assessing local extent and metastatic disease.

Rhabdomyosarcoma Rhabdomyosarcoma is a highly malignant tumor that accounts for over 50% of soft tissue sarcomas in childhood. The lesion arises from the same embryonal mesenchymal cells that give rise to striated muscle [1]. A number of different histological subgroups have been delineated. In childhood, the commonest site for these lesions is the head and neck, and the second commonest is the pelvis. Other less common sites include the extremities, trunk, retroperitoneum, and biliary tract. In the pelvis these lesions most commonly occur in the prostate, bladder, uterus, vagina, spermatic cord, and coverings of the scrotum. Occasionally, rhabdomyosarcomas or more undifferentiated sarcomas may arise from more lateral soft tissue structures of the pelvis. At times it may be difficult to determine the exact site of origin in the pelvis, particularly with large lesions.

There is no doubt from our experience that CT is the most accurate modality in the delineation of the extent of the primary lesion and metastatic disease, both at the time of diagnosis and in follow-up (Figs. 15.17–15.20). Occasionally, cystographic studies are necessary to further define the exact relationship of the mass to the urinary tract if complicated surgical procedures are contemplated.

Pelvic rhabdomyosarcomas may indeed grow to an enormous size (see Fig. 15.19). It is for this reason that they cannot be adequately assessed with sonography. The lesions have an attenuation value of soft tissue and occasionally enhance a little more than muscle. In the larger lesions, areas of lower attenuation are found centrally and are due to necrosis and hemorrhage. Calcification is rare at the time of diagnosis but may occur as a result of chemotherapy or radiation therapy. CT is particularly useful in defining the degree of infiltration of the tumor into surrounding muscles and bone (see Figs. 15.19, 15.20). Infiltration into bone, however, is not common. As has been indicated elsewhere in the text, the diagnosis of invasion into adjacent soft tissues can be difficult even with CT. This information is particularly important when considering surgery. Siegel [24, 25] has pointed out that the presence of fat planes between the neoplasm and adjacent structures indicates lack of invasion, but the absence of fat planes may well be normal or may be due to adherence or invasion.

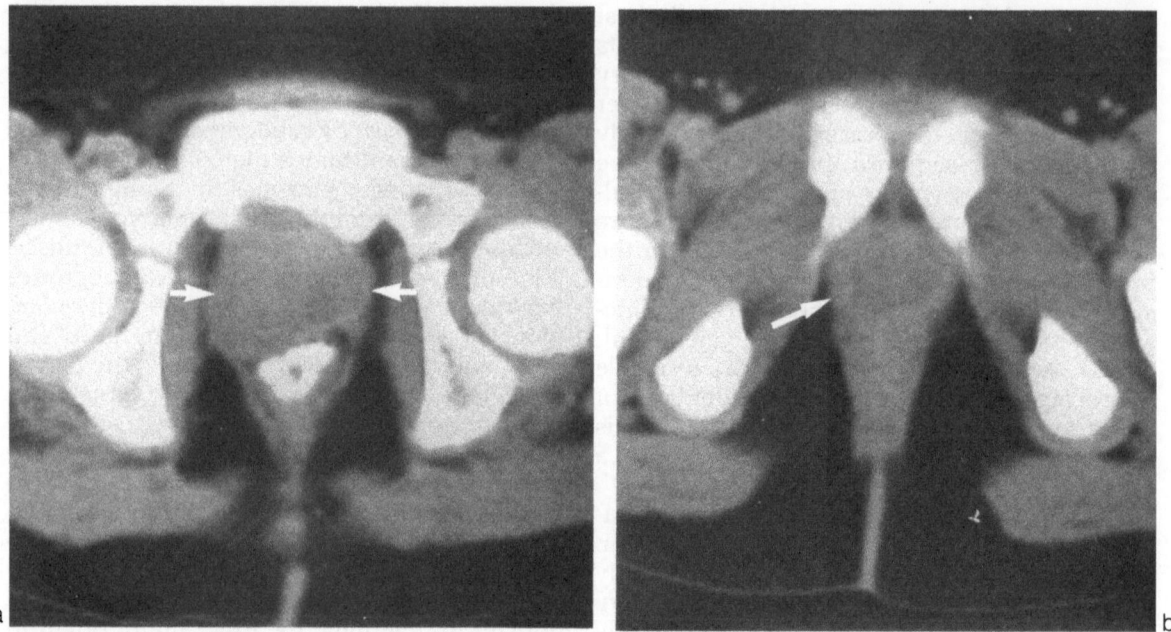

Fig. 15.17a,b. An 8-year-old girl with uterine rhabdomyosarcoma (*arrows*) seen in scan **a** lying behind the bladder and in front of the rectum. The mass extends down into the vagina in scan **b**.

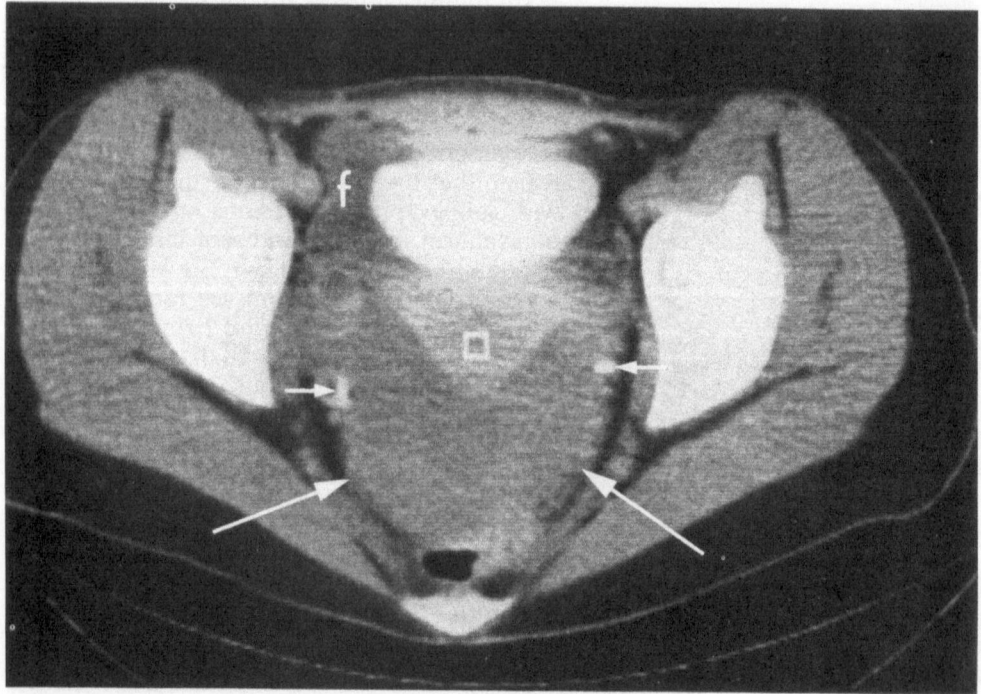

Fig. 15.18. A 12-year-old girl with a pelvic rhabdomyosarcoma (*long arrows*). The mass lies behind the uterus, which is indicated by the *cursor*. A small amount of fluid is noted lateral to the bladder on the right (*f*). The ureters (*short arrows*) lie lateral to the mass.

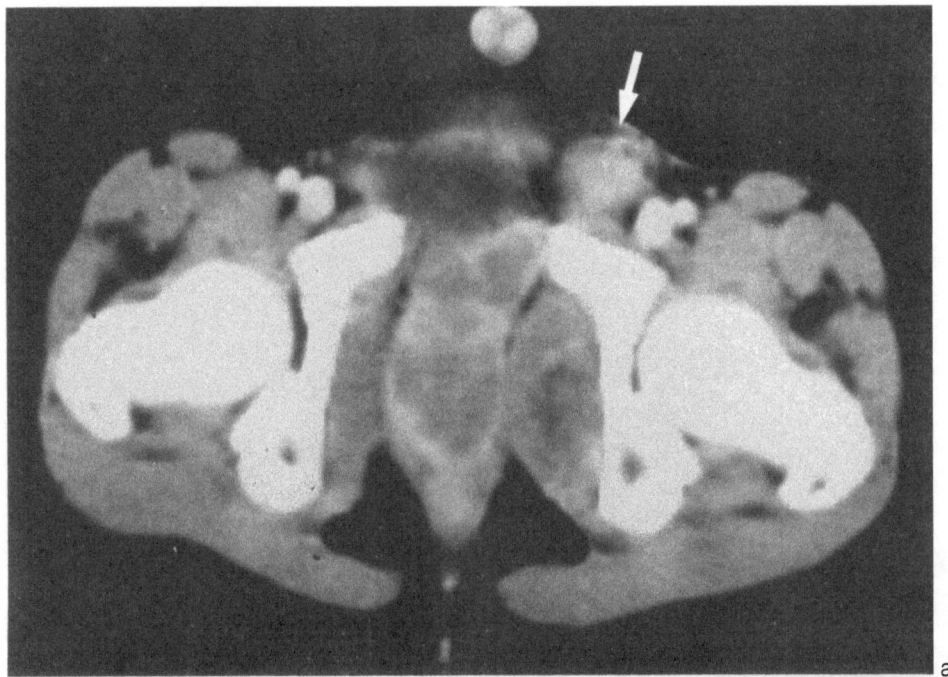

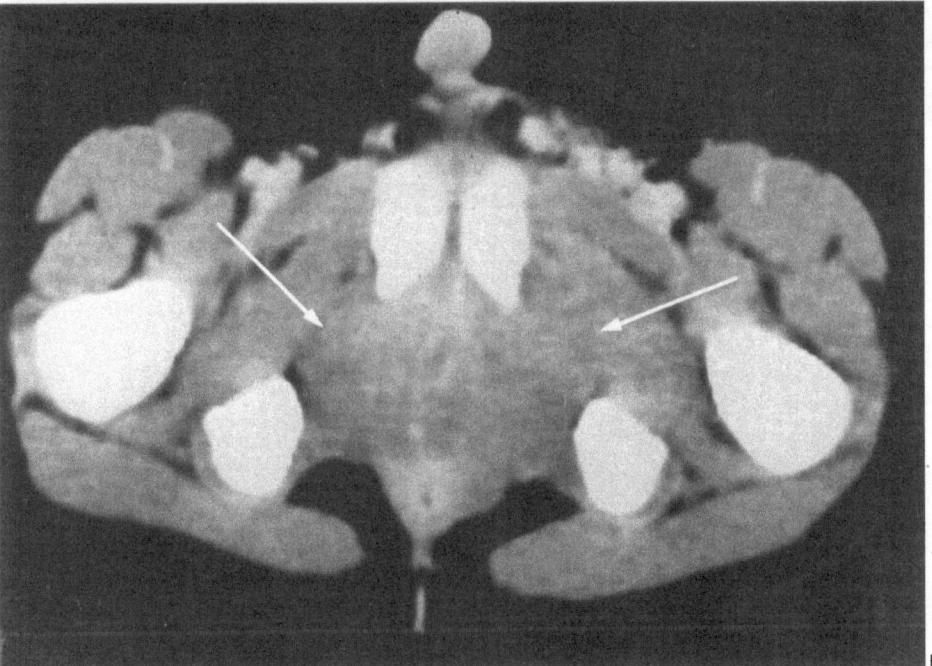

Fig. 15.19a–d. A 9-year-old boy with prostatic rhabdomyosarcoma. **a** A large mass with inhomogeneous enhancement is noted filling the central portion of the lower pelvis in the region of the prostate. Metastatic disease is present along the lateral pelvic wall on the left as well as in the left inguinal nodes (*arrow*) just medial to the femoral vein. **b** In this lower scan extension of the mass into the perineum is noted as well as extension through the obturator foramina with displacement of the obturator externus muscles laterally (*arrows*). The fat planes between the muscle and the mass are not clearly visualized on the left, suggesting infiltration of the muscle. **c** After an initial response to nonoperative therapy the child again presented with a recurrent mass in the central pelvis with extension into and destruction of the left pubic bone (*arrow*). **d** Following further radiation and chemotherapy the scan shows postradiation changes to the pubic bones and a decrease in the size of the central pelvic mass. In both scans **c** and **d** some calcification is noted in the mass, and the low attenuation centrally in scan **d** is probably related to areas of necrosis. (**Fig. 15.19c,d** *overleaf*)

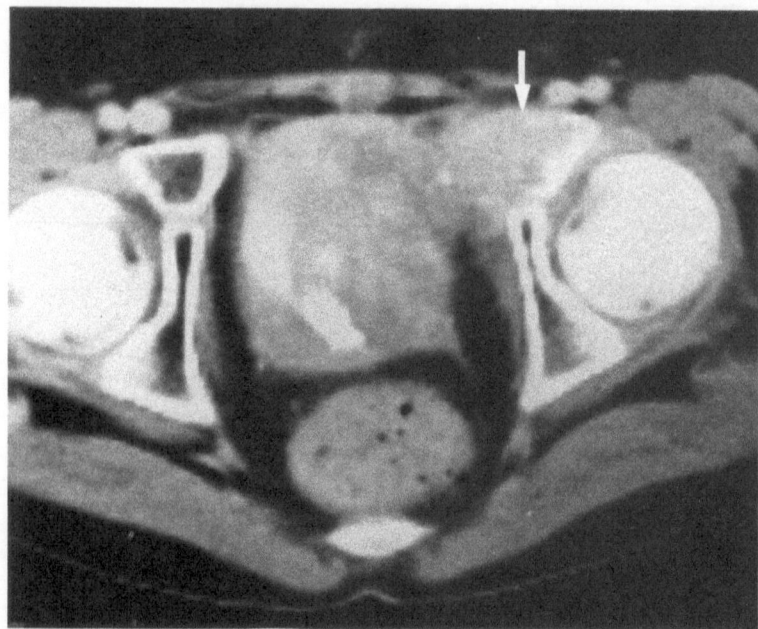

Fig. 15.19c

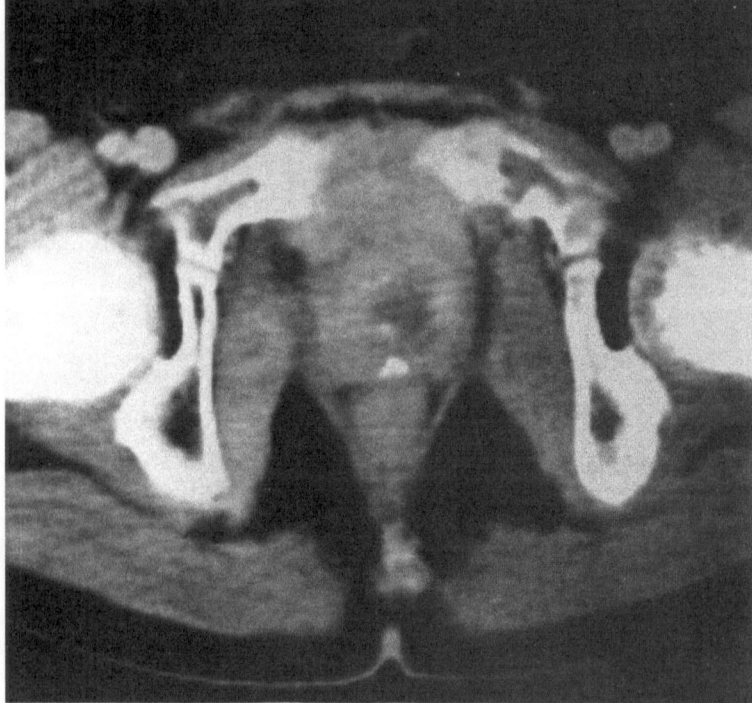

Fig. 15.19d

Lateral Pelvic Masses

Masses occurring along the lateral pelvic wall are most commonly lymphadenopathy caused by lymphoma or rhabdomyosarcoma and other undifferentiated sarcomas (Figs. 15.20, 15.21).

Lymphoma of the pelvic nodes is usually found in association with involvement higher in the retroperitoneum and has been discussed in more detail in Chapter 8 (see p. 98). Lymphomas may also cause mass lesions in the prostate or ovaries.

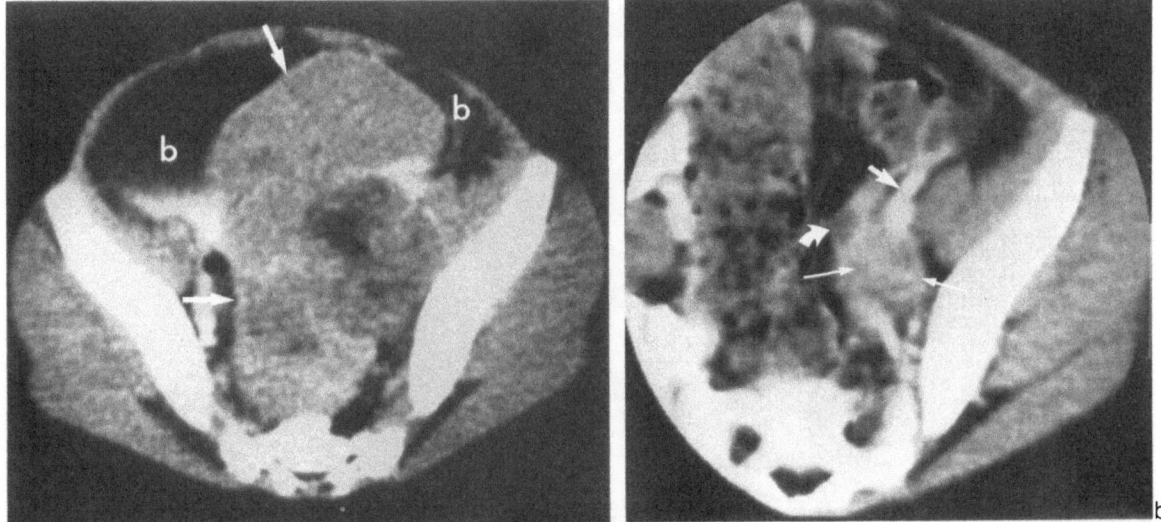

Fig. 15.20a,b. A 6-year-old girl with a rhabdomyosarcoma arising from the lateral pelvic wall. **a** The mass (*arrows*) extends backward to the sacrum and projects into the back wall of the bladder (*b*). There is no definitive line of demarcation between the mass and the psoas muscle on the left. **b** Following radiation and chemotherapy the mass has become markedly smaller in size (*small arrows*) and is seen to lie posterior to the left common iliac artery and vein (*larger arrow*). *Curved arrow* indicates dilated unopacified left ureter. The CT has accurately followed the size of this mass and its response to therapy and has outlined in detail its extent and relationship to adjacent vital structures. This information facilitated the subsequent surgical removal of the mass.

Abscesses

At the Hospital for Sick Children, Toronto, we have used sonography extensively and with great success not only to diagnose and follow up pelvic abscesses but also to localize these lesions for drainage procedures. Most of the cases that we have studied in this way involved complications related to appendicitis, inflammatory bowel disease, or the postoperative period. We have only had to use CT in children suspected of having a pelvic abscess on rare occasions when sonography has been nondiagnostic or equivocal. In this regard we have found CT extremely useful and accurate.

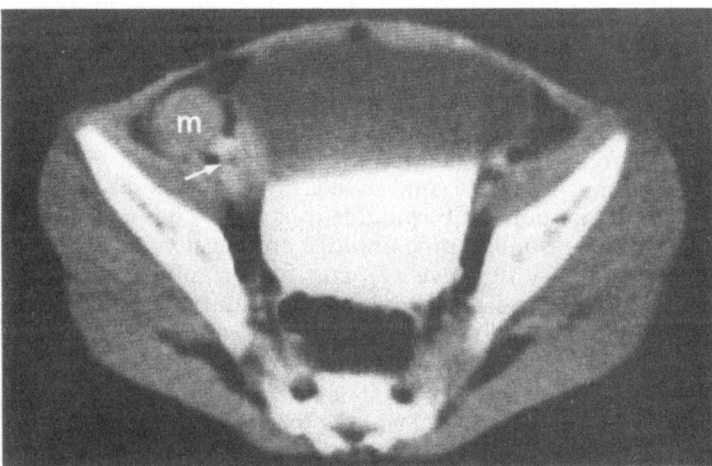

Fig. 15.21. A 6-year-old girl with Hodgkin's disease shows a large mass of lymph nodes (*m*) in the right iliac fossa. These lie anterior to the common iliac artery and vein (*arrow*). Further slightly enlarged nodes are also noted between the iliac vessels and the bladder wall on the right.

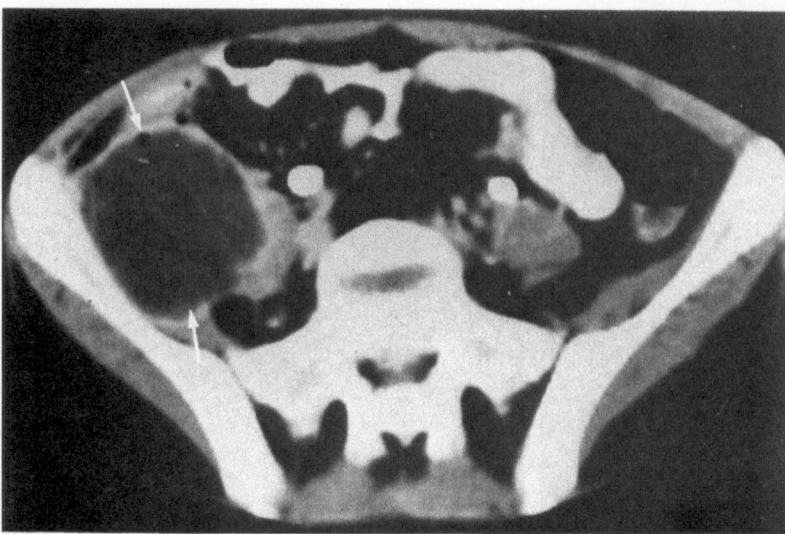

Fig. 15.22. A 14-year-old boy with Crohn's disease. CT scan after intravenous contrast enhancement shows a large abscess (*arrows*) in the right iliac fossa. A thin rim of enhancement is noted in the wall of the abscess. The central area shows no enhancement, and a small bubble of air is present in the upper part of the abscess adjacent to the *arrow*.

Abscesses appear as masses with soft tissue attenuation (Figs. 15.22, 15.23). Usually a thick irregular wall is present which usually shows marked enhancement. Obliteration of tissue planes around the lesion is also noted. Air bubbles or an air fluid level are characteristic findings of abscesses (Figs. 15.22, 15.23). If these features are absent, the lesion may mimic other types of soft tissue masses, and clinical correlation or aspiration is required to make the diagnosis.

Hematomas

Pelvic and retroperitoneal hematomas may be localized or diffuse. Most pelvic hematomas that we have seen have been in children with severe blunt abdominal trauma or with pelvic fracture. Hematomas may well mimic other mass lesions but show no enhancement. Their attenuation diminishes in time, as they resolve. Psoas muscle hematomas in hemophiliacs are usually adequately evaluated and followed with sonography.

Nonpalpable Testes

Incompletely descended testes may be found anywhere from the renal hilum to the inguinal canal or along the course of the normal spermatic cord. Accurate localization of testes that are not palpable in the scrotum is important for directing the surgical approach because the risks of infertility and malignancy are higher in undescended testes [15, 36].

At the Hospital for Sick Children, Toronto, we have used real-time sonography as the modality of choice in attempting to locate such testes as the vast majority will be located in the inguinal area or lower pelvis. In 1980, Wolverson et al. [36] compared the value of CT with high-resolution real-time sonography in the localization of nonpalpable undescended testes in 20 patients between the ages of 3 and 23 years. These authors found that CT was more sensitive than sonography. However, they recommended the use of real-time sonography as the modality of choice for this procedure because it is simple, accurate, and avoids the use of ionizing radiation. CT should thus only be used if the sonographic findings are negative or equivocal. A negative CT and sonographic examination does not, however, exclude very small testes, but angiography and venography should rarely become necessary.

Undescended testes appear as a soft tissue mass on CT and may be round or oval in shape depending on their orientation to the transverse axial CT scans (Fig. 15.24b). Their attenuation values are slightly lower than the adjacent non-fatty soft tissues and show no appreciable

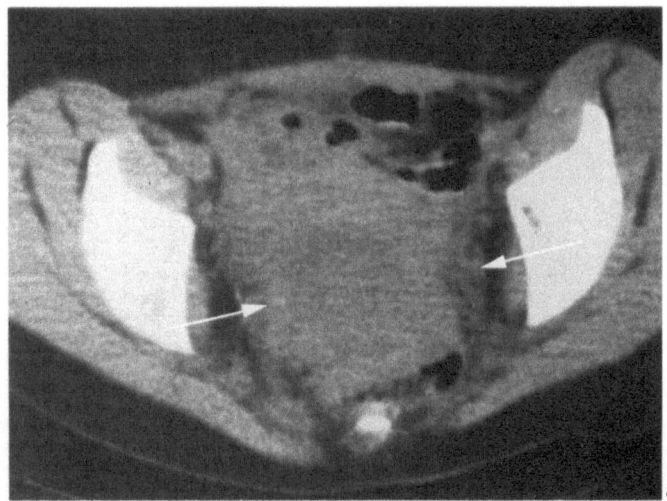

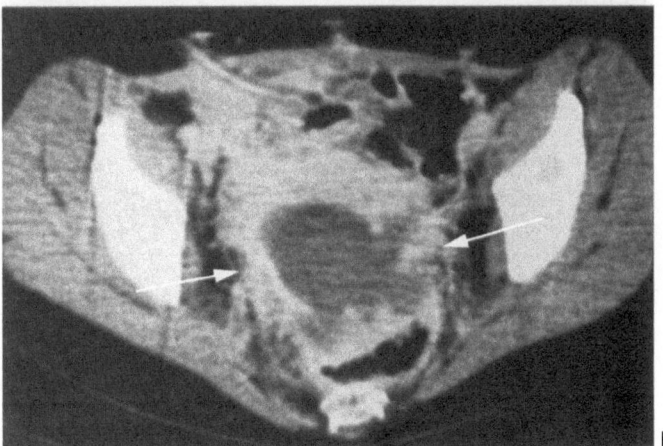

Fig. 15.23a,b. CT scans before (**a**) and after (**b**) intravenous contrast enhancement in a 12-year-old girl who developed fever following an ileocecocystoplasty. A large mass (*arrows*) of lower attenuation is noted in the central portion of the pelvis, and there is marked irregular enhancement of the periphery of the mass after contrast administration in scan **b**. This lesion was an inflammatory mass with a large amount of pus in the central area which has failed to enhance in scan **b**. A suprapubic catheter is noted passing anteriorly into the abdomen in scan **b**.

enhancement following intravenous contrast administration. These testes are usually smaller than normally descended testes, and their outline may not be as well defined. An adjacent curvilinear density may represent the vascular pedicle supplying the testis [36]. The testicle is found in the expected course of normal testicular descent, but the vast majority lie in the external inguinal ring or in the superficial inguinal pouch (Fig. 15.24b). Less commonly they may occur in an intra-abdominal site, usually in the lower pelvis, where they are located on the medial surface of the external iliac vessels.

An undescended testis or absent testis may be associated with absence of cord structures on images in the inguinal canal, or below if descent has not occurred to this site (Fig. 15.24a). Occasionally, if a testis is absent, spermatic cord remnants or an inguinal hernial sac may be noted on CT as linear thickening of the anterior abdominal wall in this region [36].

We have also had success with CT in localizing undescended testes in the inguinal region in children, as the amount of adipose tissue in this site allows for adequate delineation of the testis. However, we have had no success in localizing testes higher in the pelvis and abdomen, probably because testes in these higher sites are extremely small, and the lack of fat makes differentiation from adjacent bowel, vessels, and nodes difficult. An interesting case of a teratoma in an undescended testis is illustrated in Fig. 15.24c.

Renal Transplants

CT has been used to assess tranplanted kidneys and the complications resulting from transplant

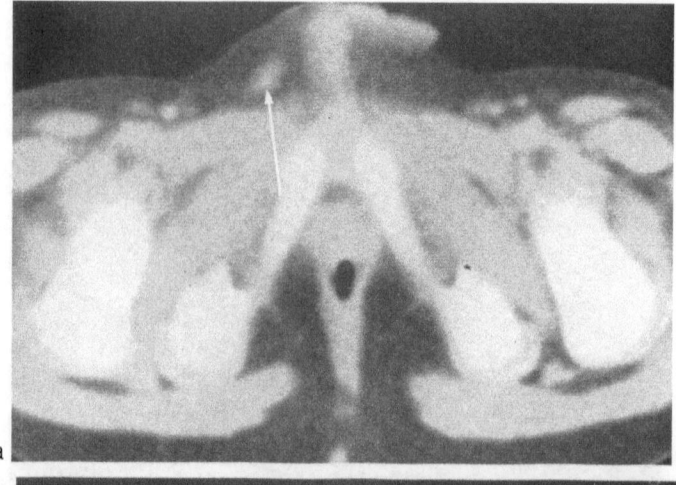

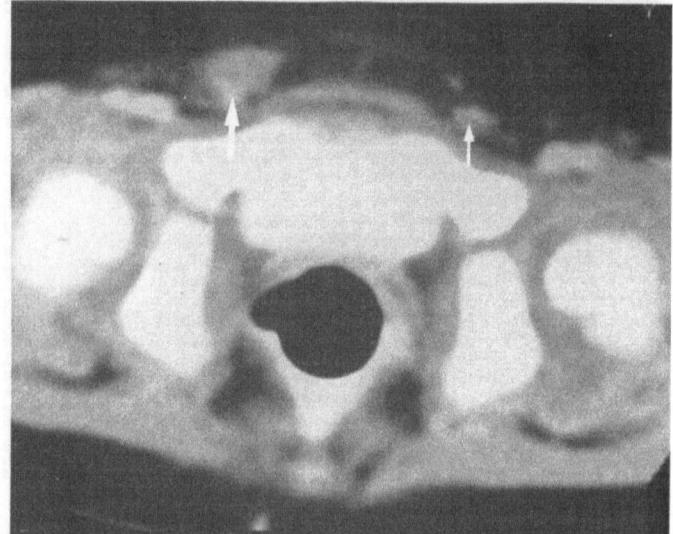

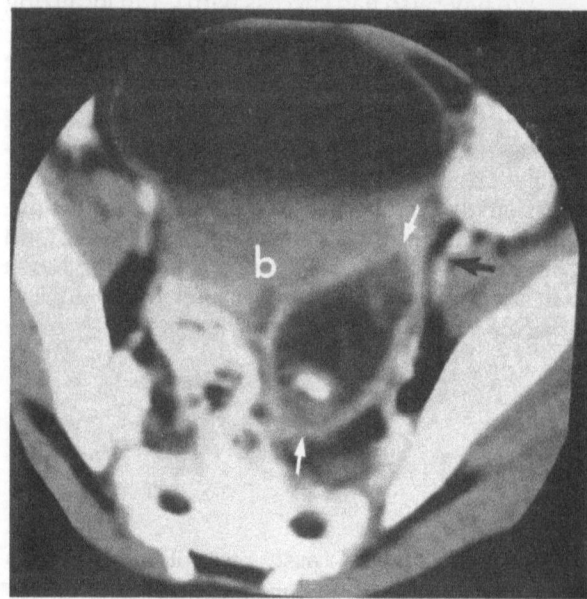

Fig. 15.24. a Normal right spermatic cord (*arrow*) and absence of spermatic cord on the left associated with undescended testicle. **b** Undescended right testicle lying in the inguinal canal (*large arrow*). Normal left spermatic cord (*small arrow*). **c** A 4-year-old boy with undescended left testicle presented with left iliac fossa pain. CT shows a 4×2 cm oval mass (*white arrows*) lying posteriorly in the left side of the pelvis There is enhancement of a rim of tissue around the periphery of this mass with calcification in the posterior part. At operation this was found to be the undescended left testicle containing a teratoma that had undergone torsion. *b*, bladder. *Black arrow* indicates left external iliac artery and vein.

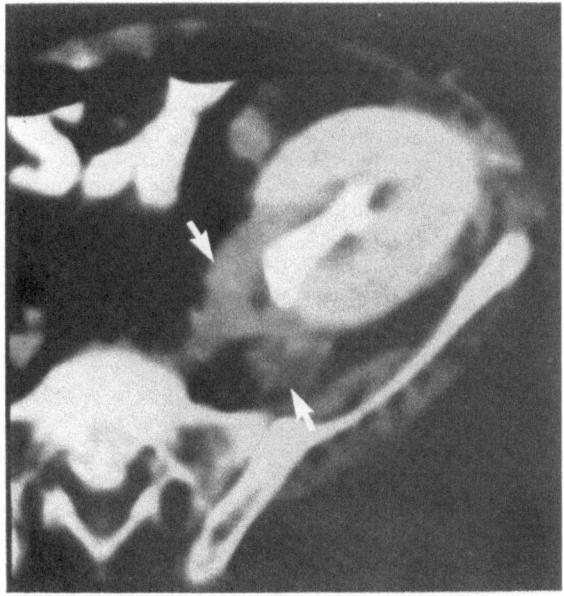

Fig. 15.25. A 14-year-old boy with fever and a transplanted kidney in left iliac fossa. The CT shows the position of the kidney, which is functioning normally. Some ill-defined soft tissue around the hilum of this kidney was felt to represent an area of hemorrhage with superimposed infection, being the cause of the fever.

operations at other hospitals [25] and, to a limited extent, at the Hospital for Sick Children, Toronto (Fig. 15.25). However, we have relied heavily and very successfully on sonography and radionuclide renal scans for the investigation of patients with renal transplants and feel that CT has little more to offer in this regard.

References

1. Altman AJ, Schwarz AD (1983) The soft tissue sarcomas. In: Malignant diseases of infancy, childhood and adolescence. Saunders, Philadelphia, pp 423–444
2. Benson RC Jr, Segira JW, Carney JA (1978) Primary yolk sac (endodermal sinus) tumor of the prostate. Cancer 41:1395
3. Brasch RC, de Lorimier AA, Herzog RJ, Van Natta FC (1978) Extragonadal endodermal sinus (yolk sac) tumor. Angiographic findings and literature review. Pediatr Radiol 7:115
4. Chapman P, Linggood RM (1980) The management of pineal area tumors:a recent reappraisal. Cancer 46:1253
5. Chretien PB, Milan JD, Foote FW, Miller TR (1970) Embryonal adenocarcinomas (a type of malignant teratoma) of the sacrococcygeal region. Cancer 26:522
6. Fox MA, Vix VA (1980) Endodermal sinus (yolk sac) tumors of the anterior mediastinum. AJR 135:291
7. Friedman AC, Pyatt RS, Hartman DS, Downey EF Jr, Olson WB (1982) CT of benign cystic teratomas. AJR 138:659–665
8. Gonzalez-Crussi F (1979) The human yolk sac and yolk sac (endodermal sinus) tumors. A review. Perspect Pediatr Pathol 5:179
9. Grosfeld JL, Ballantine VN, Lowe D, Baehner RL (1976) Benign and malignant teratomas in children:analysis of 85 patients. Surgery 80:297
10. Hart WR (1975) Primary endodermal sinus (yolk sac) tumor of the liver. First reported case. Cancer 35:1453–1458
11. Huntington RW Jr, Morgenstern NL, Sargent JA, Giem RN, Richards A, Hanford KC (1963) Germinal tumors exhibiting the endodermal sinus pattern of Teilum in young children. Cancer 16:34–37
12. Huntington RW, Bullock WK (1970) Yolk sac tumors of extragonadal origin. Cancer 25:1368
13. Juckes AW, Fraser MM, Dexter D (1979) Endodermal sinus (yolk sac) tumors in infants and children. J Pediatr Surg 14(5):520
14. Kenney PJ, Siegel MJ, McAlister WH (1982) Congenital intraspinal neuroblastoma: a treatable simulant of myelodysplasia. AJR 138:166–167
15. Lee JKT, McClennan BL, Stanley RJ, Sagel SS (1980) Utility of computed tomography in the localization of the undescended testis. Radiology 135:121–125
16. Mackinnon AE, Cohen SJ (1978) Archenteronoma (yolk sac) tumors. J Pediatr Surg 13(1):21
17. Norris HJ, Bagley GP, Taylor HB (1970) Carcinoma of the infant vagina. Arch Pathol 90:473
18. O'Sullivan P, Daneman A, Chan HSL, Smith C, Robey G, Fitz CR, Martin DJ (1983) Extragonadal endodermal sinus tumors in children:a review of 24 cases. Pediatr Radiol 13:249–257
19. Pileri S, Martinelli G, Bazzocchi F, Grigioni FW, Govoni E, Severi B (1979) Tumore del seno entodermico. Pathologica 71:663
20. Rao, NR, Veliath GD, Srinivasan M (1964) An unusual case of sacrococcygeal mesonephroma (Schiller). Cancer 17:1604
21. Rao TV, Rajakumari K, Reddy CRR (1974) Extragonadal endodermal sinus tumor of Teilum. Oncology 30:23
22. Roth LM, Panganibar WG (1976) Gonadal and extragonadal yolk sac carcinomas. Cancer 37:812
23. Schey WL, Shkolnik A, White H (1977) Clinical and radiographic considerations of sacrococcygeal teratomas: an analysis of 26 new cases and review of the literature. Radiology 125:189–195
24. Siegel MJ, Glasier CM, Sagel SS (1981) CT of pelvic disorders in children. AJR 137:1139–1143
25. Siegel MJ (1983) Computed tomography of the pediatric pelvis. CT 7:77–83
26. Smith CR, Baumal R, Mancer K (1982) Endodermal sinus tumors of infancy and childhood. Lab Invest 46:78A
27. Talerman A, Haije WG, Baggerman L (1980) Serum alpha fetoprotein (AFP) in patients with germ cell tumors of the gonads and extragonadal sites. Cancer 46:381–385
28. Tavcar D, Robboy SJ, Chapman P (1980) Endodermal sinus tumor of the pineal region. Cancer 45:2646
29. Teilum G (1959) Endodermal sinus tumor of the ovary and testis. Cancer 12:1092
30. Teilum G (1978) The concept of endodermal sinus (yolk sac) tumor. Scand J Immunol [Suppl] 8:75
31. Thiele J, Castro S, Lee KD (1971) Extragonadal endodermal sinus tumor (yolk sac tumor) of the pelvis. Cancer 27:391

32. Tsuchida Y, Kaneko M, Saito S, Endo Y, Urano Y, Ohmi K, Asaka T (1978) Clinicopathological aspects of endodermal sinus tumor in childhood with reference to PAS-positive hyaline globules observed in tissue culture. Scand J Immunol [Suppl] 8:137
33. Tsuchida Y, Kaneko M, Yokomori K, Saito S, Urano Y, Asaka I, Takeuchi T (1978) Alpha-fetoprotein pre-albumin, albumin, alpha-1-antitrypsin and transferrin as diagnostic and therapeutic markers for endodermal sinus tumors. J Pediatr Surg 13:25

34. Ungerleider RS, Donaldson SS, Warnke RA, Wilbur JR (1978) Endodermal sinus tumor. Cancer 41:1627
35. Weedon D, Musgrave J (1974) Endodermal sinus tumor of the face. Pathology 6:365
36. Wolverson MK, Jagannadharao B, Sundaram M, Riaz MA, Nalesnik WJ, Houttuin E (1980) CT in localization of impalpable cryptorchid testes. AJR 134:725–729
37. Zaczek T (1963) Mesonephric carcinoma of cervix uteri in an 11-month-old girl treated by hysterectomy. Am J Obstet Gynecol 85:176

Chapter 16

Approach to Abdominal and Pelvic Masses, Inflammation, and Trauma

Masses

The purpose of radiographic investigations in a child with an abdominal mass is to define as accurately as possible the exact site of origin and extent of the mass as well as characterizing the type of lesion present. Radiographic studies are also essential to determine whether metastatic disease is present in the abdomen and chest. This information is vital for the correct management of such children as it will influence not only whether further studies are necessary, but also the type of therapy that will be instituted, whether this be conservative, surgical, radiotherapy, or chemotherapy.

Causes of Abdominal Masses

The causes of abdominal masses in neonates and older children are summarized in Tables 16.1 and 16.2 respectively. The commonest site for mass lesions in children is the retroperitoneum. Those in the neonatal period tend to be benign, while malignancy is much more common in older children. The appearances of these various masses on CT has already been described in detail in Chapters 8–15.

This chapter outlines our general approach to children with abdominal masses, including those arising from the pelvis. The chapter outlines the difficulties that both clinicians and radi-

ologists may have when choosing the initial modality as well as when deciding on the correct sequence of subsequent modalities in the investigation of a particular child with an abdominal mass lesion.

In neonates, the causes of abdominal or pelvic masses are as follows: approximately 55% arise in the kidney, and of these approximately 25% are due to hydronephrosis and 15% due to multicystic dysplastic kidneys; 15% are of genital origin and 15% of gastrointestinal origin; 10% are due to nonrenal retroperitoneal lesions; and 5% are due to hepatosplenobiliary causes [5].

In infants and older children, the causes are as follows: 55%, as in neonates, are due to renal masses, and in this age group 22% are due to Wilms' tumor and 20% due to hydronephrosis; 23% are due to nonrenal retroperitoneal lesions, the commonest in this group being neuroblastoma followed by teratoma; 18% arise from the gastrointestinal tract, of which 10% are appendiceal abscesses and 6% hepatobiliary disease; and 4% are genital in origin [5].

Older Investigative Modalities

In the past, the choice of modalities was limited and the management of these children was thus extremely easy. Any child with an abdominal mass had an abdominal radiograph together with an excretory urogram, and in many cases this was followed by angiography.

Table 16.1. Abdominal and pelvic masses in neonates

1. *Renal masses:*
   hydronephrosis — UPJ obstruction
   multicystic dysplastic kidney
   renal vein thrombosis
   ectopic kidney
   mesoblastic nephroma
   nephroblastomatosis
   Wilms' tumor
   polycystic disease

2. *Nonrenal retroperitoneal masses:*
   neuroblastoma
   adrenal hemorrhage
   teratoma
   adrenal abscess

3. *Hepatobiliary masses:*
   hemangioendothelioma
   hepatoblastoma
   metastatic neuroblastoma
   hepatic cyst
   choledochal cyst
   hydrops of gallbladder

4. *Pelvic masses:*
   distended bladder and ureter
   hydrometrocolpos
   ovarian cyst
   presacral germ cell tumor
   presacral neurogenic tumor

5. *Gastrointestinal masses:*
   duplication cyst
   mesenteric/omental cyst
   complicated meconium ileus
   volvulus
   dilatation proximal to atresia
   pyloric stenosis

6. *Miscellaneous:*
   splenic cyst
   hematoma
   abscesses
   lipoblastoma

Table 16.2. Abdominal and pelvic masses in infants and older children

1. *Renal masses:*
   Wilms' tumor
   Wilms' tumor variants
   renal cell carcinoma
   leukemia and lymphoma
   hydronephrosis
   adult polycystic disease
   solitary cysts
   other congenital malformations
   abscess

2. *Nonrenal retroperitoneal masses:*
   neuroblastoma
   adrenal carcinoma and adenoma
   pheochromocytoma
   retroperitoneal teratoma
   retroperitoneal sarcomas and lymphomas

3. *Hepatobiliary masses:*
   hepatoblastoma
   hepatocellular carcinoma
   simple cysts
   echinococcal cysts
   hepatic abscesses
   leukemia and lymphoma
   choledochal cyst

4. *Gastrointestinal masses:*
   appendiceal abscesses
   Crohn's disease
   duplication cysts
   neoplasms — lymphoma and carcinoma
   intussusception

5. *Genital masses:*
   hydrometrocolpos
   ovarian cysts
   ovarian teratoma
   ovarian solid tumors
   genital rhabdomyosarcoma

6. *Miscellaneous:*
   abscesses
   hematomas
   splenic cyst
   abdominal wall neoplasms

Plain Abdominal Radiograph

The plain abdominal radiograph offers limited information. The general location of the mass is usually indicated by the displacement of adjacent gas-filled loops of bowel and more rarely by associated adjacent soft tissue deformity and bony erosion. The range of densities visualized on plain radiographs is limited. However, the presence of calcification (suggesting a tumor such as a neuroblastoma), fat (suggesting a dermoid or a lipoma), and air in the mass (suggesting an abscess) may well be defined.

Excretory Urography

In the past, excretory urography has served as the gold standard as the initial study of choice in children with abdominal masses. Most pediatric abdominal masses arise in the retroperitoneal area or pelvis and the vast majority cause some deformity or displacement of different parts of the urinary system. Excretory urography thus often supplies valuable information regarding the site of origin of these masses. Distortion of the collecting system, *greater* than displacement, is characteristic of intrarenal masses. Displacement *greater* than distortion is characteristic of extrarenal masses. However, occasionally large masses in or adjacent to the kidney may not affect the renal outline or collecting system.

Newer Investigative Modalities

With the introduction of the newer modalities has come a better resolution of small structures within the abdomen as well as a greater discrimination of attenuation values of various structures. More sophisticated recent nuclear medicine studies have also been added to our armamentarium, and nuclear medicine angiograms, venograms, blood pool studies, and static scans often add useful information when investigating these patients. To a large extent at present, sonography has replaced the excretory urogram as the initial modality of choice in the investigation of patients with abdominal masses. The information obtained from these newer modalities as well as the pitfalls in their use are described below.

Sonography

Like CT, sonography has the ability to define multiple organ systems and vessels within the abdomen and pelvis. However, sonography is a relatively cheap nontraumatic imaging modality with no known harmful effects that requires no contrast medium injection. It is a technique ideally suited to small and thin individuals as the beam will not penetrate fat easily. Pediatric patients are thus ideally suited to examinations with this modality. For these reasons, sonography has come to replace excretory urography as the initial imaging modality in the evaluation of the vast majority of children with abdominal mass lesions at most pediatric institutions.

Abdominal sonography can define the site of origin of a mass and determine its extent and relationship to surrounding viscera and vessels, including infiltration of tumor into the inferior vena cava. Sonography can define the effect of the mass on adjacent viscera such as the renal collecting system and biliary tract. It can determine the integrity of other organs, for example by defining the presence or absence of metastatic disease. Based on the echo pattern of the mass, sonography can determine the consistency and type of lesion present. During respiration movement of mass lesions relative to adjacent viscera

can be observed with real-time sonographic equipment. This may give valuable information regarding the site of origin of the mass and whether there is infiltration of adjacent viscera.

However, sonography does have certain specific drawbacks:

1. Obese, and very large children may be difficult to examine as the beam will not penetrate fat or long distances well.

2. Ultrasound cannot penetrate bone, and therefore lesions of bone or adjacent to bone are better studied with CT.

3. The ultrasound beam will not penetrate gas, and therefore gastrointestinal gas acts as a barrier. This is a problem with small masses, as these will often be completely hidden by overlying gas, and it is of particular importance in the mid abdomen and upper pelvis. Larger masses tend to displace the gas and are usually easily delineated.

4. At the other end of the spectrum, however, a problem does arise with extremely large masses. In this situation, the true site or viscus of origin of the mass may be difficult to define, the great vessels of the abdomen may be difficult to locate, and the surrounding viscera may be so compressed that their appearance on sonography may be impossible to recognize.

5. The sonographic appearances of various masses may occasionally be atypical, making characterization of the lesion difficult.

6. Sonography does not assess function or vascularity of the lesion.

7. Clinicians find it more difficult to interpret sonographic studies than other modalities. (This may be regarded as an advantage by some radiologists!)

8. It is extremely difficult for a radiotherapist to plan radiation fields accurately from the sonography hard copy film.

At the Hospital for Sick Children, Toronto, we have used abdominal sonography as the initial imaging modality in the investigation of the vast majority of cases of children presenting with abdominal or pelvic mass lesions. In many instances the sonographic study may be the definitive study. This is particularly true in patients with benign lesions and includes those lesions that involve the biliary tract such as choledochal cysts and hydrops of the gallbladder, splenic cysts, pancreatic pseudocysts, ovarian cysts, hydrometrocolpos, inflammatory masses, and cerebrospinal and other fluid collections.

Sonography is often also the definitive modality in many solid lesions in the neonatal period.

In other cases further studies may be required as sonography cannot supply the extra information necessary for adequate patient management. Children found to have hydronephrosis or renal cystic disease will require nuclear medicine renal scans, excretory urography, or cystography, depending on the clinical situation and the sonographic findings.

Sonography is also particularly useful as the initial study in cases of malignant mass lesions. Based on the clinical and sonographic findings the correct diagnosis can be made in most patients. However, at our institution, all cases of malignant solid lesions are then investigated with a CT study (see below). CT is also necessary in those cases in which one of the drawbacks of sonography that have been listed above prevent adequate delineation of the lesion being studied.

Sonography is particularly helpful as the initial study in investigation of malignant abdominal masses as this modality usually defines the site of origin of the mass; this information is useful prior to the performance of CT as the CT study can then be tailored in accordance with the type of lesion that is present. For example, if a paraspinal mass is noted, such as a neuroblastoma, the CT should be performed with intrathecal metrizamide injection. Sonography is also the modality of choice in the assessment of tumor invasion of the inferior vena cava. This is usually a simple technique and can be done extremely rapidly. In the presence of extremely large masses the cava may be so displaced and compressed that it is difficult to locate and in these situations changing the position of the patient may well allow the mass to fall away from the cava causing it to open up somewhat. If this is not possible, venography is indicated if the patient has a tumor that has a propensity to grow into the cava. We have found that sonography has been more useful than CT in the assessment of the cava since delineation of the cava with CT depends on adequate enhancement of the vessel, which may not always be possible, and flow defects from the nonopacified blood from the renal and hepatic veins may make assessment difficult at times. The ability to scan in numerous different planes with sonography is an advantage, as cleavage planes may be more easily delineated with longitudinal or oblique scans than the transverse scans of CT. In this regard, sagittal and coronal reconstruction images are not as helpful as sonography performed in various planes. Tumor movement with respiration can also be assessed on real-time sonography [3]. This technique may also add some information regarding the site of origin of the lesion and its invasion on the few occasions when CT may not be able to achieve this.

Nuclear Medicine

Nuclear medicine studies have been used widely in the evaluation of children with abdominal masses. Because the studies are more organ specific than sonography and CT they have a more limited role generally; however, they may be invaluable and are even mandatory in specific instances.

Gallium-67 (^{67}Ga) may be taken up in both neoplastic and inflammatory processes. However, it is extremely useful in the delineation of the extent of disease in patients with lymphoma and also when attempting to differentiate benign from malignant neoplasms when inflammatory processes are not being considered, on the basis of the clinical picture.

^{99m}Tc-MDP is mandatory in all children suspected of having a lesion that may metastasize to bones. In addition to the value of this radiopharmaceutical in such instances, it is also taken up by various malignant neoplasms, most commonly neuroblastoma. Unfortunately, this uptake is nonspecific, and we have also seen uptake by adrenal carcinoma, hepatoblastoma, and Wilms' tumor.

^{99m}Tc-sulfur colloid liver/spleen scans are extremely useful in the differentiation of hyperplastic liver nodules from neoplasms. This modality, however, is not as sensitive as sonography or CT in the detection of metastatic disease and is often too nonspecific to determine whether the primary lesion is intra- or extrahepatic. Dynamic nuclear imaging studies do provide valuable information regarding the vascularity of lesions, and in this regard these studies may occasionally be diagnostic of hemangioendothelioma of the liver. Unfortunately, some vascular hepatic neoplasms may also be extremely vascular, and this modality is often nonspecific.

Renal imaging may offer more information regarding renal function, but the various renal radionuclide studies do not offer more anatomical information than sonography or CT and thus are extremely limited in their evaluation of renal masses. Technetium-labelled iminodiacetic acid derivatives may be useful for the delineation of biliary masses such as choledochal cysts, but these lesions are generally adequately studied with sonography and intraoperative chole-angiography.

Computed Tomography

We have found CT to be the most accurate modality in defining the exact site or origin of abdominal and pelvic masses and their relationship to adjacent viscera and vessels. It is the most accurate modality in defining metastases within the abdomen as well as in the chest. However, CT should not be considered a completely noninvasive study, but rather a less invasive one, because it uses ionizing radiation, sedation is often necessary, and intravenous contrast injection is usually required for studies of the abdomen. Filling of the gastrointestinal tract with contrast is mandatory, and in many younger children this means the positioning of a feeding tube with the tip in the stomach or proximal jejunum. Rectal contrast may also be necessary. For these reasons CT should not necessarily be used in all children with abdominal masses. It should only be used in those patients in whom the superior anatomical detail provided by CT will provide essential information either preoperatively or during follow-up. Guidelines for the way in which CT should be used in masses of the abdominal and pelvic viscera have been outlined in Chapters 7–15. A general overview of the value and disadvantages of CT in abdominal and pelvic masses will be outlined here.

It should be always remembered that in order to obtain an adequate study of the abdomen meticulous attention should be paid to technique with regard to the adequate filling of the gastrointestinal tract with contrast and the delineation of the major abdominal vessels by rapid bolus injection of contrast. If this is not done, the results of the examination may be suboptimal; indeed, in such instances more information may be obtained from other modalities such as sonography (Fig. 16.1; see also Fig. 9.9, p. 116). In some children specific techniques may be required, such as intrathecal injection of metrizamide in children with paraspinal neuroblastoma. For this reason it is always helpful to have a study from a less invasive modality such as sonography in an attempt to determine whether the patient has a lesion that will require investigation by a myelogram as well. Having this information from other modalities will enable one to tailor the CT study to suit the special needs of each particular patient.

At the Hospital for Sick Children, Toronto, we have found that CT is of greatest value in the delineation of malignant tumors both at the time of initial presentation and during follow-up. CT is the most accurate modality for determining the extent of these lesions preoperatively. Our extensive experience has also shown that CT is the most accurate modality in assessing tumor response to radiotherapy and/or chemotherapy. The size of the tumor and its relationship to adjacent structures is more accurately defined with CT than other modalities. Even when neoplasms do not shrink in size following such therapy, a dramatic change in attenuation values may be seen in follow-up scans, indicating that the lesion has become necrotic or fibrotic (see Fig. 11.13, p. 160). This is an important facet of the evaluation of response to therapy, which cannot be made clinically.

We have also used CT successfully to assess the tumor bed following surgical excision. Postoperative CT offers a superior visualization of the abdomen in patients who have had malignant disease removed. This is mainly because the region of the mass becomes occupied by bowel gas postoperatively and therefore this area may often be difficult to image with sonography. We recommend that CT of the tumor bed be performed between 4 and 6 weeks following surgery in all children with a malignant lesion with a known propensity for local recurrence or if there is known local invasion, tumor spillage, or incomplete surgical resection. This scan serves as a baseline for follow-up studies. Postoperative changes such as fibrosis, hematoma, and abscess may also simulate tumor recurrence. The presence of such masses in a tumor bed should be compared with the initial baseline CT done postoperatively, and any increase in size should be considered as tumor recurrence unless there is clinical evidence of infection or hemorrhage in that area. Unfortunately, in a number of children that we have seen, clinical symptoms or elevation of tumor markers such as serum alpha-fetoprotein may well indicate the presence of local recurrence when no definite changes are evident on CT.

We have found CT to be the single most useful modality in the detection of metabolically active nonpalpable abdominal tumors. Children with these lesions present with the distant effects of the neoplasms, and in this regard CT has helped dramatically to alter the management of these patients. These lesions are usually 1–2 cm in size

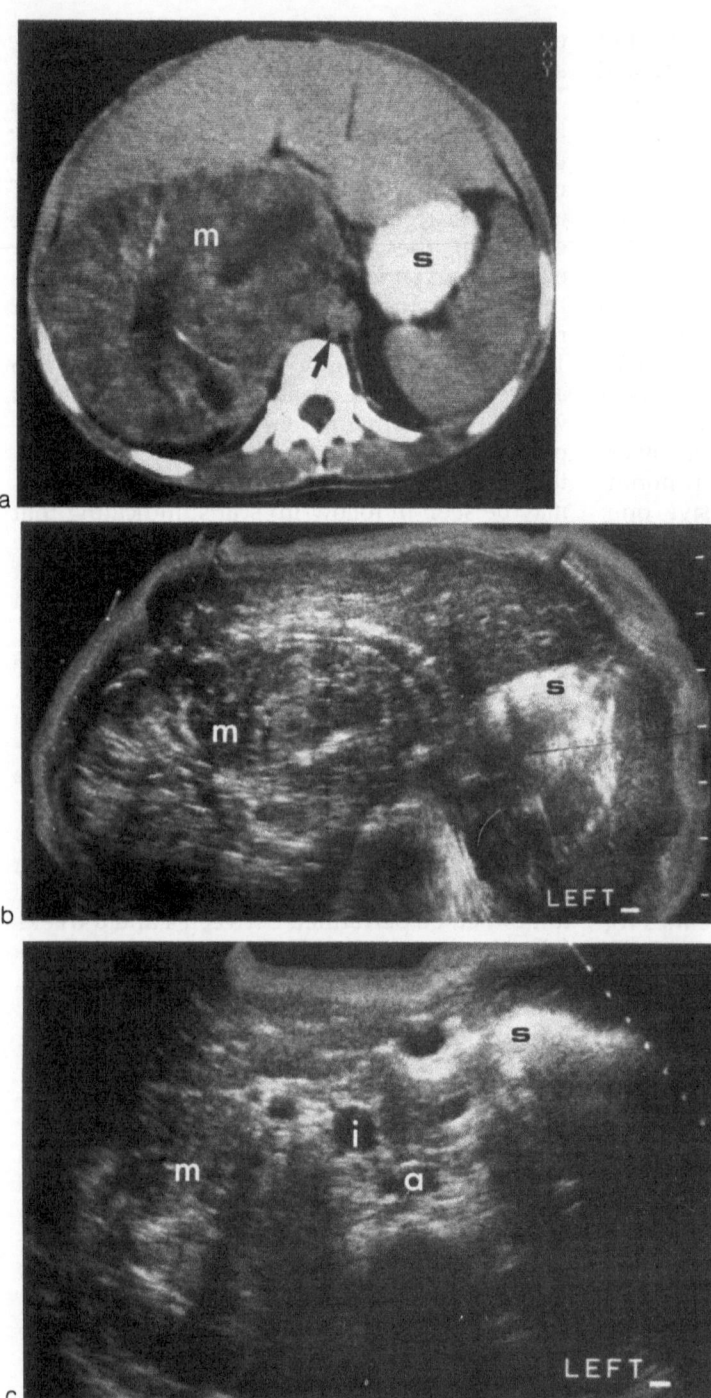

Fig. 16.1a–c. A 9-year-old girl with right adrenal carcinoma. **a,b** CT scan and transverse sonogram (**b**) show the large right-sided mass (*m*) crossing the midline and displacing the aorta (*arrow*) a little more to the left. *s*, stomach. The inhomogeneous attenuation noted on CT and the mixed echo pattern on sonography reflect the areas of hemorrhage and necrosis that are commonly seen in these large adrenal carcinomas. Calcification is also well seen on the CT scan. **c** Further transverse sonography reveals the more detailed relationship of the mass (*m*) to the inferior vena cava (*i*), which is displaced a little forward, and the aorta (*a*). The relationship of the mass to the adjacent structures was better defined with sonography than with the CT study, which was performed following the injection of intravenous contrast. Had the CT been performed during rapid bolus injection of contrast material, that modality might well have displayed the relationships of the mass far better. These two studies in this patient illustrate the value of meticulous technique when attempting to delineate the anatomy of the upper abdomen in children.

when they present as the result of their distant effects, and, because CT does not rely on organ displacement but rather on its great spatial and density resolution, it is an ideal modality for early detection of these lesions. In certain instances CT can be used as the initial and only modality. This is particularly the case when one knows from the clinical data what part of the abdomen should be examined (e.g., adrenal carcinoma) or if the lesions are of a type that may be multiple (e.g., pheochromocytoma). In contrast, however, in other instances other less invasive modalities such as sonography are extremely useful prior to the use of CT. Thus, sonography may provide valuable information so that the CT study can be tailored to suit the needs of a particular patient, e.g., the injection of intrathecal metrizamide for paraspinal neuroblastoma. In patients with nonspecific symptoms such as fever of unknown origin or a raised ESR, or in those patients with a suggestion of neuroblastoma because of the presence of opsomyoclonus, where the primary is usually solitary, sonography may delineate the presence of the lesion; thus the subsequent CT scan can be limited to that region rather than the entire abdomen. Because time on our CT machine is at such a premium, sonography plays a major role in this regard by decreasing the time spent in examining these patients with CT.

The scout radiograph is an extremely useful facet of the examination of the abdomen in patients with abdominal masses. At the end of the examination the transverse scans that mark the limits of the tumor can be posted on the scout radiograph. This depiction of the anatomy is extremely useful for radiotherapists, enabling them to plan radiation fields accurately. Further accurate measurements of such lesions may be made with the cursor on the transverse scan.

Computed tomography has also proved extremely useful in those instances where the patient is too large or obese, or where the lesions are partially hidden by bowel gas or bone and cannot be adequately examined by sonography. In these situations CT delineates the entire sectional anatomy of the abdomen and pelvis as fat, bone, and bowel gas do not act as barriers to visualization of all the viscera. However, CT is not without its limitations and pitfalls:

1. The lack of meticulous technique may lead to false interpretations. Unenhanced bowel loops or vessels may simulate soft tissue masses such as neoplasms or abscesses in this situation.

2. The concept that CT is not a completely noninvasive study has already been stressed.

3. CT is relatively less available than sonography and more expensive, although a CT study may well cost less than numerous other studies which may not supply all the information.

4. Despite meticulous technique CT may not add any further information about masses in the abdomen and pelvis of neonates. These patients are ideally suited to study with high-frequency sonographic transducers; indeed in most of the neonatal masses sonography is usually the definitive procedure. The lack of retroperitoneal fat limits the role of CT in these neonates, and often CT studies have little further to offer than sonography.

5. In the presence of extremely large lesions it may be difficult or impossible at times to determine the exact site of origin of a mass (Fig. 16.2). This applies to lesions that may arise in the kidney, retroperitoneum, adrenal gland, or liver. In this situation the direction of displacement of the surrounding viscera and vessels may aid in localization of the origin of the lesion. For example, right adrenal lesions displace the inferior vena cava and pancreatic head forward. Posteromedial displacement of the inferior vena cava is usually seen with hepatic masses.

6. Although infiltration of the tumor into surrounding muscles and bone is much better evaluated with CT than other modalities, it should be stressed that the diagnosis of invasion can indeed be extremely difficult at times, even with this modality. This information is extremely important when considering surgery. The presence of fat planes between structures will rule out invasion, but the absence of fat planes may be either normal or due to adherence or invasion of the tumor into an adjacent structure. The question of invasion is also difficult at the superior and inferior limits of the tumor, where the transverse axial scans cut the lesion tangentially. At these sites averaging of the tumor with the adjacent organ may produce images that give one the appearance of local invasion (Fig. 16.3; see also Fig. 10.12, p. 139, and Fig. 11.14, p. 161). This is particularly a problem in extrahepatic masses of the upper abdomen that occasionally appear to be invading liver. In our experience the vast majority of these lesions are not invading the liver and at very most are merely adherent to it.

7. Sonography has the advantage that scans can be made in any plane, and in some patients certain lesions and their surrounding viscera and

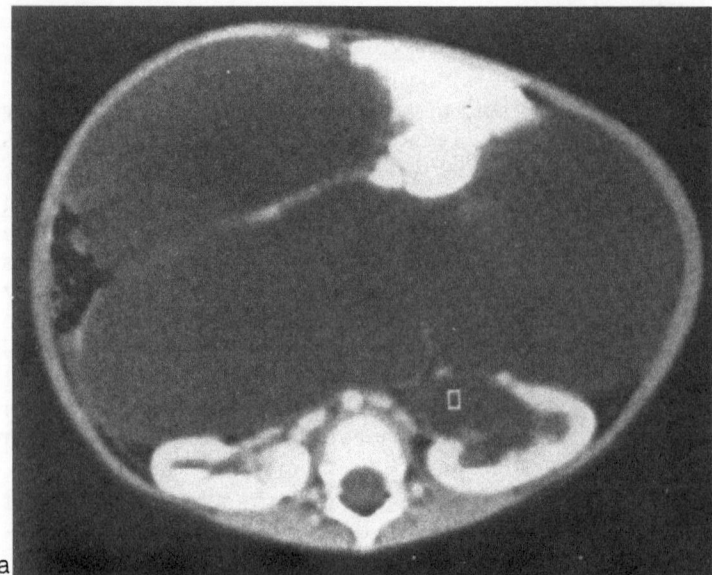

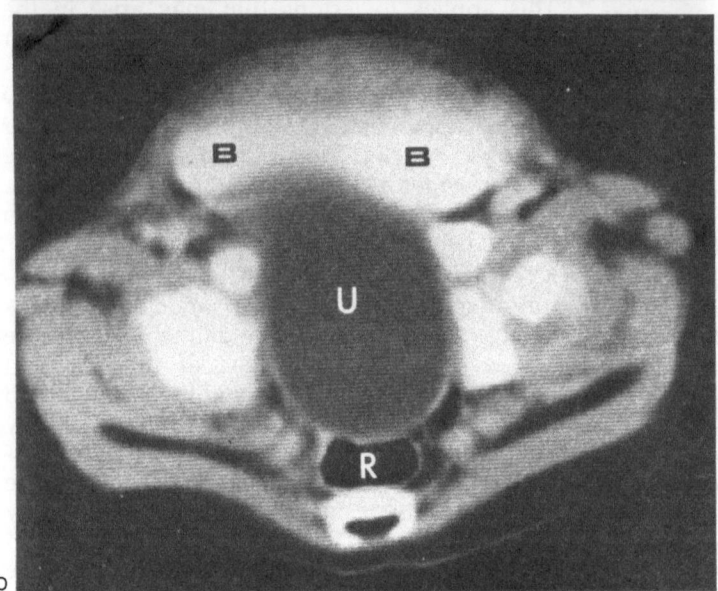

Fig. 16.2a,b. A 1-year-old boy with abdominal distension. Abdominal sonography revealed that the abdomen was filled with cystic masses. Although a left hydronephrosis was noted, the relationship of these fluid-filled structures to the kidney could not be delineated. **a** CT shows that the abdomen is filled with fluid-filled structures and delineates the relationship of these to the collecting system of the left kidney (*square cursor*). These masses represent exceptionally severe hydronephrosis of an upper pole of a left duplex kidney. **b** The ureter (*U*) fills the pelvis and displaces the bladder (*B*) anteriorly and compresses the anterior wall of the rectum (*R*).

vessels may be better delineated by longitudinal or oblique scans. Although newer CT machines can reconstruct images in coronal, sagittal, or oblique planes, the resultant images lack the spatial resolution of the original transverse scan. True coronal and sagittal scans can be obtained by placing small children in the scanner in the appropriate positions, but this is not always feasible with older children. It has been our experience that the use of these types of scan adds little further meaningful information beyond that obtained with the transverse scans. These views, however, are occasionally particularly appreciated by clinicians, who often cannot reconstruct the pathological anatomy from the transverse scan.

8. Delineation of the inferior vena cava is extremely important in those patients with tumors that have a propensity to grow into the large veins and up the inferior vena cava. A potential pitfall in CT is misinterpreting flow defects from the less opacified blood from the renal or hepatic veins flowing into the more opacified blood of the inferior vena cava. These defects should be traced in adjacent scans to their origin in the respective veins, and in this way their true nature will be appreciated.

In summary, we have found CT to be the single most accurate modality in the delineation of the origin and extent of abdominal masses, and its greatest value is in the delineation of malignant lesions both at the time of diagnosis and during follow-up. It is also extremely useful in the delineation of small metabolically active nonpalpable masses and is more accurate than other modalities in delineating small and multiple lesions in the liver and kidneys. It is also extremely useful for the detection of tumor calcification and enlarged lymph nodes. The images are not degraded by fat, bone, or bowel gas as are those of sonography, and in this regard CT is extremely accurate in delineating lesions that arise in or adjacent to bone and those that have intraspinal extension. Nevertheless, CT does have certain disadvantages. Lack of retroperitoneal fat limits the value of CT in the study of masses in neonates, in whom sonography usually supplies all the necessary information. Invasion of adjacent viscera may be

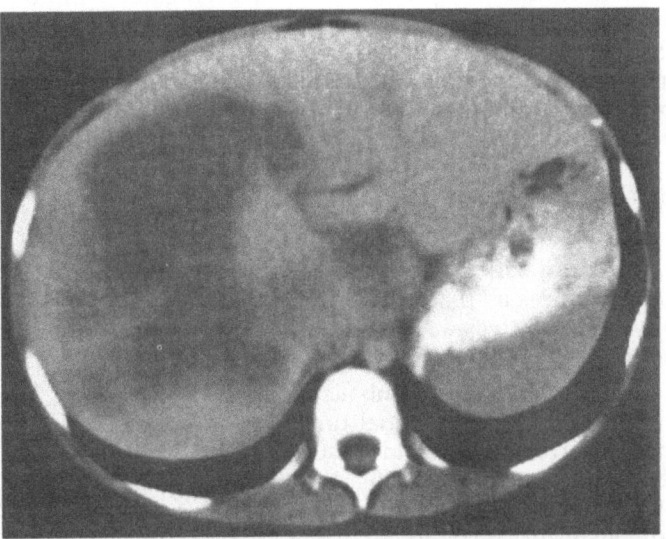

a

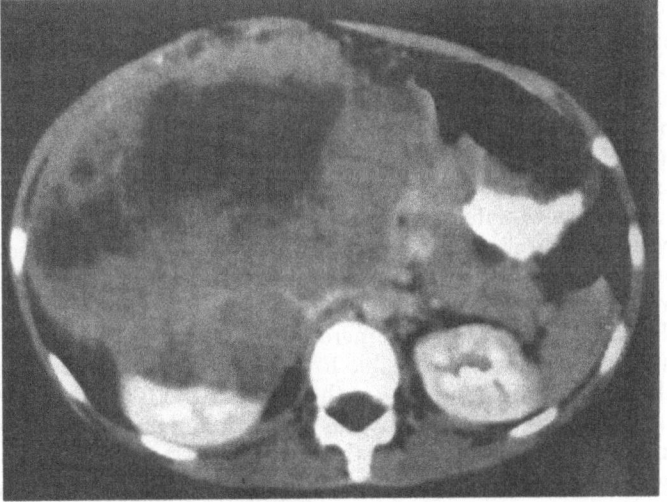

b

Fig. 16.3a,b. An 8-year-old boy with huge right flank mass. **a** The mass is of lower attenuation than the surrounding liver. The line of demarcation between this tissue and the liver is ill defined, particularly posteriorly in the right and caudate lobes. This suggests liver invasion. **b** A lower scan shows the mass crossing the midline from the right flank and its relationship to the anterior surface of the right kidney. It was uncertain whether this relationship represented a lesion arising in the anterior part of the kidney or invading this kidney. At operation the mass was noted to arise in the kidney but there was no liver invasion — merely compression. Biopsy revealed a Wilms' tumor. This case illustrates how difficult it may be at times to delineate the exact site of origin of large solid masses which appear to be invading several structures.

difficult to delineate, and it may be impossible to determine the site of origin of huge abdominal or pelvic masses. Finally, flow defects in the inferior vena cava should not be misinterpreted as tumor thrombi. Therefore, although CT is of immense value in the delineation of abdominal and pelvic masses, its pitfalls and limitations should be well understood so that its role in the investigation of any particular lesion can be adequately evaluated.

Angiography

Prior to the advent of sonography and CT most children with abdominal masses, particularly those that were malignant, were evaluated with angiography. In the hands of an experienced pediatric angiographer this is a safe and accurate procedure and does provide information regarding the site of origin, extent, and vascularity of the mass. Today, the vast majority of abdominal masses can be adequately studied with sonography and CT and in many cases angiography has become redundant.

The indications for abdominal angiography at present can be summarized as follows:

1. Children with large tumors in whom the surgeon requires a "road map" of vascular geography preoperatively. A "road map" may also be required in bilateral Wilms' tumor.

2. When preoperative embolization is required. Embolization of abdominal tumors is not commonly performed in children. Occasionally, this technique is useful, particularly in hemangiomas of the liver when these do not involute spontaneously or respond to more conservative measures.

3. Liver tumors. The angiographic appearances of many benign and malignant liver lesions may appear similar, but the great value of angiography is its use in determining the resectability of hepatic masses. The most important feature that angiography may determine is whether the tumor has violated the important surgical line between the medial and lateral divisions of the left lobe of the liver. This has been the main indication for angiography in hepatic tumors in the past. However, our increasing experience has shown that it is possible to determine operability of a hepatic mass on the basis of the CT scan, because angiography has not supplied any further information about the extent of lesions when compared with scans performed on newer generation CT machines. Despite this, the geographic arterial anatomy, particularly the definition of anomalous vessels, is sufficient indication for continuing to use angiography in the preoperative evaluation of liver tumors.

Venous sampling is a highly accurate method of documenting the site of metabolically active tumors. It is of particular value in the localization of pheochromocytomas and functioning adrenocortical tumors. Experience with fast scan CT examinations has made these venous sampling procedures extremely uncommon as the vast majority of small metabolically active tumors can be easily located within the abdomen and pelvis by CT.

Inferior vena cavography has been mandatory in the past in patients in whom the tumor has a propensity to invade the inferior vena cava, but more recently this has been replaced by sonography, which is highly sensitive and noninvasive.

Magnetic Resonance Imaging

Magnetic resonance imaging has been recently used in a number of centres for the delineation of mass lesions not only in the abdomen but elsewhere in the body as well. Its role in the investigation of pediatric abdominal masses is still undefined. It may well replace CT in many instances. Its major advantages over CT are that it does not involve ionizing radiation and does not require the injection of intravenous contrast material. Moreover, images can be taken in any plane without repositioning of the patient.

Summary

Sonography is the modality of choice in the investigation of children with abdominal masses. It is relatively inexpensive and does not use ionizing radiation. In many instances sonography may provide the definitive diagnosis, combined with sufficient information for adequate management. This is particularly true in neonates, in whom high-frequency transducers can be used, and also in cystic lesions and benign lesions of the biliary and genital tracts. In other instances sonography may not be able to provide all the information and other studies may be required. This is particularly true in patients with renal disease, who may require renal isotope scans or urography and cystography.

CT plays a major role in the delineation of the origin and extent of malignant lesions both at the time at diagnosis and during follow-up. It is also useful for the delineation of metastatic disease in the lungs as well as of small metabolically active tumors. It is also of great benefit in those patients where sonography cannot adequately delineate the lesion because of fat, bone, or bowel gas. CT is the modality of choice in delineating lesions arising from or adjacent to bone and for the detection of intraspinal extension.

Nuclear medicine and angiography have a limited role in the investigation of abdominal masses, and the role of magnetic resonance imaging has yet to be defined.

Inflammation

The evaluation of children with known or suspected inflammatory disease or abscess formation of the abdomen and pelvis is an extremely common problem. Most of these children have inflammatory lesions involving the bowel, such as appendicitis or Crohn's disease, or have had previous abdominal surgery, such as laparotomy or peritoneal dialysis. Many of the children investigated for suspected abdominal inflammation may be immunodeficient on a congenital or acquired basis.

These children may present in a variety of ways depending on the site of the inflammatory process or abcess and its severity and extent. Symptoms and signs may make localization of the lesion easy, but in many instances localizing symptoms and signs are absent, making the clinical problem a difficult one. In such children general symptoms and signs of an inflammatory process are the only ones present, with no definite abnormality indicating that the disease is originating in the abdomen or pelvis. The evaluation of the abdomen and pelvis in these children includes a meticulous evaluation of the peritoneal cavity, retroperitoneum, and major abdominal viscera, including the liver, spleen, kidneys, pancreas, and bowel.

When no localizing abdominal or pelvic symptoms or signs are present, conventional abdominal and chest radiographs are extremely important. Obvious inflammatory processes may be noted in the chest. Abdominal inflammatory processes may lead to gaseous distention of loops of bowel, air fluid levels, the presence of soft tissue masses caused by fluid-filled loops of bowel or abscesses, and extraluminal air, which may collect within an abscess. Subphrenic abscesses may be associated with an elevated hemidiaphragm and pleural effusion.

At the Hospital for Sick Children, Toronto, we have used sonography with great success in the search for abdominal and pelvic inflammatory processes and abscesses. We have found that in conjunction with plain radiographs sonography is extremely helpful in the vast majority of patients with intra-abdominal inflammatory processes as it defines the site and extent of disease well. Sonography is an invaluable noninvasive modality for the follow-up of such processes and is also our modality of choice for guidance of abscess and fluid drainage as well as visceral biopsy.

Sonography does, however, have some limitations in this regard. The presence of a large amount of bowel gas may obscure smaller lesions. Large dilated loops of bowel may occasionally simulate abscesses when peristaltic activity is lost. The presence of abdominal wounds, dressings, and abdominal tenderness limits access to parts of the abdomen and pelvis. The echo pattern of abscesses may occasionally be nonspecific and may mimic hematomas or neoplasms.

[67]Ga citrate has been used extensively, as this radiopharmaceutical is taken up by leukocytes at sites of inflammation. It has the advantage that the entire body can be examined, particularly in patients with no localizing findings. However, the study takes 24–72 h to complete, and excretion into the colon may limit the accuracy of the study as collections in the colon may mimic abscesses. Poor anatomical detail is provided by gallium scans, and total body irradiation is involved. Uptake is nonspecific, as neoplasms may also take up gallium, as well as incisions following operation.

Computed tomography is extremely useful in the evaluation of the abdomen and pelvis for inflammatory processes [1]. However, in order to obtain an adequate study, meticulous attention must be paid to the adequate opacification of bowel with orally or rectally administered water-soluble contrast material. Injection of intravenous contrast is also useful to delineate the major vessels and viscera. Fluid-filled loops of bowel may mimic abscesses. However, with intravenous contrast injection the wall of the bowel which enhances is noted to be thin in comparison with abscess cavities, which tend to have a much thicker and irregular outline. Occasionally, it may be necessary to rescan certain areas where there are unopacified bowel loops in order to differentiate the two.

Abscesses appear centrally as low-attenuation areas that fail to enhance on contrast administration. Fluid and air may be present in the centre of an abscess. The wall of the abscess usually enhances quite dramatically and occasionally it may be difficult to differentiate this from a large necrotic tumor. Inflammatory processes or abscesses in the viscera such as the liver, spleen, or kidneys usually appear as areas of lower attenuation which are better defined after the injection of intravenous contrast (see Fig. 11.9, p. 154, Fig. 11.10, p. 155, Fig. 12.9, p. 184, and Fig. 12.10, p. 184).

The major advantages of CT over sonography in the investigation of these patients are (1) that CT offers better anatomical details, (2) it is unimpeded by gas or bone, and (3) it can be performed if the patient has abdominal wounds, incisions, drains, dressings, or tenderness (see Fig. 16.6). However, it is a more difficult procedure to perform than sonography as meticulous attention has to be paid to adequate opacification of the bowel and vessels.

Therefore, CT should not be used as an initial diagnostic modality in patients with suspected abdominal or pelvic inflammatory disease or abscesses but should be reserved for specific instances when plain radiography and sonography cannot adequately answer the clinical question. CT has proved useful in those patients in whom there is a high clinical suspicion of an inflammatory process but the gallium or sonographic studies are equivocal. CT is also useful in delineating lesions that may be difficult to interpret on sonography (Fig. 16.4), and in defining inflammatory processes in unusual sites, particularly when their relationships to adjacent structures cannot be well determined by sonography (Fig. 16.5). CT appears to be more accurate than sonography in the detection of extremely small lesions, particularly of the viscera (Fig. 16.6; see also Fig. 12.9, p.184). CT is also useful in documentation of inflammatory processess with wide extension that cannot be adequately delineated by sonography (Fig. 16.7). We have occasionally used CT to guide aspiration of abscesses when these lesions are not readily accessible by sonography.

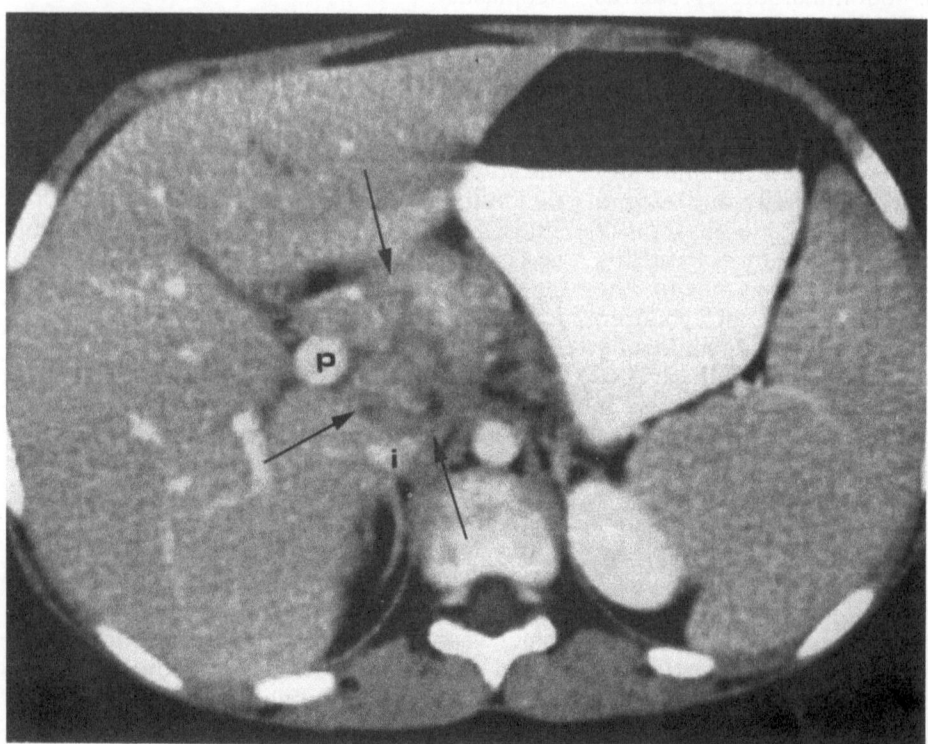

Fig. 16.4. An 8-year-old girl with fever. CT shows a mass (*arrows*) with inhomogeneous enhancement to the right of the midline separating the inferior vena cava (*i*) and portal vein (*p*). At operation this mass was noted to represent a group of necrotic lymph nodes and no organism was cultured from these. The spleen also appeared slightly enlarged.

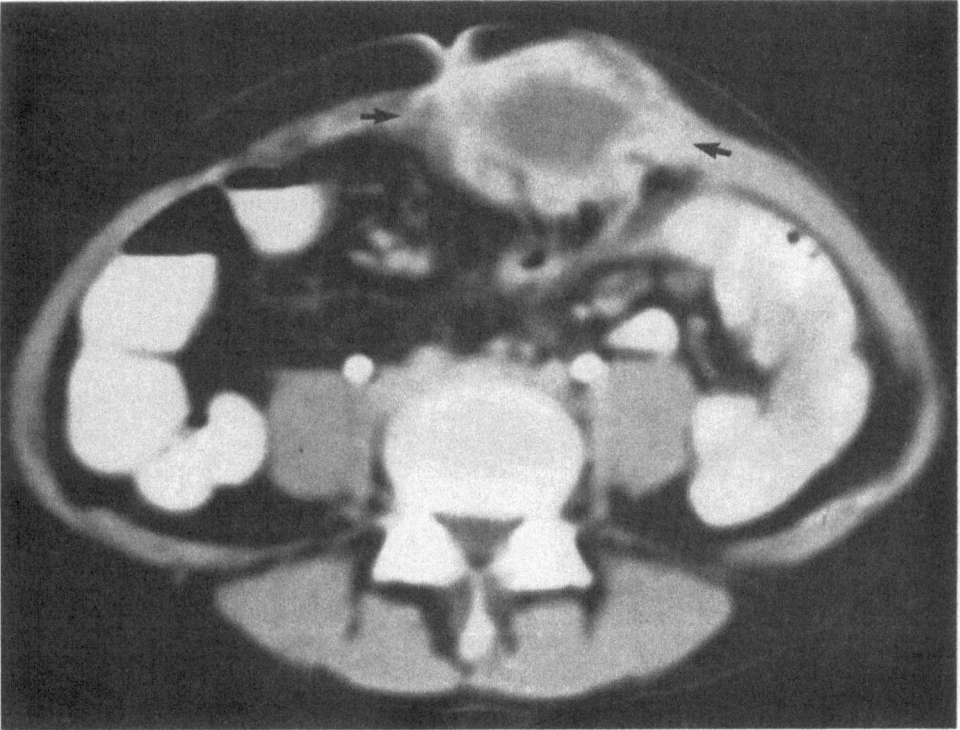

Fig. 16.5. A 15-year-old boy with known Crohns' disease. CT shows a large abscess (*arrows*) replacing the left rectus abdominis muscle. This mass enhances peripherally and has no enhancement centrally because of the presence of pus. Note the relationship of the mass to underlying bowel. This abscess had occurred postoperatively following bowel resection.

Trauma

Computed Tomography

Computed tomography has been successfully used for the evaluation of the abdomen following blunt trauma in both adults and children [4, 6]. However, there is limited published experience regarding the value of this modality in children. In 1981, Kuhn and Berger [6] described the value of CT in 18 children and, in 1984, Kaufman et al. [4] reported their experience with the use of CT in 100 children with clinical evidence of serious blunt abdominal injury. In the latter study the usefulness of CT was compared with liver/spleen scintigraphy and abdominal sonography. These authors showed that CT has fewer false negative and false positive results than the other two modalities and provides the most information of any single diagnostic imaging test available [4]. However, these authors went on to state that it would take additional time and further study to determine whether CT truly affected patient outcome.

Our own experience at the Hospital for Sick Children in Toronto has also shown the great value of CT in blunt abdominal trauma, as well as in other extracranial trauma. During the one-year period from June 1983 to June 1984, only 19 patients with extracranial trauma were studied with CT; 7 of these patients had follow-up studies, making a total of 26 studies. The regions that were studied were as follows: abdomen 9; skeletal 8 (sacroiliac joints 6, hips 1, feet 1; see Chap. 23); larynx 1; chest 1. Of the 26 studies, 18 were done on an elective basis and only 8 were performed as emergencies. Abnormalities were found in 22 of the 26 studies. Only in four studies were results normal. In these four patients head CT was also performed, and the abdomen was studied because of the suspicion of abdominal trauma. In all four the normal appearances on abdominal CT obviated the necessity of using other modalities.

At the Hospital for Sick Children, Toronto we have attempted to formulate guidelines for the use of the various modalities in children with blunt abdominal trauma [2]. We believe that this is the most efficient and cost-effective method for

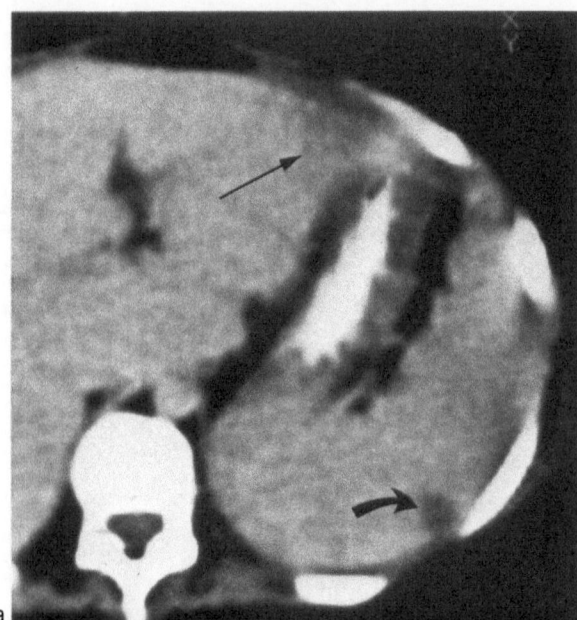

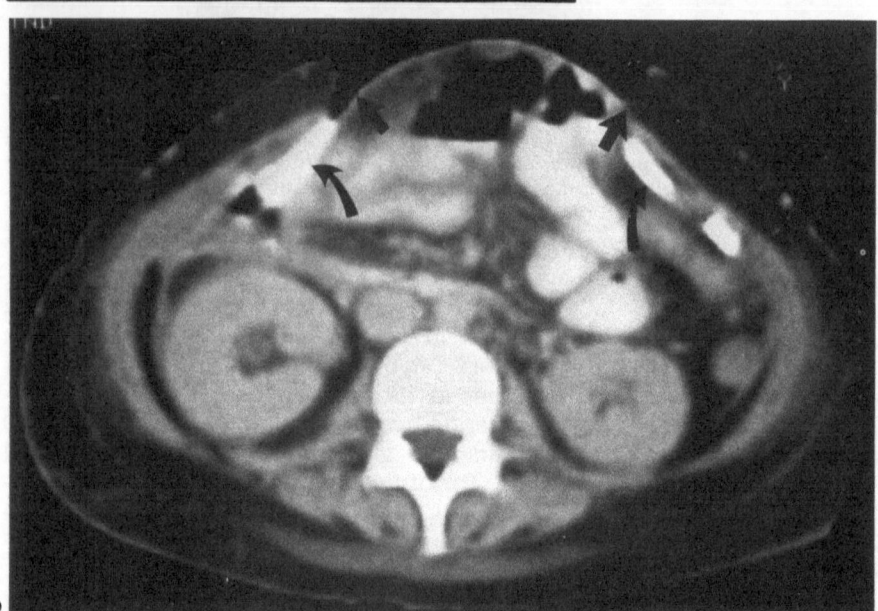

Fig. 16.6a,b. A 13-year-old girl with previous bowel resection for Crohn's disease. **a** CT shows abscess in anterior aspect of left lobe of liver (*arrrow*) and small abscess in the spleen (*curved arrows*). **b** lower scan shows dehiscence of the wound. (*arrows*). Patients with this complication are difficult to examine sonographically, and in this situation CT is a valuable modality in delineating the presence of intra-abdominal inflammatory processes. *Curved arrows*, drains

the initial evaluation of patients suspected of intra-abdominal injury. In this way the modalities used are chosen according to the clinical situation and are tailored to meet the individual patient's needs. Even though CT may be the ideal modality for the documentation of intra-abdominal injury, we believe it is not necessary in every case. Many patients can be quite adequately managed after investigation with other modalities without any significant injuries being overlooked.

At our institution the prime indications for abdominal CT are as follows:

1. Severely injured but stable patients suspected of having injuries to multiple intra-abdominal organ systems or when clinical symptoms and signs are not typical of involvement of any one organ system

2. Patients with open wounds or with an extremely tender abdomen who cannot be examined with sonography

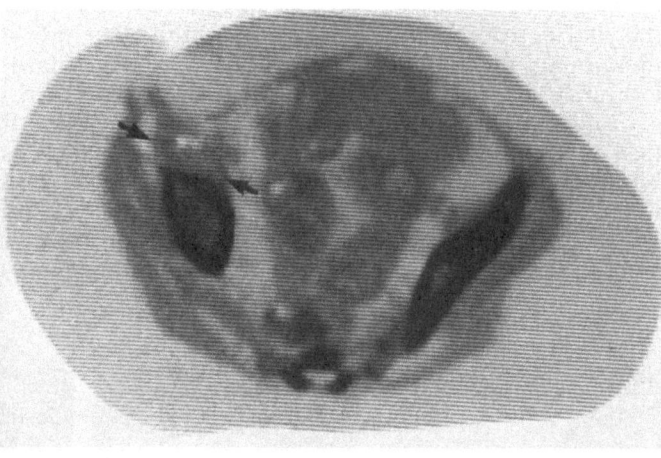

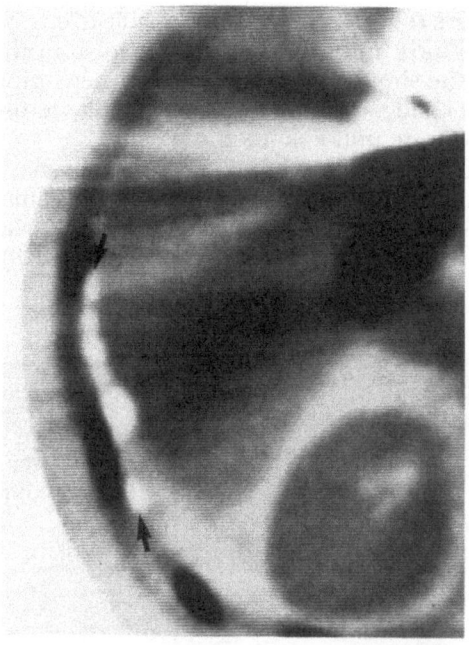

a

b

Fig. 16.7a,b. A 6-year-old girl with known collagen vascular disease and fever. **a** Bubbles of air (*arrows*) are noted along the lateral aspect of the right lobe of the liver. **b** An abscess (*arrows*) is noted in the region of the iliopsoas tendon on the right. Small bubbles of air are noted within the abscess anteriorly. In this patient CT accurately defined the presence of free gas and an abscess that had developed following a silent perforation of a peptic ulcer.

3. Patients with head injury having head CT should have an abdominal CT if abdominal trauma is suspected in order to avoid wasting time organizing another modality on an emergency basis and to limit movement of the patient within the radiology department

4. Patients with abdominal trauma who have been studied with other modalities and in whom the results of those other modalities are either equivocal or unusual and a traumatic lesion is still suspected.

Patients who are hemodynamically unstable or uncooperative and cannot be adequately restrained or sedated are not considered candidates for body CT studies.

In order to obtain a meaningful CT study meticulous attention to technique is extremely important. Patients should be adequately restrained and sedation and analgesia given as required (see Chap. 2, p. 10). All patients should receive adequate doses of dilute water-soluble contrast material orally as outlined in Chapter 7 (see p. 85) unless there is a contraindication to giving fluids orally. Often it is easier to administer this via a nasogastric tube in severely injured patients. If the tube causes undue artifacts dur-

ing scanning it can be withdrawn so that its tip lies in the esophagus. Later, it can readvance into the stomach and an attempt made to withdraw the residual gastric content at the end of the examination.

Once the patient has been adequately positioned and immobilized a digital radiograph of the abdomen is obtained. Adjacent transverse axial scans 1 cm thick are then obtained from the level of the domes of the diaphragm to the level of the aortic bifurcation during rapid bolus injection of contrast material intravenously; 2 ml/kg Hypaque 60% is usually adequate. Further scans through the pelvis may be necessary in those patients with suspected pelvic trauma, whether this be soft tissue or skeletal. Repeat scans through the upper abdomen may be indicated if bowel loops fail to fill with contrast material and differentiation from hematoma is difficult. A change in the pattern of gas, contrast, and bowel fluid on the repeat study will confirm the presence of bowel rather than hematoma, which remain unchanged. Repeat digital radiographs or plain abdominal films at the end of the study may help display the appearance of the entire urinary tract but seldom add significant further information. It must be emphasized that the vital signs of traumatized patients should be monitored at regular intervals during the examination.

Children with severe abdominal trauma who may also have other associated brain and skeletal injuries should not be kept in the scan room any longer than is required to obtain an adequate study. Preparation for the scan should be made prior to the child arriving in the room so that the procedure runs as smoothly as possible to ensure that the most information is obtained from the scan in the shortest possible time, thus ensuring that the child can be moved back quickly to the intensive care unit if so required.

On CT, abdominal hematomas usually have an attenuation value lower than that of the adjacent viscera (see Fig. 8.12, p. 102, Fig. 11.24a, p. 169, Fig. 12.20, p. 195, and Fig. 14.10, p. 219).

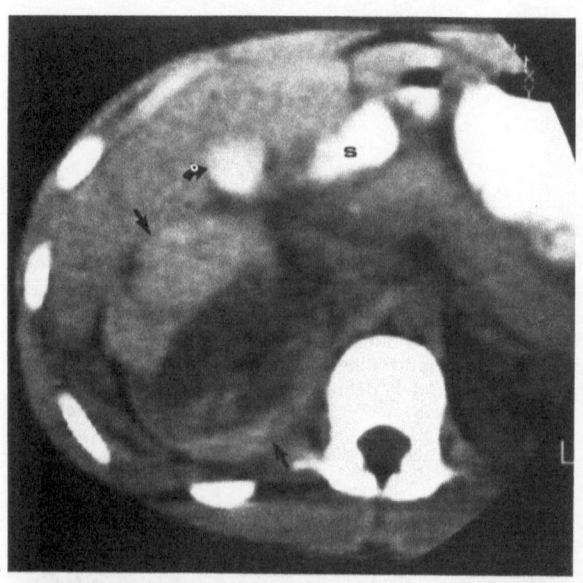

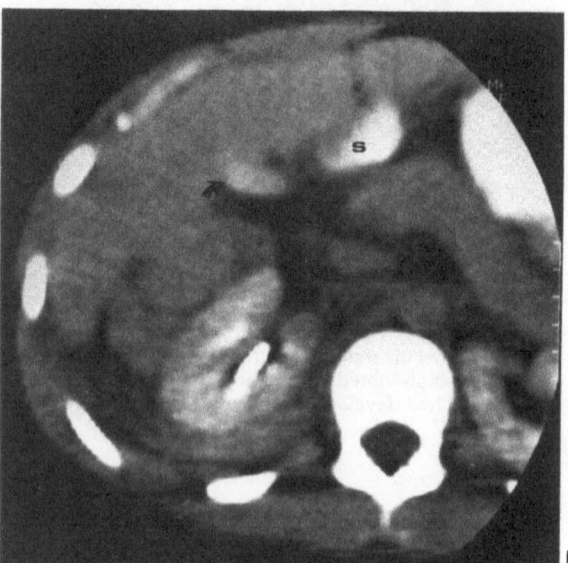

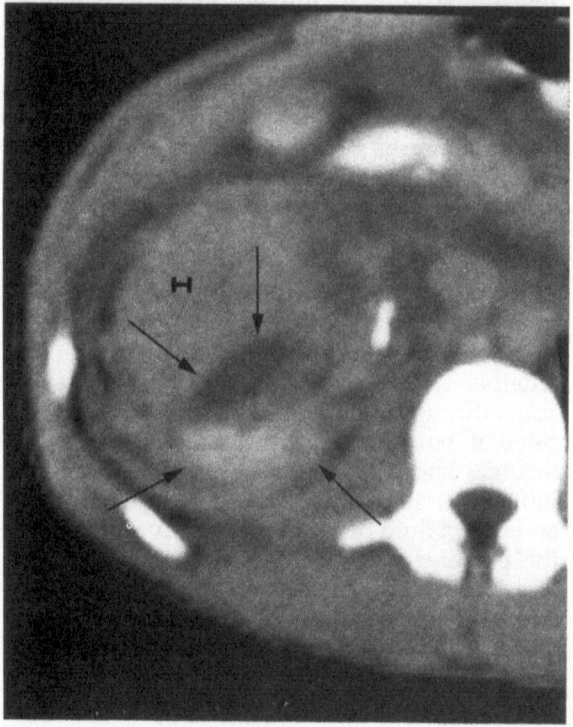

Fig. 16.8a–c. An 8-year-old boy following a motor vehicle accident. Scans before (**a**) and after (**b**) intravenous contrast administration. **a** A large perirenal hematoma (*arrows*) is noted around the right kidney. The hematoma has a higher attenuation value than the underlying kidney. Two triangular areas of high attenuation are noted in the posterolateral aspect of the kidney and represent intrarenal hematomas. The high attenuation values of these hematomas is due to the fact that they are recent, as the child was studied within hours after the injury. *Curved arrow*, blood within the gallbladder; *s*, Gastrografin in the stomach. **b** Following the injection of intravenous contrast material the upper portion of the right kidney has enhanced well and is functioning normally. The perirenal hematomas now have a relatively lower attenuation than the enhancing kidney. The intrarenal hematomas are no longer visualized. **c** Another scan through the lower pole of the kidney (*arrows*) after contrast injection shows normal enhancement of the posterior aspect of the kidney but no enhancement anteriorly as this portion of the kidney was not perfused. This was confirmed at operation. *H*, perirenal hematoma

However, occasionally when CT is performed within a short time after the traumatic incident hematomas may have a higher attenuation than the abdominal viscera (Fig. 16.8). A similar appearance is seen in rare instances when CT is performed during active bleeding and intravenously injected contrast material leaks directly from the vascular system into the hematoma (Fig. 16.9). Hemorrhage into the gallbladder may have a high attenuation, probably as the result of clot retraction and water absorption (see Chap.

13, p. 202). High attenuation values are also seen in instances of urinary tract trauma when contrast-bearing urine leaks into interstitial spaces (Fig. 16.10) or into urinomas (see Fig. 11.24b, p. 169). Small leaks are much more easily appreciated on CT than on conventional radiographic techniques. In scans through the upper abdomen the lower lung fields should always be assessed for evidence of small hemothoraces or pneumothoraces (Fig. 16.11). The presence of pneumothoraces may flatten the usual convex

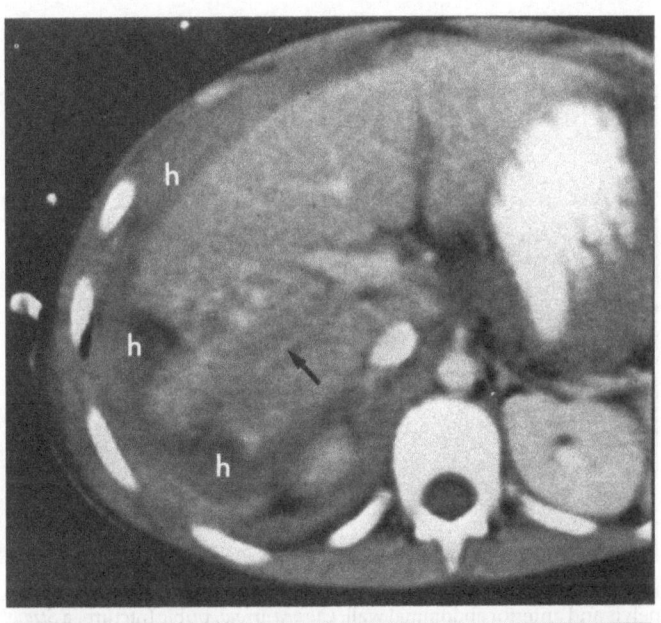

a

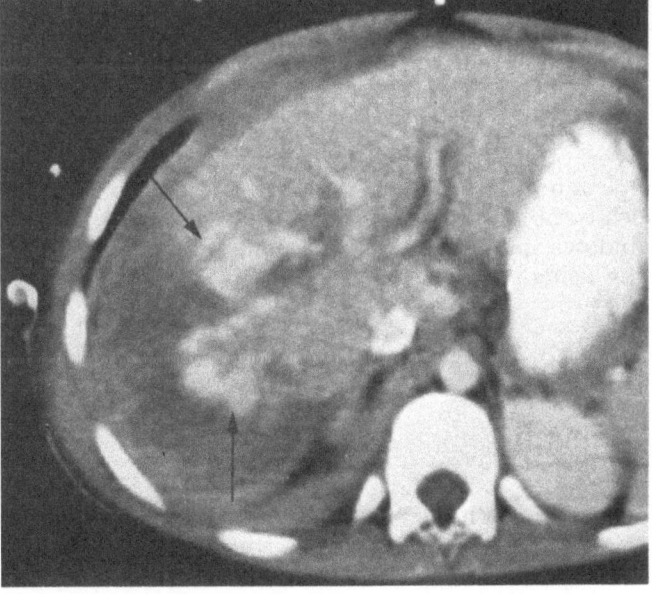

b

Fig. 16.9a,b. A 4-year-old boy with large hepatic hematoma following motor vehicle accident. Scans were performed during the rapid bolus injection of intravenous contrast material. **a** Posterior branch of right portal vein (*arrow*) is noted coursing directly toward the area of maximal liver injury, where there is both intrahepatic and subcapsular hemorrhage (*h*). **b** Lower scan shows area of high attenuation (*arrows*) within the liver caused by contrast leak from the portal vein directly into the hematoma. The rapid blood loss into this hematoma was the cause for the child's instability clinically.

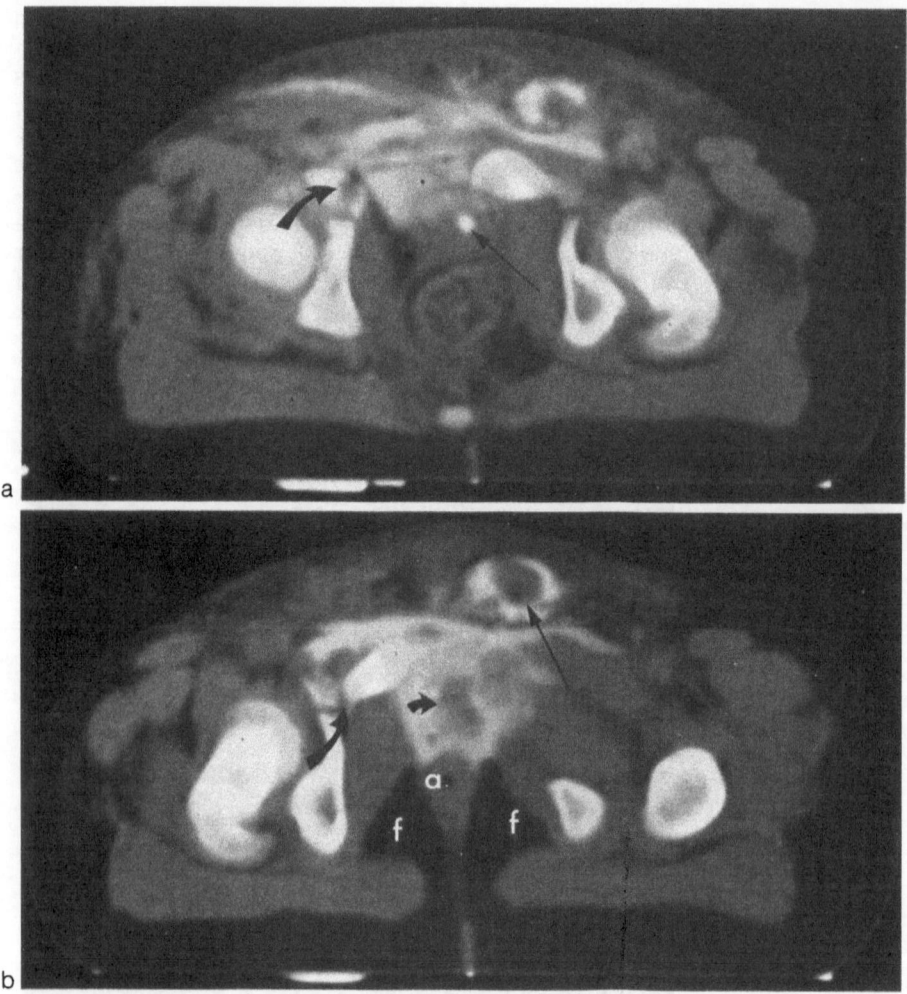

Fig. 16.10a,b Scans through pelvis on a 14-year-old boy with pelvic trauma show leak of contrast into the soft tissues of the pelvis and anterior abdominal wall. *Curved arrow*, pubic fracture. **a** *Straight arrow* indicates contrast in bladder neck surrounded by the triangular soft tissue of the prostate. **b** The triangular prostate (*small curved arrow*) is surrounded by dense extravasated contrast material. *Straight arrow* indicates left testis lying in inguinal canal and surrounded by contrast material. Note the edema and hematoma of the anterior abdominal wall. *a*, anus; *f*, ischiorectal fossa.

upper outline of the liver and spleen. This appearance should alert one to the presence of such complications when images are viewed at windows suited to the abdomen rather than the lung fields.

Other Modalities

Plain Radiographs

Plain radiographs of the abdomen remain the basic mandatory starting point in the investigation of patients with blunt abdominal trauma.

Although the information afforded by this type of study may be limited, it provides essential information regarding the bowel gas pattern, fat planes, and soft tissues, as well as any possible associated skeletal injuries. All of these may provide clues to the nature and site of any more serious underlying visceral injuries and will help direct the clinician and radiologist in the sequence of use of subsequent modalities.

Plain radiographs of the chest are particularly valuable in patients with more than just minor trauma to the upper abdomen. Associated lung contusions, hemopneumothoraces, and fractures may give hints to the side and site of associated abdominal injuries.

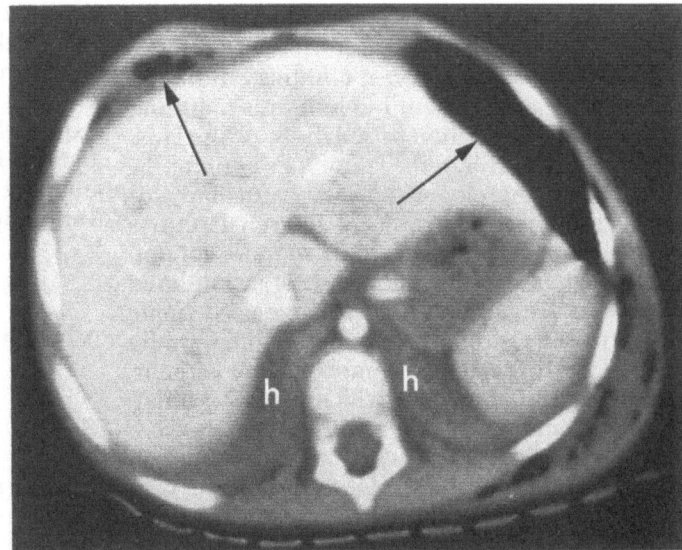

Fig. 16.11. A 9-year-old boy following a motor vehicle accident. CT shows bilateral retroperitoneal hemorrhage (*h*) and pneumothorax (*arrows*) bilaterally. A small amount of fluid is also noted in the right pleural cavity. Note the unusual position and shape of the left lobe of the liver caused by the compression by the left pneumothorax.

Excretory Urography

Excretory urography, like CT, provides both anatomical and functional information about the kidneys and adjacent structures. However, even when combined with nephrotomography, excretory urography is not capable of defining the anatomy of the urinary tract and adjacent structures in the same detail as CT. However, we have used excretory urography in those children with hematuria who have relatively minor injuries (see below). In this situation the functional and anatomical information obtained can be complemented by the anatomical information afforded by abdominal sonography.

Sonography

At the Hospital for Sick Children, Toronto, we have not routinely used sonography to assess children with blunt abdominal trauma at the time of presentation. Like others [4] we have found that sonography is not as accurate as CT and often underestimates the size of visceral hematomas, particularly in the spleen, liver, and kidneys. Sonography also provides no functional information, which is particularly important in patients with suspected renal injury. Sonography has further drawbacks as it cannot be used in patients with significant abdominal tenderness, or in the presence of abdominal wall injuries, dressing, and drains. The presence of ileus, which often accompanies severe trauma,

and bowel gas may make an adequate examination of the abdomen and pelvis impossible.

However, sonography may have a role to play in certain emergency situations. Mobile real-time equipment is valuable for examination of unstable patients in the trauma unit or intensive care unit. This is particularly valuable for the documentation of even small amounts of free intraperitoneal fluid. Sonography is the modality of choice in those children in whom only a pancreatic injury is suspected. It may also provide further anatomical information in those children with minor renal injuries who have already been studied with excretory urography or renal scintigraphy. However, the special value of sonography is in the follow-up of abdominal traumatic lesions that have already been documented by other modalities.

Scintigraphy

The major drawback of scintigraphic studies is their organ specificity. Multiple scintigraphic studies or other modalities are thus required in children in whom trauma to multiple organ systems is suspected. The necessity of using other modalities may waste valuable time and add to the cost of the investigation of children with blunt abdominal trauma when a single meticulously performed abdominal CT may cost less and provide all the necessary information. However, Kaufman et al. [4] have pointed out certain advantages of scintigraphy over CT which should always be considered. Scintigraphy is easier to perform than CT as it does not require intravenous or oral contrast administration and is affected less by patient motion, thus requiring less patient cooperation or sedation. At the Hospital for Sick Children, Toronto, scintigraphic studies have therefore been used particularly for the evaluation of liver, spleen, and renal injuries as an alternative approach to CT in those circumstances when the indications for CT (as outlined on p. 258) are not present. We have used single photon emission computed tomography (SPECT), which has vastly improved the examination of multiple organs, which usually overlap in planar images [2]. Our approach includes a 5-min renal flow study which, if normal, is followed by a SPECT liver/spleen study and a continuing renal study. This technique has provided a significant improvement in detection of lesions over planar images. It provides an easy, accurate, and cost-effective approach in the investigation of some children with blunt abdominal trauma. The only drawbacks are that it takes longer than an abdominal CT scan and the radiation dose delivered to the organ studied is slightly greater than with CT.

Angiography

Angiography is a time-consuming and invasive modality that does not delineate the extent of abdominal trauma to the same degree as CT. Angiography may thus delay the time in which diagnosis is made and therapy instituted and carries a not inconsiderable morbidity. For these reasons its use in abdominal trauma has decreased dramatically since the advent of CT; indeed, it is now only rarely used in this clinical situation. Angiography is helpful, however, for the delineation of renal pedicle injuries (see p. 265) and extremely rarely for the demonstration of the exact site of bleeding or for therapeutic intervention (e.g., embolization).

Peritoneal Lavage

In 30 of 100 children with suspected intra-abdominal trauma, Kaufman et al. [4] found free intraperitoneal fluid on both CT and sonography. These imaging modalities documented an organ injury in 28 but failed to find a source of bleeding in 2. Of all of the children in the series with one or more injured organs, 46% had evi-

dence of free intraperitoneal fluid. Because extremely small quantities of free intraperitoneal fluid can be easily documented by sonography or CT, the necessity for peritoneal lavage is thus extremely rare. It may be useful in the unstable patient in whom there may be no time for an imaging procedure such as bedside real-time sonography.

Visceral Injuries

Spleen

Splenic injury is the commonest visceral injury in children with blunt abdominal trauma and was found in 25% of the patients studied by Kaufman et al. [4] (see also Chap. 14, p. 219). Plain radiographs are neither specific nor sensitive [6], but the presence of rib fractures, pneumothorax, elevation of the left hemidiaphragm, enlargement of the splenic shadow, and signs of free intraperitoneal fluid may hint at a splenic lesion.

Kaufman et al. [4] found that sonography had a 50% rate of false negative results in children with splenic trauma. This modality should thus not be used as the modality of choice for the investigation of splenic trauma, but rather for follow-up. These authors found that spleen scintigraphy was almost as accurate as CT. In 24 patients with splenic trauma, CT had no false negative results and 4 false positive results [4]. These latter related to irregularities of the inferior splenic margin, normally inhomogeneous enhancement of the spleen, and intraperitoneal fluid misinterpreted as a subcapsular hematoma. These minor abnormalities were felt to have limited clinical consequences.

With splenic scintigraphy, false positive results may be as high as 10%, most of which are due to shape variation, congenital clefts, pure subcapsular hematoma, and masses adjacent to the liver and spleen, while false negative results tend to be due to small lesions [4, 6].

Liver

Of the 100 children studied by Kaufman et al. [4], 20% had liver injuries and in all the liver enzymes were elevated. CT had fewer false positive and false negative results than scintigraphy. Sonography proved less accurate than CT. Artifact over the liver from bowel gas and ribs may give the liver a heterogeneous appearance which may simulate or mask traumatic lesions. If the study is done in a meticulous manner these artifacts are minimal and lesions that are missed will usually be small and of no clinical consequence (see also Chap. 12, p. 193).

Kidneys (see also Chap. 11)

In children suspected of having renal injuries, it is imperative to obtain anatomical and functional information about both kidneys. This combined information is extremely important in order to determine which patients have renal pedicle injuries. The vast majority of parenchymal injuries can be treated conservatively but pedicle injuries require operative therapy.

Plain radiographs are nonspecific and may merely hint at the site and side of injury. Sonography, we have found, may underestimate the extent of parenchymal disruption and unfortunately supplies no functional information whatsoever. However, sonography is helpful for follow-up of previously documented renal lesions and may be useful in the acute phase by providing additional anatomical information in those patients who have minor degrees of renal injury and who have already been studied by excretory urography or renal scintigraphy. Although both excretory urography and scintigraphy provide valuable functional information regarding the kidneys, they do not provide the detailed anatomical delineation of the kidneys and perirenal tissues afforded by CT. We have therefore used CT as the modality of choice in children with more severe renal injuries or those suspected of having multiple intra-abdominal visceral injuries. Kaufman et al. [4] found renal injuries in 11% of the 100 children with blunt abdominal trauma that they had studied and showed that CT had fewer false positive and false negative results than sonography. Angiography is essential in those patients with renal pedicle injuries and may play a role in those few children with continued massive hemorrhage.

Pancreas (see also Chap. 9)

Trauma to the pancreas is found much less commonly than other visceral injuries in children and was seen in only 3 of the 100 patients studied by Kaufman et al. [4]. In children suspected of having only pancreatic injury, sonography is usually the modality of choice as traumatic pancreatic lesions and complications are usually easily defined with this modality (see Chap. 9, p. 112). However, CT is extremely valuable for the delineation of pancreatic lesions, particularly in those children with abdominal tenderness or ileus in whom sonography may not be able to delineate the gland and also in those children with suspected multiple organ injuries. Changes which may be seen on CT or sonography include swelling of the gland, hematomas, lacerations, and pseudocysts as a late complication.

Other Injuries

Traumatic lesions involving the gallbladder are rare and have been discussed in Chap. 13 (see p. 201). Retroperitoneal and pelvic hematomas have been discussed in Chapters 8 (p. 102) and 15 (p. 240), respectively. Lesions of the gastrointestinal tract are also rare and were found in only 3 of the 100 patients studied by Kaufman et al. [4]. These lesions include duodenal hematoma, mesenteric hematoma, and perforation. In many of these patients contrast studies of the gastrointestinal tract may better define the lesion than CT, particularly with regard to the site of perforation and hematoma. Free intraperitoneal fluid is usually associated with visceral trauma, which can be easily documented on CT.

Summary

Plain radiographs are essential in the investigation of all patients with abdominal trauma. The sequence of subsequent modalities should be tailored to suit the needs of the individual patient, and should be governed by the clinical and plain radiographic findings. CT is the single most accurate modality for the investigation of children with blunt abdominal trauma. It is especially valuable in severely injured patients who are stable and who are suspected of having multiple organ involvement or when symptoms and signs are not typical of any one particular organ involvement. This is particularly important when one considers that 18% of children with visceral injury will have another associated viscus traumatized as well [4].

An alternative approach is the combination of renal and liver/spleen scintigraphy, as used at our institution [2] (see p. 264). Excretory urography or renal scintigraphy are adequate in children with minor renal injuries. Sonography appears to underestimate the extent of parenchymal damage and provides no functional information regarding the kidneys. However, it is extremely valuable for follow-up. Angiography and peritoneal lavage are rarely required.

References

1. Afshani E (1981) Computed tomography of abdominal abscesses in children. Radiol Clin North Am 19:515–526

2. Gilday DL, Ash JM, Reilly BJ, Alton DJ (1984) Childhood abdominal trauma — an easy and efficient approach. Paper presented at the 27th Annual Meeting of the Society for Pediatric Radiology, Las Vegas, April 1984

3. Haller JO, Bass IS, Slovis TL, Friedman AP, Kuhns LR, Watts FB (1984) Difficulties in delineating upper abdominal masses with CT and ultrasound in children. Paper presented at the 70th Annual Meeting of the Radiological Society of North America, Chicago, November 1984

4. Kaufman RA, Towbin R, Babcock DS, Gelfand MJ, Guice KS, Oldham KT, Noseworthy J (1984) Upper abdominal trauma in children: imaging evaluation. AJR 142:449–460

5. Kirks DR, Merten DF, Grossman H, Bowie JD (1981) Diagnostic imaging of pediatric abdominal masses: an overview. Radiol Clin North Am 19:527–545

6. Kuhn JP, Berger PE (1981) Computed tomography in the evaluation of blunt abdominal trauma in children. Radiol Clin North Am 19:503–513

Chapter 17

Miscellaneous

Abdominal Wall

The anterior abdominal wall consists of skin, subcutaneous fat, fascia, anterolateral and midline muscle groups, and peritoneum. In younger children with little abdominal wall fat these individual structures are difficult to discern on CT. Lesions of any of the layers of the abdominal wall may be studied with CT, and the appearances of lesions such as hernias, hematomas, neoplasms, and inflammatory processes have been previously reported, mainly in adults.

We have seldom used CT to define lesions of the abdominal wall in children. However, we have found CT to be particularly useful in defining the extent of both benign and malignant mass lesions of the abdominal wall such as hemangiomas and rhabdomyosarcomas. CT is also useful in defining the size of the lesion following therapy. Examples of abdominal wall lesions are shown in Figs. 17.1, 17.2 and 17.3.

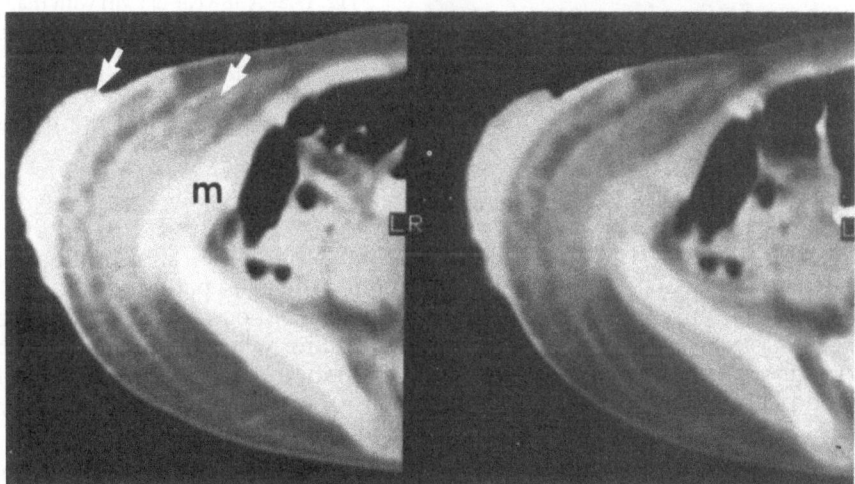

Fig. 17.1. A 2-year-old boy with a hemangioma over the right iliac crest. An enhancing lesion is noted in the skin and subcutaneous tissues (*arrows*). The muscles of the anterior abdominal wall (*m*), however, are not involved. The hemangiomatous tissue of the skin and subcutaneous tissue showed good enhancement following the injection of intravenous contrast material.

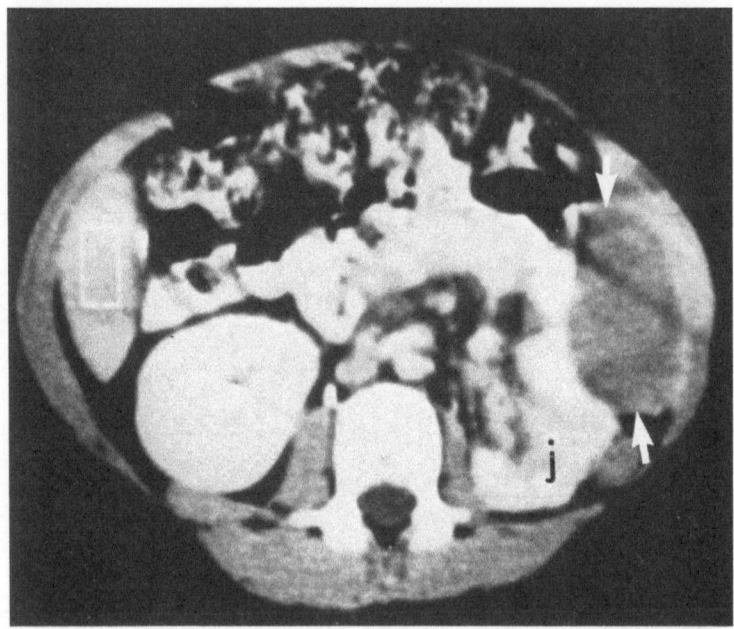

Fig. 17.2. A 6-year-old girl with previous left nephrectomy for Wilms' tumor. Four years after chemotherapy and radiation therapy a CT scan reveals a soft tissue mass (*arrows*) deep to the muscles of the anterolateral abdominal wall on the left. This was a benign fibroma, and its etiology was thought to be related to the previous radiation. Note the jejunum (*j*) lying in the left renal bed. *Rectangular cursor* marks the liver.

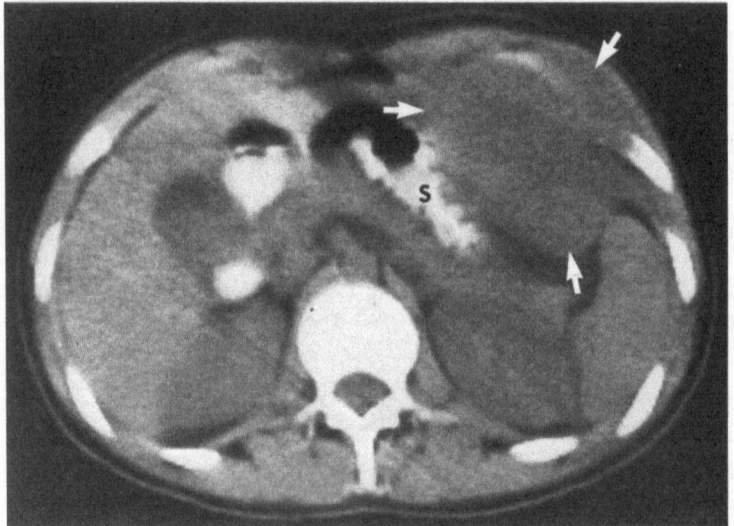

Fig. 17.3. A 16-year-old girl with rhabdomyosarcoma of the anterior abdominal wall (*arrows*). The scan shows the degree of extension of the mass externally and the greater extent of the mass internally, with displacement of the stomach (*s*).

Ascites

Sonography is very much more sensitive than both clinical examination and plain radiographs in the detection of ascites. We have used sonography with great success to evaluate children in whom small volumes of ascitic fluid are known to be present or are suspected within the peritoneal cavity. With this modality it is easy to determine whether fluid collections are loculated or free by scanning the patient in a number of different positions. The echo pattern of the ascitic fluid is nonspecific but occasionally it may be helpful in determining whether the fluid is an exudate rather than a transudate. Low-level echoes or linear strands within the fluid may indicate either infection, hemorrhage, or malignant disease. Occasionally, sonography may define the cause for the ascites, which may not be evident clinically. We have also used sonography with great success to localize fluid collections for drainage.

When the clinical, laboratory, and sonographic findings fail to determine the cause of ascites, abdominal CT may be helpful. However, we have used abdominal CT specifically for this purpose only on rare occasions. Small amounts of fluid within the peritoneal cavity are readily visualized on CT. The attenuation values of the fluid are usually low: 0–20 HU. However, it is difficult to determine the type of fluid present on the basis of the CT numbers alone. By scanning the patient in two different positions it is possible to determine whether the fluid is loculated or free. Unless loculated, the fluid accumulates in the dependent areas of the peritoneal cavity, which vary with the position of the patient.

Fluid starts to accumulate in the pelvis in the pouch of Douglas. In this situation the uterus will be delineated even in young children between the fluid-filled bladder anteriorly and the ascitic fluid posteriorly (see Fig. 15.2, p. 222). Fluid may also be found in the pararectal fossa and the anterior paravesical area, where it may mimic a mass adjacent to the bladder (Fig. 17.4).

In the abdomen, the fluid initially accumulates in the paracolic gutters and extends on the right up into Morrison's pouch between the liver and right kidney. With increasing volumes the fluid extends into the subphrenic spaces, around the whole liver and spleen, and then anterior to the small and large bowel, which become compressed into the central portion of the abdomen (Figs. 17.5, 17.6). Fluid anterior to the liver outlines the falciform ligament, which is clearly visualized as it passes to the liver from the anterior abdominal wall (Fig. 17.6). Small volumes of ascites may surround the gallbladder separating it from the liver and making the wall of the gallbladder easily visible (see Fig. 13.1, p. 198). With large collections, fluid is often seen in the lesser sac posterior to the stomach and anterior to the pancreatic body and tail, which may appear to be squashed posteriorly (Fig. 17.6).

When performing scans through the lower chest and upper abdomen it is occasionally very difficult to determine whether large fluid collections are indeed part of an ascites or part of a large pleural effusion that has caused inversion of the diaphragm. By following the adjacent superior and inferior scans it is usually possible to determine the location of the fluid collection. Pleural fluid may indeed by visualized lying lateral to the liver or spleen (Fig. 17.7). In the presence of ascites, the margins of the liver and spleen tend to remain sharp, but in the presence of a large pleural effusion the margins are more indistinct (Figs. 17.6, 17.7). Pleural fluid also tends to extend further medially than ascites and will be found to be lying between the vertebral column and the crus of the diaphragm, which will be displaced laterally. Fluid anterior to the crus is due to ascites.

Occasionally, the cause for the ascites will be evident on CT. For example, diffuse parenchymal liver disease and complications related to portal hypertension may be easily visualized. Our experience with two recent interesting children who presented with ascites are illustrated in Figs. 17.5 and 17.6.

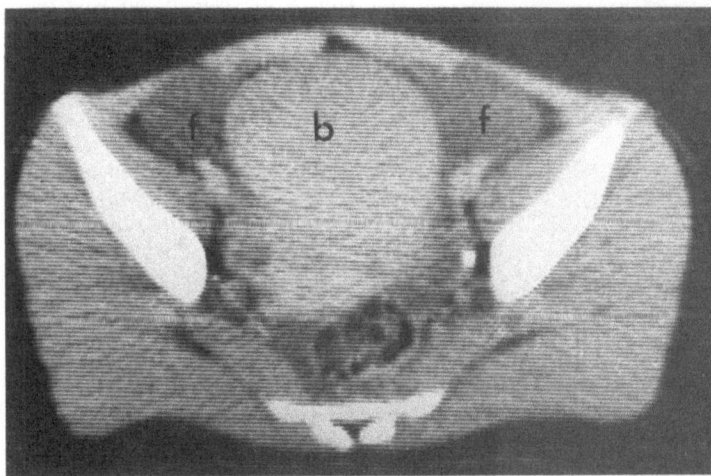

Fig. 17.4. CT in patient with ascites shows collections of fluid (*f*) on either side of the bladder (*b*). This fluid may masquerade as pelvic mass lesions.

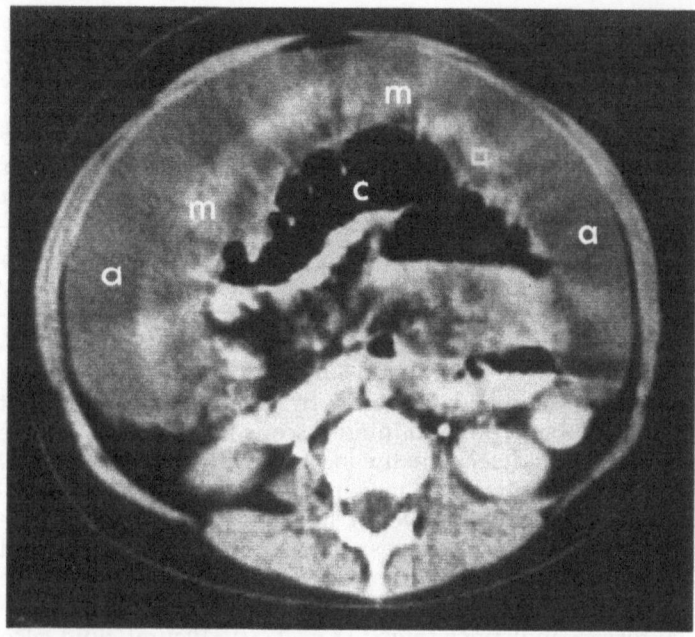

Fig. 17.5. A 15-year-old girl with ataxia telangiectasia who presented with ascites (*a*). CT shows areas of soft tissue attenuation in the region of the omentum (*m*) anterior to the transverse colon (*c*). These masses were found to be metastases from an adenocarcinoma. The origin of the adenocarcinoma was never documented.

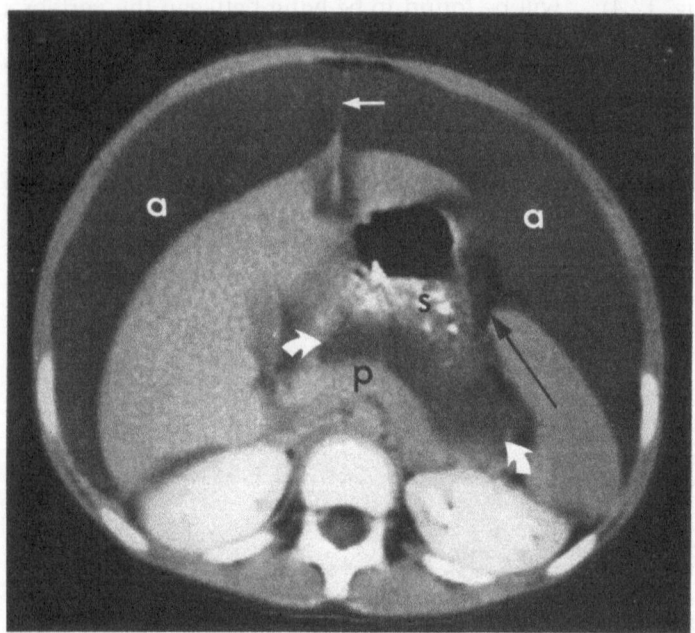

Fig. 17.6. A 12-year-old girl who presented with ascites (*a*). The fluid in the greater peritoneal sac outlines the ligamentum teres anteriorly (*white arrow*). Fluid is also noted in the lesser sac (*curved arrows*) between the stomach (*s*) anteriorly and the pancreas (*p*) posteriorly. Note the omental fat (*black arrow*) between the stomach and spleen contrasted against the ascitic fluid.

Omentum and Mesentery

Omental and mesenteric lesions are uncommon in children. The omental fat is usually not readily visualized, but in the presence of ascites the fat may be easily seen because of its lower attenuation than the adjacent fluid (see Fig. 17.6). However, CT is extremely useful in the definition and follow-up of children with mass lesions of these areas. Examples of such lesions are shown in Fig. 17.5 and Figs. 17.7–17.10. These lesions may be benign or malignant processes and include hemorrhages, hemangiomas, lymphangiomatosis, mesenteric cysts, and carcinomas.

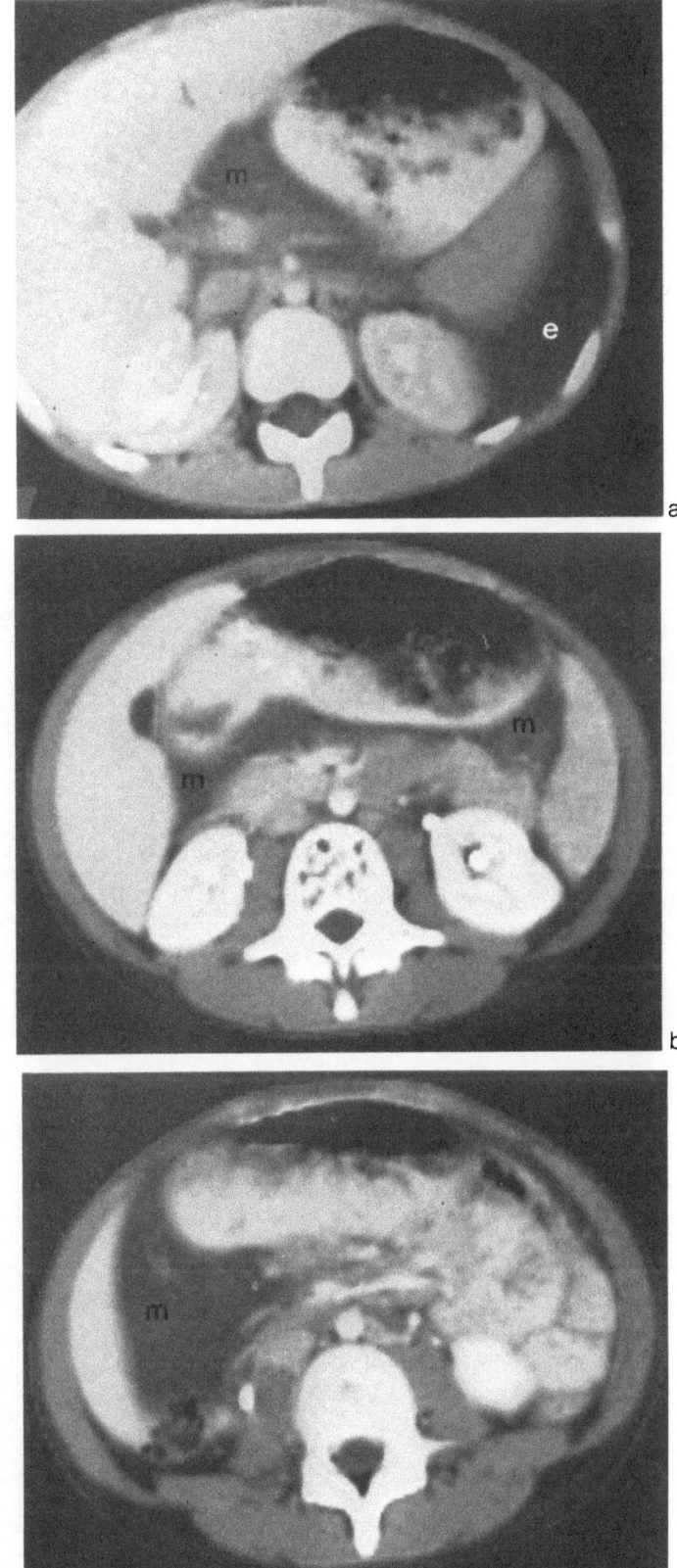

Fig. 17.7a–c. A 12-year-old girl who presented with respiratory distress. **a** Scan of the upper abdomen showed cause to be a large pleural effusion (*e*). All three scans show extensive areas of soft tissue attenuation (*m*) extending across the transverse mesocolon and into the omentum. These changes were all related to congenital lymphangiomatosis. Note the vertebral body involvement with the same pathological process in scan **b**.

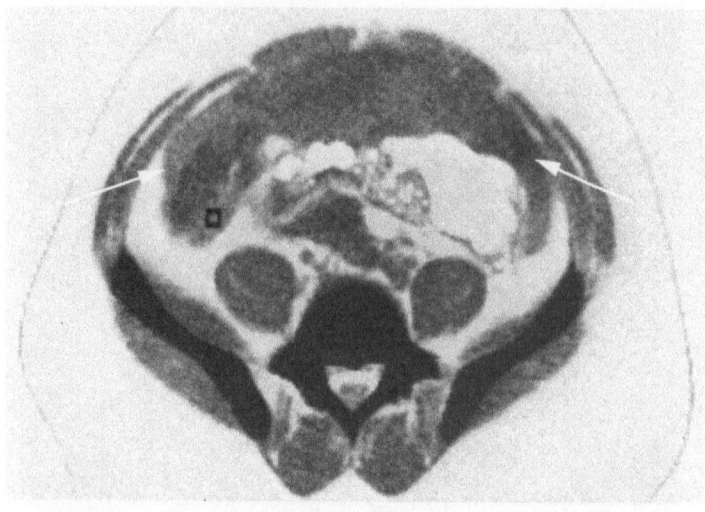

Fig. 17.8. A 12-year-old boy with hemophilia and a bleed into the omentum. This hemorrhage is seen as thickening of the omentum (*arrows*).

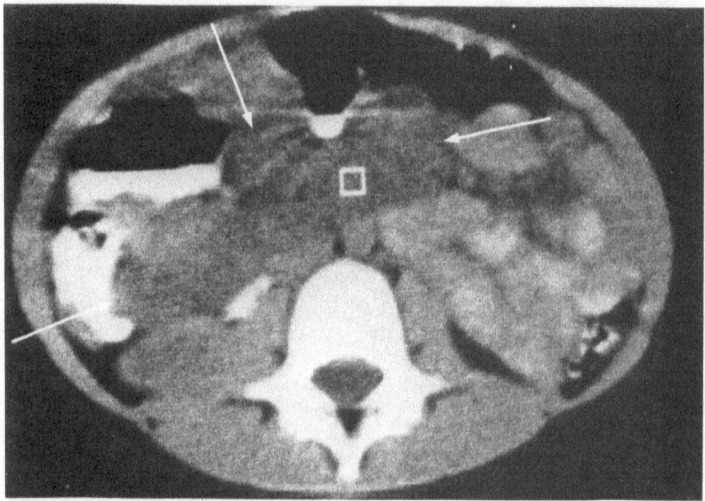

Fig. 17.9. An 8-year-old girl with a large retroperitoneal and mesenteric neurofibroma (*arrows*). CT shows the mass extending from the retroperitoneum anterior to the aorta and inferior vena cava up into the mesentery and displacing small and large bowel loops.

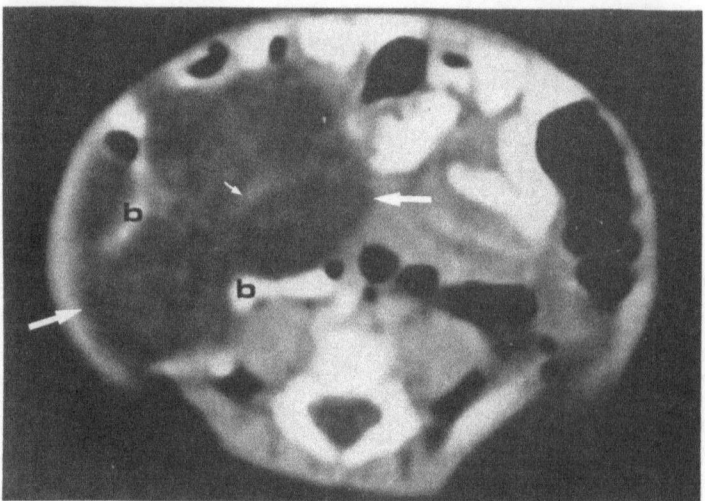

Fig. 17.10. A 3-week-old boy with a right flank mass. CT shows the large mass extending from the flank into the mesentery, up to the midline (*arrows*). The mass has a low attenuation and only shows enhancement in linear fashion in certain areas (*small arrow*) because of vascular septa in the mass. The CT shows the relationship of the mass to adjacent bowel loops (*b*), which have enhanced following the administration of dilute oral contrast material. This mass was a lymphangioma of the mesentery.

Gastrointestinal Tract

Barium studies and endoscopy remain the prime methods of evaluating the esophagus, stomach, and small and large intestines. These modalities define the internal surface of the gastrointestinal tract and provide indirect evidence regarding intramural and extrinsic abnormalities. CT can define the mucosa of the gastrointestinal tract in less detail, but the gastric rugae and the valvulae conniventes (see Fig. 8.3, p. 93), of the small bowel are often visualized. Larger mucosal lesions may well be visualized on CT. The major contribution of CT is in the evaluation of the wall of the gastrointestinal tract and adjacent structures, and in this regard CT may often reveal important information necessary for correct patient management.

In adults, the value of CT has been documented in a variety of gastrointestinal abnormalities [5, 8, 11]. These include mainly neoplastic and inflammatory processes. CT may also be useful in the delineation of the cause of gastrointestinal displacement as well as in the delineation of intussusception, obstruction, and hernias [5, 8].

In our pediatric experience we have rarely used CT to define a lesion of the gastrointestinal tract. However, CT has been useful in a few children with lesions involving the bowel wall. In this regard CT plays an important role in defining the degree of involvement as well as in the assessment of spread (Figs. 17.11, 17.12; see also Fig. 15.14, p. 234). CT has also been useful in the definition of lesions arising adjacent to the gastrointestinal tract and thought to be invading it (Fig. 17.10).

It has been mentioned previously that fluid-filled bowel loops may masquerade as soft tissue masses on CT (see Fig. 7.2, p. 87, and Fig. 7.3, p. 88). Furthermore, scans performed during or just after intravenous contrast administration show enhancement of the bowel wall surrounding the intraluminal fluid (see Fig. 15.10, p. 232). Occasionally, this appearance may simulate abscess formation. These pitfalls apply particularly to the small bowel. It is for these reasons that the administration of oral contrast material is mandatory prior to the vast majority of abdominal CT studies. Large bowel is usually filled with formed or semiformed stool mixed with air and less commonly simulates masses and abscesses. Rectally administered contrast is thus less commonly required to differentiate colon from mass lesion.

Small bowel contents, apart from bowel gas, usually have an attenuation slightly higher than water. However, colonic and gastric contents often have a much higher attenuation. Indeed, we have not uncommonly found material of extremely high attenuation within the stomach of children who have not received oral contrast (see Fig. 14.3, p. 212). This high-attenuation material is due to normal dietary intake and should not be mistaken for unusual ingested foreign material or fresh blood within the stomach.

Conjoined Twins

The term "conjoined twins" denotes twins that are physically connected to each other. This connection varies and ranges from a superficial connection of connective tissue to a significant sharing of major internal structures. The degree to which major organs are shared is the deciding factor in determining the operability of a set of twins.

The overall incidence of conjoined twins stillborn or alive has been estimated at 1 in 50 000–60 000 births [12]. The incidence of conjoined twins amenable to surgical separation has been estimated at five to six per year worldwide by Aird [1].

Conjoined twins are classified by combining the anatomical area of union with the Greek work *pagos* (that which is fixed) — hence the anatomical descriptions of thoracopagus, xiphopagus, and omphalopagus. These three types account for approximately 73% of conjoined twins. A further 19% are joined posteriorly buttock to buttock (pygopagus) and 6% are joined side by side at the hip (ischiopagus). Craniopagus is the rarest at 2% [3,13].

The ischiopagus types can be further subdivided according to the number of lower extremities present. Of these the most common is the ischiopagus tripus, with one normal lower extremity possessed by each twin and a third, often malformed or vestigial, limb shared by both from a rudimentary acetabulum formed at the point of fusion of the bony pelvis. Tetrapus and bipus types make up the remainder of this subcategory [3].

Thoracopagus twins have a high incidence of associated cardiac defects. Of these twins, 75% have conjoined hearts and 90% have a common

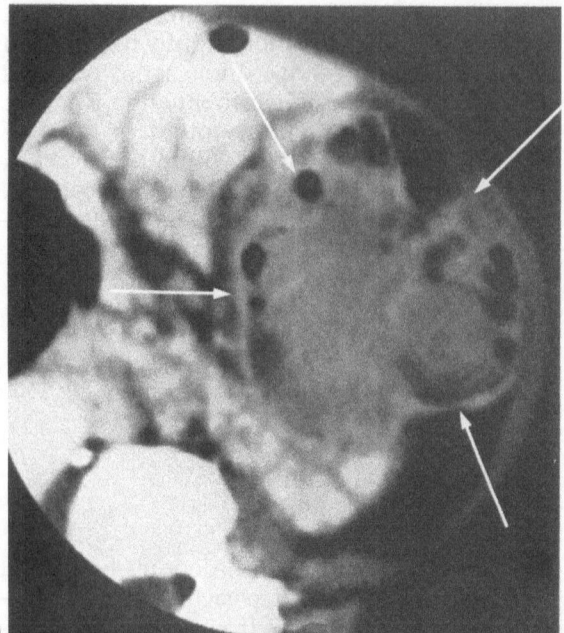

a

Fig. 17.11a–c. Examples of the value of CT in gastrointestinal mass lesions. **a** A 12-year-old girl with a left upper quadrant mass (*arrows*). This mass is shown to be arising in bowel and projecting into the lumen of the bowel. The mass is surrounded by bubbles of air in the lumen of the bowel and was found to be a carcinoid tumor. CT excluded local spread and metastasis at the time of diagnosis. **b,c** A 10-year-old boy with 1 month's history of vomiting and weight loss. CT shows a large mass (*arrows*) in the right upper quadrant and flank. Note the concentric circles of varying attenuation in the mass, particularly in scan **c**. The stomach (*S*) is filled with Gastrografin and air. Note the relationship of the stomach to the mass in **b**, as indicated by the *long arrow*. This represents the site of an intussusception originating in the gastric antrum and passing distally into the jejunum. It shows how the stomach becomes incorporated into the central portion of the mass in **b** and the concentric circular pattern of the intussusception (noted in **c**). At operation there was marked thickening of the muscle of the antrum, duodenum, and jejunum from the chronic intussusception. The lead point was a hamartoma in the gastric antrum. There was no history of polyps elsewhere in the bowel or a family history or clinical findings to suggest a clinical syndrome.

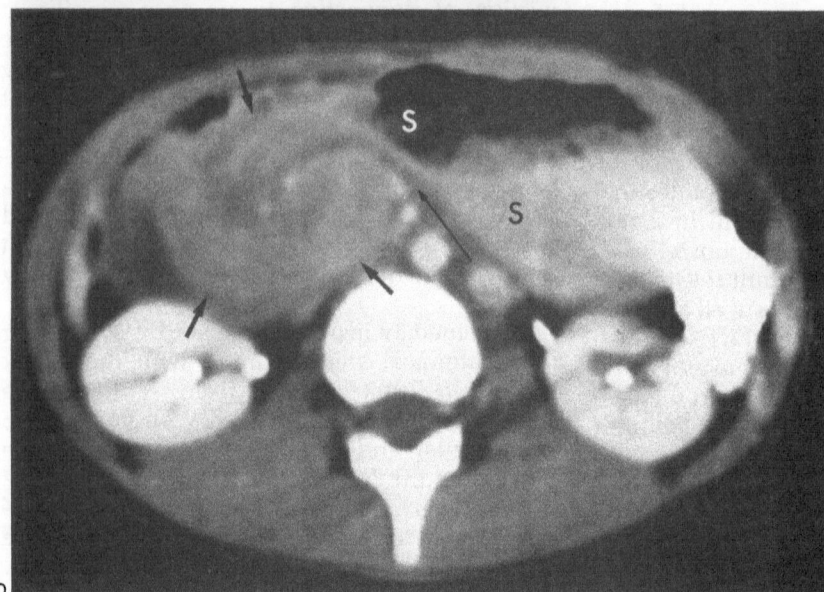

b   **Fig. 17.11c** (*opposite*) ▶

pericardium [10]. The operability of these twins is determined by the degree to which these major structures are shared. A classification has been proposed by Izukawa and his colleagues [6] to assess the cardiac findings and to place these twins into one of three classes:

Class A — pericardial union only

Class B — atrial connection but ventricular separation

Class C — ventricular connection, usually associated with multiple cardiac defects

The hearts of Class A twins are frequently normal, while those of Class C are associated with significant defects. Although one case of successful separation of Class B thoracopagus twins joined at the right atria has been recently described [14], there have been no reported cases of successful separation of twins of the Class C type.

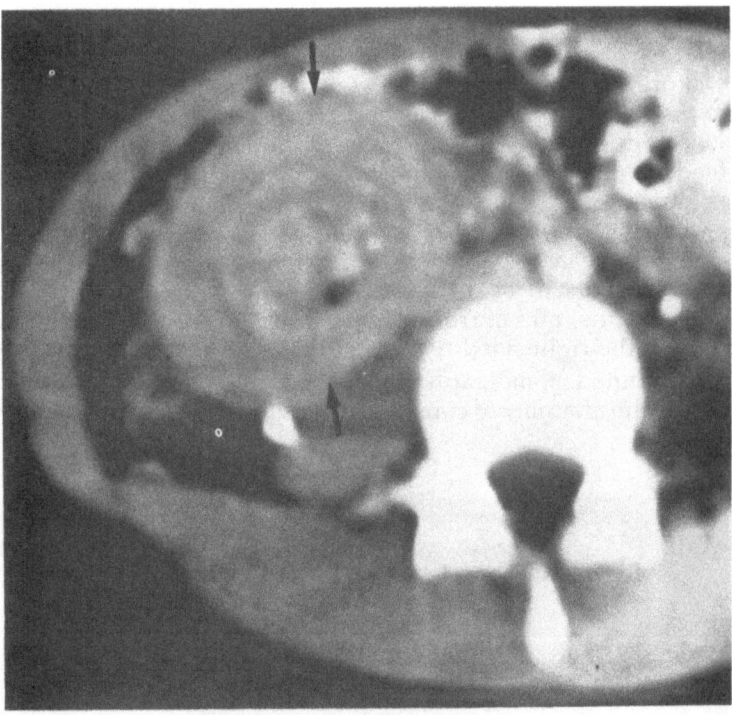

Fig. 17.11c

The internal anatomy of ischiopagus and omphalopagus twins is quite variable and depends on the degree of joining. A bridge of liver tissue is common in twins joined across the upper abdomen. The upper gastrointestinal tracts are usually normal with the distal small bowels joined to form one terminal ileum. A single colon often terminates in a single anal orifice. Each twin commonly has at least one kidney and one bladder supplied by the ureter from that respective twin. The urethrae are ordinarily separate. Septate vaginas, bicornate uteri, or cloacal problems are not uncommon. The bony pelvis is often formed by the fusion of each twin's open "C"-shaped pelvis with that of the other to form a common pelvic ring. The lower extremities often lie at right angles to the body axis. The major abdominal arterial trunks

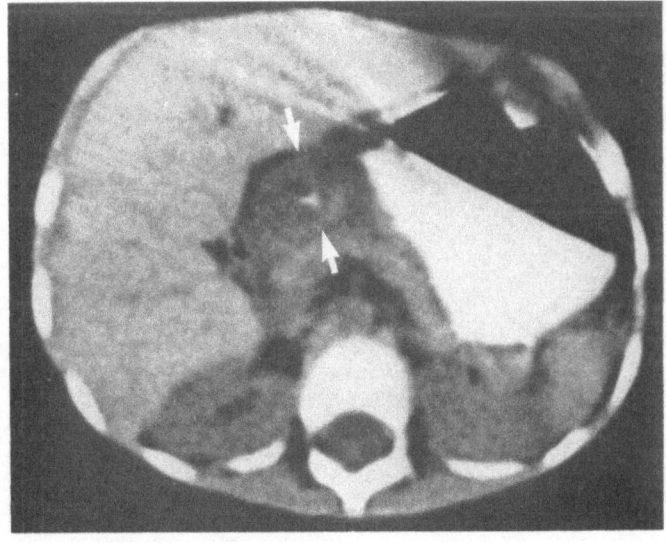

Fig. 17.12. A 4-year-old boy with chronic granulomatous disease and vomiting. CT scan performed to follow-up the size of previously documented liver abscesses shows at this time marked thickening of the gastric antrum (*arrows*). A small fleck of dilute water-soluble contrast is noted in the lumen of the antrum, which is markedly compressed by the thickened antral walls as a result of chronic granulomatous disease.

are usually the same as in a normal baby [9]. In the case of an ischiopagus tripus twin, one twin will provide the majority of the vascular supply to the third leg [9]. This fact becomes important when deciding which twin will receive a skin flap made from the third leg and assessing possible postoperative viability of this flap. The formation and viability of a skin flap is often crucial when covering the large postoperative abdominal wall defects. Situs inversus occurs in 73% of conjoined twins, and mirror imaging is more common in the right-sided twin [2].

Computed tomography has been used to assess the anatomy of conjoined twins [4, 7, 14].

We have had the opportunity to study three sets of conjoined twins [15]. All three were studied with dynamic CT scans. These studies provided valuable information which helped determine management. In an example of thoracopagus, dynamic CT delineated fused ventricles with a common atrial canal. This finding confirmed the inoperability of these twins. The other two sets we studied were examples of omphalo-ischiopagus. In one set, four lower limbs were present, and in the other, three (Fig. 17.13). Imaging modalities are exceedingly important in defining three groups of problems in this type of conjoined twin:

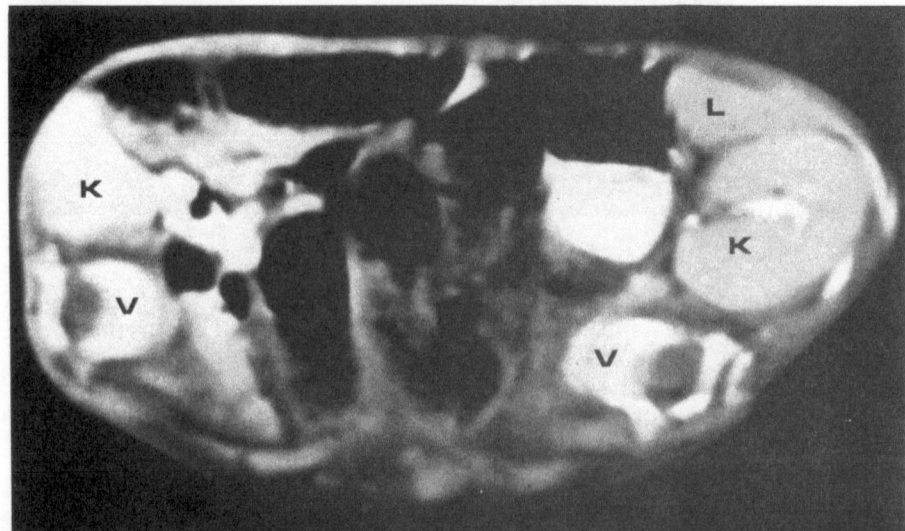

Fig. 17.13a

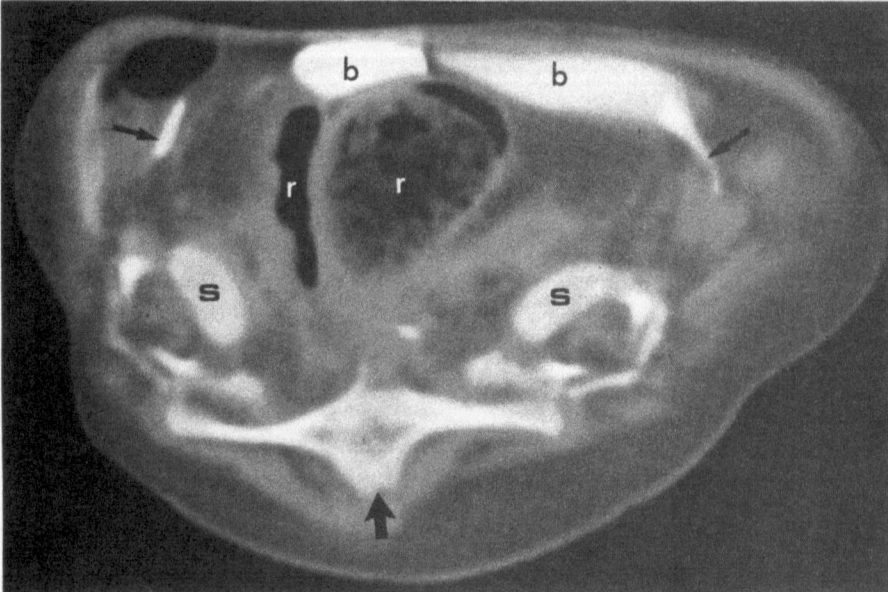

Fig. 17. 13b

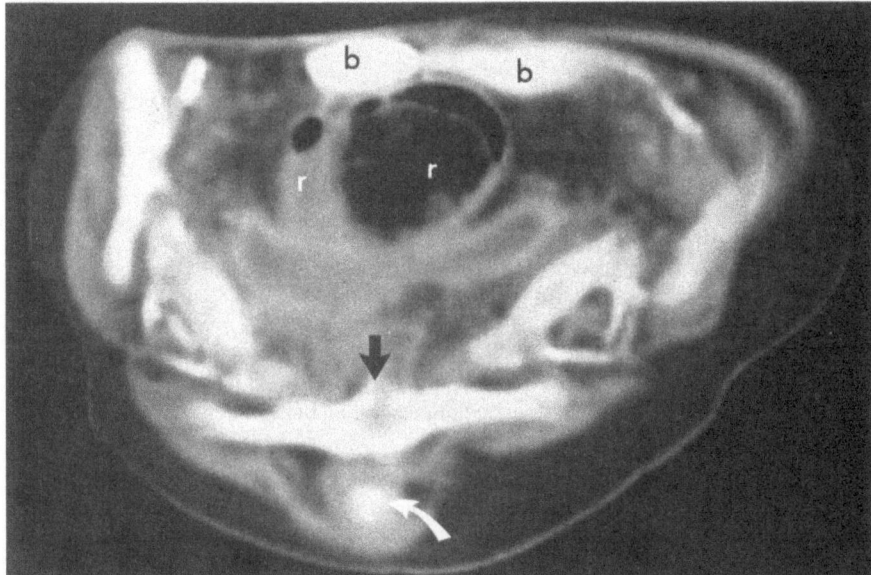

Fig. 17.13c

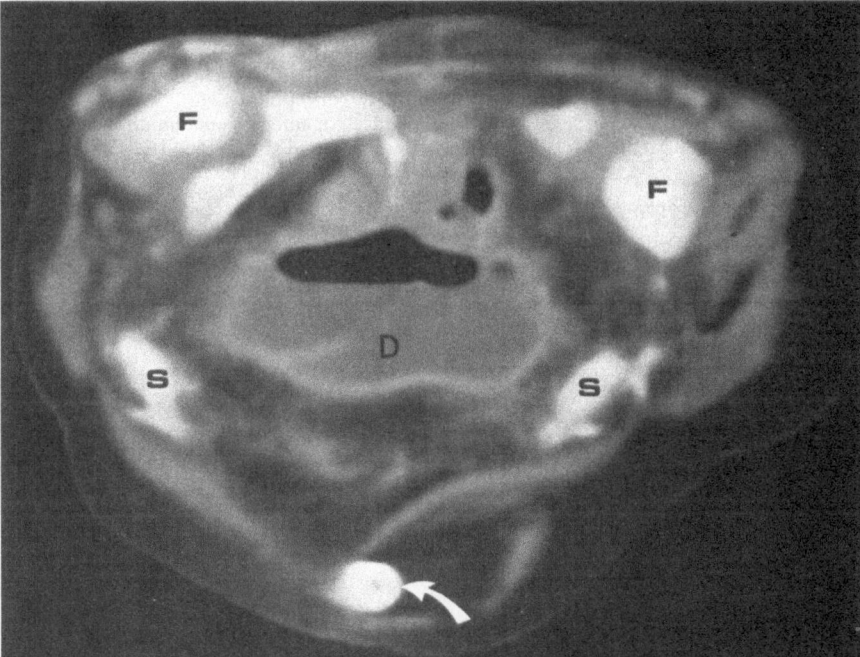

Fig. 17.13d

Fig. 17.13a–d. Examples of the value of CT in conjoined twins. The twins were 2½ years old and were joined at the pelvis (ischiopagus tripus). **a** Scan through the upper abdomen shows the two separate vertebral columns (*V*) and one kidney (*K*) anterior to each vertebra. *L*, part of transverse liver. The kidney on the left of the image was perfused sooner than the kidney on the right because the injection of contrast was made into a foot of the ipsilateral twin and perfusion to the opposite side was slower. The number, site, and anatomical configuration of the kidneys was not adequately delineated by other modalities because of the position of the kidneys relative to the vertebral columns and the large amount of bowel gas, as well as the presence of bladder duplication. **b, c, d** Scans through the pelvis show each sacrum (*S*) and fusion of the adjacent iliac wings posteriorly (*large black arrow*). The ureters (*small black arrows*) are noted passing toward the bladder, which is duplicated (*b*). The rectum (*r*) also shows duplication, with a large posterior duplication-type cyst (*D*) with an air-fluid level noted in image **d**. The femoral heads (*F*) of the two normal lower extremities are noted anterolaterally, and the third vestigial limb is noted posteriorly (*curved white arrow*). The anatomical relationships, particularly in the pelvis, were best defined with CT and provided essential preoperative information for the attention of general, urological, and orthopedic surgeons. Angiography was deemed unnecessary. The twins have been successfully separated and each has only one limb. The skin from the third limb was used to cover the abdomen on one of the twins.

1. Skeletal fusion. The transverse axial scans provided by CT delineate the relationships of the musculoskeletal system of the lower spine, pelvis, and hips without overlap. CT is the study of choice for the delineation of these areas as the overlapping structures are difficult to evaluate with conventional radiography. In the neonatal period, however, poor ossification of the skeleton makes interpretation somewhat difficult at times.

2. Visceral fusion. Dynamic CT proved much more helpful than renal radionuclide studies or excretory urography in the assessment of the kidneys, major vessels, the retroperitoneum and pelvis, and also in delineating the relationships between duplicated organ systems and a dermoid cyst in one set. Delineation of the vascular supply to a vestigial limb is extremely useful prior to surgery, as described above. However, CT proved limited in its ability to define the exact anatomy of the liver and the number of spleens present, as examination of the upper abdomen was made difficult because of the abundant bowel gas and respiratory motion artifacts in both sets of twins. In this regard, radionuclide sulfur colloid liver/spleen scans were indispensable.

3. Fusion of the distal genitourinary systems and anorectal malformations are common in these type of twins. CT plays little role in the delineation of the anatomy of this particular area. In this regard cystourethrograms, vaginograms, and loopograms are vitally important.

In summary, CT is extremely useful in the evaluation of the musculoskeletal and visceral anatomy in conjoined twins. Dynamic scans help to delineate the sites of the major vessels and to assess the amount of cross-flow between the two twins. These findings preclude the need for further more invasive procedures such as angiography. However, the limitations of CT in the areas described above demand that the CT findings be correlated with the results of other imaging modalities that are used specifically to delineate the liver and spleen and the distal genitourinary and gastrointestinal tracts.

References

1. Aird I (1959) Conjoined twins: further observation. Br Med J I:1313–1315
2. Cywes S, Block C (1964) Conjoined twins, a review with a report of a case. S Afr Med J 38:817–821
3. Eades J, Thomas C (1966) Successful separation of ischiopagus tetrapus conjoined twins. Ann Surg 164:1059–1072
4. Halwa S, Wojtowics J, Gradzki J, Wojciechowski K, Solawa M (1979) Computed tomography in preoperative diagnosis of conjoined twins. J Comput Assist Tomogr 3(3):411–412
5. Iko BO, Teal JS, Siram SM, Chinwuba CE, Roux VJ, Scott VF (1984) Computed tomography of adult colonic intussusception: clinical and experimental studies. AJR 143:769–772
6. Izukawa T, Kidd B, Moes C, Tyrrell M, Ives E, Simpson J, Shandling B (1978) Assessment of the cardiovascular system in conjoined thoracopagus twins. Am J Dis Child 132:19–24
7. Kelekis L, Kelekis D, Mameletzis K, Kelemouridis B, Artopoulos J (1980) Thoracopagus twins studied with computed tomography. J Comput Assist Tomogr 4(3):405–406
8. Mauro MA, Koehler RE (1983) Alimentary tract. In: Lee JKT, Sagel SS, Stanley RJ (eds) Computed body tomography. Raven, New York, pp 307–340
9. Muller T (1970) Ischiopagus: an anatomical study of two cases, tripus and tetrapus. S Afr Med J 44:136–147
10. Nichols B, Blattner R, Rudolph A (1967) General clinical management of thoracopagus conjoined twins. Birth Defects 3:38–51
11. Plojoux O, Hauser H, Wettstein P (1982) Computed tomography of intramural hematoma of the small intestine. Radiology 144:559–561
12. Potter E (1961) Pathology of the fetus and the infant. In: Medical year book, vol 2. Year Book Medical Publishers, Chicago, pp 203–233
13. Robertson EG (1953) Craniopagus parietalis — report of a case. Arch Neurol Psychiatry 70:189–205
14. Rossi P, Cozzi F, Iannaccone G (1981) CT for assessing feasibility of separation of thoracopagus twins. J Comput Assist Tomogr 5(4):574–576
15. Ward K, Daneman A, Stringer DA (1985) Conjoined twins: the value of dynamic CT. (submitted for publication)

Section IV:

NECK

Chapter 18

Technique and Anatomy

Introduction

CT is used far less frequently for evaluation of the neck than for evaluation of the chest, abdomen and pelvis, or musculoskeletal system. At the Hospital for Sick Children, Toronto, the two commonest indications for evaluation of the neck with CT are the investigation of laryngeal abnormalities and for the delineation of neck masses. These topics are discussed in detail in Chapters 19 and 20 respectively.

Technique

The general principles of CT technique, as outlined in Chapter 2, apply to the technique of neck CT just as they do to the remainder of the body. However, because many of the patients being studied have laryngeal abnormalities, and because others have neck masses that may impinge on the airway or spinal canal, certain facets of our technique are worth stressing [2].

Sedation and Airway Control

Many of the patients (with laryngeal lesions in particular) are young and require sedation. The decision to sedate a child with respiratory distress is made only after adequate consultation with the clinicians caring for the patient. The following guidelines should be observed:

Patients under 2 months of age are scanned after they have fallen asleep after being bottle fed.

Older patients who are uncooperative receive a maximum of 6 mg of Nembutal/kg intramuscularly.

If it is felt that sedation may make the child a greater respiratory risk, an anesthetist is requested to stand by during the examination in case intubation is required.

In those children who are already intubated the anesthetist can be instructed when to withhold ventilation during the time of scanning.

Meticulous tracheostomy care is imperative in those children with tracheostomies who are sedated. A nurse knowledgeable in techniques of tracheostomy toilet is a valuable member of the team for this procedure.

Scan Technique

The child is best positioned with the neck fully extended. To achieve this a pillow or sponge should be placed under the shoulders and the head allowed to fall back gently. In babies it is sufficient to place a rolled-up diaper under the shoulders. If this is uncomfortable for the patient or interferes with respiration or sedation, a less extended position may have to be accepted.

A lateral scout radiograph of the neck in extension is then obtained (Fig. 18.1). This radiograph enables one to delineate valuable landmarks in the neck such as the vertebrae, mandible, hyoid bone, epiglottis, vocal cords, and airway. One can then accurately choose the limits of the transverse axial scans from this scout radiograph. In smaller children, and particularly for lesions of the larynx, 5-mm thick adjacent scans are obtained through the area of interest with a scan time of 2 s. In much larger patients with large masses 1-cm thick adjacent scans may be satisfactory. The axial scans are performed during quiet respiration, as the vast majority of patients are sedated. Those who are cooperative should be studied during inspiration. Scans should be viewed at several window settings to enable one to assess the soft tissues and bony and cartilagenous elements. The lines of the transverse scans that show the limits of the lesion can then be posted on the scout radiograph, and this enables one to appreciate the limits of a lesion with respect to the previously mentioned easily visible landmarks. Coronal reconstruction is extremely useful in those patients in whom an abnormality of the larynx is noted on the axial scan.

Intravenous contrast injection is only used if a mass lesion is present or suspected but is unnecessary for the examination of intrinsic laryngeal abnormalities. The injection of intra-thecal metrizamide prior to the study is extremely valuable if a mass lesion with suspected intraspinal extension is being evaluated.

In using these techniques, particularly with regard to the meticulous attention to sedation care and airway control, we have had no respiratory complications in any of the children we have studied. Excellent CT scans were obtained in all but three examinations where poor quality was caused by respiratory motion because of the patients' respiratory distress. In these few instances CT was not able to provide much help.

Anatomy

The reader is referred to figures in Chapters 19 and 20 for appearances of normal cervical anatomy.

Posterior

Posteriorly the vertebral column forms a valuable landmark in all scans of the neck. Posterolateral to the vertebrae is the musculature of the erector spinae muscles. A detailed anatomical knowledge of the various posterolateral

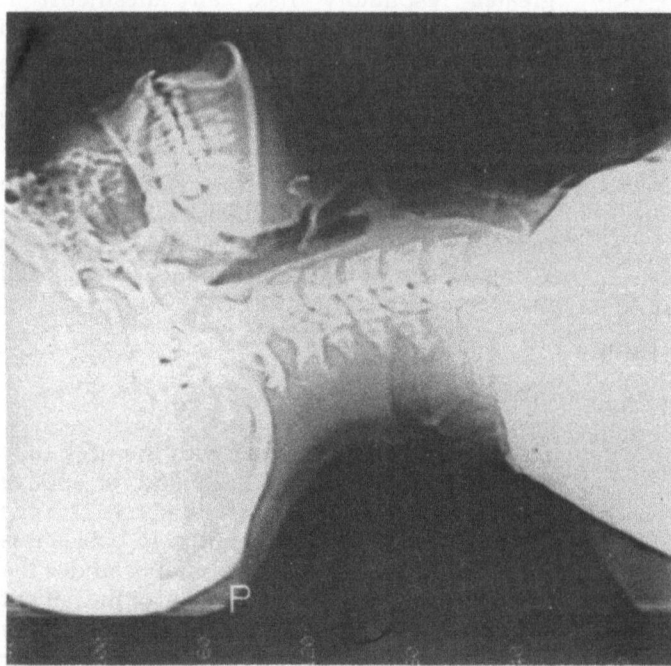

Fig. 18.1. Lateral computed radiograph of the neck. Note extension of neck with pillow under shoulders. The vertebrae, mandible, hyoid bone, epiglottis, vocal cords, and airway serve as valuable landmarks. These enable one to choose accurately the limits of the transverse axial scans one wishes to perform. Posting the lines of the transverse scans on this radiograph enables one to appreciate the limits of a lesion with respect to these easily visible landmarks.

muscle groups is unnecessary. However, it is useful to have the patient lying straight in the gantry, so that the symmetry of the muscles on either side of the midline can be evaluated and abnormalities easily detected. In the lower portions of the neck the trapezius muscle can be seen posterolaterally. The commonest abnormalities evaluated in this area are mass lesions (see Fig. 20.2, p. 297, and Fig. 20.3, p. 298). Masses involve this area less commonly than the anterior and lateral aspects of the neck.

Anterior

The anatomy anterior to the vertebral column is much more complex, and a thorough understanding of this area is required in order to evaluate abnormalities adequately [3, 4].

Suprahyoid

Superiorly the mandible and hyoid bone serve as useful landmarks. Both are well ossified in the newborn and are therefore easily visualized at all ages. The body of the hyoid is seen in the midline with the greater cornua extending posterolaterally, forming a semicircular arch. The muscles of the floor of the mouth pass anteriorly from the hyoid to the mandible. Anterolateral and a little superior to the hyoid lie the submandibular glands. Posterior to the hyoid lies the upper airway and in this region the valleculae, base of tongue, epiglottis, and pyriform sinuses may be seen (see Fig. 20.9, p. 303). Lateral to the hyoid lie the internal and external carotid arteries and the internal jugular vein posterolaterally. The sternocleidomastoid muscle extends from the region of the sternoclavicular joint to the mastoid. It is therefore a constant landmark in all scans of the neck. Superiorly it lies laterally as it approaches the mastoids (see Fig. 20.2, p. 297, and Fig. 20.7, p. 301).

Infrahyoid

In the infrahyoid part of the neck the sternocleidomastoid muscle comes to lie progressively more anteriorly as it passes inferiorly. It is an important landmark as it marks the anterior border of the posterior triangle and the posterolateral boundary of the anterior triangles (see Fig. 20.1, p. 294, Fig. 20.7, p. 301, and Fig.

20.9, p. 303). The external jugular vein is seen lying on the superficial surface of the muscle (see Fig. 20.1, p. 294). The muscles lying in the anterior aspect of the vertebral bodies are the paired longus colli muscles. In the lower portions of the neck the scaleni lie on either side of the vertebral bodies.

The thyroid cartilage forms a useful landmark below the hyoid. In children, however, it is poorly calcified, particularly in infants (see Fig. 19.3, p. 288, and Fig. 19.4, p. 289). Nevertheless, its characteristic shape, which is an arch-like structure resembling a triangle without a base, can certainly be recognized. Within the arch lies the laryngeal vestibule with the pyriform sinuses on either side (see Fig. 20.9, p. 303). Posteriorly lies the esophagus. Lateral to the thyroid cartilage are the structures in the carotid sheath (the carotid artery medially and the internal jugular vein laterally). Anterior to the thyroid cartilage lie the strap muscles of the neck together with the anterior jugular veins. The shape of the airway in the region of the lower part of the thyroid cartilage is somewhat elliptical, with the long axis in the anteroposterior direction. This shape is due to the presence of the vocal cords at this level.

Inferiorly to the thyroid lies the cricoid cartilage, which forms a complete circle. This too is poorly calcified in children, but its circular shape can usually be well appreciated.

Below the level of the cricoid the extrathoracic segment of the trachea is seen. This has a somewhat horseshoe shape with the straighter surface of the membranous part of the trachea directed posteriorly. Occasionally, in scans performed during deep inspiration the trachea may have a more rounded appearance. The individual tracheal cartilages are not visualized. The esophagus lies behind the trachea anterior to the vertebral bodies (see Fig. 20.1, p. 294, and Fig. 20.4, p. 299). Occasionally, it may appear to indent the membranous part of the trachea. The esophagus usually appears as a rounded soft tissue density with a central lucency and occasionally may have a figure of eight appearance if the lumen is collapsed centrally. In children, air may often be present within the lumen of the esophagus normally and is easily visualized behind the trachea. Occasionally, the esophagus is positioned off the midline slightly toward the left.

In the lower part of the neck the thyroid gland can be easily seen. The thyroid lobes have a pyramidal shape in cross section and lie lateral to the trachea (see Fig. 20.1, p. 294, and Fig. 20.6,

p. 301). Often the isthmus of the gland may be identified anterior to the trachea joining the two lobes (see Fig. 20.1a, p. 294). The isthmus lies between the trachea and the anterior strap muscles over which the anterior jugular veins course. In children, the normal thyroid gland contains sufficient iodine so that the attenuation values are extremely high. Indeed, the normal thyroid appears to be enhanced even when no intravenous contrast has been administered. In 1983, Iida et al. [1] measured the attenuation values in adult thyroids. They found that the attenuation values in normal controls were significantly higher than in patients with diseased thyroids. In children the normal attenuation values of the thyroid are between 100 and 120 HU. We have seen decreases in thyroid attenuation values in both diffuse and focal thyroid disease (see Fig. 20.1, p. 294).

Posterolateral to the thyroid lobes lie the common carotid artery medially and the internal jugular vein laterally (see Fig. 20.1, p. 294, and Fig. 20.9, p. 303). The jugular veins are frequently asymmetrical; indeed, one may be twice as large as the opposite vein. In unenhanced scans these structures may masquerade as lymph nodes. In the lower portions of the neck the vertebral arteries are noted to be positioned outside the foramina transversaria lying between the vertebral bodies and the scalene muscles. In the lower neck the sternocleidomastoid muscles lie medially compared with higher levels, and the scalene and trapezius muscles show a much larger mass.

In children, the paucity of fat in the neck makes delineation of soft tissue structures difficult in scans without intravenous contrast administration. However, certain anatomical landmarks are usually easily visualized and help in the orientation of the scans. These useful anatomical landmarks include the well-ossified hyoid bone, the epiglottis, the airway, the normal shape of the poorly calcified thyroid and cricoid cartilages, and the thyroid gland with its normal high attenuation. In scans designed to assess the airway intravenous contrast is usually not necessary. However, scans performed during bolus injection of intravenous contrast material are desirable for accurate localization and determination of the extent and character of cervical masses. These type of scans are extremely useful for determining the correct management of individual patients. However, the paucity of fat still makes the delineation of normal lymph node chains and nerves in children extremely difficult.

References

1. Iida Y, Konishi J, Harioka T, Misaki T, Endo K, Torizuka K (1983) Thyroid CT number and its relationship to iodine concentration. Radiology 147:793–795
2. Liu P, Daneman A (1984) Computed tomography of intrinsic laryngeal and tracheal abnormalities in children. J Comput Assist Tomogr 8(4):662–669
3. Mancuso AA, Harnsberger HR, Muraki AS, Stevens MH (1983) Computed tomography of cervical and retropharyngeal lymph nodes: normal anatomy, variants of normal, and applications in staging head and neck cancer. Radiology 148:709–714
4. Reede DL, Whelan MA, Bergeron RT (1982) Computed tomography of the infrahyoid neck. Radiology 145:389–395

Chapter 19

Larynx

Introduction

In children with suspected pathology of the larynx, plain radiographs in the frontal and lateral projections are essential and invaluable. While plain film findings may not be specific they often give sufficient information to allow the correct treatment to be instituted. However, when these studies are nondiagnostic or the findings are unusual in appearance or equivocal, other imaging methods are indicated. Fluoroscopy with spot films is useful, particularly if positioning of the child's head is difficult. Barium swallow is useful to rule out the presence of esophageal foreign bodies as the cause for respiratory distress and also to delineate the posterior pharyngeal wall. More recently high kilovoltage techniques, magnification views, and digital radiography have been used to demonstrate the details of the larynx in greater detail [4]. Positive contrast laryngography is contraindicated in patients with respiratory distress and is difficult to perform in pediatric patients.

The use of CT in the evaluation of adult patients with laryngeal carcinoma and trauma has been well documented [1, 2, 6, 8, 9, 10]. However, use of CT in the evaluation of intrinsic abnormalities of the larynx in children has not been previously assessed. We have used CT in patients with respiratory distress who were suspected of having laryngeal lesions in an attempt to learn three things:

1. Could CT provide enough information in some patients to obviate the necessity for more invasive endoscopy with its attendant risks?
2. Could CT provide extra information that could not be obtained by endoscopy?
3. Could CT provide useful information prior to endoscopy?

During the 3-year period 1981–1983, inclusive, 34 children underwent CT of the larynx at the Hospital for Sick Children, Toronto. In 1984, Liu and Daneman reviewed the clinical, plain radiographic, computed tomographic, and endoscopic findings in these children [7]. This study has proved the value of CT in the assessment of intrinsic laryngeal abnormalities.

Case Material

Of the 34 patients with respiratory distress with suspected or known laryngeal lesions there were 22 males and 12 females, and the age at the time of examination ranged from 10 days to 17.5 years. We divided these patients into four groups depending on whether there had been previous intubation or not and whether there was a previously documented subglottic stenosis.

In the first group of 12 patients (age range 10 days to 3 years) there was no previous history of intubation. Of importance is the fact that in seven of these patients the CT findings of an adequate caliber larynx provided adequate information for the clinician and thus obviated the necessity for endoscopy. Another patient in this group was a child with chondrodysplasia punctata in whom CT showed a minor degree of asymmetry and narrowing of the subglottic area with some calcification in the wall of the larynx (Fig. 19.1).

The next group of nine patients (age range 6 weeks to 16 years) had previous prolonged intubation during the neonatal period for respiratory distress. CT revealed a normal larynx in two, minor narrowing in six and was nondiagnostic in one because of the tracheal tug related to the severe respiratory distress. In three patients in whom there was minor narrowing, the CT findings obviated the necessity for endoscopy. In the other three with more marked narrowing CT provided extremely important information which facilitated endoscopy. In two of these the narrowing was in the form of a subglottic web (Fig. 19.2), and in one of these two a further supraglottic web causing fusion of the aryepiglottic folds was noted (Fig. 19.3). In a third the subglottic region was almost completely obliterated.

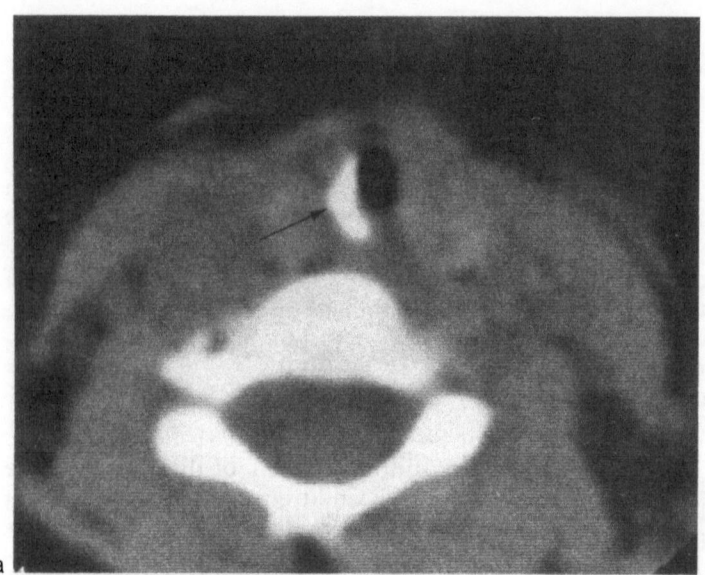

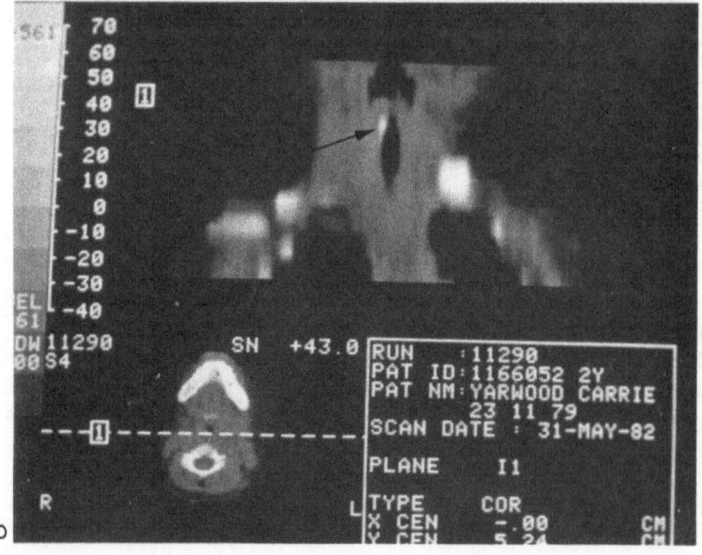

Fig. 19.1a,b. A 3-year-old girl with chondrodysplasia punctata. Axial scan (**a**) and coronal reformatted image (**b**) demonstrate crescentic calcification (*arrow*) adjacent to segment of mild congenital subglottic stenosis. (Liu and Daneman 1984 [7])

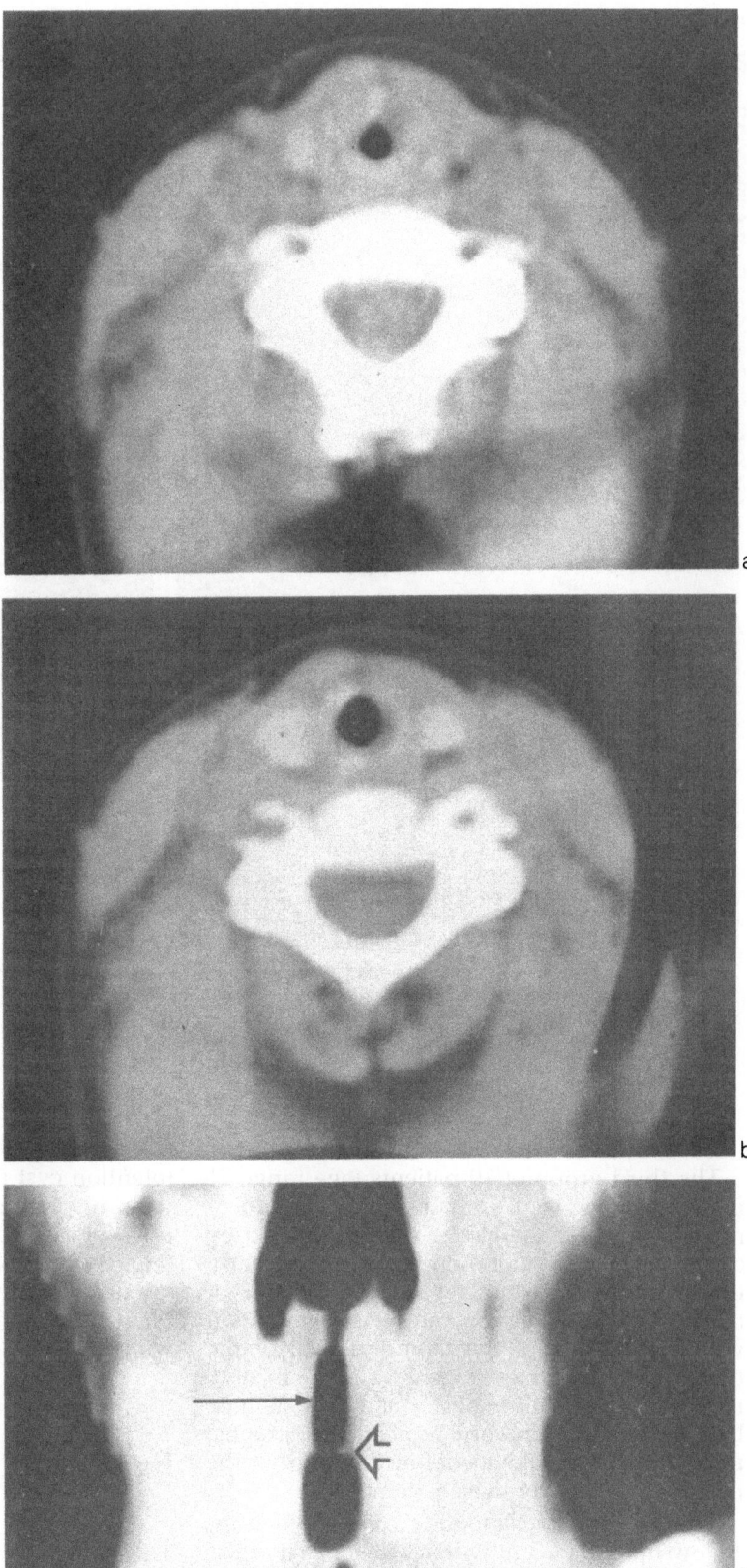

Fig. 19.2a–c. A 12-year-old boy with a past history of laryngeal intubation. Axial scans show laryngeal lumen to be rounded in shape because of subglottic stenosis (**a** and **b**). Coronal reformatted image (**c**) confirms subglottic narrowing (*arrow*). At the lower limit of this narrowing a membrane is noted (*open arrow*). This was confirmed endoscopically. (Liu and Daneman 1984 [7])

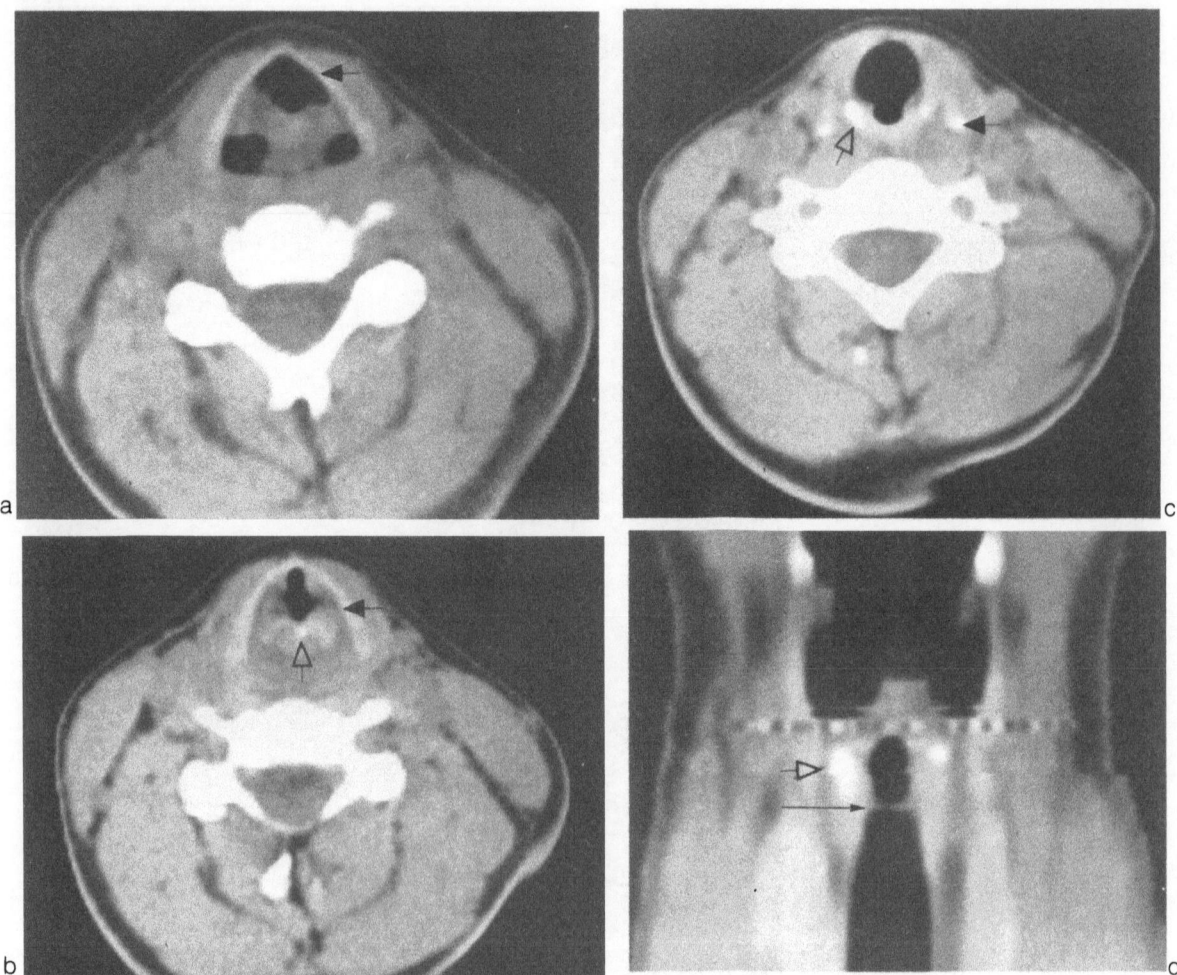

Fig. 19.3a–d. A 17-year-old girl with a past history of laryngeal intubation. Axial scans demonstrate markedly thickened tissue fused across upper larynx extending inferiorly from aryepiglottic folds (**a**), irregularly shaped vocal cords with airway narrowing and calcification (*open arrow* in **b**), and posterior irregularity (**c**). Immediate subglottic membrane (*arrow* in **d**) shown in coronal reformatted image. *Short arrow*, thyroid cartilage. (Liu and Daneman 1984 [7])

The third group of 10 patients (age range 21 months to 11¼ years) had previously documented acquired subglottic stenosis caused by earlier prolonged intubation. Eight of these had a tracheostomy. CT showed varying degrees of laryngeal narrowing or complete obliteration with calcification of the laryngeal wall or the tissue filling the lumen (Figs. 19.4, 19.5). In all 10 the anatomical abnormality was better defined by CT than by endoscopy or plain radiographs, and endoscopy could not define the length of the narrowing in any of these patients.

The fourth miscellaneous group included the follow-up of a patient with a previous laryngeal rhabdomyosarcoma, an infant with a laryngeal retention cyst (Fig. 19.6) and a 16-year-old boy with respiratory distress caused by a hypopharyngeal web following previous lye ingestion (Fig. 19.7). In all three CT revealed more anatomical detail of the larynx and adjacent tissues than plain films and supplied valuable information which facilitated endoscopy.

Summary

The commonest abnormality that we have studied in the larynx is that of subglottic stenosis.

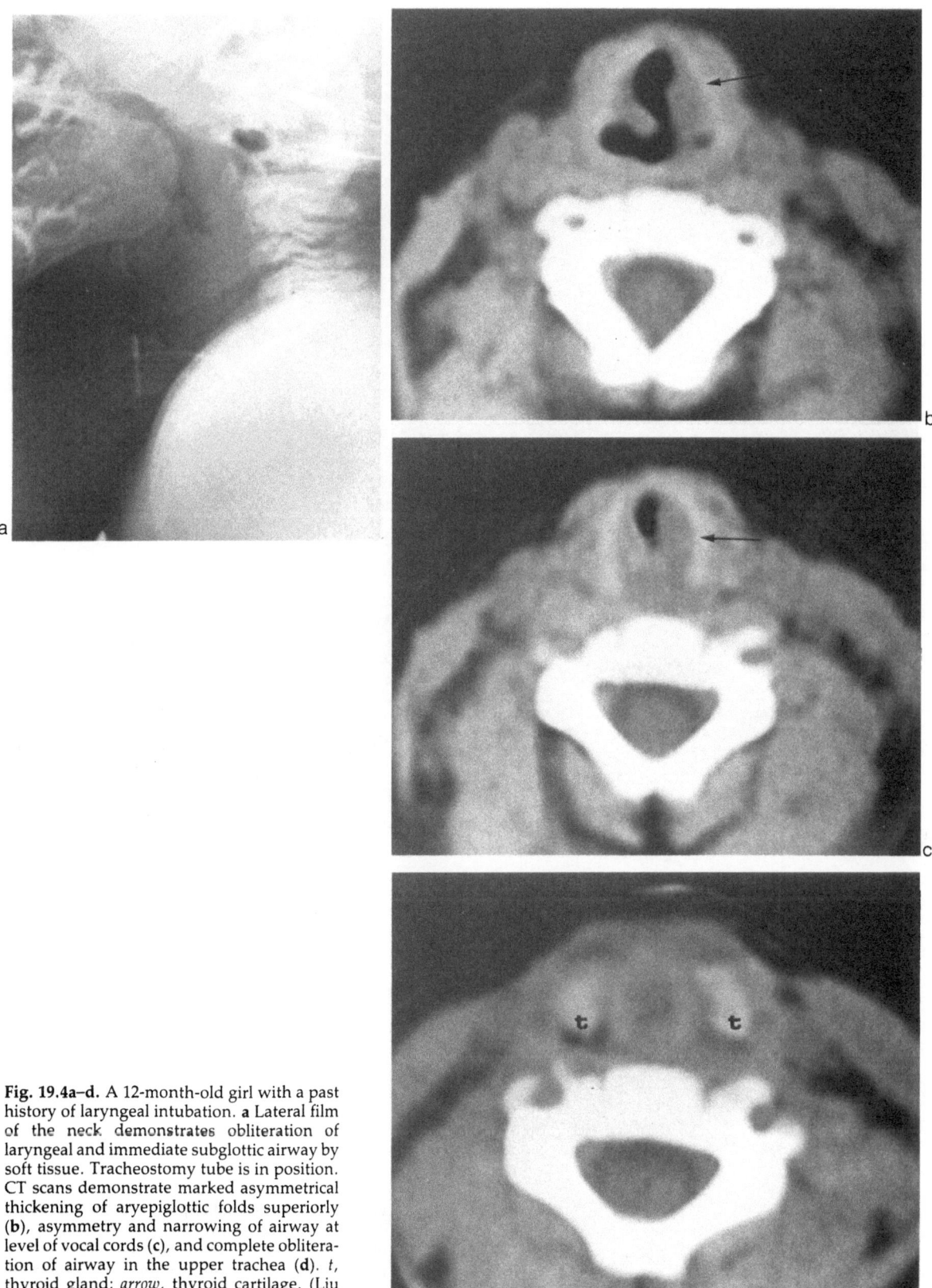

Fig. 19.4a–d. A 12-month-old girl with a past history of laryngeal intubation. **a** Lateral film of the neck demonstrates obliteration of laryngeal and immediate subglottic airway by soft tissue. Tracheostomy tube is in position. CT scans demonstrate marked asymmetrical thickening of aryepiglottic folds superiorly (**b**), asymmetry and narrowing of airway at level of vocal cords (**c**), and complete obliteration of airway in the upper trachea (**d**). *t*, thyroid gland; *arrow*, thyroid cartilage. (Liu and Daneman 1984 [7])

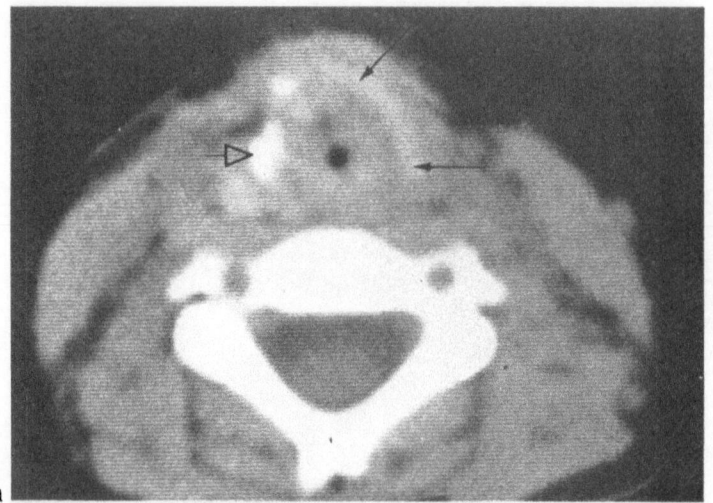

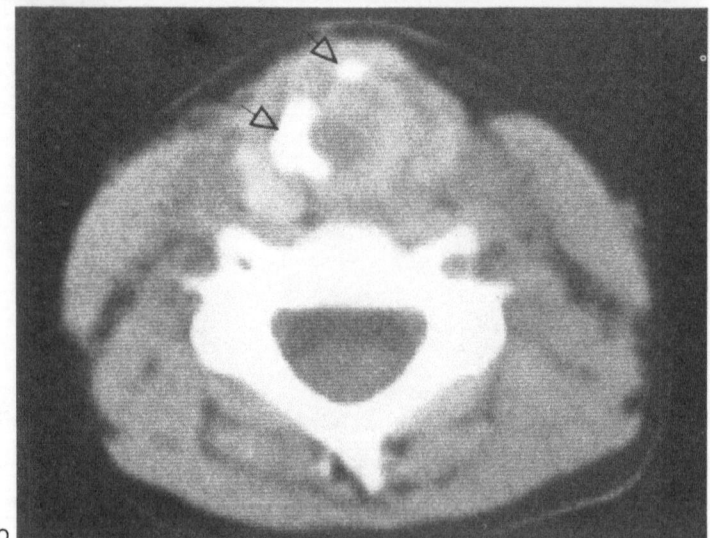

Fig. 19.5a,b. A 4-year-old girl with a past history of laryngeal intubation. CT scans demonstrate severe subglottic stenosis (**a**), progressing to complete obstruction on the more inferior scan (**b**). Note the dystrophic calcifications (*open arrows*) in the adjacent soft tissues on the right and anteriorly. *Arrows*, thyroid cartilage. (Liu and Daneman 1984 [7])

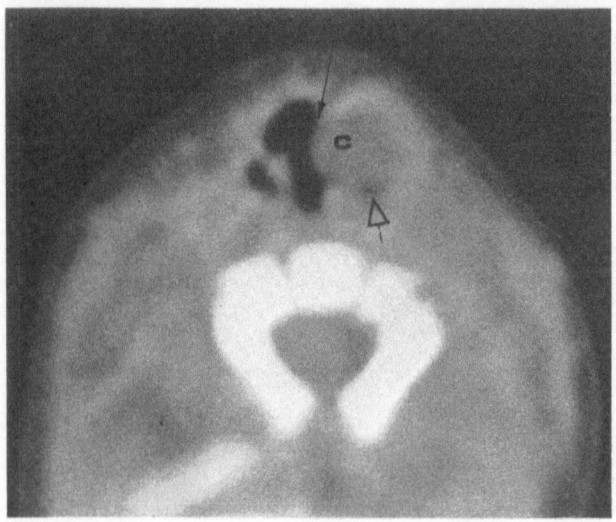

Fig. 19.6. A 6-week-old boy with stridor. Axial scan demonstrates laryngeal retention cyst (*c*) almost obliterating the left pyriform sinus (*open arrow*), pushing the epiglottis and aryepiglottic folds toward the right, and compressing the laryngeal airway (*arrow*). (Liu and Daneman 1984 [7])

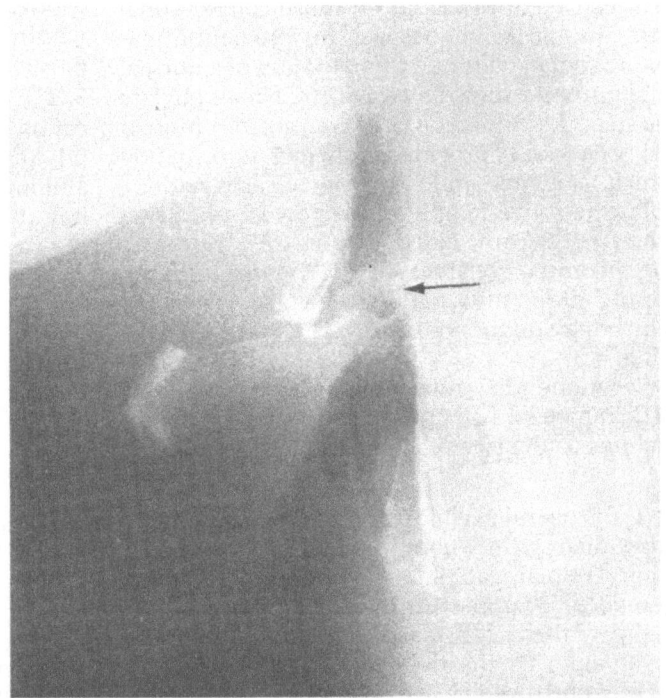

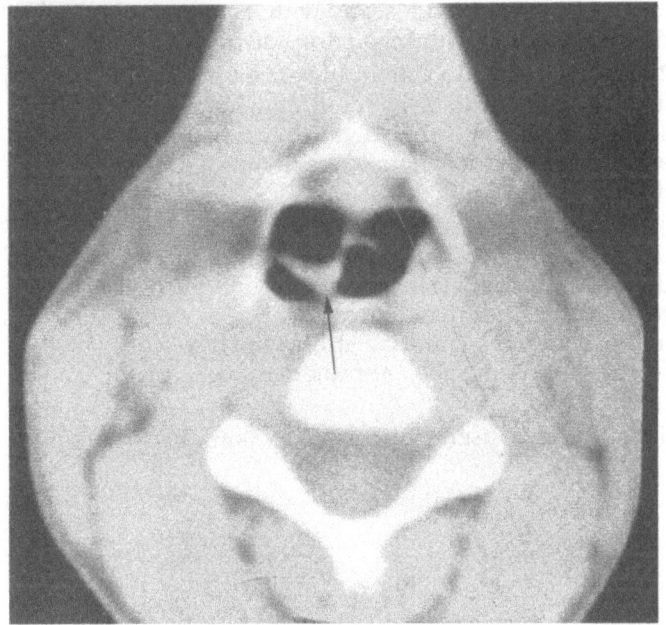

Fig. 19.7a,b. A 15-year-old boy with a past history of lye ingestion who presented with respiratory difficulty. **a** Upper gastrointestinal tract swallow demonstrates hypopharyngeal web (*arrow*). **b** CT scan reveals fusion of the web with right aryepiglottic fold (*arrow*). (Liu and Daneman 1984) [7])

Stenosis in the subglottic region is most commonly a result of prolonged intubation, usually in the neonatal period [5]. We have also used CT to assess the larynx in children who have had no previous intubation but in whom an anatomical abnormality of the larynx is suspected, based on clinical and plain radiographic findings.

We have found CT to be extremely useful in the delineation of intrinsic laryngeal lesions. CT accurately defines the caliber of the airway and documents the site and extent of narrowed segments as well as giving detailed information about the tissues adjacent to the airway. CT may delineate more subtle changes in airway caliber than can be appreciated on more conventional radiographic techniques and can also define anatomical detail better. Documentation of a normal or slightly narrowed airway on CT may obviate the need for endoscopy, as was seen in nine of our cases. CT provided valuable information which facilitated endoscopy in 14 cases and CT delineated the length of narrowed segments when endoscopy failed to do so in 10 cases. Sagittal and coronal reconstruction images often supply added information (see Figs. 19.2, 19.3), which may not be well appreciated on the transverse scan.

Recommended indications for performing CT to delineate known or suspected intrinsic abnormalities of the larynx in children are as follows:

1. CT is useful in children with stridor or respiratory distress in whom it is felt, on the basis of clinical or plain radiographic findings, that a congenital or acquired intrinsic anatomical abnormality of the airway exists. In this situation CT is invaluable, as the delineation of a normal or sightly narrowed airway may obviate the necessity for diagnostic endoscopy with its attendant risks in children with respiratory distress.

2. CT will easily document the extent of airway involvement in those children in whom endoscopy reveals airway narrowing but in whom the endoscope cannot negotiate the involved area to determine its length.

3. CT provides excellent anatomical delineation of the airway and surrounding tissues in children with mass lesions of the larynx, such as retention cysts or rhabdomyosarcoma, as well as in those with respiratory distress who have confusing or unusual appearance on plain radiograph.

4. CT is also useful on rare occasions in the delineation of the presence of foreign bodies within the lumen of the airway or those that may have eroded through the airway [3].

5. CT has been shown to be useful in the delineation of traumatic lesions of the larynx in adults [8] and is probably also useful in children, although we have not had the opportunity to use it in this situation.

References

1. Archer CR, Yeager VL (1979) Evaluation of laryngeal cartilages by computed tomography. J Comput Assist Tomogr 3 (5):604–611
2. Archer CR, Sagel SS, Yeager VL, Martin S, Friedman WH (1981) Staging of carcinoma of the larynx: comparative accuracy of CT and laryngography. AJR 136:571–575
3. Berger PE, Kuhn JP, Kuhns L (1980) Computed tomography and the occult tracheobronchial foreign body. Radiology 134:133–135
4. Brown DM, Enzmann DR, Hopp ML, Castellino RA (1983) Digital subtraction laryngography. Radiology 147: 655–657
5. Fearon B, Crysdale WS, Bird R (1978) Subglottic stenosis of the larynx in the infant and child. Methods and management. Paper presented at the Meeting of the American Laryngological Association, Palm Beach, Florida, 22–23 April, 1978
6. Hoover LA, Hanafee WN (1983) Conventional and computed tomography of the larynx and upper airway. Appl Radiol 12:99–111
7. Liu P, Daneman A (1984) CT of intrinsic laryngeal and tracheal abnormalities in children. J Comput Assist Tomogr. 8:662–669
8. Mancuso AA, Hanafee WN (1979) Computed tomography of the injured larynx. Radiology 133:139–144
9. Mancuso AA, Calcaterra TC, Hanafee WN (1978) Computed tomography of the larynx. Radiol Clin North Am 16:195–208
10. Silverman PM, Korobkin M (1983) High-resolution computed tomography of the normal larynx. AJR 140:875–879

Chapter 20

Neck Masses

Introduction

Neck masses in children are a frequent occurrence. The differential diagnosis includes congenital, inflammatory, and malignant lesions. By obtaining a detailed history and doing a careful physical examination, the clinician may often arrive at a proper diagnosis which may be confirmed with appropriate laboratory tests. However, in many instances the diagnosis may not be possible clinically, and radiological investigations are required both for diagnostic and management purposes.

In 1984, Donoghue et al. [2] reviewed the clinical and radiological findings of the 127 children with a palpable or visible neck mass who required radiological investigation at the Hospital for Sick Children, Toronto, during the 6-year period 1978–1983, inclusive. This was a retrospective review designed to assess the value and limitations of the newer imaging modalities in the evaluation of neck masses in children. The causes and relative incidence of these neck masses are summarized in Table 20.1. There were 75 females and 52 males, and the age range was 3 days to $17\frac{1}{2}$ years at the time of initial presentation. The diagnosis was confirmed histologically in 79. In the others the diagnosis was based on a combination of clinical, laboratory and radiographic findings. This chapter describes and illustrates patients from this series and also illustrates some further examples of neck masses seen subsequent to the study (see Figs. 20.1, 20.9, and 20.10).

Clinical clues to the diagnosis of a neck mass include the age of presentation of the patient and the presence or absence of associated local or generalized signs of inflammation. Furthermore, certain cystic and solid lesions may be diagnosed by their characteristic location in the neck. For example, masses in the position of the normal thyroid which move with swallowing are most likely thyroid in origin; thyroglossal duct cysts and dermoid cysts are usually in or closely adja-

Table 20.1. Causes of neck masses in children from the Hospital for Sick Children, Toronto, during the 6-year-period 1978–1983 (Donoghue et al. 1984 [2])

Diagnosis	No. of cases	Percentage
Thyroid masses	43	33.85
Lymphadenitis	18	14.17
Cystic hygroma	10	7.87
Abscess	11	8.66
Rhabdomyosarcoma	8	6.30
Thyroglossal duct cyst	6	4.72
Lymphoma	5	3.93
Hemangioma	5	3.93
Branchial cleft cyst	4	3.15
Neuroblastoma	3	2.36
Dermoid cyst	3	2.36
Neurofibroma	2	1.57
Lymphoepithelioma	1		
Endodermal sinus tumor	1		
Schwannoma	1		
Angiofibroma	1		
False aneurysm	1	9	7.09
Osteosarcoma	1		
Pharyngeal duplication	1		
Undifferentiated sarcoma	1		
Ectatic internal jugular vein	1		

cent to the midline; branchial cleft cysts typically lie anterior and medial to the sternocleidomastoid muscle and lateral to the lobes of the thyroid, and may extend between the internal and external carotid arteries. However, two patients of ours had branchial cleft cysts in atypical locations. A parotid cyst was thought to be an anomaly of the first branchial cleft and a suprasternal cyst probably represented a third branchial cleft anomaly. Both of these are extremely rare. Cystic hygromas usually occur posterior to the sternocleidomastoid muscle but may have quite wide extensions.

Solid lesions include lymphomas, which usually arise in the posterior triangle of the neck, and rhabdomyosarcomas and angiofibromas,

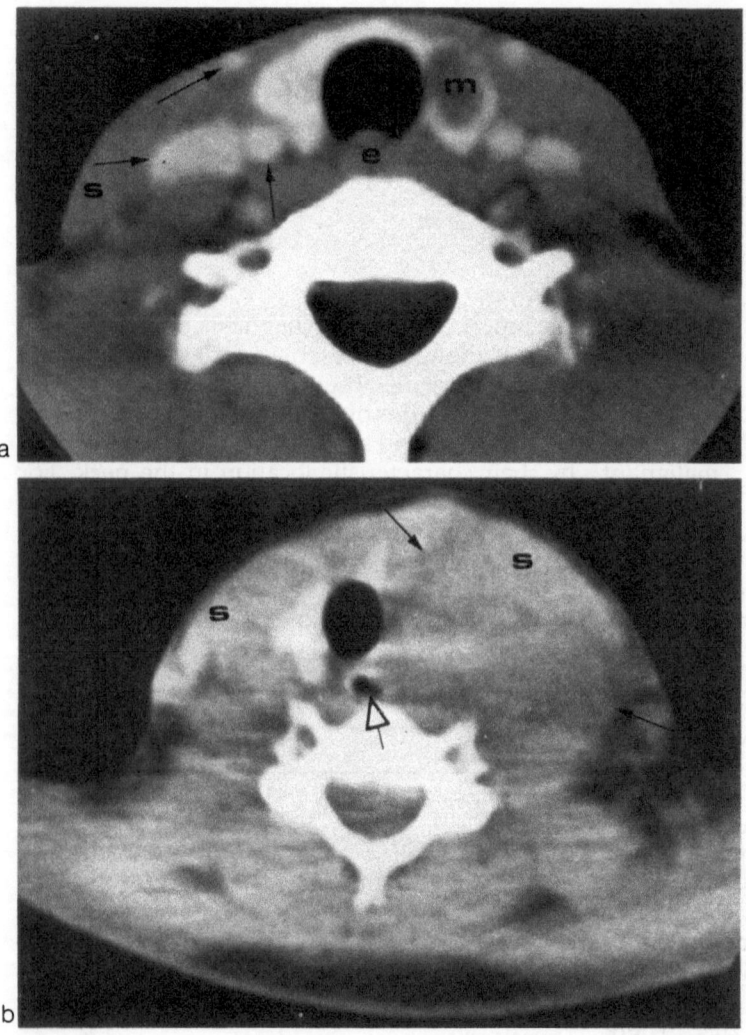

Fig. 20.1. a A 12-year-old boy who received previous mediastinal and cervical radiation for Hodgkin's disease presented with a small left-sided lower cervical mass. Cervical CT during intravenous contrast administration shows an oval lesion in the left lobe of the thyroid gland (*m*). The attenuation of this mass is lower than the adjacent normal thyroid parenchyma, which is compressed posterolaterally around the mass. The right lobe and the isthmus are easily visualized. The histology of this lesion is uncertain as further investigations have been refused. *Lower arrow*, right common carotid artery; *middle arrow*, right internal jugular vein; *upper arrow*, right external jugular vein; *s*, right sternocleidomastoid muscle; *e*, esophagus. Note the normal asymmetry between the two internal jugular veins and the horseshoe shape of the trachea, with slight internal convexity of the posterior membranous portion of the trachea. **b** A 10-year-old girl with a large follicular carcinoma (*arrows*) replacing the left lobe of the thyroid. The right lobe of the thyroid remains intact. *s*, sternocleidomastoid muscle; *open arrow*, esophagus. Note the displacement of the trachea to the right, with slight narrowing of the lumen. The scan was performed without contrast administration and thus the vessels are not well visualized, and differentiation of the carcinoma from the adjacent sternocleidomastoid muscle on the left is difficult.

which usually arise in the nasopharynx. Neurofibromas and Schwannomas may occur anywhere along nerve sheaths. Lymphadenitis and abscess formation may also occur in any part of the neck, and often the clinical findings may not be suggestive of an inflammatory process.

Plain Radiographs

Plain radiographs of the neck were of extremely limited value. In 39 of 42 children who had this study, the radiograph merely confirmed the presence of the soft tissue mass and showed airway narrowing in those patients already known to have clinical evidence of airway compromise.

In only three children did plain radiographs add extra useful information. A neonate with a large pharyngeal duplication had an air-fluid level within the mass suggesting that the lesion communicated with the gastrointestinal or respiratory tracts (see Fig. 20.4); in one child with a rhabdomyosarcoma and another with an osteosarcoma, bone destruction was evident adjacent to the mass.

We feel that plain radiographs of the neck are only indicated in cases of neck masses in which it is felt that the lesion is of bony origin or invading bone, or if there is clinical evidence of airway compromise and a CT scan is not deemed necessary for adequate management.

Sonography

Sonography has both advantages and disadvantages in the evaluation of neck masses. Like CT it can demonstrate normal cervical anatomy as well as delineate the exact site, size, extent, and relationship of a mass to surrounding normal cervical structures, particularly the thyroid gland and vessels. Because it does not use ionizing radiation it is an ideal screening modality in many instances. It is pertinent here to describe in broad general terms the capabilities of sonography rather than describing the detailed sonographic appearances of the various neck masses.

Ninety-seven (76.6%) children in our group had sonography of the neck. Sonography was accurate in determining whether diffuse thyroid disease or a solitary or multiple focal thyroid lesions were present in all 43 children who had clinical evidence of a thyroid mass. However, sonography is of limited benefit in defining the cause of diffuse thyroid disease. In one of our patients with a focal follicular carcinoma that was found to be the only active thyroid tissue on radionuclide scan, sonography documented the presence of adjacent normal thyroid tissue. Completely echo-free thyroid masses were found to be benign cysts. However, it should be stressed that there are no sonographic criteria to differentiate benign from malignant echogenic thyroid lesions, and solitary cystic lesions may rarely be malignant [1].

In the 54 children with extrathyroidal lesions sonography accurately delineated the site of the lesion and documented the presence of a normal thyroid gland separate from the mass. These lesions included lymphadenitis, abscesses, cystic hygromas, hemangiomas, dermoid, thyroglossal and branchial cleft cysts, ectatic internal jugular vein, submandibular rhabdomyosarcoma, and neuroblastoma.

In 28 of these 54 patients the correct clinical diagnosis was made prior to sonography, and this modality showed features consistent with the diagnosis. In ten patients a clinical diagnosis could not be made, and sonography could not provide the exact diagnosis because of its nonspecific echo pattern, although it provided sufficient information for correct management. In only one patient did sonography provide an exact diagnosis not suspected clinically. This patient had an ectatic internal jugular vein. In 15 children the initial clinical diagnosis was not adequately documented; therefore, we could not retrospectively assess the role played by sonography in these patients.

Completely echo-free extrathyroidal masses were all found to be benign cysts. Two thyroid and ten extrathyroidal masses with mixed echogenicity or low-level echoes were also found to be benign cystic lesions. Echoes within these masses were related to hemorrhage, infection, cholesterol or mucoid material. The extrathyroidal lesions in this group included cystic hygromas, and dermoid, thyroglossal, and branchial cleft cysts. Based on the echo pattern alone, differentiation of enlarged inflamed lymph nodes from abscesses, hemangiomas, cystic hygromas and solid neoplasms may be impossible. In these instances, differentiation of solid from cystic lesions may thus be impossible.

In all 43 children with thyroid lesions and in 48 of the 54 with extrathyroid masses, sonography supplied sufficient information regarding the site, extent, and relationship of the mass to surrounding structures to ensure correct management of the patient. However, in these patients the exact diagnosis of the mass could not always be made on the basis of its echo pattern alone as this was nonspecific. When this information was combined with the clinical findings and the site of the mass the list of possibilities was narrowed somewhat. In a review of 17 children with non-inflammatory neck masses in 1983, Friedman et al. [3] found that the correct diagnosis was obvious clinically prior to sonography in 8, and in the remaining 9 sonography did not provide the exact diagnosis.

Sonography is thus a useful noninvasive modality in the investigation of neck masses. In the delineation of thyroid as well as many benign extrathyroidal lesions sonography may be the definitive modality. However, the sonographic appearances of various cystic and solid neck masses are nonspecific.

Computed Tomography

Although sonography is the ideal screening modality in the evaluation of the majority of pediatric neck masses, there are a number of instances when CT is essential. CT is capable of defining the extent of neck masses in greater detail than sonography and may provide further information concerning the character of these lesions by assessing their vascularity following intravenous contrast medium administration. CT can also delineate changes in adjacent tissue planes more accurately than can sonography. However, the appearances of most neck neoplasms on CT are nonspecific.

Thirty-four patients (27.3%) underwent CT of the neck, which was used to delineate both benign and malignant lesions. The appearances of these lesions are listed below. In 28 of these patients, CT was performed following clinical examination or previous plain radiography of the neck. The other six patients had sonography

prior to CT. These included three children with cystic hygroma, two with hemangioma, and one with branchial cleft cyst. In these six, CT was required to give better definition of the extent of the lesions, which were adjacent to or destroying bone, adjacent to the airway, or extending into the chest.

Benign Lesions

Cystic Lesions

Cystic Hygroma   Cystic hygromas are thought to result from an abnormal development of the lymphatic sacs in the jugular region. In 80% of cystic hygromas there is neck involvement, and in 10% there is an extension into the mediastinum. Less commonly the entire mass may be found within the chest. In 65% of patients the mass is present at birth. Although some cystic hygromas may not become apparent until adulthood, the vast majority usually present by the end of the second year of life. In two cases described by Silverman et al. [7] these lesions appeared to have attenuation of water on CT. Som et al. [8] described the CT appearance in two children, one of whom showed a high-attenuation area caused by hemorrhage. In our group, six of the ten patients with cystic hygromas required CT examination. Sonography had been performed previously in three of these, and the findings correlated with the CT appearance.

In six patients the attenuation values of the contents of the cystic hygroma were lower than that of muscle prior to intravenous contrast medium administration. In one of these there was a single area of increased attenuation with a fluid-fluid level which was shown to be an area of hemorrhage at operation (Fig. 20.2). In three children there were visible septa in the mass lesion which were better visualized after intravenous contrast medium administration. There were some areas of enhancement in the mass in one patient. The diagnosis in this case was based on the clinical examination and a strong family history of cystic hygromas.

➤

Fig. 20.2a–c. An 18½-month-old boy with a cystic hygroma. **a,b** CT scans before (**a**) and after (**b**) intravenous contrast medium administration. There is a large right septated soft tissue mass with attenuation values lower than muscle. The septations are better seen after contrast administration. The fluid-fluid level (*open arrow*) in one of the loculi represented a recent hemorrhage. There is airway displacement. *Square cursor* in **a** shows extension of mass behind hyoid bone (*h*) and pharynx (*p*). *Upper arrow*, right jugular vein; *lower arrow*, right common carotid artery. Anterior to the hyoid are the muscles of the floor of the mouth. **c** CT scan shows extension of the mass anterior and posterior to the right clavicle but not into the thoracic cavity. CT shows the anatomical extent of this lesion far better than sonography. (Donoghue et al. 1984 [2])

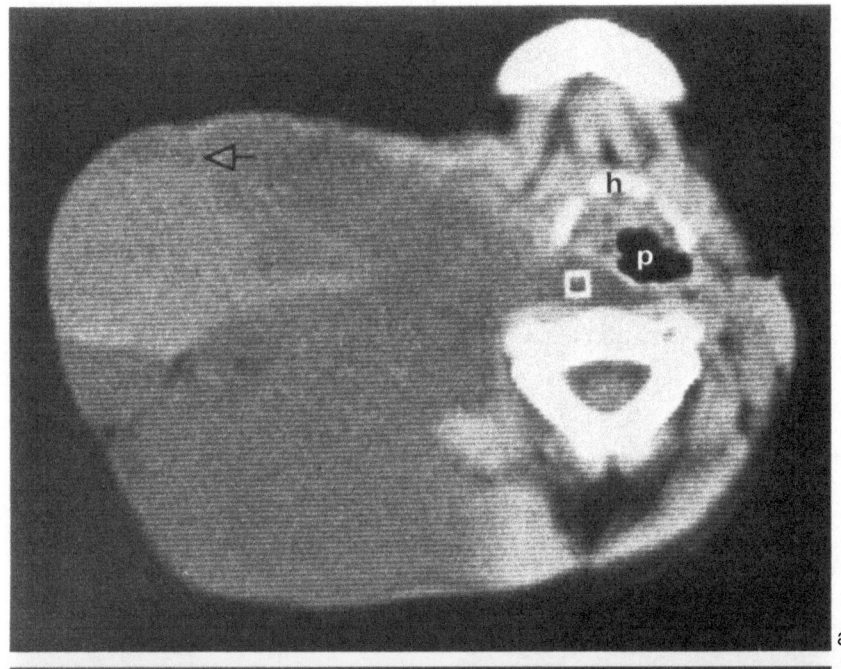

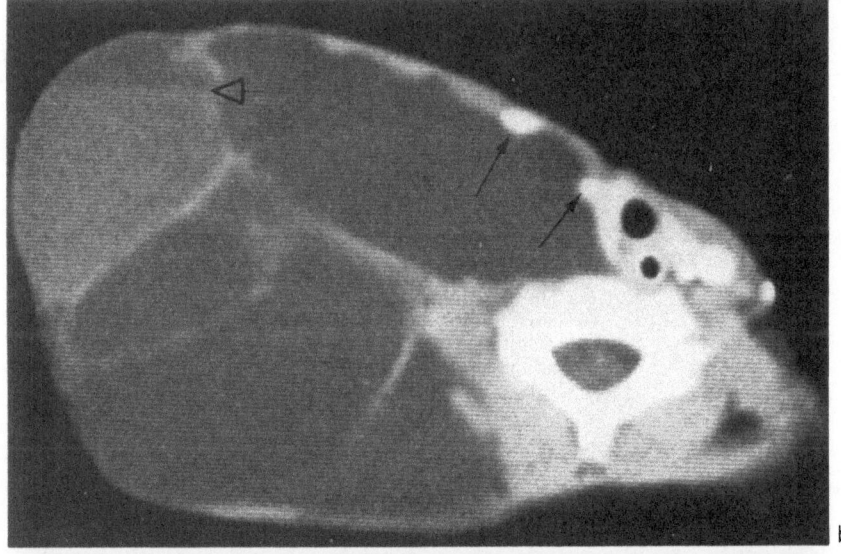

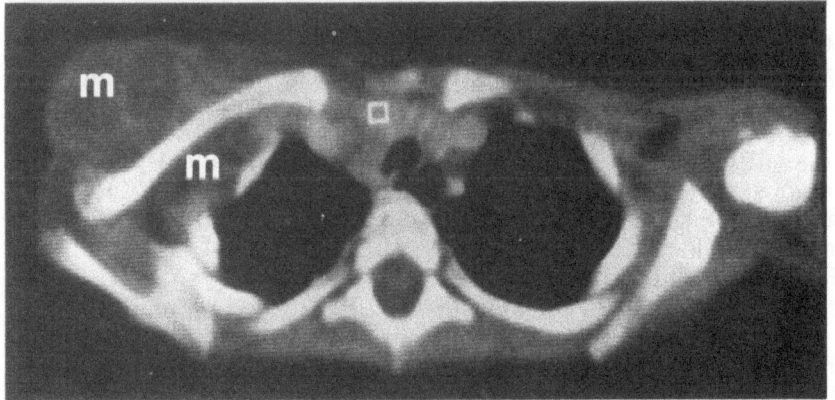

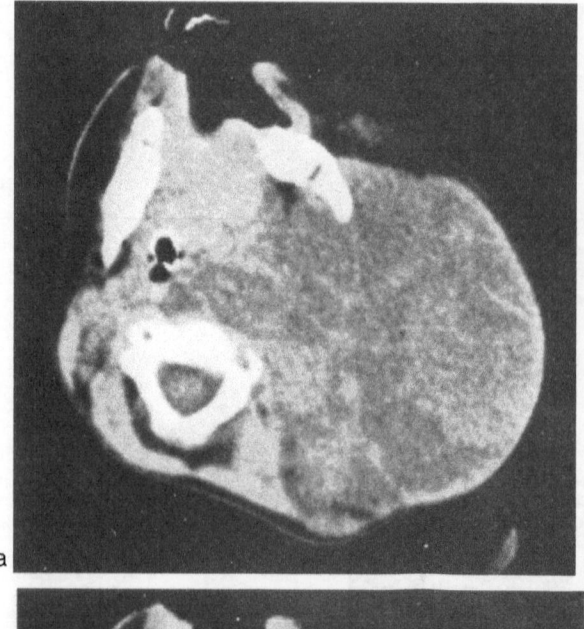

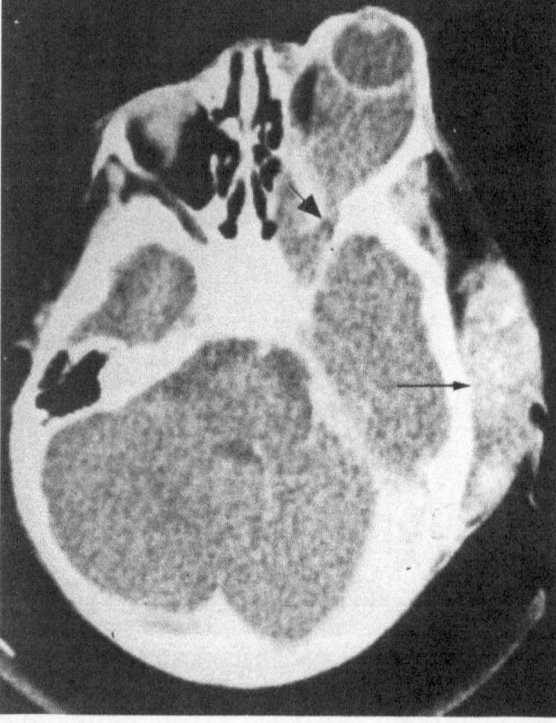

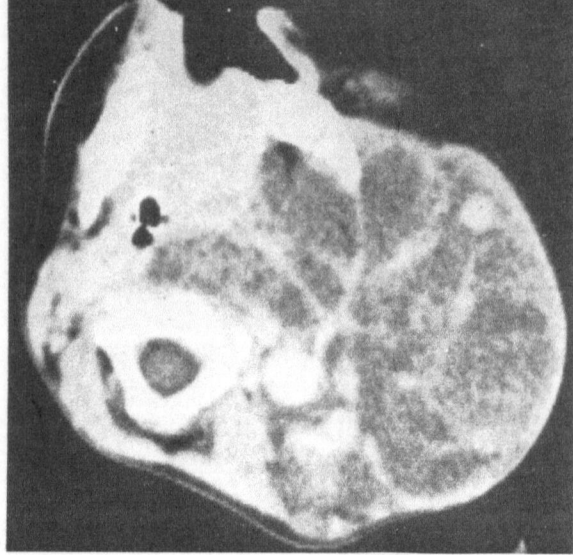

Fig. 20.3a–c. A 1-year-old girl with a cystic hygroma. **a** CT shows a large soft tissue mass of lower attenuation than the surrounding muscle with visible septa. There is airway displacement. **b** After intravenous contrast medium administration the septa are more easily visible. **c** There is extension of the mass into the left retro-orbital region with left-sided proptosis and extension through the posterior wall of the orbit into the left temporal fossa (*short arrow*). There is also left facial involvement (*long arrow*). (Donoghue et al. 1984 [2])

In seven of our patients the lesion was confined to the neck, including the nasopharynx. One patient had bilateral neck masses, and another had a lesion which was located anterior to the sternomastoid and crossed the midline. Two other patients had lesions which also involved the face, and in another CT showed extension through the floor of the middle cranial fossa and into the left orbit (Fig. 20.3). In another patient the mass was confined to the right suboccipital region. In a more recent patient CT showed a large extension into the anterior mediastinum. In the two children reported by Som et al. [8], facial paralysis caused by extension into the parotid gland was present. In all of these patients CT played a major role in defining the extent of the lesion better than other modalities. CT should thus be used in patients with cystic hygromas when the extent and effects of the mass have not been adequately defined by sonography.

Branchial Cleft Cyst The second branchial arch normally grows caudally to cover the third and fourth arches and clefts and fuses with underlying tissue. Incomplete obliteration of the underlying epithelial lined clefts results in the development of a branchial cleft cyst [4]. Since the second arch grows so far caudally it is most predisposed to this type of anomaly. These lesions usually become evident in adulthood and may present with a neck mass, often with superimposed infection.

Only one of our four patients with a branchial cleft cyst had a CT scan, and this demonstrated a cystic lesion anterior to the sternocleidomastoid muscle. Silverman et al., in 1983 [7], reported two cases in which this type of lesion appeared as a cystic mass, with a thick wall and septation in one. Both lesions were involved with an inflammatory process. Kriepke et al. [4] have reported similar appearances in three patients. CT is only required to delineate these lesions when their extent is inadequately defined by sonography.

Miscellaneous Cystic Lesions An air-fluid level was noted in the neonate with the large phar-

yngeal diverticulum, but the communication to the pharynx could not be demonstrated by CT or on barium studies (Fig. 20.4).

The CT appearances of other cystic neck lesions have been described [7]. These include thyroglossal duct cysts and "complicated" laryngocele. Thyroglossal duct cysts usually present in the first decade as a mass, occasionally with associated infection. They are a remnant of the thyroglossal duct, which represents the connection between the thyroid gland and the foramen cecum at the base of the tongue. On CT these lesions appear as midline fluid-filled cystic structures and may have a thickened wall if inflamed [7]. CT is of value in defining extension of the mass superiorly toward the tongue as this may be difficult with sonography. Documentation of the existence of a normal separate thyroid gland is mandatory prior to removal of these lesions and is achieved simply with sonography. Laryngoceles represent an abnormal sacular dilatation of the appendix of the laryngeal

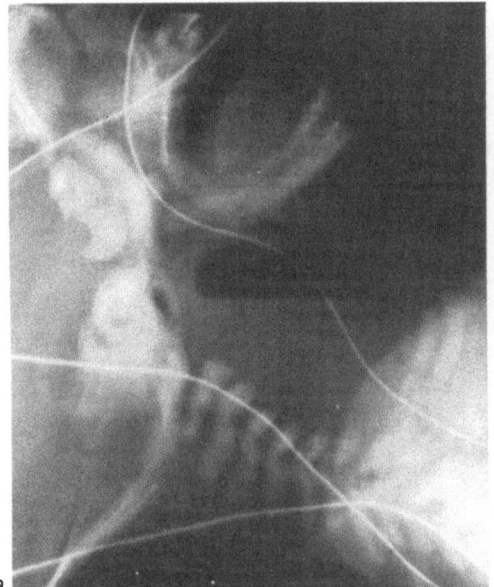

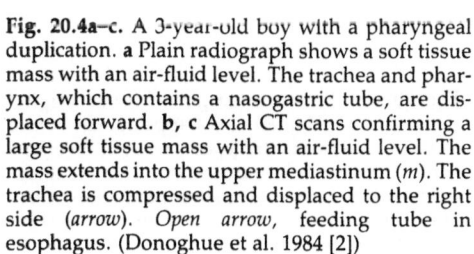

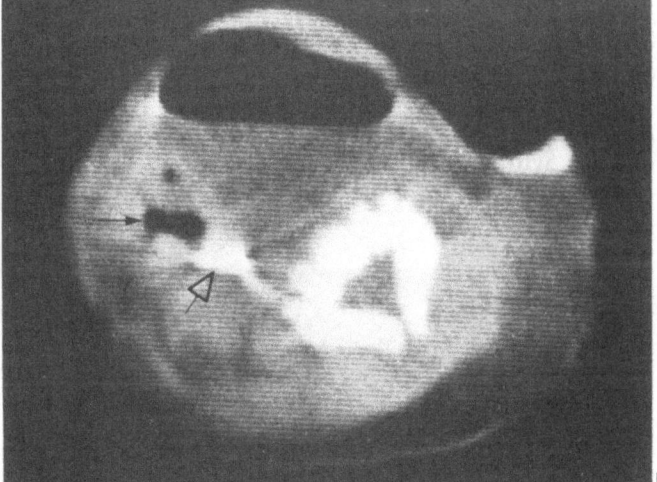

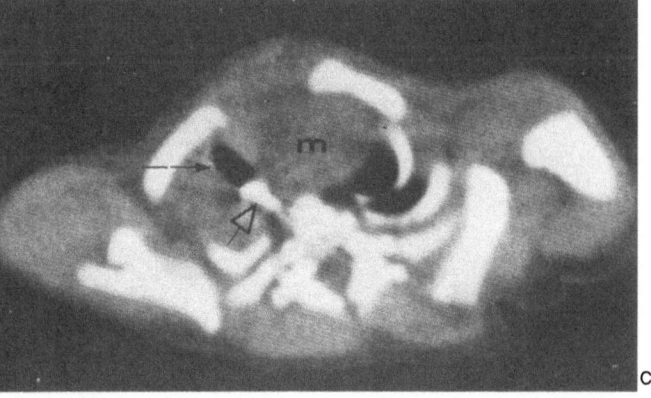

Fig. 20.4a–c. A 3-year-old boy with a pharyngeal duplication. **a** Plain radiograph shows a soft tissue mass with an air-fluid level. The trachea and pharynx, which contains a nasogastric tube, are displaced forward. **b, c** Axial CT scans confirming a large soft tissue mass with an air-fluid level. The mass extends into the upper mediastinum (*m*). The trachea is compressed and displaced to the right side (*arrow*). *Open arrow,* feeding tube in esophagus. (Donoghue et al. 1984 [2])

ventricle [7]. They are usually air filled, and the communication with the larynx can be documented on CT. Occasionally, they may become completely or partially filled with fluid and appear as cystic structures [7].

Solid Lesions

Hemangioma In our study the group with hemangiomas included four females and one male, with ages ranging from 6½ months to 14 years. In two patients the hemangioma was of low attenuation prior to contrast medium administration. In one of these lesions there was no enhancement, and in the other patchy areas of enhancement followed intravenous contrast administration. In two patients the lesions had an attenuation value similar to that of the surrounding muscles, and each lesion showed a significant increase in the attenuation (approximately 60 HU) after intravenous contrast administration (Figs. 20.5, 20.6). One patient had some airway narrowing not evident on plain films. In another the lesion extended into the maxillary antrum and orbit. ⁹⁹ᵐTc-pertechnetate scans were performed in two patients, and both scans demonstrated vascular lesions.

Neurofibroma Neurofibromas are usually well defined with nonspecific features on CT. En-hancement may be limited. We have studied two girls with neurofibromas of the neck. In both, the attenuation of the lesion was similar to that of surrounding muscles after contrast administration (Fig. 20.7). These lesions may be multiple, and associated findings such as enlargement of adjacent neural foramina or atrophy of the innervated muscles are occasionally seen on CT [6] (see also Chap. 21, p. 319)

Miscellaneous Solid Lesions The single examples of Schwannoma and angiofibroma appeared as soft tissue masses with attenuation similar to that of surrounding muscles without contrast enhancement. The false aneurysm of the right common carotid artery showed enhancement after intravenous contrast administration, and the mass subsequently became partially filled with contrast medium. Patients with suspected lymphadenitis or abscesses were not studied with CT in our original series (see below).

Malignant Lesions

Lymphoma Approximately 65% of children with lymphoma at the Hospital for Sick Children, Toronto, have cervical adenopathy at the time of presentation. Only five children with such neck masses had radiological examination of the neck. There were four males and one

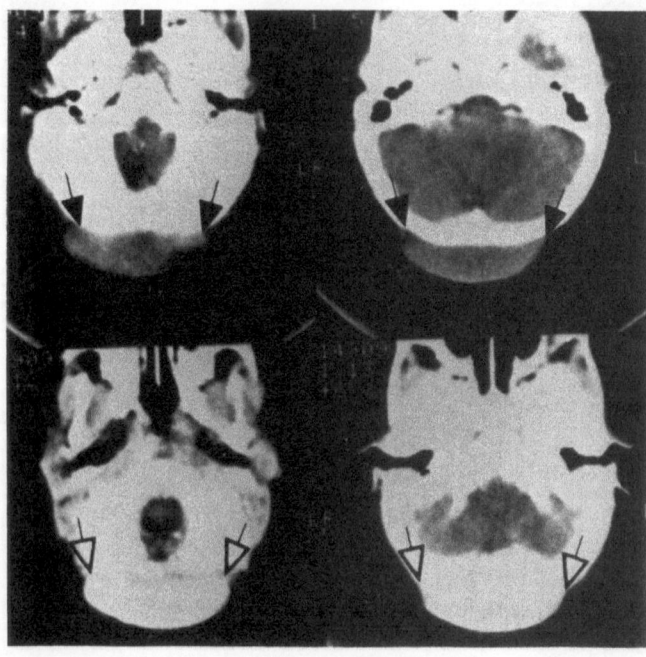

Fig. 20.5. A 9-month-old girl with suboccipital hemangioma. Hemangioma appearances before (*closed arrows*) and after (*open arrows*) intravenous contrast medium adminstration. There is a significant diffuse increase in the attenuation values after intravenous contrast medium administration. (Donoghue et al. 1984 [2])

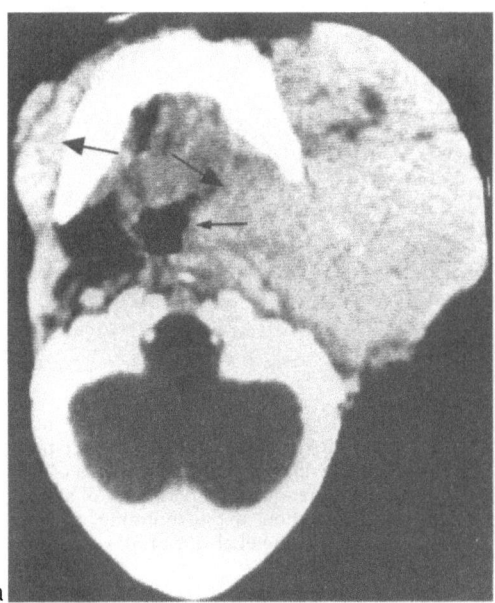 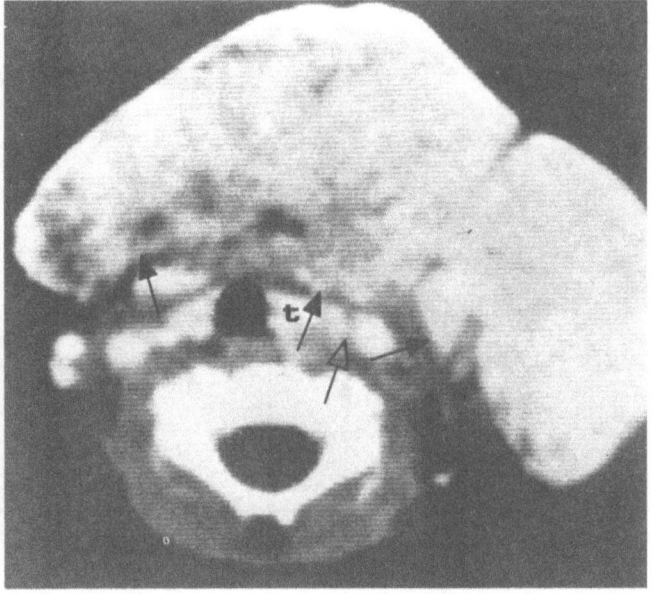

a   b

Fig. 20.6a,b. A 6½-month-old girl with a neck and facial hemangioma (*short arrows*). CT scans after intravenous contrast medium administration. These confirm the very large enhancing mass, which extends medially to involve the left side of the nasopharynx (*small arrow*). There is some airway distortion. *t*, thyroid gland; *open arrow*, between left common carotid and internal jugular vessels. (Donoghue et al. 1984 [2])

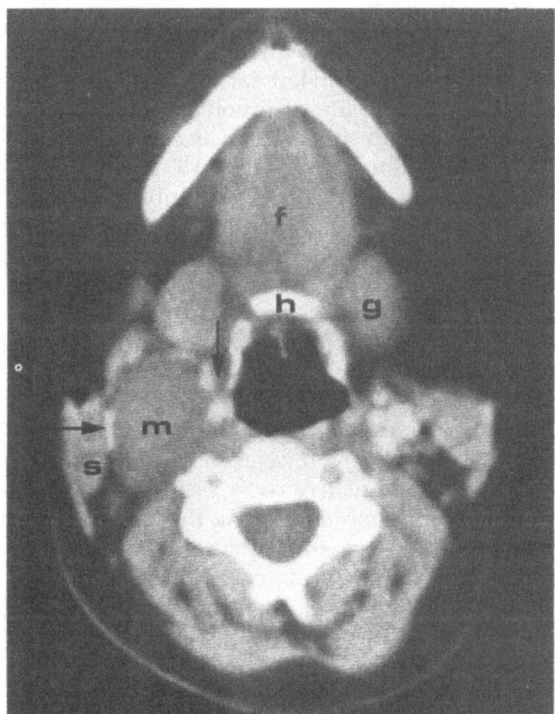

Fig. 20.7. A 13-year-old girl with cervical neurofibroma. CT scan shows a well-defined homogeneous mass (*m*) deep to the sternocleidomastoid muscle (*s*), displacing the neck vessels (*arrows*); *h*, hyoid bone; *g*, left submandibular gland; *f*, muscles of floor of mouth. (Donoghue et al. 1984 [2])

female between 5½ and 15 years of age. All five cases were histologically proven to be non-Hodgkin's lymphoma.

In all five cases CT scans were performed to define the extent of the disease within the neck. In three, the lesions had a central area of low attenuation with a periphery of similar attenuation to the surrounding muscles (Fig. 20.8). In the other two, the lesions were homogeneous, with attenuation values similar to the muscles. Four patients received intravenous contrast material. Two of these showed slight generalized enhancement, one showed peripherally uniform rim enhancement, and one showed no enhancement. Extension of the mass into the upper mediastinum in one case and into the extradural space at the level of the first cervical vertebra in another was exquisitely demonstrated with CT. Sonography was not performed in any of these cases. More recently we have studied a case of cervical Hodgkin's disease. CT showed diffuse and rim enhancement in extensive lymphadenopathy deep to both sternocleidomastoid muscles (Fig. 20.9).

Reede et al. [6] found that the most useful characteristic in separating inflammatory nodes from those involved with malignancy is the pattern of enhancement. Regular uniform rim enhancement and/or uniform enhancement sug-

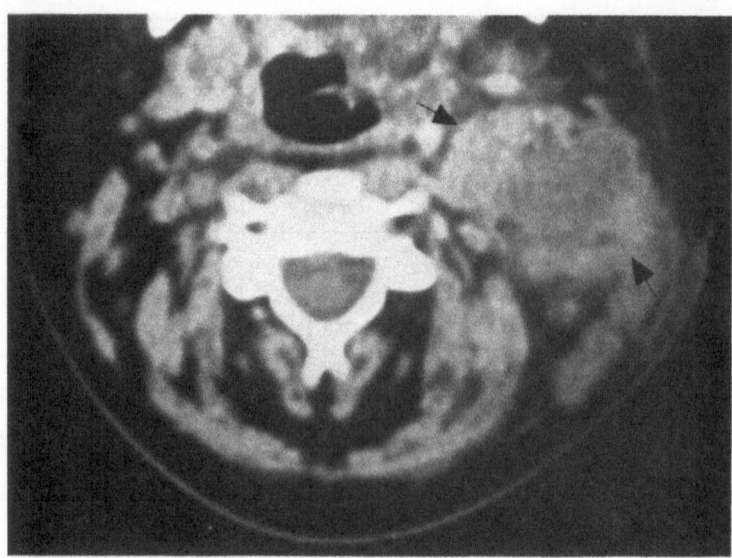

Fig. 20.8. A 14-year-old boy with non-Hodgkin's lymphoma. The left neck mass (*arrows*) has a central area of low attenuation and a periphery of similar attenuation to surrounding muscle. (Donoghue et al. 1984 [2])

gest neoplastic involvement with lymphoma, while thick irregular rim enhancement suggests inflammation. These authors also found that nodes involved with non-Hodgkin's lymphoma were hypodense compared with muscle. This characteristic may be useful in distinguishing such lesions from Hodgkin's lymphoma. The appearance of fascial planes may also be useful, as obliteration of these planes is seen with inflammatory processes, whereas preservation is more consistent with neoplastic disease.

No use was made of CT in any of the 18 cases of lymphadenitis or 11 cases of cervical abcesses in our original group. The results of the clinical and sonographic examinations of these inflammatory masses revealed sufficient information to ensure correct management. We have subsequently studied the case of a boy with previously treated cervical Hodgkin's disease who presented with a recurrent neck mass. CT showed thick irregular rim enhancement with loss of the adjacent tissue planes. This was proven to be a cervical abscess (Fig. 20.10). CT is thus useful for defining the extent of cervical masses thought to be enlarged lymph nodes in those patients in whom there is no local or general signs of inflammation and in patients with proven malignant lymphadenopathy when knowledge of the exact extent of the nodes is imperative for adequate radiation therapy (see Fig. 20.9).

Rhabdomyosarcoma Rhabdomyosarcomas in childhood are most commonly found in the head and neck and pelvis. In the region of the neck

the commonest site of occurrence is the nasopharynx, although lesions may occur more rarely in other sites such as the larynx. Eight patients in our group had rhabdomyosarcoma, and these included seven males and one female, with an age range of 2½ months to 5 years. Five patients had symptoms of nasal obstruction, four had cranial nerve signs, and one patient had hemorrhage from the left ear. The nasopharynx was the primary site of involvement in seven, and in the eighth the lesion was confined to the left submandibular region. All seven nasopharyngeal lesions were of the embryonal type.

All eight patients had plain radiographs of the neck, and in five a soft tissue mass was visualized. Left mastoid destruction was noted in one nasopharyngeal lesion, and in another no abnormality was evident. The lesion in the left submandibular area appeared echogenic on sonography, but none of the nasopharyngeal lesions were studied with this modality. CT was performed in all seven cases of nasopharyngeal lesions and showed a soft tissue mass with attenuation values similar to the surrounding muscle both before and after contrast enhancement (Fig. 20.11). In six cases there was associated involvement of the sinuses, with bone destruction in five. Intracranial extension of the tumor was found in four (Fig. 20.11). In all of these cases the lesion was easily visualized because of its greater attenuation than the adjacent brain. Orbital extension was found in one case and left mastoid extension in another. Six patients had follow-up CT scans after treatment with radiotherapy and chemotherapy, and in

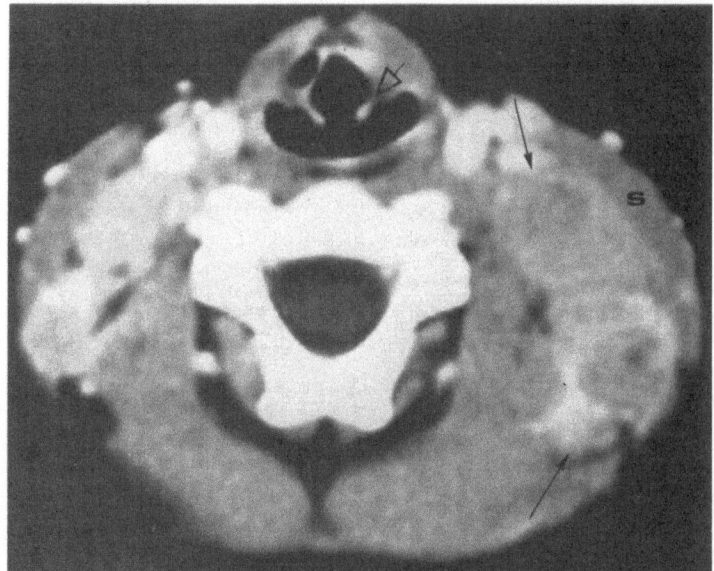

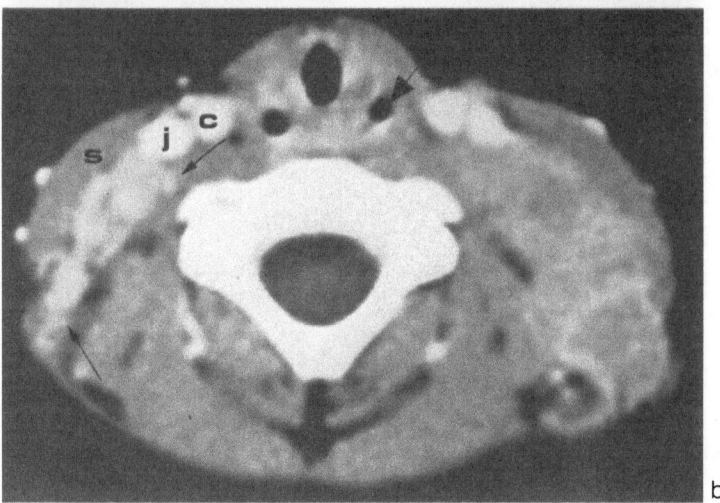

Fig. 20.9a,b. A 5-year-old boy with bilateral cervical masses caused by Hodgkin's disease. CT scans following intravenous contrast administration show enhancing nodes (*long arrows*) deep to sternocleidomastoid muscle (*s*) bilaterally. Note rim enhancement, particularly in left mass. The extent of the nodes was better defined with CT than sonography. Note aryepiglottic folds (*open arrow*) and pyriform fossae (*short arrow*). *c*, common carotid artery; *j*, internal jugular vein.

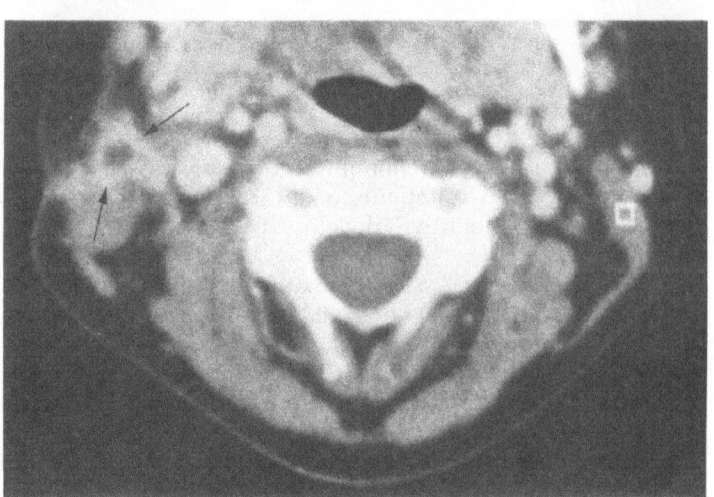

Fig. 20.10. A 12-year-old boy with right cervical abscess (*arrows*). Note rim enhancement and loss of adjacent tissue planes compared with the left side.

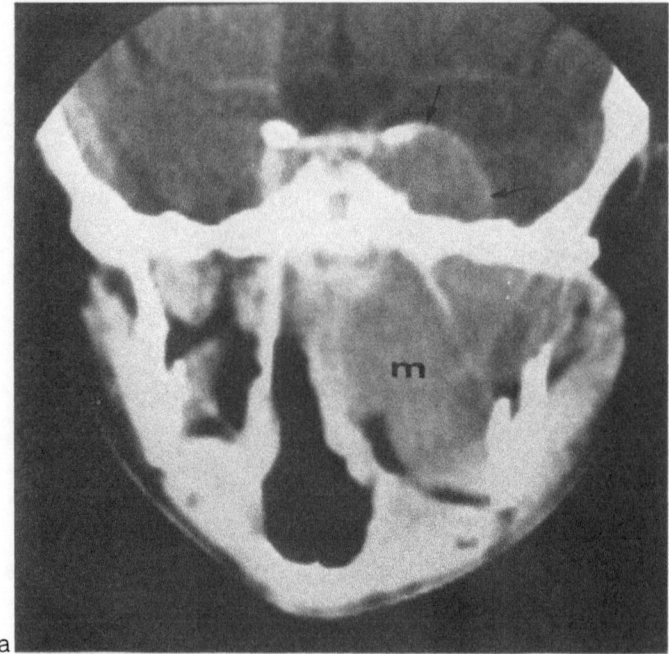

a

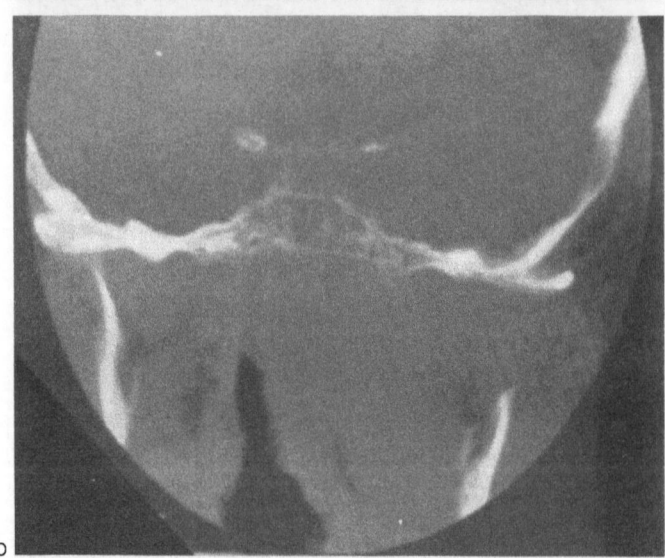

b

Fig. 20.11a,b. A 9-year-old girl with nasopharyngeal rhabdomyosarcoma. Coronal CT scans following intravenous contrast administration. **a** Scan shows a large left nasopharyngeal soft tissue mass (*m*) with extension through the floor of the middle cranial fossa into the left cavernous sinus (*arrows*). The attenuation values are similar to surrounding muscle and greater than adjacent brain. **b** Note the bone destruction. (Donoghue et al. 1984 [2])

each case a marked reduction in tumor size was noted. However, two patients with intracranial extension subsequently developed distant metastases.

Our experience has shown that CT is the investigative modality of choice in suspected or proven rhabdomyosarcomas of the head and neck because of their tendency for rapid growth and invasion of neighboring structures, including the sinuses, orbits, nasal cavity, middle cranial fossa, and mastoids. The exact extent of the lesions arising in parameningeal sites is extremely important because these lesions have a propensity to metastasize distantly within the central nervous system.

Neuroblastoma Neuroblastomas of the cervical region are very much less common than those occurring in the abdomen and chest. These patients may present with a Horner's syndrome or changes in the color of the iris. In our group there were three such patients, including two males and one female, with ages ranging from 3½ to 13 years. Two patients had a primary cervical

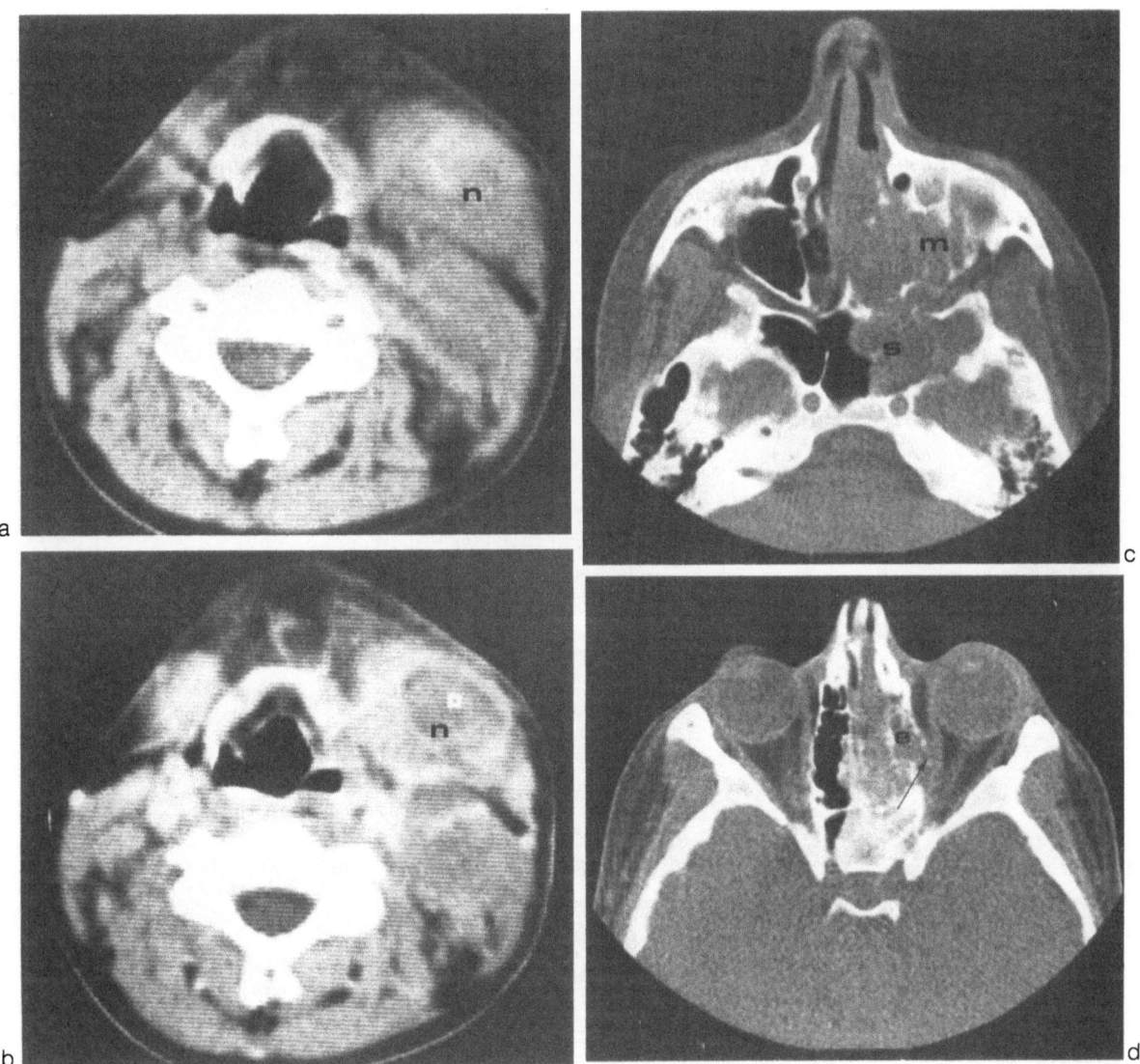

Fig. 20.12a–d. A 13-year-old girl with stage IV neuroblastoma. **a** Unenhanced CT scan showing a left-sided soft tissue mass (*n*) which is infiltrating surrounding tissues and is of similar attenuation to surrounding muscle. **b** After intravenous contrast medium administration there is some peripheral patchy enhancement. **c, d** Scans showing invasion into the left ethmoid (*e*), sphenoid (*s*), and maxillary (*m*) sinuses. There is also left orbital extension causing displacement of the medial rectus muscle (*arrow*). (Donoghue et al. 1984 [2])

tumor and one had a metastatic lesion. All three had stage IV disease at presentation. Sonography in one showed an echogenic lesion. In both the other two patients CT scans showed lesions with attenuation values similar to the surrounding muscles and only slight patchy enhancement after intravenous contrast administration. In one patient with a primary lesion, extension into the chest with some calcification was noted, and in the other there was direct extension into the sinuses and left orbit (Fig. 20.12).

In the initial diagnosis and follow-up of cervical neuroblastoma CT is the modality of choice as it gives the best delineation of the extent of the lesion and its relationship to adjacent structures.

Miscellaneous Malignant Lesions The group of patients with miscellaneous malignant lesions included one with an undifferentiated sarcoma that had an attenuation value similar to that of the surrounding muscles without contrast administration. Three further lesions, including a lymphoepithelioma, nasopharyngeal endodermal sinus tumor, and mandibular osteosarcoma showed the presence of soft tissue masses with attenuation similar to that of muscle both before and after intravenous contrast administration. The extent of these lesions was well delineated with CT. The recurrent endodermal sinus tumor was shown to be invading the nasal cavity and sinuses with bone destruction (see Fig. 20.15) [5].

The osteosarcoma was noted to have associated mandibular destruction (Fig. 20.14). The undifferentiated sarcoma was shown to have a large component of extradural extension with widening of the involved intervetebral foramen (see Fig. 20.13). The extent of these miscellaneous malignant lesions is best delineated by CT, particularly when the lesion arises in, is adjacent to, or invades bones.

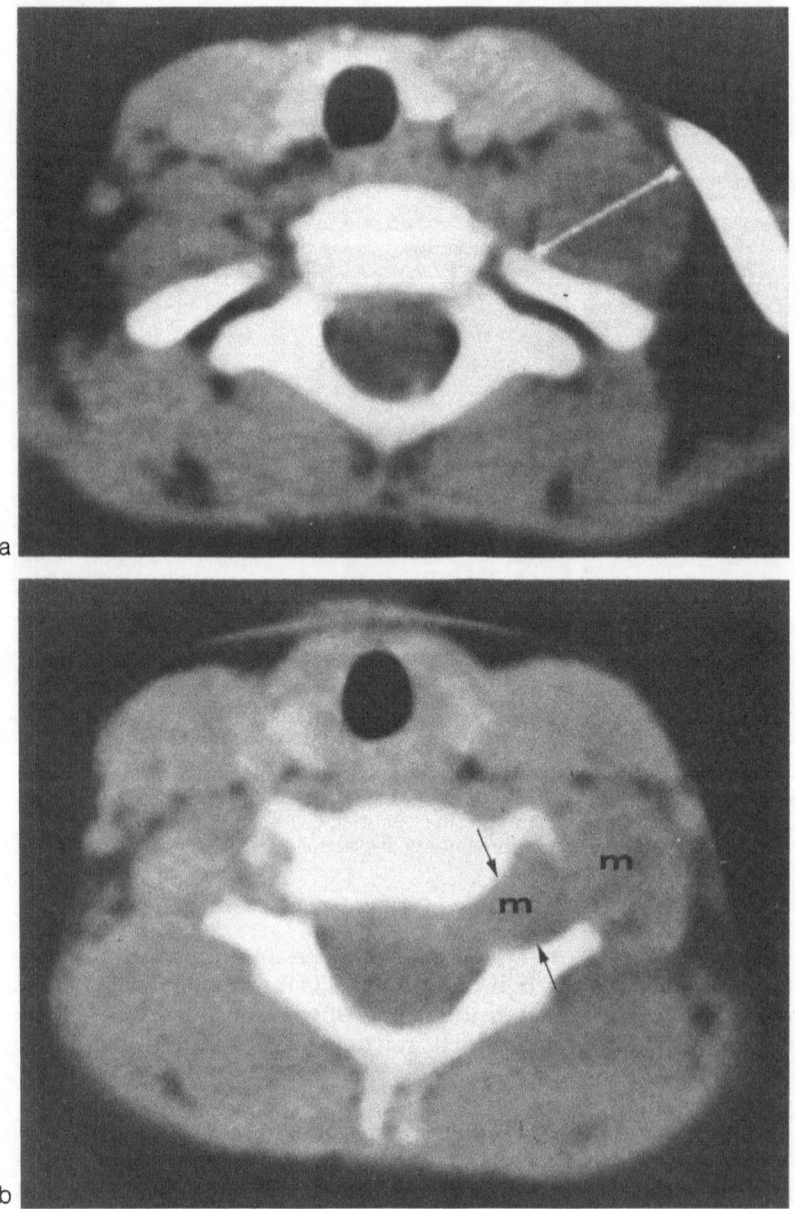

Fig. 20.13a,b. A 3-year-old boy with an undifferentiated sarcoma. **a** CT scan without contrast administration shows a left neck mass (*between cursors*). **b** Intraspinal extension of the neck mass (*m*) through a widened left intervertebral foramen (*arrows*). (Donoghue et al. 1984 [2])

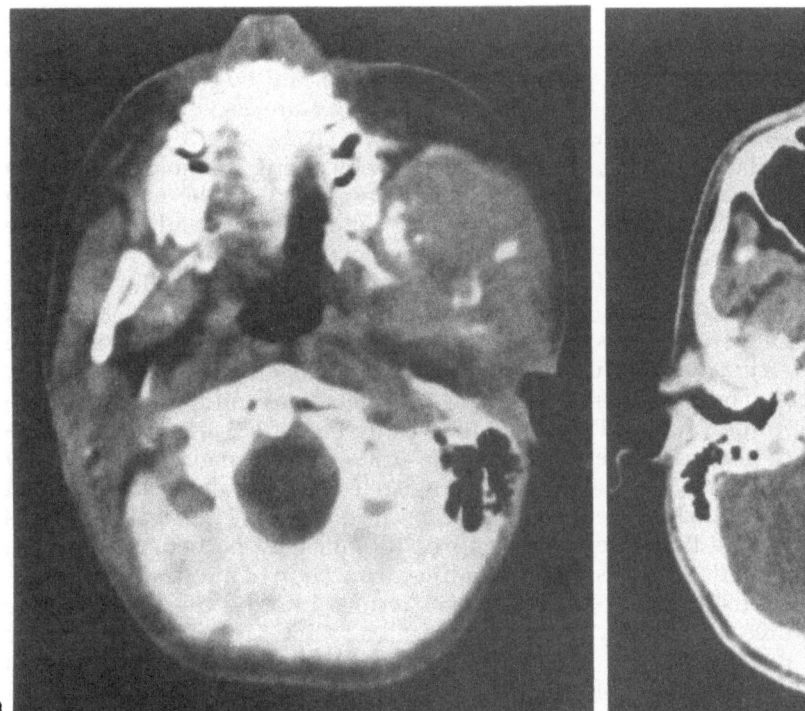
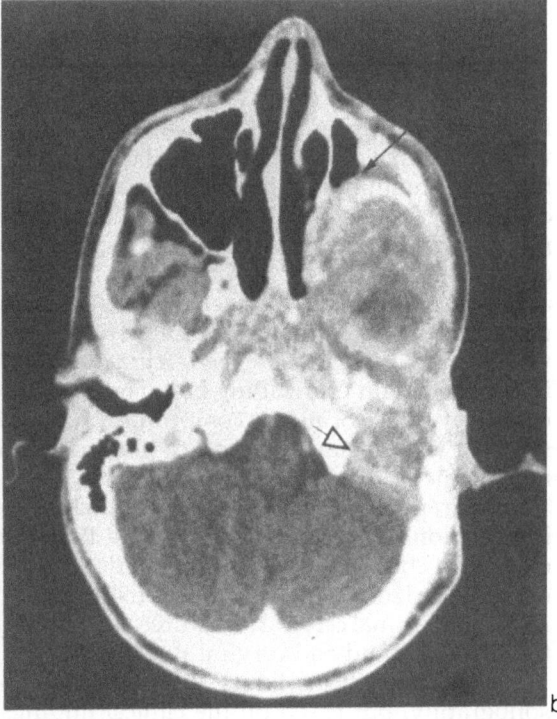

a   b

Fig. 20.14a,b. An 11-year-old boy with a left mandibular osteosarcoma. **a** CT scan showing left mandibular destruction with an adjacent soft tissue mass which contains some areas of ossification. **b** Extension of tumor into the temporal fossa, petrous bone (*open arrow*), and through the posterior wall of the left maxillary sinus (*arrow*). (Donoghue et al. 1984 [2])

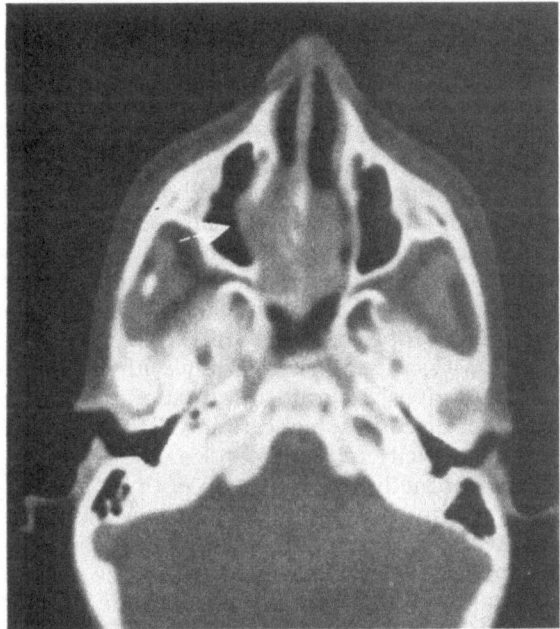

Fig. 20.15. A 3½-year-old girl with recurrent nasopharyngeal endodermal sinus tumor. CT scan shows extension of tumor into right maxillary antrum and nasal cavity. *Arrow* shows bone erosion. (O'Sullivan et al. 1983 [5])

Other Modalities

Nuclear medicine studies did not play a major role in the investigation of patients in our series. ^{67}Ga citrate scans proved sensitive but non-specific. In seven there was uptake of gallium in the mass and these included rhabdomyosarcoma, lymphoma, neuroblastoma, osteosarcoma, and lymphoepithelioma. Gallium uptake may also be seen in inflammatory masses. Radionuclide ^{99m}Tc and ^{131}I scans were not as sensitive as sonography in the evaluation of multiple focal thyroid lesions but may be useful, though non-specific, in determining the activity of focal thyroid abnormalities.

Angiography was performed as an aid to surgery in four patients, one with nasopharyngeal endodermal sinus tumor, one with angiofibroma, one with osteosarcoma of the mandible, and the fourth with a false aneurysm of the right common carotid artery.

Summary

Plain radiographs are of little value in children with a neck mass. The presence of calcification, fat or air within the mass or adjacent bone destruction are helpful findings but are not commonly present. Airway narrowing is only evident in those children with clinical evidence of airway compromise. We feel that plain radiographs of the neck are only indicated in patients with neck masses in whom it is felt that the lesion is of bony origin or invading bone, or if there is clinical evidence of airway compromise and a CT scan is not deemed necessary for adequate management.

Sonography and CT both yield much more information than plain radiographs. Both are capable of characterizing a mass and defining its exact site, size, extent, and relationship to surrounding normal cervical structures, particularly the thyroid gland and cervical vasculature.

Lack of specificity limits the usefulness of sonography, but based on the clinical findings, site, and echo pattern of the mass this modality is often useful in narrowing down the list of possible causes for the mass. The main use of sonography is in the differentiation of diffuse from focal thyroid lesions and in the accurate localization of small and moderate-sized extrathyroidal masses and the delineation of their relationship to normal structures. Sonography is able to define the anatomy of the thyroid gland independently of the functional state of the tissue and thus may provide information not obtained by radionuclide scan. However, sonography is limited in the delineation of the extent and anatomical relationships of huge neck masses, as the entire anatomy of the neck is impossible to delineate in single images, and the grossly distorted anatomy may be difficult to recognize. Lesions associated with bone or airway are also inadequately defined by sonography.

The use of sonography in the evaluation of lesions involving vessels of the neck has been well documented in adults. Although sonography has limited application in children, it is helpful not only in delineating the relationship of a mass to the adjacent vessels but also as the initial modality in delineating lesions derived from the cervical vessels. Scans during Valsalva maneuver are useful in defining ectatic internal jugular veins.

Sonography is the ideal initial screening modality in the evaluation of most pediatric neck masses, but there are a number of instances where CT is essential. Although the appearances of mass lesions on CT are also not always specific, this modality may be able to characterize a lesion more fully by giving valuable information regarding the vascularity of the mass. CT can also delineate alterations in adjacent tissue planes in more detail than sonography.

The greatest value of CT is its ability to define the detailed anatomical extent of mass lesions of the neck, particularly those that arise from or are adjacent to bone or the airway (see Figs. 20.11, 20.12, 20.14). Intracranial and intraspinal extension of the soft tissue masses are exquisitely displayed by CT. Intracranial extension of nasopharyngeal lesions is best depicted in direct coronal scans (see Fig. 20.11), and intraspinal extension of tumors may be better delineated after intrathecal injection of metrizamide. Extension of neck lesions into the chest is also more clearly delineated with CT than sonography (see Fig. 20.2). Primary bone tumors rarely occur in the neck, but CT is just as valuable in their evaluation as it is with their counterparts in the rest of the body (see Fig. 20.14). The exact relationship of masses to the airway is best delineated by CT as air does not degrade the CT image. Even minor alterations in airway caliber (see Fig. 20.2), which may not be appreciated on plain radiographs, will be easily documented by CT. CT plays a major role in the delineation of huge lesions, the extent of which cannot be adequately assessed with sonography (see Fig. 20.2). In addition, CT enables accurate detection of associated nonpalpable lymph nodes, especially if they lie deep to the sternocleidomastoid muscle, and thus improves the accuracy of staging neoplasms [6] (see Fig. 20.9). Finally, CT offers the most accurate means of follow-up of patients who have received radiation treatment and/or chemotherapy. It is of particular value in the postradiation period, when it is frequently difficult to assess the neck clinically with accuracy. CT thus gives accurate information regarding extent of disease, while certain CT features add some specificity to the diagnosis.

Nuclear medicine studies do not play a major role in the investigation of neck masses, as these are usually nonspecific. Both inflammatory lesions and a wide variety of neoplastic masses may take up ^{67}Ga citrate. Radionuclide thyroid scans are not as sensitive as sonography in the evaluation of multiple focal thyroid disease but may be useful, although nonspecific, in determining the activity of focal abnormalities.

Angiography is only necessary in uncommon instances as an aid to the surgeon or as an interventional modality in the therapy of malignant and vascular tumors.

Although the echo pattern of neck masses is nonspecific, sonography is the ideal screening modality in the majority of pediatric neck masses. When sonographic findings are combined with clinical findings sufficient information is available to give adequate treatment to children with inflammatory and small benign cystic lesions and small solid lesions. Large cystic lesions and large solid lesions are more adequately assessed by CT as their extent is more accurately defined with this modality. This is particularly true of lesions associated with bone or the airway. Plain radiographs, radionuclide studies, and angiography are uncommonly required and should be reserved for specific situations.

References

1. Bachrach LK, Daneman D, Daneman A, Martin DJ (1983) Use of ultrasound in childhood thyroid disorders. J Pediatr 103:547–552
2. Donoghue V, Daneman A, Fitz CR (1984) The radiological investigation of neck masses in children: a review of 127 patients. Paper presented at the Meeting of the European Society for Pediatric Radiology, Florence, April 1984
3. Friedman AP, Haller JO, Goodman JD, Nagar H (1983) Sonographic evaluation of non-inflammatory neck masses in children. Radiology 147:693–697
4. Kreipke DL, Lingeman RE (1984) Cross-sectional imaging (CT, NMR) of branchial cysts: report of three cases. J Comput Assist Tomogr 8 (1):114–116
5. O'Sullivan P, Daneman A, Chan HSL, Smith C, Robey G, Fitz C, Martin DJ (1983) Extragonadal endodermal sinus tumors in children: a review of 24 cases. Pediatr Radiol 13:249–257
6. Reede DL, Whelan MA, Bergeron RT (1982) Computed tomography of the infrahyoid neck. Part II: Pathology. Radiology 145:397–402
7. Silverman PM, Korobkin M, Moore AV (1983) Computed tomography of cystic neck masses. J Comput Assist Tomogr 7 (3):498–502
8. Som PM, Zimmerman RA, Biller HF (1984) Cystic hygroma and facial nerve paralysis. A rare association. J Comput Assist Tomogr 8(1):110–113

MUSCULOSKELETAL SYSTEM

Chapter 21

Soft Tissues

Introduction

Computed tomography has had a major impact on the evaluation of soft tissue masses of the musculoskeletal system in children. The cross-sectional display of the soft tissues of the musculoskeletal system and the high density and spatial resolution of CT have made delineation of the origin and extent of soft tissue lesions much more accurate than with the older modalities such as plain radiography, angiography, and radionuclide studies. CT is capable of delineating lesions arising in all the components of the soft tissues including skin, subcutaneous fat, muscles, vascular channels, and nerves. In this regard CT has proved useful in many congenital, inflammatory, traumatic, and neoplastic disorders [18, 19]. The information obtained from these studies has made the use of more invasive techniques such as angiography redundant.

Another extremely valuable capability of CT is the characterization of soft tissue lesions. For example, negative attenuation values will be found in lipomas, which are uncommon in children. Abscesses may show central areas of low attenuation but surrounding areas of great enhancement because of the inflammatory reaction. Neoplasms may have central areas of low attenuation caused by areas of fibrosis or necrosis and tend to enhance along the periphery in the more vascular areas to a lesser degree than abscesses. Unfortunately, many processes may have a nonspecific appearance, and the characterization of these lesions will require correlation with clinical findings and appearances on other imaging modalities. This applies to both benign and malignant processes.

Sonography has also proved extremely useful in the delineation of soft tissue lesions but is somewhat limited in its ability to define the exact extent of larger lesions and cannot delineate associated bony erosion or reaction. Both CT and ultrasound are valuable for the guidance of biopsy of soft tissue lesions and for drainage of fluid collections.

However, CT is not without its limitations in the assessment of abnormalities of the soft tissues of the musculoskeletal system. The paucity of fat and concomitant poor visualization of tissue planes in children, particularly in the legs and forearms, often makes the precise delineation of the margins of soft tissue masses and their relationship to vascular bundles difficult. This is particularly true with malignant lesions, when it may be impossible to differentiate whether the lesion has infiltrated or merely compressed adjacent muscles. In contrast, benign mass lesions tend to be better defined, and the plane of separation between the mass and the adjacent muscles may be more easily visualized on CT. Differentiation of benign from malignant mass lesions is difficult, however, and one should not rely entirely on the appearance of the margins of the mass. Scans performed during the intravenous injection of contrast material will help to delineate the major neurovascular bundles and their relationship to the mass. Occasionally, differential enhancement between the mass and surrounding musculature will help to define the margins of the mass better.

The limitations of CT in the evaluation of soft tissue masses may be listed as follows:

1. Small masses or those that are isodense with muscle may be better delineated with sonography.
2. If there is asymmetry of the two sides of the body a mass may be overlooked.
3. The relative paucity of fat in children may make delineation of the extent of the lesion difficult.
4. Adjacent bone changes may not be due to bony invasion but may simply represent reaction.
5. Adjacent edema should not be considered part of the lesion.
6. Adjacent bony resorption, particularly in the medulla, may be either due to disease or vascular hyperemia.

Despite these limitations we have still found CT to be the most accurate imaging modality in the assessment of soft tissue masses of the extremities in children. This is particularly true of lesions that lie deep and/or are adjacent to bone. CT defines the radial and longitudinal extent of the mass exquisitely and easily confirms or excludes bony involvement or reaction.

Technique

Uncooperative or very young patients should be sedated in order to obtain an adequate study. Even if the patient is cooperative, it is usually helpful to tape the patient's extremities in position in order to prevent small degrees of movement during the scans. It is extremely important to tape the extremities in as symmetrical a position as possible so that the appearances of an abnormal extremity can be compared with the opposite side. This is also very valuable when studying soft tissue lesions around the pelvis or shoulder girdle. When examining lesions of the upper extremities the arms should be extended above the head and taped in position. In those patients who cannot move their arms into this position because of pain, or because of a mass or the presence of a prothesis, the study should be performed with the arms alongside the chest. This is a less desirable position as soft tissue

detail is difficult to obtain with a large scan aperture to include the entire chest and arms. Patients are usually studied in the supine position, but if a soft tissue lesion is on the posterior aspect of the trunk or extremities it is often better to examine the patient prone so that the lesion is not distorted by being in the dependent position (see Fig. 2.2, p. 13).

An initial computed radiograph should be obtained of the area to be examined and this is usually performed in the anteroposterior view. From this radiograph the limits of the scan can be chosen. We have found it most useful to perform studies during the intravenous bolus injection of contrast material, but in selected instances scans prior to contrast or after contrast administration may be useful. The bolus technique is extremely useful for delineation of the major vascular bundles and also helps to define the vascularity of the lesion and thus its character.

The transverse axial scans should be used to assess the radial and longitudinal extent of the mass and its relationship to bone, neurovascular bundles, and joints. The scans should be viewed at both soft tissue and bone windows, and numerous soft tissue attenuation values should be measured in various parts of the lesion.

Once the transverse scans are completed the lines marking the limits of the mass can be posted on the scout radiograph. Reconstruction of images has not proved helpful as the resolution is poor, and we have seldom used the technique. It is occasionally useful, however, to demonstrate lesions in this way as clinicians often find it facilitates interpretation of the anatomy. Direct coronal and sagittal scans of the extremities or the torso can be obtained, particularly in younger children, who can fit into the gantry more easily in these unusual positions, but in our experience these scans have seldom given us extra useful information.

Edema, Hematomas, and Infection

Computed tomography is certainly not the modality of choice for the detection of edema. There is usually clinical evidence if the superficial tissues are involved, and involvement of deeper structures may be shown by conventional radiography. Edema appears as thickening of the soft tissue septa, blurring of adjacent muscle and ligamentous edges, and changes in

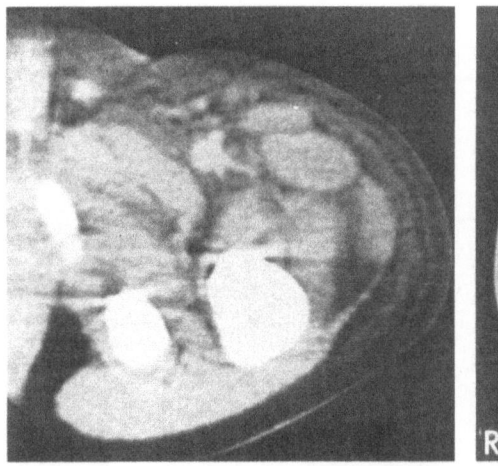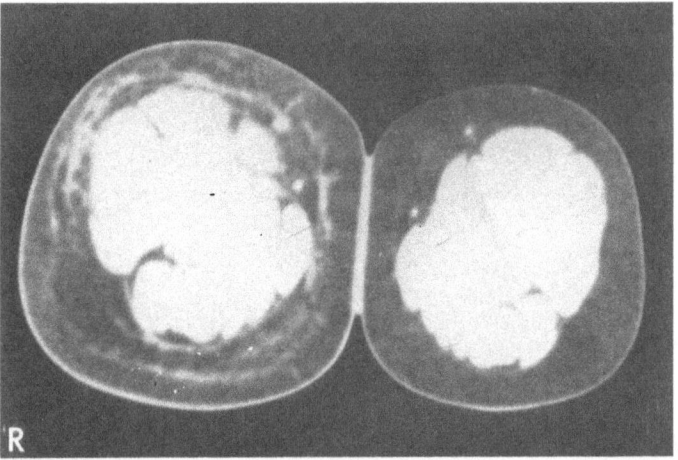

a
b

Fig. 21.1a. A 12-year-old boy with large pelvic rhabdomyosarcoma causing obstruction of venous return from the left lower limb. Edema is present in the subcutaneous tissues mainly anteriorly and laterally at the level of the greater trochanter. This manifests as an irregular increase in attenuation of the fatty tissues and can be compared with the normal fat of the subcutaneous tissue posteriorly. **b** A 14-year-old girl with congenital lymphedema of the right lower limb. Note that the size of the right thigh is larger than the left. There is tissue of irregular outline and increased attenuation in the subcutaneous tissues encircling the limb on the right, representing lymphedema and dilated lymphatic channels. This can be compared with the normal subcutaneous tissue on the left. The study was performed to assess the exact extent of this process for adequate plastic operation.

the negative attenuation values of fat, which may indeed become positive. (Fig. 21.1). However, edema does occur in association with other focal soft tissue lesions such as abscess or neoplasms. It is important in these situations not to misinterpret the edematous changes with those of the adjacent neoplasms. The changes that are seen with edema are somewhat nonspecific and may be also seen in some patients with lymphangiectasia (Fig. 21.1) or diffuse hemorrhage into the soft tissues.

Hematomas may occasionally appear as somewhat diffuse increased attenuation of the soft tissues but more frequently appear as more focal mass lesions (Fig. 21.2). Hematomas are nonenhancing lesions, and their attenuation values will depend on the age of the hematoma. Recent lesions will have attenuation values higher than

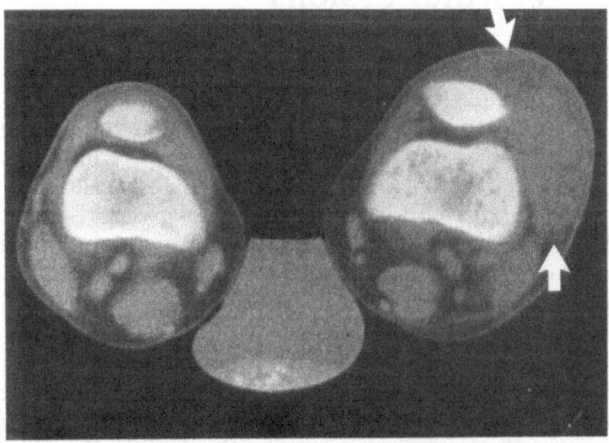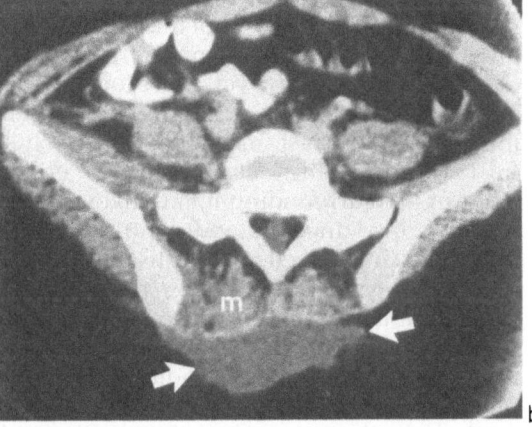

a
b

Fig. 21.2a. A boy with hemophilia and hematoma (*arrows*) of the vastus lateralis muscle on the left. The knee joint is spared. The hematoma blends with the surrounding muscle and its attenuation is similar to that of the muscles. **b** Localized hematoma (*arrows*) posterior to the back muscles (*m*) at the lumbosacral junction following pelvic trauma. Note that the attenuation of the hematoma is less than that of the adjacent muscles.

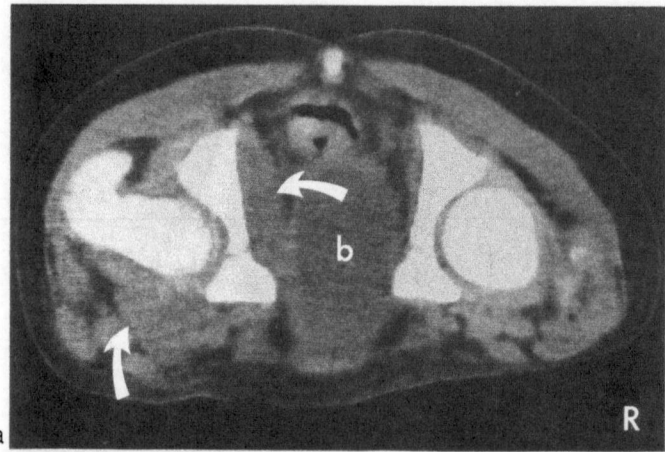

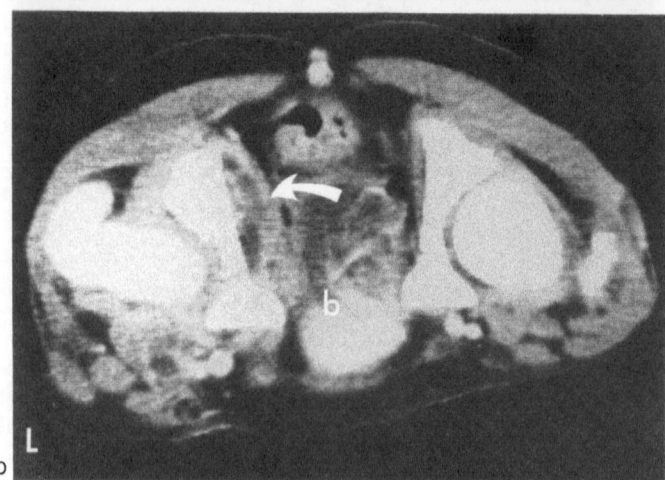

Fig. 21.3a,b. A 12-year-old boy with septic arthritis of the left hip. Scans before (**a**) and after (**b**) intravenous contrast administration were performed with the patient in the prone position. Note the enlargement of the soft tissues adjacent to the left hip (*curved arrows*) both superficially and internally. Following contrast administration there has been enhancement of the peripheral portions of this tissue; the unenhanced central areas represent areas of pus. The CT showed the exact extent of the soft tissue involvement adjacent to the left hip more accurately than any other modality. *b*, bladder

the adjacent muscle, but older lesions will have lower values.

Inflammatory processes of the soft tissues may give changes on CT which mimic those of edema described above. However, more focal abscesses will appear as mass lesions (Fig. 21.3). The use of intravenous contrast injection is extremely useful to delineate these lesions, as the enhancement of the surrounding inflammatory tissue is usually quite dramatic and contrasts with the nonenhancing central necrotic tissue. The extent of such lesions is much better shown after contrast administration. In the presence of inflammatory lesions of the soft tissues it is always important to evaluate the adjacent bone with images taken at bone windows to assess any cortical reaction or erosion. Attenuation values of the medullary cavity should also be obtained to assess whether the fatty marrow has been replaced by inflammatory tissue.

Vascular Lesions

In scans performed without contrast enhancement the superficial veins in the subcutaneous tissue are usually easily seen in many individuals. Because of the paucity of fatty planes in younger children the deeper vascular bundles may be difficult to visualize and may only be easily seen during intravenous bolus contrast administration. Such an injection should be done into a limb that is not within the scanner gantry. This will ensure homogeneous dilineation of both the arteries and veins of the limb being studied. Injection into the superficial veins of the limb under examination will lead to very high enhancement of these veins, and the deeper vascular structures may not show as much enhancement.

The commonest type of vascular lesions that we have studied with CT are the hemangiomas and related lesions of soft tissue. We have reviewed 19 such lesions seen in 17 children over a 5-year period at the Hospital for Sick Children, Toronto [14]. There were 12 females and 5 males, and the age at the time of presentation ranged from 2 months to $17\frac{1}{2}$ years. In 11 patients the diagnosis was confirmed histologically, but in the remaining 6 the diagnosis was based on clinical findings. These lesions occurred in the extremities, chest wall, abdominal wall, and neck.

The classification of vasoformative lesions is beset with a confusing nomenclature which has evolved, at least in part, from a lack of understanding of their pathophysiology. Capillary hemangiomas form the largest group of these benign lesions and clinically are characterized by rapid growth in the neonatal period followed by slow involution [8]. The early proliferative lesion is formed of plump endothelial cells with slit-like lumina and moderate numbers of mitotic figures. During the involuting phase the vascular channels dilate and the endothelial lining becomes flattened. Interstitial fibrosis and thrombus formation may also occur at this time. Cavernous hemangiomas occur less frequently. Often they are larger and less likely to undergo involution. They have a great tendency to be found in deeper locations, where they may compress or destroy neighboring structures. Microscopically they are composed of dilated channels lined by flattened endothelium. Thrombus is not infrequent, and organizing thrombi may demonstrate dystrophic calcification (Fig. 21.4).

On CT hemangiomas have a varying appearance [14]. We have not studied this group of lesions with time density curves, but in general these lesions tend to show marked enhancement after intravenous contrast injection. The enhancement may be homogeneous or extremely inhomogeneous. The homogeneous enhancement probably correlates with the growth phase of the hemangioma, whereas involuting lesions have a more inhomogeneous appearance with increased amounts of fibrous and fatty tissue and phleboliths as compared with those in the proliferative phase. Illustrations in previous chapters have shown examples of these lesions in the proliferative phase (see Fig. 17.1, p. 267) and also in the involuting stage (see Fig. 6.1, p. 71). In our group of patients phleboliths were noted in only six, all of whom had lesions in the involuting phase. The fibrofatty component of the hemangiomas is easily delineated on CT as sep-

arate from the enhancing more vascular areas. Hemangiomas usually have a somewhat ill-defined outline but occasionally may be well defined.

Hemangiomas may also occur in deeper structures such as muscle. In this location they are often accompanied by a large amount of adipose tissue, which may represent replacement of the affected muscle by fat [1, 9]. This lesion may be called an angiolipoma, but we prefer the term "intramuscular cavernous hemangioma" (Fig. 21.5). These lesions are often extremely ill defined, and the negative attenuation values of the fat are easily measured. Their invasive-like character often makes operative removal difficult.

Similarly, lymphangiomas may be capillary, cavernous, or cystic in type and are usually seen in the upper portion of the body. The cystic type (cystic hygroma) are usually well circumscribed, but the capillary and cavernous types are not as easily delineated clinically and have a tendency to recur. Occasionally, involvement of adjacent bone is seen. It may be difficult on microscopy to differentiate lymphangiomas from hemangiomas. Lymphangiomas have a paucity of smooth muscle with loose aggregates of lymphoid tissue. However, hemorrhage into a lymphangioma may make it appear as a hemangioma. On CT the lymphangiomas appear as better defined lesions, usually with larger cystic spaces which fail to enhance (see Fig. 4.34, p. 52). Trabeculae between the cystic components may show enhancement. Occasionally, small lesions may be ill defined with a nonspecific, nonenhancing appearance (Fig. 21.6).

Because hemangiomas and related lesions can arise in a variety of sites and bear differing constituent elements their appearance and enhancement may be expected to vary on CT (see Figs. 21.4, 21.5; see also Fig. 17.1, p. 267, and Fig. 6.1, p. 71). Most cutaneous vascular lesions can be diagnosed by their characteristic clinical features, but their extent may be difficult to assess clinically and at surgery. The important role of CT is in the definition of the extent of these lesions as a guide for the surgeon or for conservative follow-up.

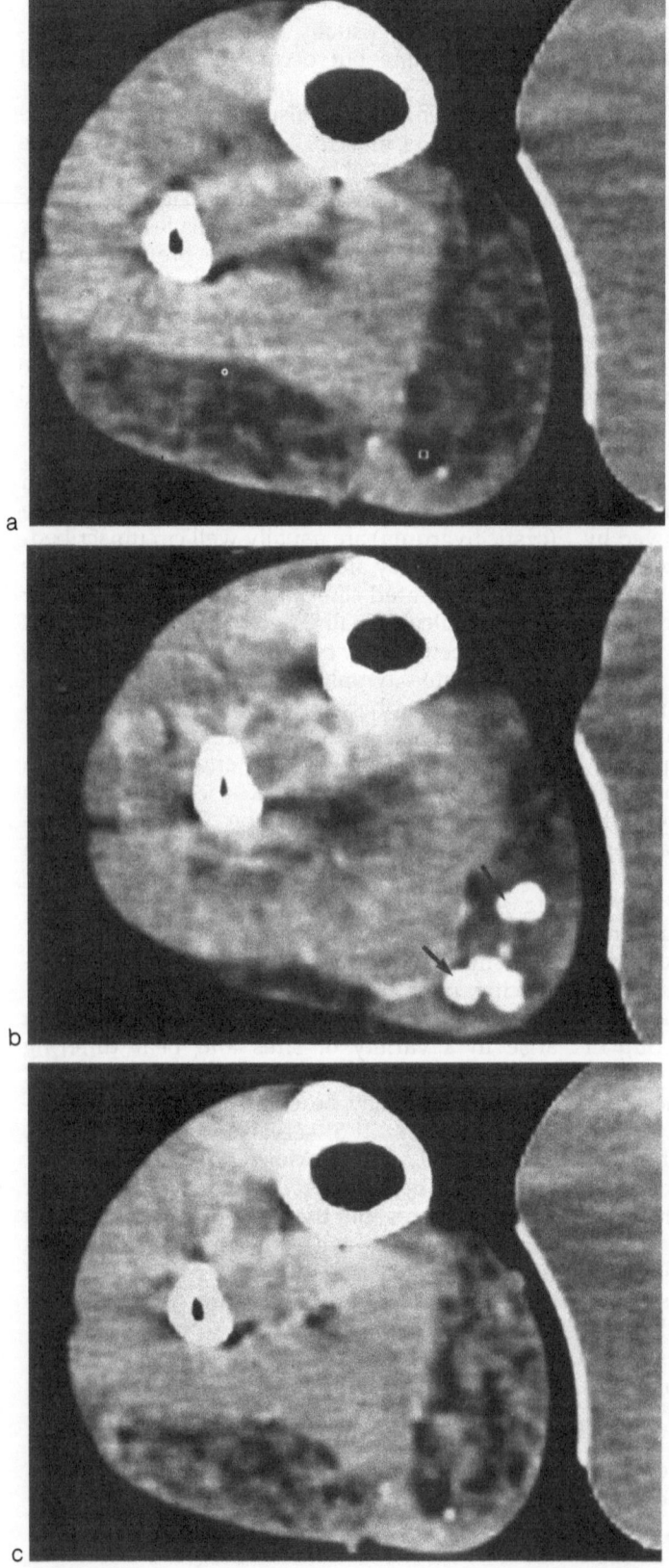

Fig. 21.4a–c. A 10½-year-old boy with clinical diagnosis of hemangioma of the calf. **a, b** Nonenhanced scans show that the entire gastrocnemius of the right leg is diffusely involved by a lesion of inhomogeneous attenuation. This contains fatty elements (*white cursor*) and phleboliths (*arrows*). **c** Inhomogeneous enhancement is seen following contrast administration. (Liu et al. 1985 [14])

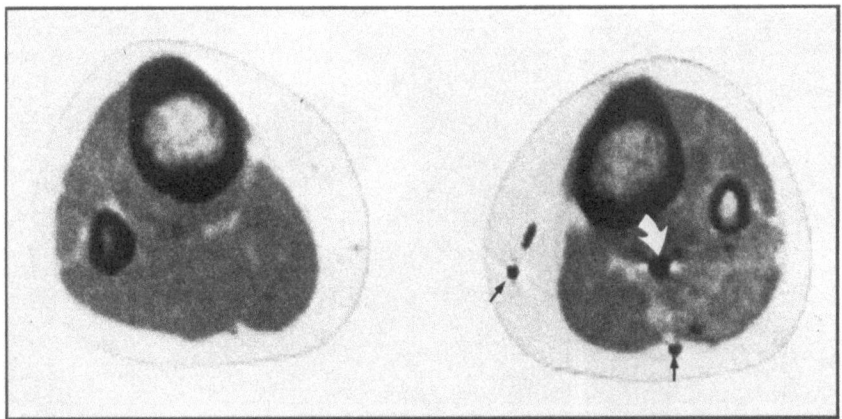

Fig. 21.5. A 13-year-old girl with angiolipoma. CT scan during injection of water-soluble contrast into a vein on the dorsum of the left foot. *Curved arrow*, popliteal vein; *small arrows*, superficial veins. In the lateral head of the left gastrocnemius an area of lower attenuation than the surrounding muscles is present. This area has irregular margins and it extends anteriorly into the muscles of the anterior compartment of the leg. The attenuation value of this lesion was equal to that of fat in many sites. (Liu et al. 1985 [14])

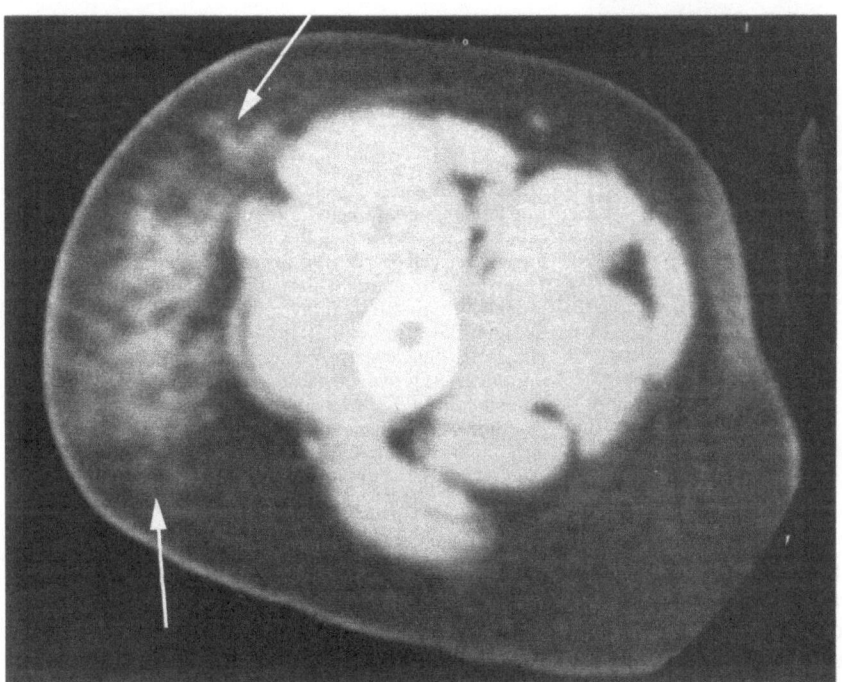

Fig. 21.6. A 1½-year-old girl with lymphangioma of the right thigh. Nonenhanced scan of the right thigh reveals an illdefined lesion (*arrows*) infiltrating the subcutaneous tissues. The underlying muscles are not involved. Postcontrast scans showed no enhancement of the lesion.

Nerve Sheath Lesions

Peripheral nerves are not usually detected on CT in children. We have had the opportunity to study one male with neurofibromatosis in whom multiple well-defined areas of low attenuation were noted in the lower limbs (Fig. 21.7) [7]. These represented fusiform enlargement of peripheral nerves because of neurofibromatous involvement. This is well known to occur in patients with neurofibromatosis. The nerves have an increased amount of endoneural myxoid matrix between the axons. The axons themselves

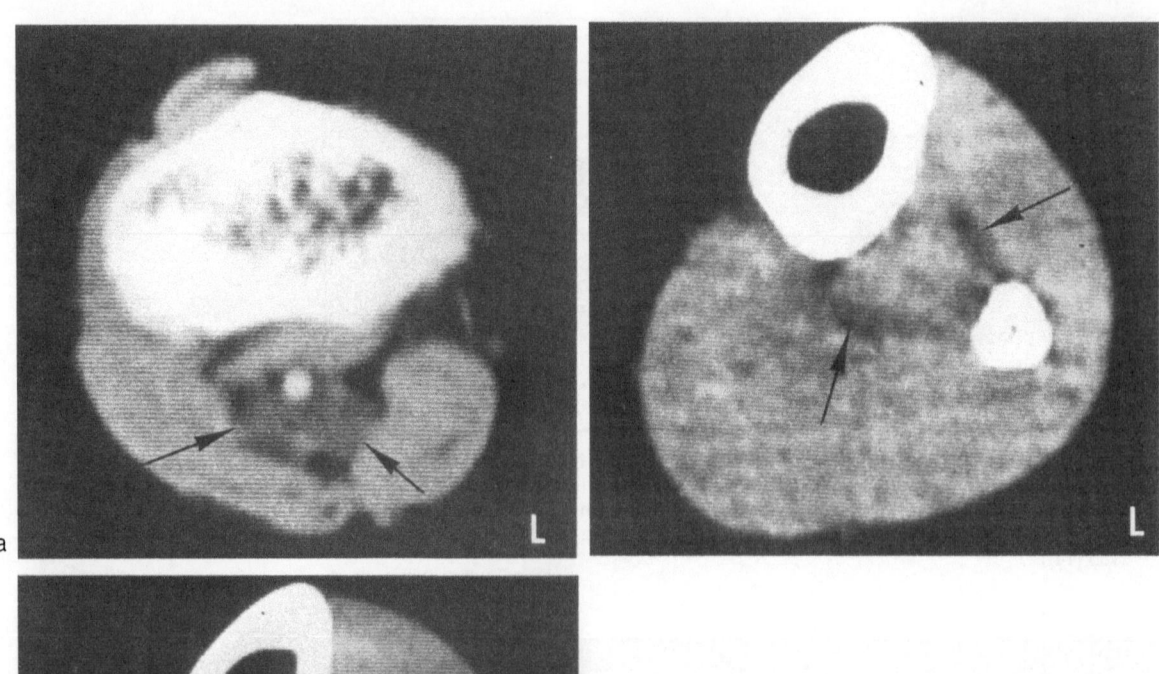

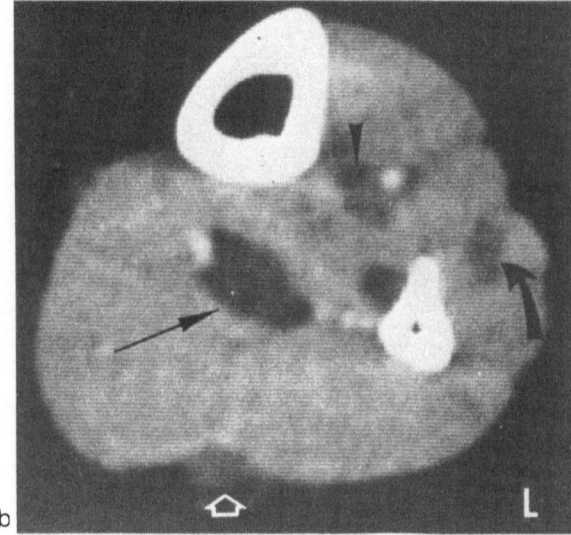

Fig. 21.7a,b. A 13-year-old boy with neurofibromatosis and previous malignant Schwannoma removed from the right calf. CT scans performed through the left popliteal fossa (**a**) and upper calf (**b**) during intravenous contrast injection. This is the same patient shown in Fig. 6.10, p. 76. Adjacent to small high-attenuation enhancing vessels are well-defined, low-attenuation enlarged nerve trunks (15–20 HU). *Long straight arrow*, posterior tibial nerve; *curved arrow*, peroneal nerve; *white arrow*, sural nerve; *arrowhead*, anterior tibial nerve. **c** CT scan through normal calf of another child at same level for comparison. Low-attenuation areas (*arrows*) measuring negative Hounsfield units represent fat planes, not nerves. (Daneman et al. 1983 [7])

retain their usual sheath of Schwann cells. Collagen fibers are present in various amounts in the matrix. The matrix is less dense in appearance, probably because of a greater amount of dissolved tissue fluid, chiefly water. This tends to spread the axons apart, thus enlarging the diameter of the nerve. Enlargement of the intercostal nerves was also noted on the chest CT in this patient (see Fig. 6.10. p. 76).

Biondetti et al. [3] have stressed three features that may be seen on CT which can be considered characteristic of neurofibromatosis. These include the presence of fluid-filled paraspinal masses (meningoceles), neurofibromas showing a homogeneous attenuation value of 30–40 HU and poor contrast enhancement, and skeletal abnormalities such as notching of the ribs and enlargement of neural foramina.

We have seen a further patient with neurofibromatosis in whom a focal neurofibroma had extremely low attenuation values (Fig. 21.8). Kumar et al. [12] described the CT findings in 15 patients with extracranial nerve sheath tumors, including Schwannomas, neurofibromas, plexiform neurofibromas, and neurofibrosarcomas. These authors correlated the appearances on CT with pathological specimens. Attenuation values of 30 HU correlated with dense bands of collagen in the specimens. However, in 11 lesions the attenuation values were significantly lower than muscle. They attributed this reduced attenuation to five factors:

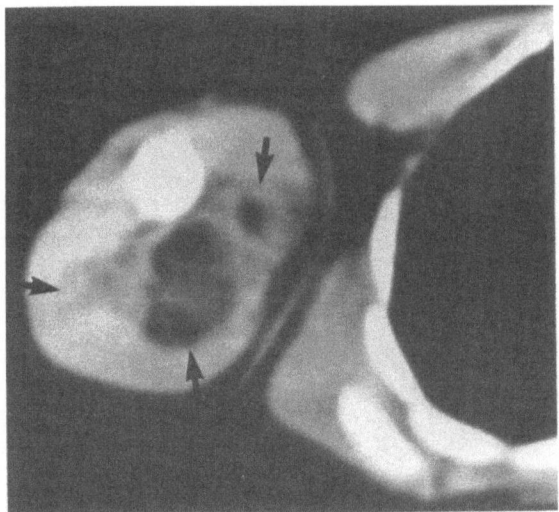

Fig. 21.8. A 14-year-old boy with neurofibromatosis. Scan through upper arm on right shows large neurofibroma in the posteromedial aspect of the arm (*arrows*).

1. A population of lipid-rich Schwann cells

2. The presence of adipocytes in neurofibromas

3. Entrapment of perineural adipose tissue by plexiform neurofibromas

4. Coalescence of interstitial fluid to form cystic spaces in Schwannomas

5. Cystic degeneration secondary to infarction or necrosis with neurofibromas and neurofibrosarcomas

These authors also stressed that the CT appearances were only moderately reliable in distinguishing benign from malignant lesions. Benign lesions tended to have distinct outlines, whereas malignant lesions tended to infiltrate. The appearance of these lesions was difficult to differentiate from abscess or metastases by CT scan alone. Our own experience with CT of extracranial structures in neurofibromatosis is limited. Examples are shown in Figs. 21.7 and 21.8 as well as in Fig. 4.28 (see p. 48), Fig. 15.12 (see p. 233), and Fig. 20.7 (see p. 301).

Perineuroma is an uncommon nerve sheath tumor. We have only seen one example of this where the entire sciatic nerve was thickened and showed marked enhancement with areas of calcification (Fig. 21.9).

Malignant peripheral nerve tumors are indeed uncommon in children. An example is shown in Fig. 21.10. In the two lesions we have studied, enhancement was noted mainly along the periphery with low-attenuation areas centrally.

Fibrous Lesions

Areas of scarring in the skin and subcutaneous tissues are often seen in patients that have suffered previous trauma or had previous surgery. These lesions appear as irregular areas of soft tissue attenuation within the subcutaneous fat. The findings are nonspecific and may be found as incidental findings.

In 1983, Campbell et al. [5] described three cases with aggressive fibromatosis that we had studied. Since that time we have had the opportunity to study two further examples. Fibromatosis was first described in 1839 by Dupuytren, who reported nodules in the palmar fascia of children [17]. In 1954, Stout [22] described 44 cases of fibroblastic lesions in children and infants and established the classification of "juvenile fibromatosis." Mackenzie [15] and Allen [1] reclassified the term "fibromatosis" with a further account of the clinicopathological features. Mackenzie defined fibromatosis as an "infiltrating fibroblastic proliferation showing none of the features of an inflammatory response and no features of unequivocal neoplasia." The term covers a broad group of fibrous lesions which have many characteristics in commmon.

The etiology of fibromatoses is unknown, and they must be differentiated from fibrosarcomas on the one hand and from benign processes in which fibroblasts occur on the other [1, 15]. These lesions may be encountered at any age and at any site and may be focal, multifocal, or diffuse [15]. They are characterized by varying numbers of well-differentiated fibroblasts separated by varying amounts of collagen and reticular fibers. The fibroblasts are uniform in size and lack anaplasia and mitotic activity [1, 15]. The lesions lack a capsule and the margins are often indistinct with extensive invasion and replacement of adjacent muscle and fat. This aggressive local behavior makes these lesions mimic fibrosarcoma; however, because of the benign histological findings and lack of metastases, patients with these lesions should not be considered as having malignant disease [1, 15]. Such lesions are usually relatively harmless but may, on rare occasions, prove fatal [15, 17].

The most effective treatment is surgical removal. To avoid recurrences, a wide margin around the palpable lesion is taken, including all areas of infiltration. Radiotherapy may play a role in the treatment of recurrences [15], or if the lesions become too large for removal. The recur-

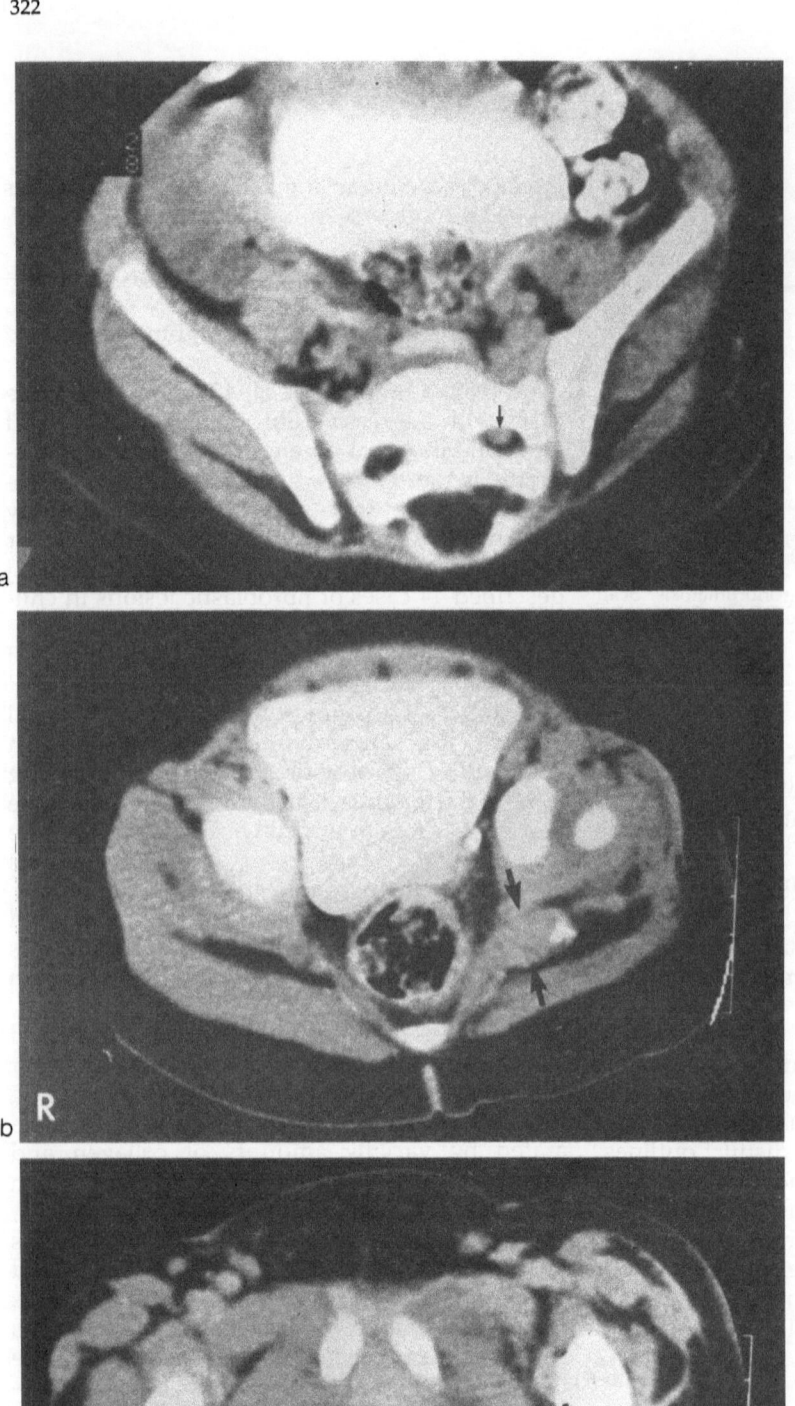

Fig. 21.9a–c. A 15-month-old girl with congenitally small left lower extremity. Note that the musculature on the left is much smaller than that on the right. **a** The nerve root in the sacral foramen on the left (*small arrow*) is much larger than that on the right. **b, c** In lower scans there is marked enlargement of the sciatic nerve (*arrows*), and calcification is noted in this mass in scan **b**. Biopsy proved the presence of a perineuroma involving the sciatic nerve.

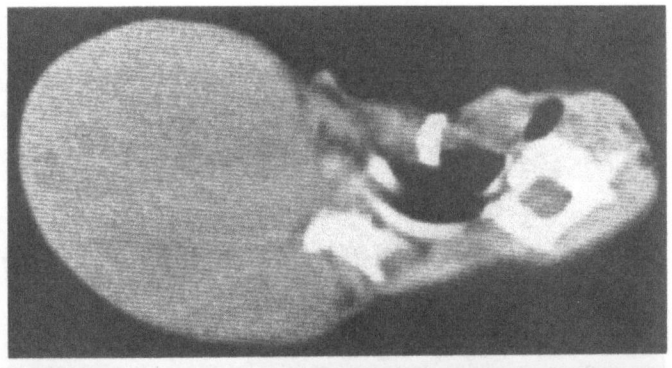

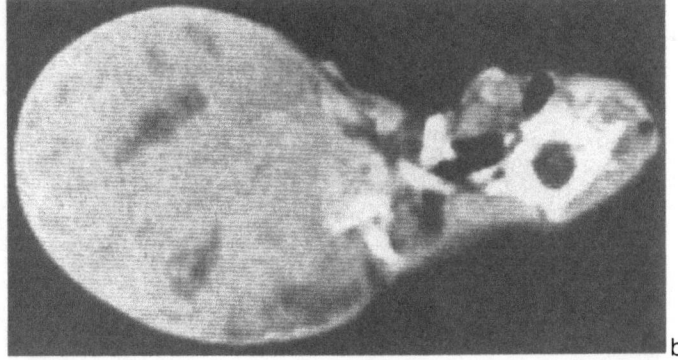

Fig. 21.10a,b. A 1-year-old boy with a large malignant neurogenic tumor of the right arm. Scans before (**a**) and after (**b**) intravenous contrast injection. Note the change in attenuation pattern, which is homogeneous before and inhomogeneous after contrast administration.

rence rate has been reported as high as 50% [17]. Bony destruction is not commonly observed, although involvement of the mandible has been described [17]. The five patients that we have examined illustrate the variability of these lesions with regards to site, size, growth rate, and rate of recurrence in these lesions [17]. Bony involvement may occasionally also be seen.

Computed tomography is the most useful modality in defining the extent of these lesions at diagnosis and in follow-up, as well as in confirming the absence of metastatic disease. These lesions are usually ill defined and have a lower density than muscle with little enhancement after intravenous administration of contrast medium (Fig. 21.11; see also Fig. 6.2, p. 72). We have been able to follow our patients closely with the use of CT scans and have been able to plan treatment accordingly.

Other Malignant Masses

Computed tomography is particularly useful for the delineation of the radial and longitudinal extent of large soft tissue masses. It is possible to differentiate between benign and aggressive masses as benign lesions usually have a smooth well-defined periphery, whereas aggressive lesions have a more ill-defined periphery and a much more heterogeneous or patchy matrix. Indeed, infiltrating lesions that may appear similar on CT are neoplasms, hematomas, and large abscesses. Malignant tumors usually have an average attenuation which may be little lower than normal for muscle and show inhomogeneous enhancement. The type of enhancement and the CT appearances have not been useful in determining the histology of these malignant lesions. At the Hospital for Sick Children, Toronto, we have used CT to delineate numerous types of malignant soft tissue lesions (Figs. 21.10, 21.12, 21.13, 21.14).

In 1984, Israels et al. [10] reported our experience with seven children with synovial sarcoma. This group included five males and two females with mean age at presentation of 4.4 years (see Fig. 21.12).

Synovial sarcoma is a soft tissue sarcoma that occurs near joints, but, despite its name, does not arise from the synovial membrane. It originates from primitive mesenchymal cells that

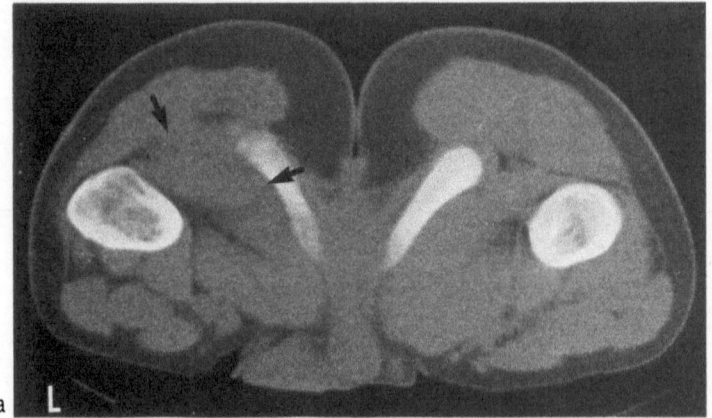

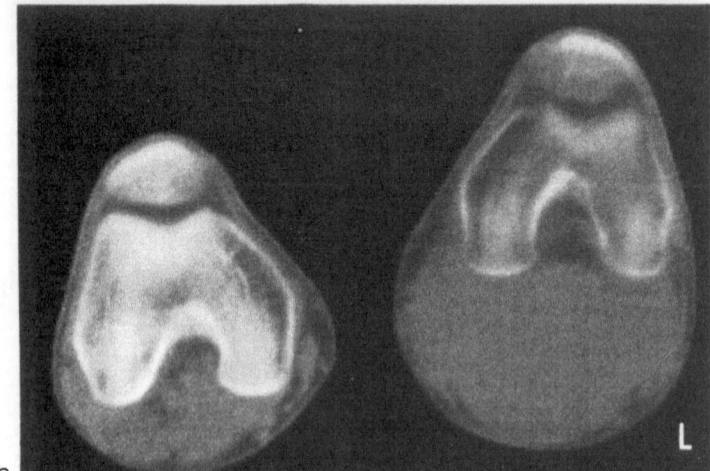

Fig. 21.11a,b. A 15-year-old boy with aggressive fibromatosis of the left buttock and leg. a CT through buttocks in prone position without contrast enhancement shows an ill-defined soft tissue mass (*arrows*) in the left buttock with atrophy of the ipsilateral muscles. The attenuation of the mass is lower than that of the muscles. b CT through level of popliteal fossa shows a large ill-defined mass on the left with an attenuation similar to that of surrounding muscles. It appears to infiltrate the muscles as the muscle margins are poorly defined. (Campbell et al. 1983 [5])

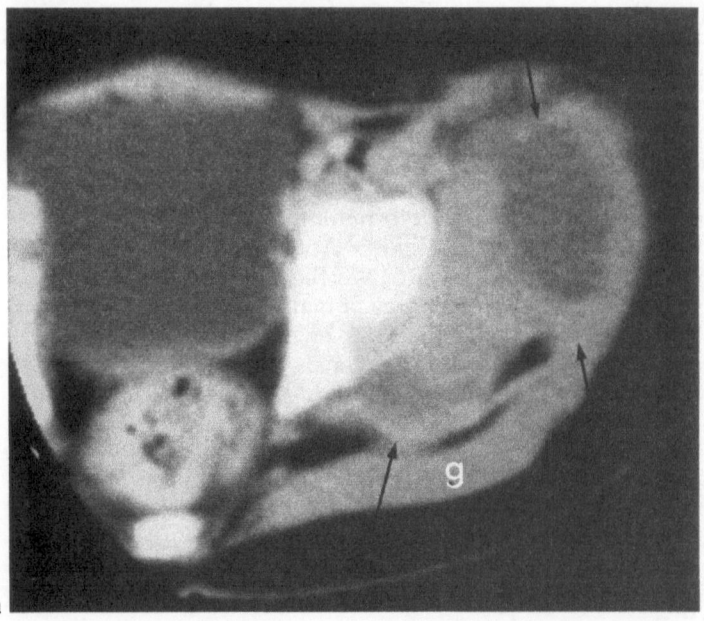

Fig. 21.12a–c. A 2-year-old boy with synovial sarcoma adjacent to left hip. a, b CT scans through pelvis and thigh during intravenous contrast injection. Mass (*arrows*) enhances peripherally and contains large areas of lower attenuation. The margins are poorly defined. It extends superiorly deep to the gluteal muscles (*g*). c Following intensive chemotherapy and radiotherapy CT scan at the same level as scan b shows much poorer enhancement because of large areas of necrosis within the tumor. The lesion is much smaller than at the time of presentation. (Israels et al. 1984 [10])

Fig. 21.12b,c *next page* ▶

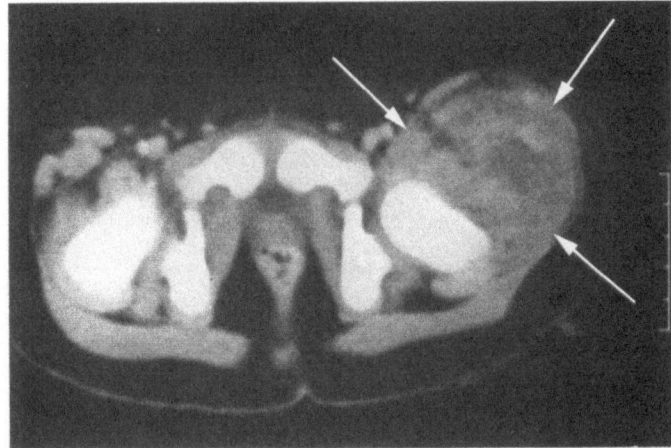

Fig. 21.12b

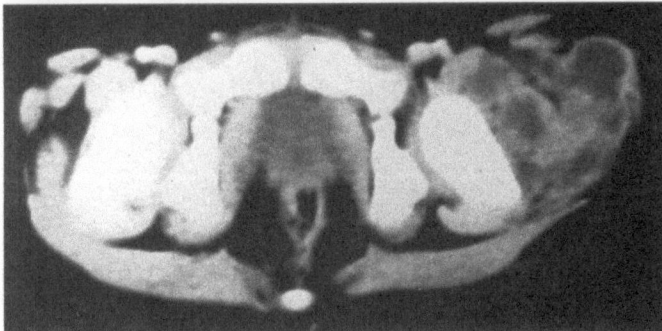

Fig. 21.12c

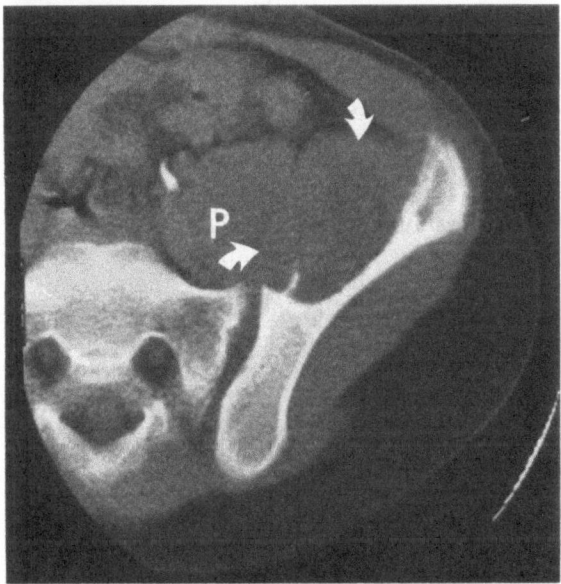

Fig. 21.13. A 12-year-old girl with a small cell anaplastic sarcoma arising in the left iliacus muscle (*curved arrows*). The psoas muscle (*P*) is displaced medially. The mass has caused some erosion and new bone formation along the medial aspect of the left ilium. An area of low attenuation in the central portion of the mass is due to an area of diminished vascularity. (Petterson et al. 1983 [18])

have differentiated sufficiently to resemble the synovium histologically [4]. The seven patients seen at the Hospital for Sick Children, Toronto, account for 2.6% of all soft-tissue sarcomas (268 cases) seen at this institution since 1919.

This tumor is characteristically seen in adults, and most cases present in the third to fifth decades of life [16]. In a review of 24 children with synovial sarcoma, Lee et al. [13] noted that one-half of their patients were 13–15 years old. As already mentioned, our patients were significantly younger, with a mean age of 4.4 years.

Typically the lesions are located in the extremities, especially in the lower extremities [4, 13]. They also occur in the abdominal and thoracic walls, but rarely in the head and neck.

Radiographic findings are nonspecific and usually show a soft tissue mass of water density [16]. In up to 30% of adult cases, there is calcification evident in the tumor mass. Extensive calcification has been suggested as indicating a more favorable prognosis [23]. Bone involvement is reported in about 20% of cases and may be due to either pressure erosion with sharp margins and reactive sclerosis or to direct invasion causing cortical destruction [16]. Plain radio-

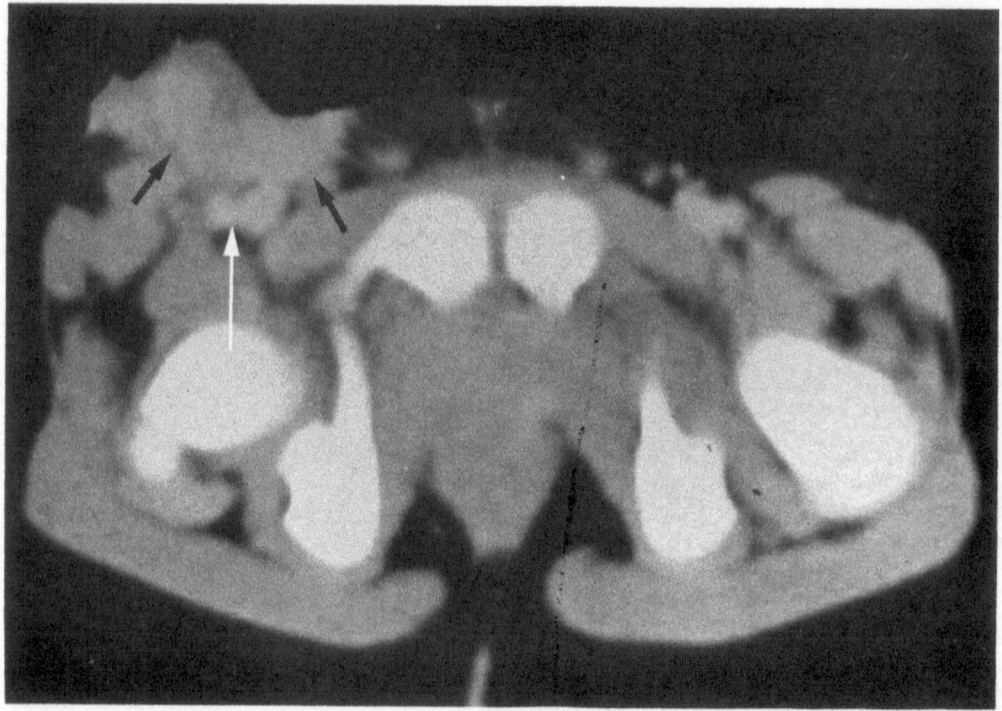

Fig. 21.14. A 10-year-old boy with Hodgkin's disease. CT shows mass of enlarged lymph nodes (*black arrows*) in the right inguinal area ulcerating through the skin. CT was performed to define the deep extent of these nodes in order to facilitate an adequate plastic operation. The *white arrow* indicates the femoral artery laterally and femoral vein medially. These are uninvolved by the tumor.

graphs of the affected parts in four of our patients showed the presence of a soft tissue mass only. No other associated abnormalities were present.

Synovial sarcoma spreads by direct extension along the myofascial planes, and the tumor is often larger than the size suspected clinically.

Metastases may occur many years after diagnosis [21]. "Limb-salvage" operations, together with radiotherapy and chemotherapy, offer the best results [6, 20, 21].

Neuromuscular Diseases

Muscle atrophy is commonly seen in association with ipsilateral congenital or acquired lesions that lead to disuse (see Figs. 21.9, 21.11, 21.12; see also Fig. 15.3, p. 223, Fig. 22.9, p. 337, Fig. 22.19, p. 345, Fig. 23.1, p. 351, and Fig. 23.19, p. 367).

Computed tomography is capable of measuring muscle mass and attenuation values. This is extremely useful in patients with neuromuscular disorders as an aid to the diagnosis and follow-up of these diseases. On CT the muscles involved show atrophy, which is manifested by fatty infiltration into the muscle. The muscles acquire a lower attenuation value because of this. CT is also helpful in delineating the sites of muscle involvement, in quantifying the amount of muscle lost, and determining the amount of fatty replacement. Riddlesberger and Kuhn [19] have stressed the value of CT in helping to establish the pattern of involvement and follow-up as well as in directing the site for biopsy. In these patients standard CT examinations include scans through five areas of the body: neck, shoulder girdle, pelvic girdle, thigh, and lower leg. The same authors have also drawn attention to the regional enlargement of muscle bundles in patients with histiocytic lymphoma and nodular sclerosing Hodgkin's disease. The etiology of this enlargement is uncertain. This is an important consideration when one finds enlarged muscles with normal CT attenuation values in these patients. The muscles revert to normal following therapy.

Foreign Bodies

The high-density resolution of CT makes it an ideal modality for the detection of foreign bodies in the soft tissues when these cannot be located with other more conventional techniques. The transverse axial scans delineate the soft tissues without any bony or gaseous overlap and will allow detection of even small low-density foreign bodies. Their relationships to vital organs and structures is easily documented.

References

1. Allen PW (1977) The fibromatoses: a clinicopathologic classification based on 140 cases. Am J Surg Pathol 1:255–270
2. Allen PW, Enzinger FM (1972) Hemangiomas of skeletal muscle. An analysis of 89 cases. Cancer 29:8–22
3. Biondetti PR, Vigo M, Fiore D, De Faveri D, Ravasini R, Benedetti L (1983) CT appearance of generalized von Recklinghausen neurofibromatosis. J Comput Assist Tomogr 7:866–869
4. Cadman NL, Soule EH, Kelly PJ (1965) Synovial sarcoma. Cancer 18:613–627
5. Campbell AN, Chan HSL, Daneman A, Martin DJ (1983) Agressive fibromatosis in childhood. Computed tomographic findings in three patients. J Comput Assist Tomogr 7:109–113
6. Carson JH, Harwood AR, Cummings BJ, Fornasier V, Langer F, Quirt I (1981) The place of radiotherapy in the treatment of synovial sarcoma. Int J Radiat Oncol Biol Phys 7:49–53
7. Daneman A, Mancer K, Sonley M (1983) CT appearance of thickened nerves in neurofibromatosis. AJR 141:899–900
8. Enzinger FM, Weiss SW (1983) Soft tissue tumors. Mosby, St Louis, pp 379–421
9. Gonzales-Crussi F, Enneking WF, Arean VM (1966) Infiltrating angiolipoma. J Bone Joint Surg [Am] 48:1111–1124
10. Israels SJ, Chan HSL, Daneman A, Weitzman SS (1984) Synovial sarcoma in childhood. AJR 142:803–806
11. King DR, Clatworthy HW (1981) The pediatric patient with sarcoma. Semin Oncol 8:215–221
12. Kumar AJ, Kuhajda FP, Martinex CR, Fishman EK, Jezic DV, Siegelman SS (1983) Computed tomography of extracranial nerve sheath tumors with pathological correlation. J Comput Assist Tomogr 7:857–865
13. Lee SM, Hajdu SL, Exelby PR (1974) Synovial sarcoma in children. Surg Gynecol Obstet 138:701–704
14. Liu P, Daneman A, Stringer DA, Smith CR (to be published) The CT appearances of hemangiomas and related lesions of soft tissues in children. A report of 17 patients. J Can Assoc Radiol
15. MacKenzie OH (1972) The fibromatoses: a clinicopathological concept. Br Med J 4:277–281
16. Murray JA (1977) Synovial sarcoma. Orthop Clin North Am 8:963–972
17. Peede LF, Epker BN (1977) Agressive juvenile fibromatosis involving the mandible. Oral Surg 43:651–657
18. Pettersson H, Daneman A, Harwood-Nash DCF (1983) Computed tomography in pediatric orthopedic radiology. In: Boijsen E, Ekelund L (eds) Computed tomography in orthopedic radiology. Thieme, Stuttgart, pp 26–48
19. Riddlesberger MM, Kuhn JP (1983) The role of computed tomography in diseases of the musculoskeletal system. CT 7:85–99
20. Rosenberg SA, Tepper J, Glatstein E (1982) The treatment of soft-tissue sarcoma of the extremities. Ann Surg 196:305–314
21. Ryan JR, Baker LH, Benjamin RS (1982) The natural history of metastatic synovial sarcoma. Clin Orthop 164:257–260
22. Stout AP (1954) Juvenile fibromatosis. Cancer 7:953–977
23. Varela-Duran J, Enzinger FM (1982) Calcifying synovial sarcoma. Cancer 50:345–352

Chapter 22

Bones

Introduction

Widespread use has been made of CT to delineate congenital, traumatic, infective and neoplastic disorders of bone [3, 7, 8, 9, 10, 13]. At our institution, the greatest impact of CT in skeletal disease is in the delineation of the extent of malignant neoplasms [7, 13].

It should be stressed that CT cannot replace plain radiographs of the skeleton; these offer vital information regarding the character of the lesion, whereas CT appearances are often non-specific. It is also important to understand the unique value of radionuclide bone scans for the detection of multiple lesions. CT should be directed at the primary skeletal process.

Technique

The technique used to study skeletal abnormalities is similar to that outlined for soft tissue lesions in Chapter 21. Adequate sedation is required for very young or uncooperative patients. Positioning of the patient in a position that is both comfortable for the patient and useful for interpretation of scans is of prime importance. Patients with skeletal lesions often have difficulty maintaining their limbs in a single position and the utmost care should be taken in an attempt to provide support for these limbs so that they are not continually moved during scanning. The limbs should be taped either together or to the table, and adequate use of pillows and sponges is desirable to support the limbs and thus maintain a stable position. An attempt should be made to position the patient as symmetrically within the gantry as possible in order that the two sides of the body may be compared. It is also important to attempt to position the patient in such a way that the transverse scans will be at 90° to the long axis of the bone being examined.

An initial anteroposterior computed radiograph is essential, as the limits of the area to be scanned can be chosen from this. Transverse axial scans are then performed through this area. These can be 1 cm thick, although thinner slices are useful for areas where greater detail is required or reconstruction is considered. Intravenous contrast injection is not necessary in all patients with skeletal abnormalities; however, if a soft tissue component is present, we have used bolus intravenous contrast injection to delineate the relationship of the mass to the larger vascular bundles and also in an attempt to differentiate the mass from surrounding muscle. A computer program giving target reconstruction of the raw data obtained during scanning may enhance the spatial and contrast resolution (as described in Chap. 2) and is particularly useful when assessing bone lesions.

The transverse axial scans should be viewed at both soft tissue and bone window settings in order that all the structures in the field can be adequately evaluated. It is extremely important to take attenuation measurements of the medullary cavity with the cursor and these should be compared with the bone in the opposite limb. In this way an accurate evaluation of the extent within the medullary cavity can be achieved. In larger patients with large lesions the transverse axial scans need not be adjacent but may be 1 cm apart.

At the end of the examination, scans following intravenous injection of contrast may be helpful to delineate certain areas that may not have been adequately outlined on the initial scans, or thinner cuts of specific areas may be helpful. The radial size of the mass can be measured with the cursor on the transverse scans.

The lines that mark the scans depicting the longitudinal limits of the soft tissue mass and medullary extent can then be posted on the initial computed radiograph. The distance of these lines to anatomical landmarks can be measured, and this information is vitally important to the orthopedic surgeon and often to the radiotherapist as well.

At the Hospital for Sick Children, Toronto, we have not found that sagittal and coronal reconstruction images or scans performed in the direct coronal or sagittal plane offer much further valuable information than the transverse scan. However, these types of images are occasionally of great benefit to the clinicians, who may be able to interpret the deranged anatomy better than from the transverse scan.

Trauma

Conventional radiography is usually adequate for the delineation of traumatic lesions of the skeleton. However, CT plays a vital role in the delineation of traumatic lesions in areas that are difficult to examine with conventional radiographs. It is beyond the purposes of this chapter to describe these uses of CT; however, in Chapter 23 the value of CT in traumatic lesions of special areas such as the hips, sacroiliac joints, feet, and spine is outlined. In Fig. 22.1 an example of a sacral fracture passing into the sacroiliac joint is shown. The joint involvement was not appreciated on plain films. This image also highlights the importance of symmetrical positioning of the patient in the gantry in order to compare the two sides (see also Chap. 23, p. 362).

Inflammation

The modality of choice for the early detection of osteomyelitis is radionuclide bone scanning. The images obtained by this technique show lesions at an earlier phase than plain radiographs. However, CT is extremely useful in patients with

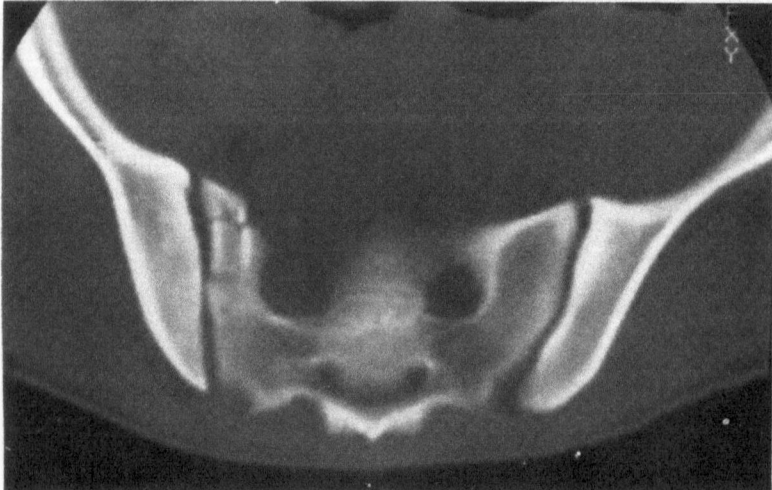

Fig. 22.1. Transverse fractures of the right side of the sacrum passing into the sacroiliac joint with minimum displacement. There is asymmetry in the size of the sacral foramina with absence of bone anterior to the foramen on the right. This asymmetry is simply related to slight patient tilt, and the scan passes directly through the anterior opening of the foramen on the right. This should not be confused with bony erosion on this side. Similar pseudo erosions may be noted in other bones when the patient is not placed straight in the gantry.

equivocal or unusual findings on plain films or radionuclide scans. In the early phases osteomyelitis may produce some demineralization of the bone with a change in the attenuation values of the medullary cavity. The medullary cavity usually has a negative value if it is filled with normal fatty marrow; however, early inflammation may cause the marrow to have an attenuation value higher than that of water. Small erosions and periosteal reaction that may not be present on plain films may well be delineated with CT. A further rare finding is that of gas within the medullary cavity as the result of infection. Associated soft tissue changes such as edema or abscess formation may also be present and, when small, may be detected on CT sooner than on conventional radiography. Other examples of osteomyelitis are illustrated in Fig. 23.12, p. 361, and Fig. 23.18, p. 366.

It should be emphasized that many of the changes that one sees on CT in skeletal disorders are nonspecific. Figure 22.2 is an example of a 5-year-old boy with a painful lesion of the proximal humerus [3]. Plain radiographs had suggested the presence of a malignant bone lesion, and CT showed features of stress fractures as reported by Somer and Meurman [12]. These features include a lucent line through the cortex

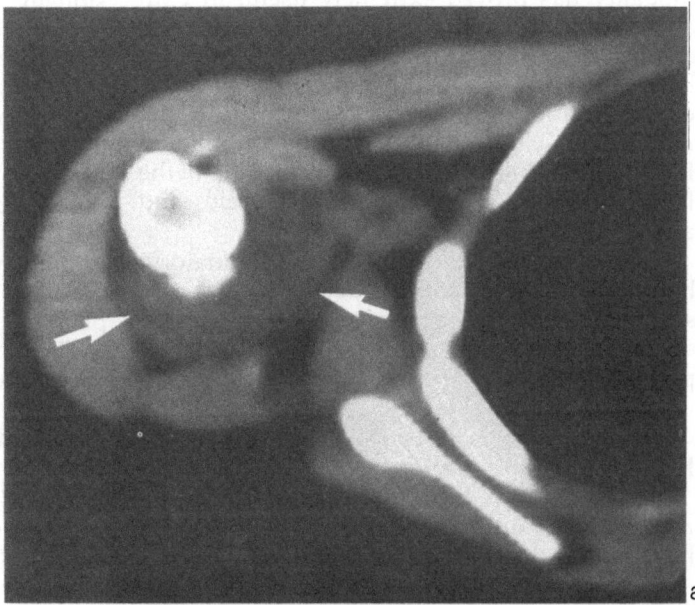

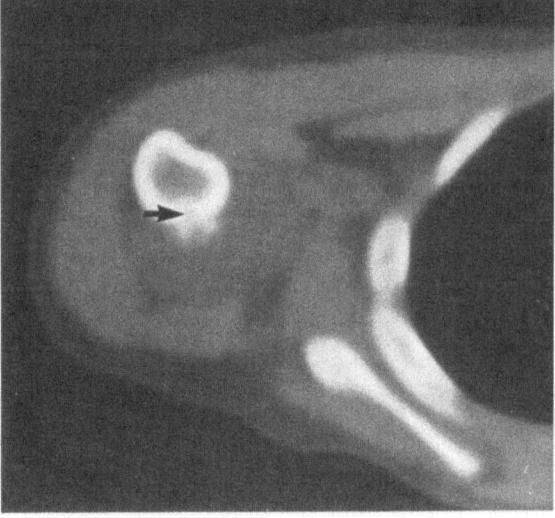

Fig. 22.2a,b. A 5-year-old boy with a painful lesion in the proximal right humerus. Plain radiographs suggested the presence of a malignant bone lesion. **a** CT shows a soft tissue mass (*arrows*) posterolateral to the humerus. **b** The same scan is viewed at bone window levels and shows a linear defect in the cortical bone (*arrow*), new bone formation projecting into the medullary cavity, and soft tissue ossification not separable from the underlying cortex. The presence of the defect in the cortical bone is similar to that described in stress fractures [12]. However, pathologically the lesion was proven to be a reactive periostitis, and follow-up CT and plain radiographs showed complete healing of the changes described. This case illustrates the need for the close correlation between clinical, radiographic, and pathological features for the diagnosis of bone lesions. (Donoghue et al. 1985 [3])

with adjacent sclerosis. However, the pathological findings were that of a reactive periostitis, and follow-up showed clinical and radiographic resolution. This patient is an example of the need for extremely close correlation between clinical, radiographic, and pathological features for the diagnosis of bone lesions.

Neoplasms

Although the appearance of various neoplasms of bone may appear nonspecific on CT, this modality has proved extremely useful in both adults and children in the evaluation of the extent of the disease process. CT can show the location of the tumor in the bone, the integrity or destruction of cortex, the extent within the medullary cavity, and the soft tissue component. It is also valuable to assess the relationship of the lesion to the vital neurovascular bundles and articular surfaces.

Conventional radiography is mandatory, however, in all patients suspected of having a skeletal tumor. The aggressiveness of the lesion and its probable histology can be assessed on plain radiographs.

Benign

At the Hospital for Sick Children, Toronto, we have found that conventional radiography has been extremely useful for both the diagnosis and treatment planning of benign skeletal tumors. CT does not usually provide any extra information regarding the character and histology of these lesions but is occasionally useful for the delineation of the extent of large lesions or those that are found in an area of complex anatomy. Figures 22.3 and 22.4 are examples of such lesions that were difficult to evaluate clinically with plain radiography. Other examples are illustrated in Chapters 6 and 23.

Osteochondromas usually have a sharply defined peripheral cortex and a less dense central medullary cavity continuous with that of the bone from which it arises (Fig. 22.3). The pedunculated cap is usually difficult to delineate. Occasionally, however, these typical findings may not be present, particularly in small lesions, and the appearances may be nonspecific (see Fig. 6.5, p. 73). We have seen many exostoses arise in areas that have been previously irradiated in children with previous malignancy. CT is particularly useful when these lesions arise in unusual sites or areas of complex anatomy (see Fig. 23.20, p. 367). CT may be helpful in determining whether exostoses are benign or have become malignant in those instances where plain radiographic findings are equivocal.

The high spatial and contrast resolution makes CT an ideal modality for the diagnosis and follow-up of osteoid osteomas. CT is particularly useful when the changes on plain radiographs are equivocal or if the lesion is small. CT is also invaluable for the documentation of lesions in areas of complex anatomy (see Fig. 23.19, p. 367) and when recurrence is suspected (see Fig. 23.7,

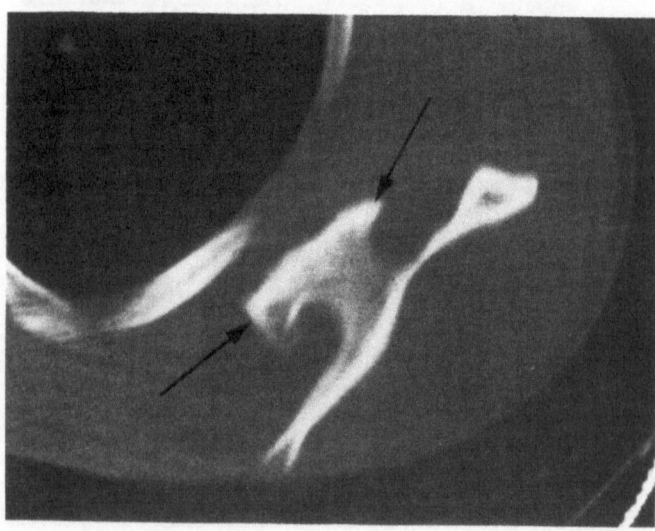

Fig. 22.3. A 16½-year-old boy who had received abdominal and chest radiation for a Wilms' tumor and pulmonary secondaries 11½ years previously. A follow-up chest radiograph revealed an exostosis on the costal surface of the left scapula, which is confirmed on the CT study (*arrows*). The CT defined the anatomy well and provided useful information preoperatively.

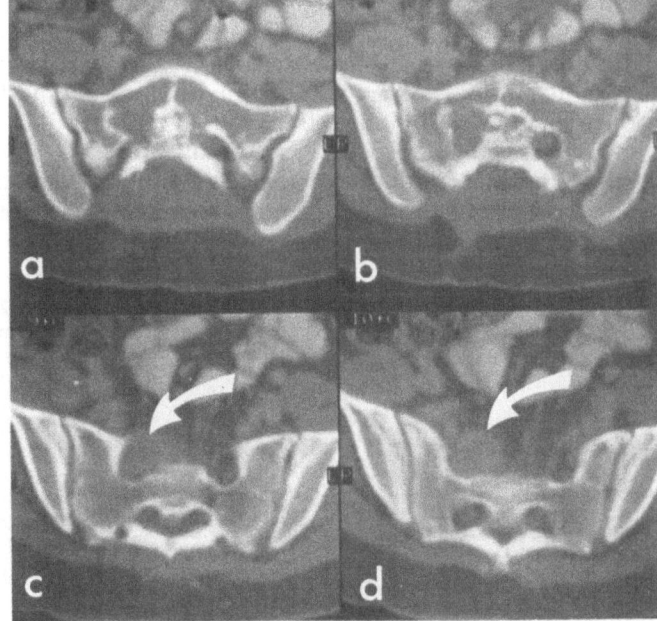

Fig. 22.4a–d. A 15-year-old girl with previous giant cell tumor of the sacrum. This had been treated with curretage and bone graft. **a** Follow-up CT shows recurrent tumor with destruction of the anterior portion of the sacrum. **b, c, d** A recurrent tumor mass is noted occupying the entire sacral foramen on the right and is noted emerging from this foramen in scans **c** and **d** (*arrows*). This recurrence could not be appreciated on plain radiographs.

p. 357). Following previous surgery a recurrence may be difficult to diagnose on plain radiographs because of the surrounding healing with sclerosis. The appearances of osteoid osteomas on CT reflect the changes described on plain radiograph. A varying amount of bony sclerosis is noted around the central nidus, which appears radiolucent. Within this nidus a small sclerotic fragment may be present.

Computed tomography is required to delineate other benign bone tumors less commonly. Its value remains in the delineation of large lesions (see Fig. 6.6, p. 73) or those occurring in sites of complex anatomy (Fig. 22.4).

Malignant

At the Hospital for Sick Children, Toronto, the greatest impact of CT on skeletal disease has been its value in the delineation of the extent of malignant bone neoplasms [7, 13]. Its value in this regard in both adults and children has been previously documented by several authors [1, 2, 4, 5, 6, 10, 11, 14].

Osteogenic and Ewing's sarcoma are the commonest primary malignant bone neoplasms in children. We have recently reviewed the plain radiographs and CT scans in 49 children with primary malignant bone tumors in order to

assess the advantages, limitations, and pitfalls of CT at the time of diagnosis, follow-up, and local recurrence, and in the search for metastases [13]. The lesions included 31 osteogenic and 18 Ewing's sarcomas, and the age at the time of presentation ranged from 4 to 17 years with a mean at 12 years. In this review we found that CT provided extra information compared with plain radiographs, particularly with regard to the extent of the soft tissue component of the lesion and the medullary extent in 56% of patients. It should be emphasized that in children suspected of having a primary malignant bone tumor plain radiographs are essential for characterization of the lesion and radionuclide bone scans for detection of multifocal disease and metastases. CT of the primary lesion is usually only performed if it is a solitary lesion. Chest radiographs are imperative prior to chest CT to define the presence or absence of metastases in the lungs. In the presence of multiple metastases, chest CT is only required for follow-up. Conventional tomography and angiography has only been performed in a few selected patients in whom it is felt that CT has not defined the full extent of the primary lesion preoperatively.

Limb-salvage procedures have become a well-accepted form of therapy for primary malignant bone tumors (in particular osteogenic sarcoma) and demand an even greater need for accurate preoperative anatomical delineation of tumor extent. In order to obtain the maximum amount of information from a CT scan, meticulous attention to technique is imperative. Our CT technique demands positioning of the patient in the gantry in a comfortable manner so that movement is kept to a minimum. The patient should be placed as symmetrically as possible to enable comparison with the opposite side from the tumor. A scout radiograph is taken and then axial scans are performed during the intravenous injection of a bolus of contrast. Adjacent scans of 5–10 mm thickness are obtained and viewed at both bone and soft tissue window. Measurements of the size of the lesion are made during these scans and attenuation values of the

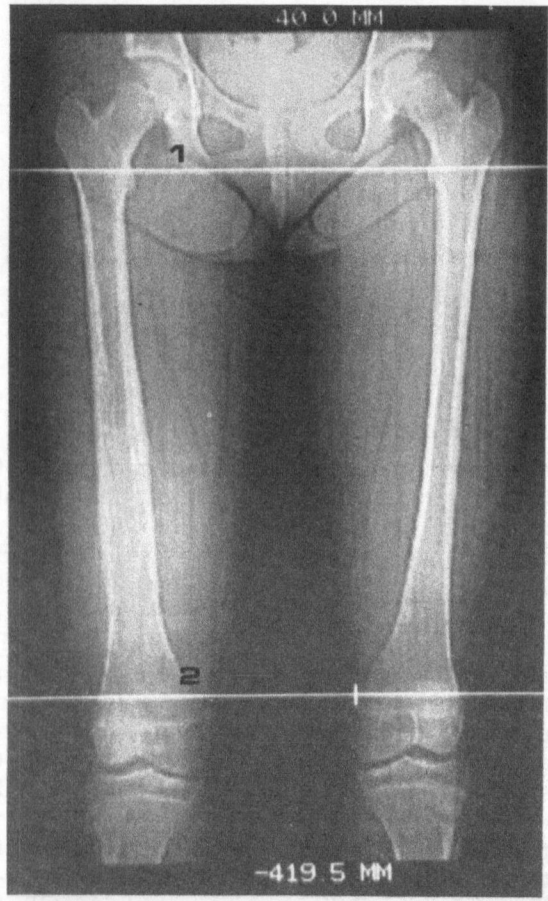

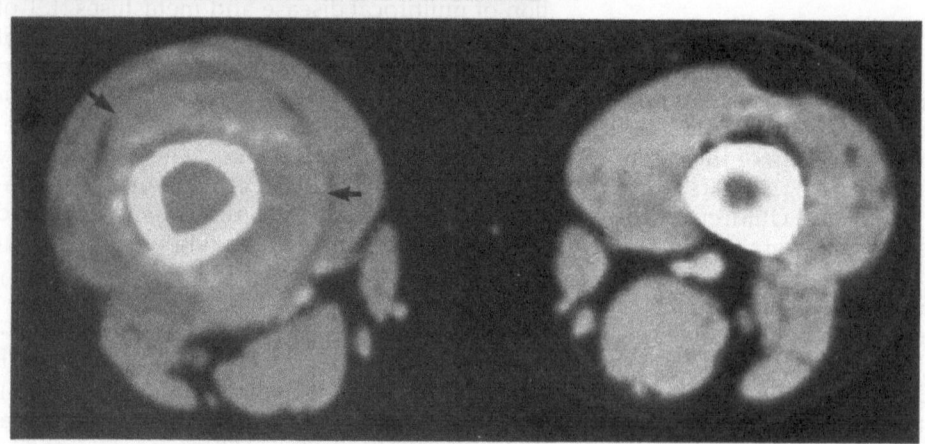

Fig. 22.5a,b. An 11-year-old girl with extensive osteogenic sarcoma of the diaphysis of the right femur. **a** Scout film shows the lesion, which is more easily seen in the lower half of the shaft. **b** CT shows thinning of the cortex, replacement of the marrow with tumor tissue, and a soft tissue mass with malignant ossification surrounding the bone (*arrows*). The mass is well defined anteriorly, laterally, and medially but is very poorly defined posteriorly, where muscular invasion is present. Following the completion of all the transverse scans the superior and inferior limits of the lesion can be illustrated on the scout view (**a**) as *lines 1* and *2* respectively. These limits of the tumor are more extensive than could be appreciated on the scout view or on plain radiographs.

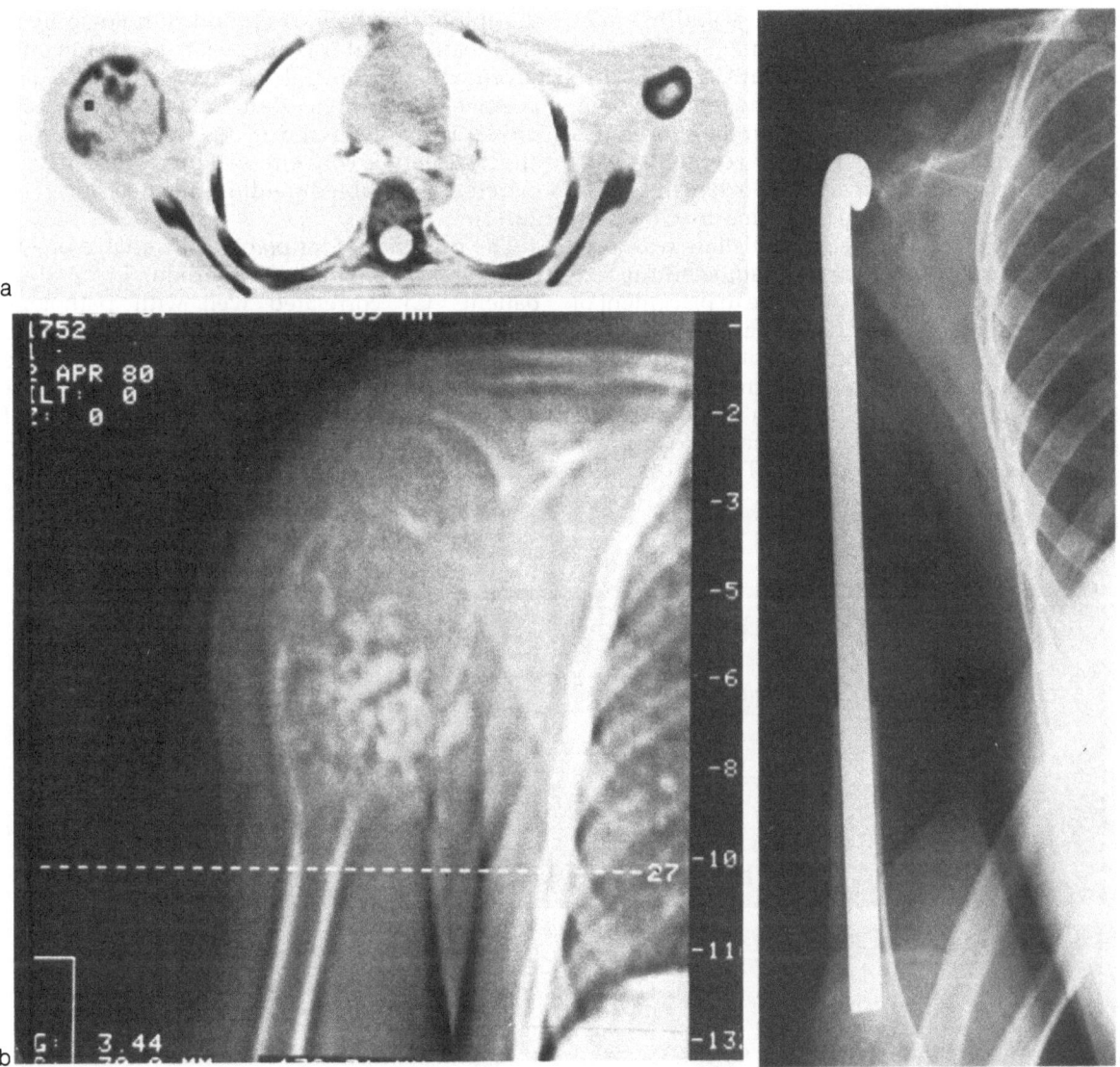

Fig. 22.6a–c. A 6-year-old girl with osteogenic sarcoma of the upper right humerus. **a** The upper humerus on the right is markedly expanded and destroyed. A small soft tissue extension of the tumor is noted posteromedially. **b** Scout radiograph shows the lesion in the upper humerus. *Line 27* indicates the lower limit of the lesion, as judged by the presence of a normal medullary cavity, cortex, and adjacent soft tissues on that scan. Using this line, the distance from the shoulder or the elbow may be measured and this will define the level to which the surgical excision should be extended. With this technique, CT is of very great benefit for the planning of surgical procedures that are aimed at limb salvage. In this way the least acceptable amount of tissue can be removed and a prosthesis inserted or a reconstructive procedure performed. **c** Postoperative radiograph shows the prosthesis replacing the humerus and connecting the lower humerus to the glenoid.

medullary cavity are compared with the opposite side in order to assess the medullary extent. The axial scan lines are then posted on the scout radiograph to delineate the extent of the lesion. Measurements from this line to normal anatomical landmarks that can be recognized at surgery are made and have proved helpful to our surgeons. Figures 22.5 and 22.6 illustrate our techniques. Sagittal and coronal reconstructed images and direct sagittal and coronal images have not proved more useful than the transverse axial scans. Figures 22.5–22.19 illustrate the CT appearances of osteogenic sarcoma and Ewing's sarcoma. Further illustrations are shown in Chapters 6 and 23.

In order to assess the accuracy of CT in the delineation of the extent of tumor we have recently correlated the CT findings with the gross and microscopic pathological findings in 21 children with osteogenic sarcoma [7]. The most important features evaluated on the transverse axial scans were the extent of the lesion in bone (Figs. 22.7, 22.8 and 22.9) and in the soft tissues (see Figs. 22.10 and 22.12). CT accurately delineated the cortical and medullary extent in 15 of 18 patients with osteogenic sarcoma in whom an accurate CT pathological correlation was possible. In two patients CT overestimated the size of the lesion: In one this was due to placement of the cursor over bony trabeculae in the metaphyseal region; in the other no attenuation measurements were taken and the medullary extent was evaluated only visually. In one patient CT underestimated the size as we failed to appreciate spread into the epiphysis. Transgression of the epiphyseal plate was found pathologically in eight patients but was appreciated on CT in only seven. CT gave one false negative and one false positive result. If one is unsure whether the epiphysis is involved and if this information may affect surgery, a conventional tomogram may be extremely valuable in aiding this decision (Fig. 22.11).

The presence of fat planes may enable one to exclude adjacent muscle invasion. In 17 of 21 patients CT correlated well with pathology regarding the presence or absence of muscle invasion. Microscopy showed invasion in three patients when CT was thought to show no invasion. CT gave one false positive result. Absence of fat planes thus makes differentiation of invasion from adherence impossible.

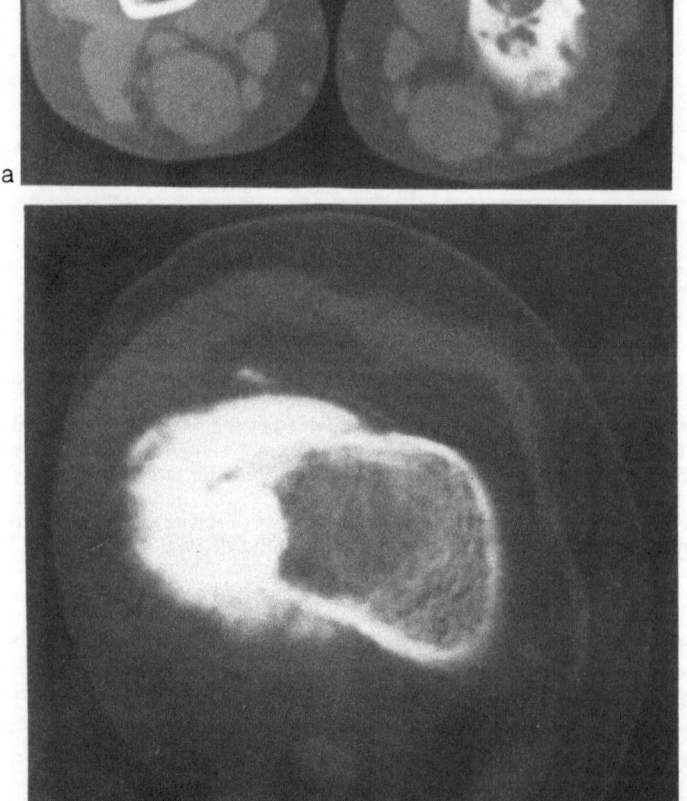

Fig. 22.7a,b. Two examples of osteogenic sarcoma of the femoral diaphysis. In both images tumor is mainly productive in nature; there is dense sclerotic tumor with destruction of the adjacent cortex and extension into the surrounding soft tissue. In each patient the lesion involves mainly one aspect of the bone rather than surrounding the entire bone. However, in **a** there is obvious extension involving the medullary cavity. In **b** there is some demineralization of the adjacent medullary bone. In neither is there any significant soft tissue mass evident beyond the limits of the bone production.

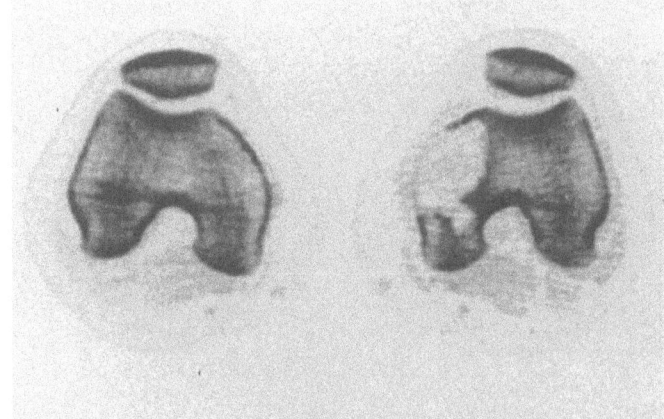

Fig. 22.8. Example of osteogenic sarcoma of the medial condyle of the left femur. This lesion is mainly osteolytic with almost no bone production and little soft tissue swelling beyond the limits of the bone, which is expanded. The edges of the lesion are ill-defined.

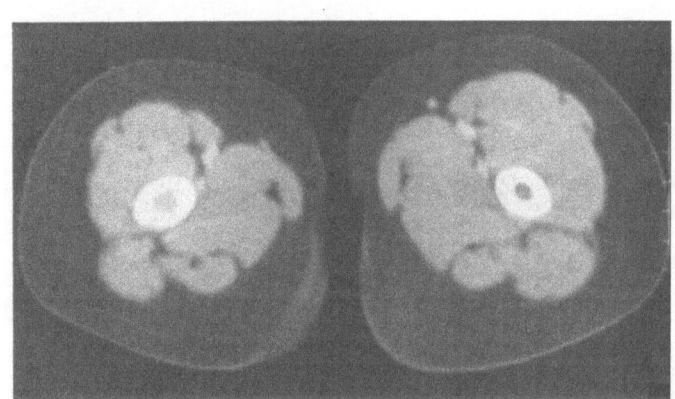

a

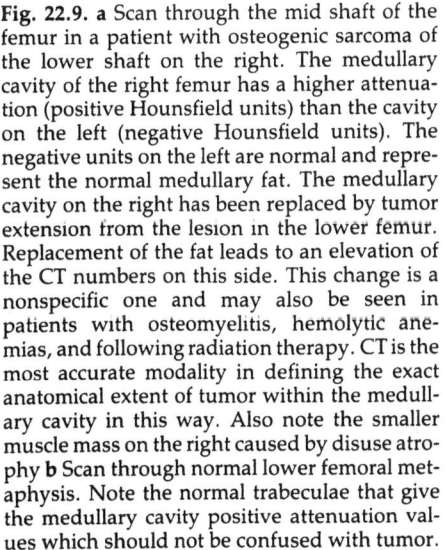

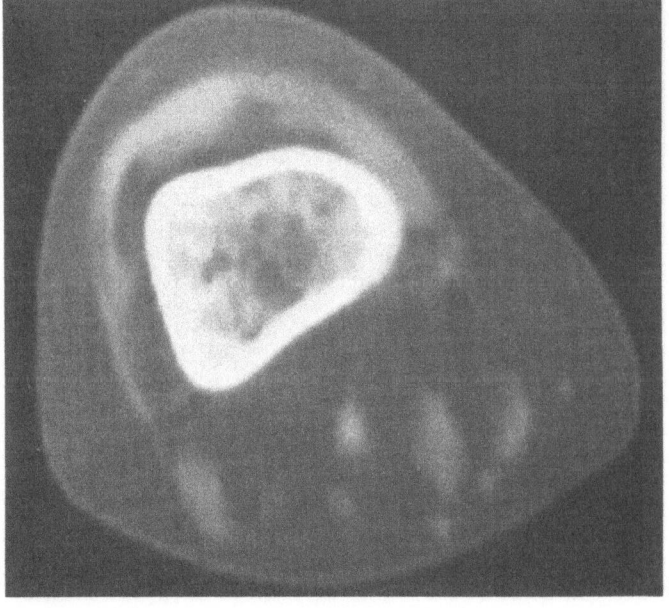

b

Fig. 22.9. a Scan through the mid shaft of the femur in a patient with osteogenic sarcoma of the lower shaft on the right. The medullary cavity of the right femur has a higher attenuation (positive Hounsfield units) than the cavity on the left (negative Hounsfield units). The negative units on the left are normal and represent the normal medullary fat. The medullary cavity on the right has been replaced by tumor extension from the lesion in the lower femur. Replacement of the fat leads to an elevation of the CT numbers on this side. This change is a nonspecific one and may also be seen in patients with osteomyelitis, hemolytic anemias, and following radiation therapy. CT is the most accurate modality in defining the exact anatomical extent of tumor within the medullary cavity in this way. Also note the smaller muscle mass on the right caused by disuse atrophy **b** Scan through normal lower femoral metaphysis. Note the normal trabeculae that give the medullary cavity positive attenuation values which should not be confused with tumor.

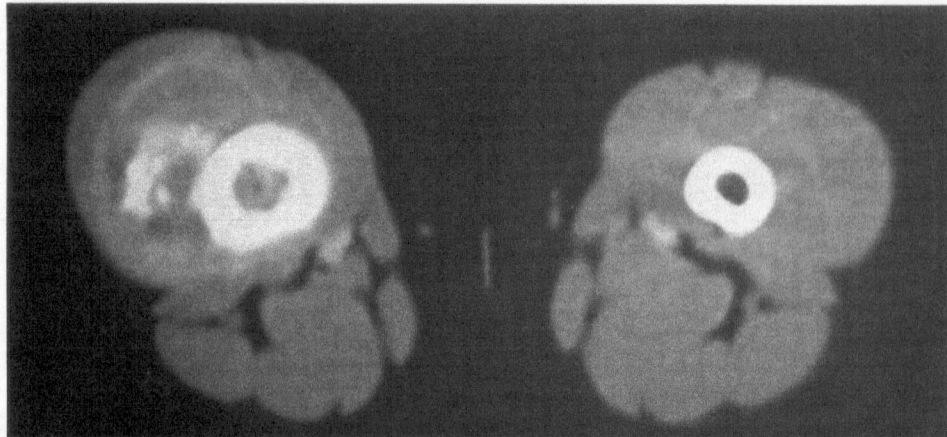

Fig. 22.10a

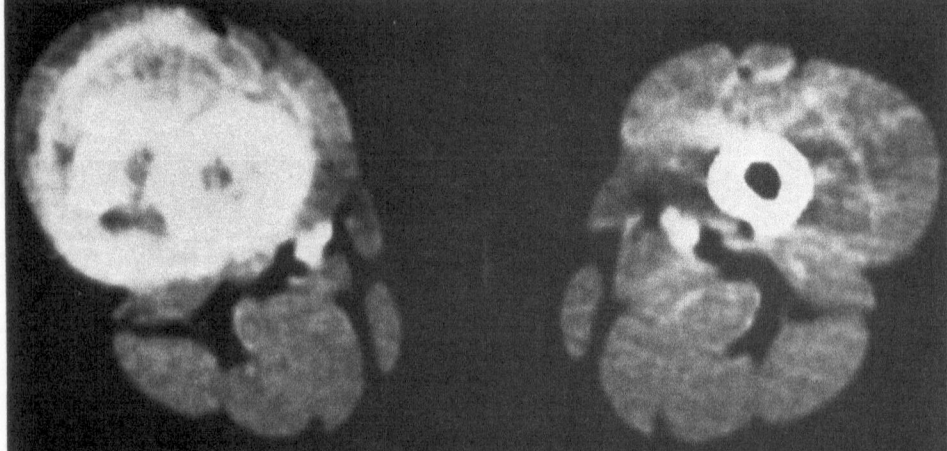

Fig. 22.10b

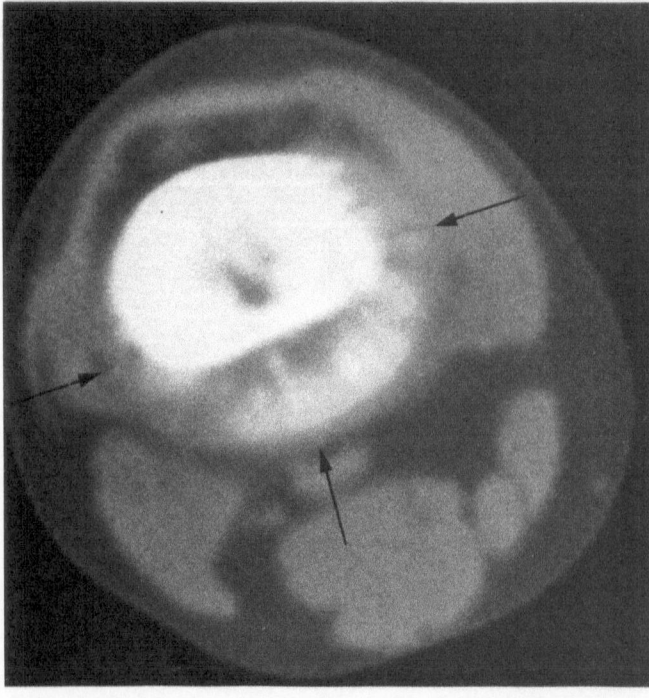

Fig. 22.10c

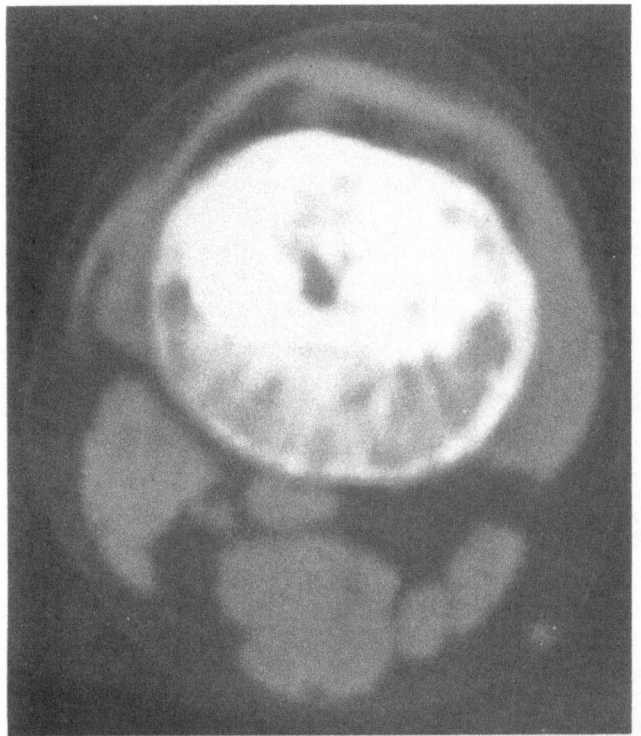

d

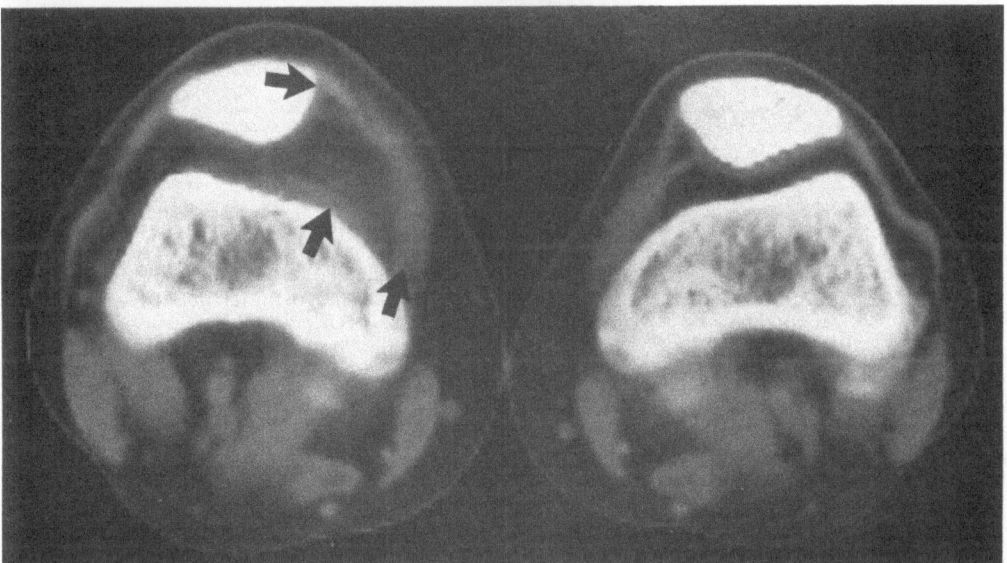

e

Fig. 22.10a,b. A 13-year-old girl with osteogenic sarcoma of the right femur. Scans at bone (**a**) and soft tissue (**b**) window settings show the thickening of the cortex, replacement of the medullary cavity, and the large soft tissue mass infiltrating into the vastus lateralis muscle. **c, d** Osteogenic sarcoma in the lower femur. Scan at the time of presentation (**c**) shows a large soft tissue mass (*arrows*) with new bone formation. It is difficult to determine whether the periosteum is intact around the somewhat hazy soft tissue mass. However, following preoperative chemotherapy scan (**d**) shows a smooth line of new bone formation has been laid down beneath the intact periosteum. At this time it is easier to predict that the periosteum is intact; indeed, it was proven microscopically. The change in appearance between the two scans enables one to predict the good response to therapy despite the lack of change in the size of the lesion. Similar changes have been shown by other authors [6, 11]. In this way CT is a valuable modality in assessing the efficacy of preoperative chemotherapy. **e** A teenage girl with a right lower femoral osteogenic sarcoma. Note the thickening and poor definition of the soft tissues medially on the right (*arrows*) compared with the left. This is due to edema adjacent to the neoplasm and should not be confused with tumor extension.

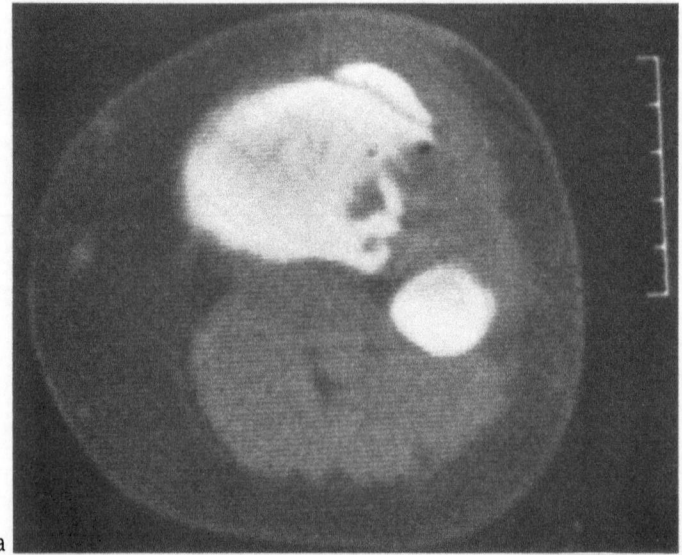

a

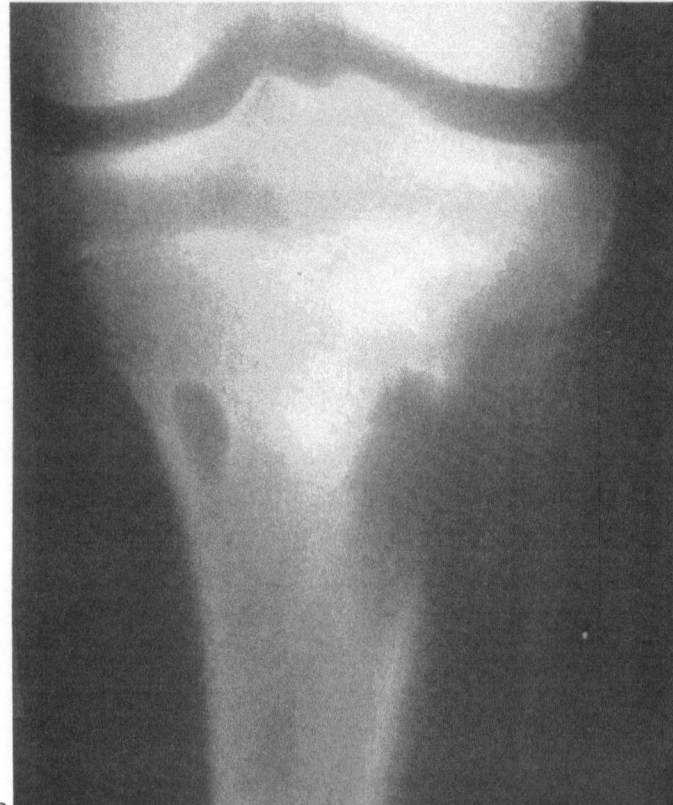

b

Fig. 22.11a,b. A 14-year-old girl with previously treated bilateral retinoblastomas who presented with a mass in the lateral aspect of the left tibia. **a** CT shows destruction of the lateral aspect of the left tibia. Because the lesion was so well localized and because the child was blind, a local resection was planned with subsequent reconstructive surgery. In order for an adequate reconstruction to be made it was important to know whether the lesion involved the epiphysis at the proximal end of the tibia. This could not be ascertained on plain radiographs or on the transverse CT scan. However, a conventional anteroposterior tomogram (**b**) clearly shows that the lateral aspect of the proximal tibial epiphysis has been invaded. This dictated the type of resection and reconstruction that was later performed. Diagnosis: osteogenic sarcoma.

The periosteum was shown to be pathologically invaded in eight patients. CT correctly showed this invasion in four patients but in the other four the periosteum was thought to be intact on CT (see Fig. 22.10). CT gave no false positive results. Irregularity of the tumor bone formation as noted in Fig. 22.7b is highly suggestive of periosteal invasion in comparison with a more regular new bone formation that is shown in Fig. 22.10c and d.

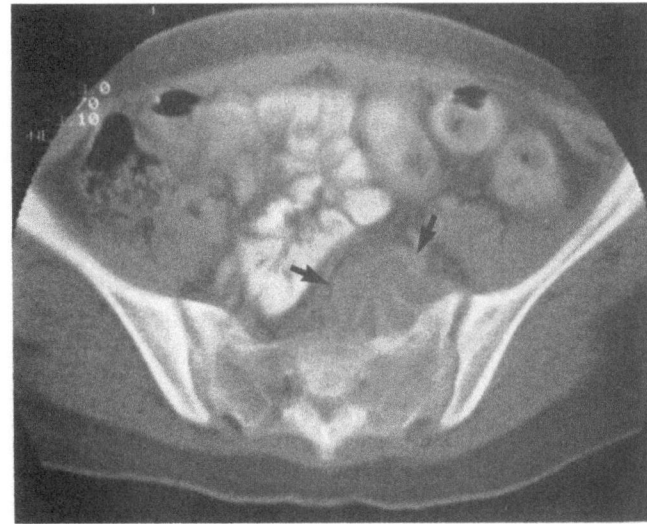

Fig. 22.12. A 16-year-old girl with osteogenic sarcoma arising in the anterior aspect of the left side of the sacrum. A soft tissue mass (*arrows*) with new bone formation is noted projecting anteriorly from the sacrum. This is an unusual site for osteogenic sarcoma. CT is invaluable in the assessment of lesions arising in the sacrum in order to plan the correct type of management.

CT correlated well with pathological findings in four patients with osteogenic sarcoma who had prominent edema adjacent to the tumor (see Fig. 22.10e). Irregularity and thickening of tissues adjacent to the tumor is usually indicative of reactive edema and should not be confused with tumor invasion. Comparison with the appearances on the opposite side may be helpful in making this distinction. The neurovascular bundles are best delineated when scans are performed during intravenous contrast injection. In none of our patients were these involved.

In those patients who have had previous local resections follow-up CT at regular intervals are imperative for the diagnosis of local recurrence (Fig. 22.13) and local spread (Fig. 22.14). In those patients treated nonoperatively for Ewing's sarcoma (Figs. 22.15, 22.16, 22.17, 22.18) or given preoperative chemotherapy for osteogenic sarcoma, baseline CT scans are invaluable in following the response of the bone and soft tissue to therapy (see Figs. 22.10c and d, 22.18, and 22.19). However, it may be difficult with CT to detect early recurrence; even if the CT shows no definite recurrent neoplasm biopsy is indicated if symptoms and signs are suggestive of recurrence (see Figs. 22.13 and 22.18.). Following radiotherapy the medullary cavity is replaced by tissue of positive attenuation often with calcification (see Fig. 22.19). It may be impossible to differentiate this from local recurrence or radiation-induced tumor in the absence of a mass. Figure 22.19c is an example of a radiation-induced osteogenic sarcoma in a femur previously treated for Ewing's sarcoma.

In summary, CT is extremely useful in delineating the bone and soft tissue extent of primary malignant bone tumors preoperatively and provides invaluable baseline information in those patients treated nonoperatively. However, in order to understand the role that CT plays in evaluating primary malignant bone tumors, the pitfalls and limitations of this modality should be clearly understood. The presence of edema adjacent to the tumor should not be confused with tumor extension. The cursor should be accurately used to assess medullary extent and enable comparison with the opposite side. It should also be understood that in the metaphyseal areas there are more bony trabeculae centrally than in the diaphysis and the cursor may well read positive attenuation values in these regions where there is no tumor infiltration. Similarly, accurate measurements cannot be made in extremely small bones or if the bone has no fat marrow normally. Involvement of the epiphysis and joint may be difficult to predict on CT and may require use of a different modality. The paucity of fat planes may make imaging in the extremities difficult, and in areas of complex anatomy muscle invasion may be impossible to predict. This is also a problem in younger children and in the distal portions of the extremity. Early local recurrence may be difficult to detect and biopsy should be dictated by clinical findings. Postradiation changes are impossible to differentiate from local recurrence or new second malignancies in the absence of a mass. Artifact from orthopedic hardware may interfere with detection of local recurrence and spread.

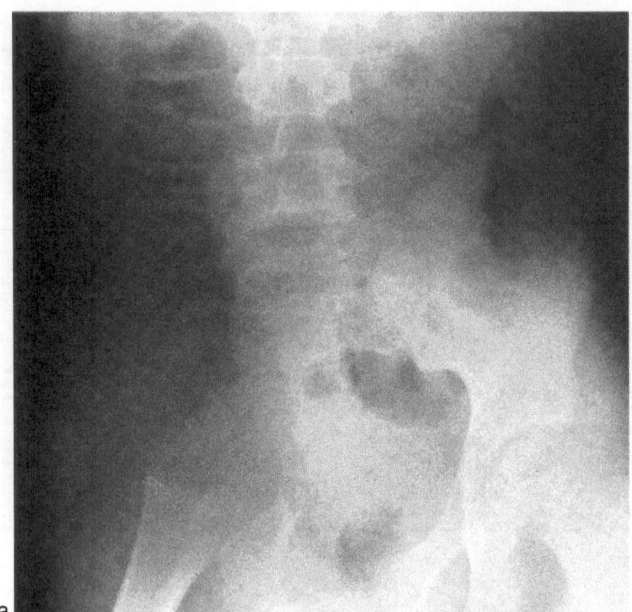

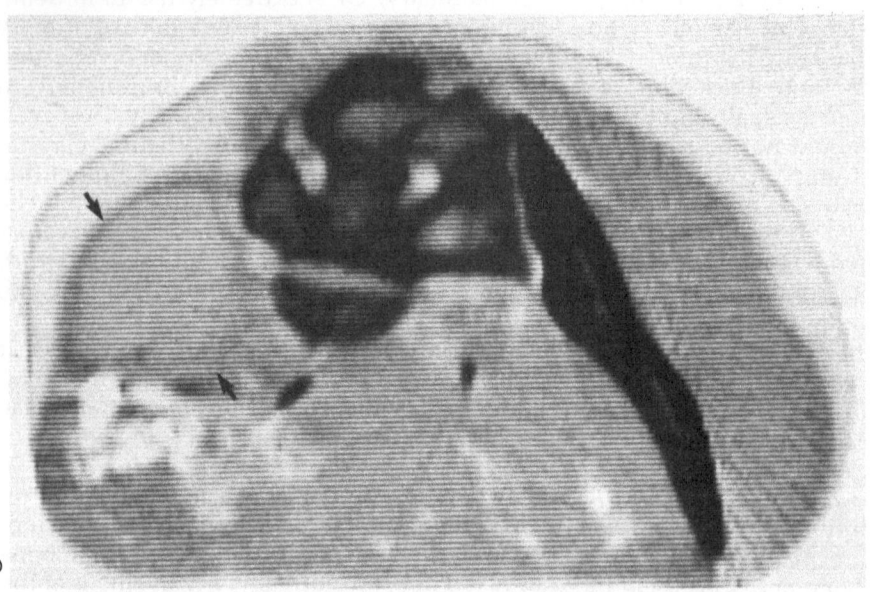

Fig. 22.13a,b. A 15-year-old boy with previously resected osteogenic sarcoma of the right ilium. **a** Plain radiograph shows local resection of right ilium and proximal femur. **b** CT performed with the patient in the prone position shows a mass (*arrows*) adjacent to the right side of the sacrum. This mass was removed and contained recurrent osteogenic sarcoma. (Pettersson et al. 1983 [9])

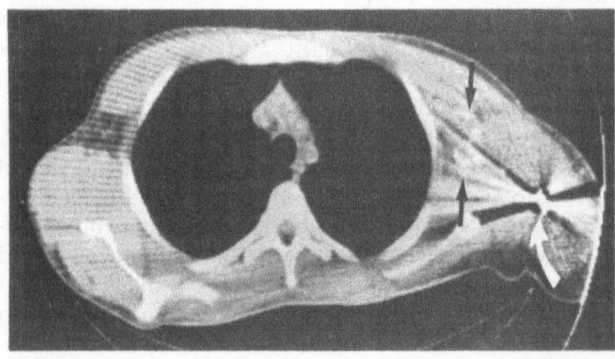

Fig. 22.14. A 17-year-old boy with previously resected osteogenic sarcoma of the upper portion of the left humerus. CT shows a prosthesis replacing the upper humerus (*curved arrow*). An artifact is noted crossing the chest from this prosthesis. The artifact partially obscures an area of high attenuation in the axilla (*black arrows*). This represents ossification of metastases which have developed in axillary lymph nodes. Despite the artifact, CT has delineated an important area of recurrent disease. This area is difficult to examine both clinically and radiographically following such procedures.

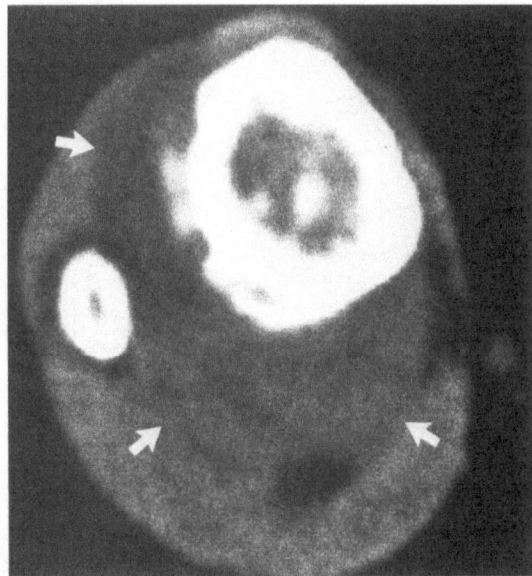

Fig. 22.15. A 12-year-old boy with Ewing's sarcoma of the right tibia. The lesion has caused irregularity of the involved cortex, has replaced the medullary fat, and has extended into the soft tissues as a large posterolateral soft tissue mass (*arrows*). A periosteal reaction is evident, and calcification within the medullary cavity is probably related to necrosis within the tumor.

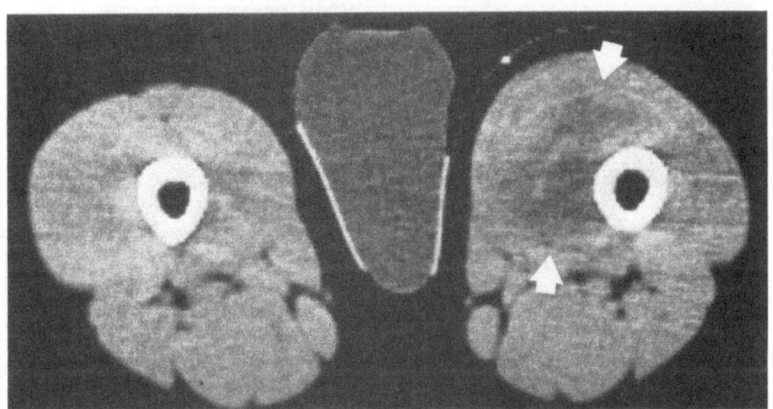

Fig. 22.16. A 13-year-old girl with Ewing's sarcoma of the left thigh. The lesion is seen as a mass (*arrows*) involving mainly the soft tissues and is very ill defined in outline. The underlying bone appears to be grossly normal on this image.

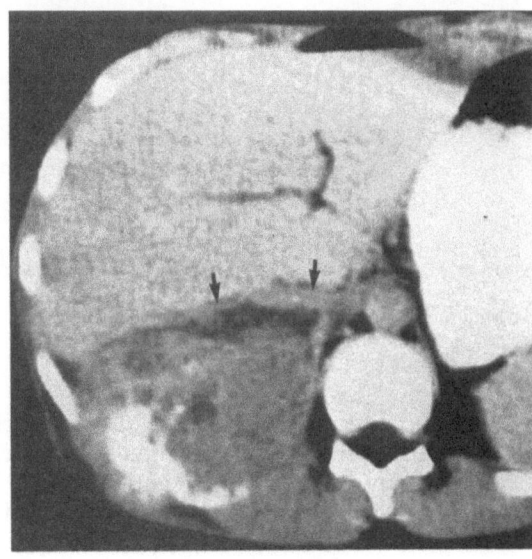

Fig. 22.17. An 11-year-old boy with Ewing's sarcoma of the right 11th rib. The bone destruction and reaction is seen on the right, and the extension of a mass anteriorly behind the crus of the diaphragm is well demonstrated. *Arrows*, diaphragmatic crus.

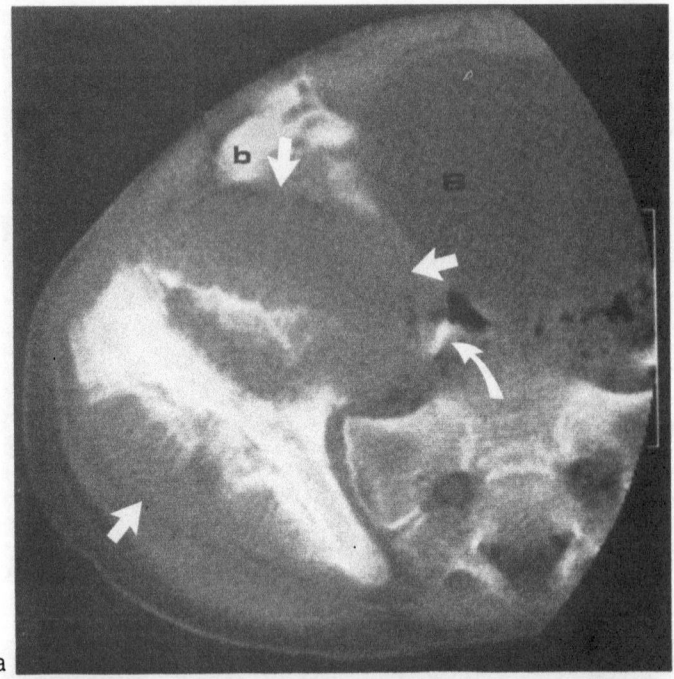

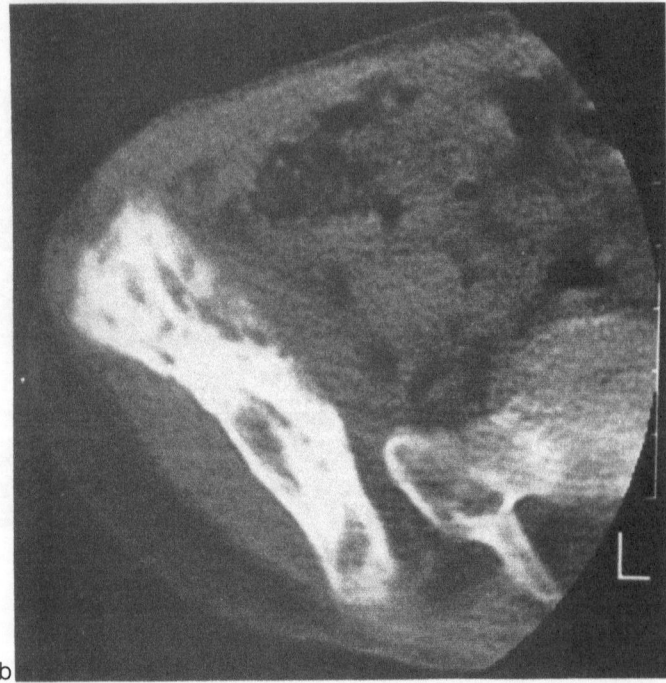

Fig. 22.18a,b. A 6-year-old boy with Ewing's sarcoma of the right ilium. **a** The bone destruction of the ilium and the adjacent bony reaction is easily seen. The soft tissue mass extends both medially and laterally (*arrows*) *Curved arrow*, right ureter; *B*, bladder; *b*, bowel. CT is extremely important in the delineation of the extent of malignant tumors arising in the pelvic bones and sacrum. The soft tissue component of such lesions is very poorly defined by other modalities, and adequate management depends upon an adequate delineation of this component of the tumor. **b** Following chemotherapy and radiotherapy, CT shows healing of the lesion with new bone formation around the ilium and resolution of the medial and lateral soft tissue masses. Repeated follow-up CT scans showed no change in this appearance even when recurrence was clinically suspected because of severe pain in the region of the right anterior superior iliac spine. A biopsy of this area revealed recurrent tissue despite no obvious change on CT.

Metastases

At our institution we have used radionuclide bone scans as the modality of choice in the detection of bony metastases. In patients with histiocytosis X, skeletal surveys are also used, as radionuclide scans may give false negative results in this disease. However, we have used CT occasionally in the evaluation of patients who are suspected of having bony metastases. This modality is only used when the findings on radionuclide scans and conventional radiography are equivocal. The earliest findings that we have seen on CT include demineralization of the

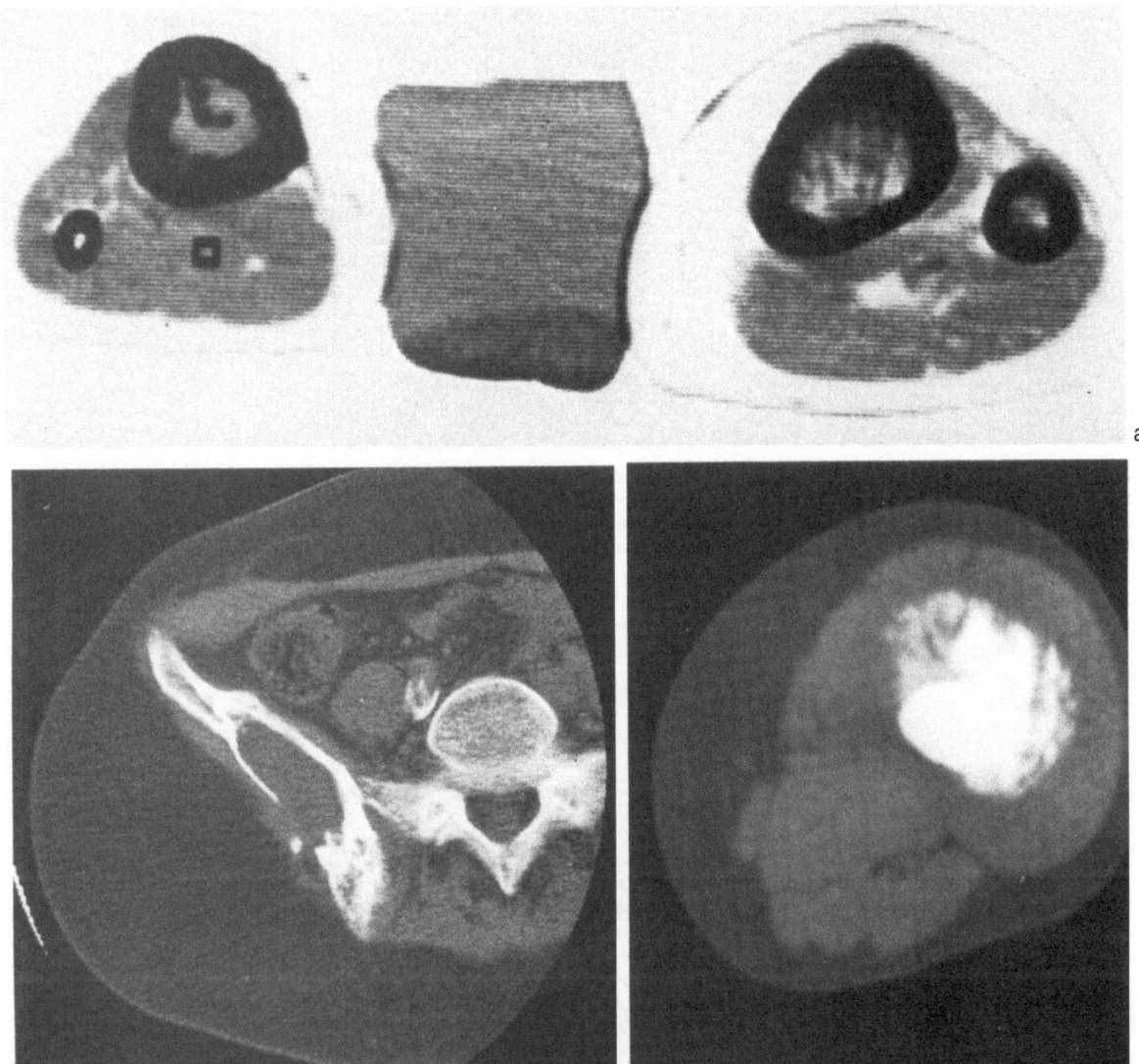

Fig. 22.19a–c. Examples of bone changes following radiation for malignant sarcomas. **a** Previously irradiated Ewing's sarcoma of right tibia. Follow-up CT showed irregularity of the cortex, replacement of the medullary fat by tissue of higher attenuation (probably representing fibrous scar tissue), and calcification. There is also atrophy of the muscles in this leg. **b** Following radiation for a right iliac Ewing's sarcoma, the bone has been replaced by tissue of attenuation which is slightly less than muscle. **c** A 17-year-old girl with radiation for left femoral Ewing's sarcoma 10 years previously. She presented at this time with pain. CT of the upper femur shows a bony mass which is easily appreciated as a radiation-induced osteogenic sarcoma. Medullary cavity changes in the lower femur were identical to that shown in **a** and were thought to represent postradiation changes but were shown pathologically to be a second site of osteogenic sarcoma. Thus without the mass effect radiation-induced osteogenic sarcoma may not be distinguishable from postradiation changes on CT. The features illustrated in these images are variations of changes noted following radiation. In the absence of a soft tissue mass or new bone destruction, recurrent lesions are extremely difficult to exclude, if these are suspected clinically.

cortex (Fig. 22.20) and trabeculae of the involved bone, but these changes are nonspecific and may be related to osteoporosis. A further finding is the presence of an intact bony cortex with replacement of the medullary cavity by tissue of positive attenuation values. Larger metastases replace the cortex as well as the medullary cavity (Fig. 22.21). The changes may be lytic or sclerotic (see also Fig. 23.23, p. 369).

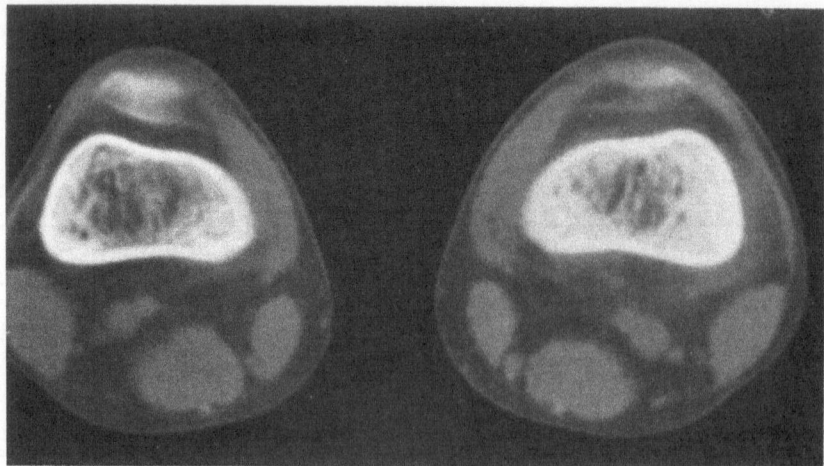

Fig. 22.20. A 12-year-old boy with previously treated undifferentiated sarcoma of C-1. Because of pain in the lower portion of the right femur a bone scan was performed and this showed increased uptake of radionuclide at the site. Plain radiographs appeared normal. This CT image illustrates a diffuse demineralization of the lower femur but no specific changes to suggest malignant disease at this site. These are the early changes of metastases within a bone, and more florid changes of metastatic disease were later seen on plain radiographs.

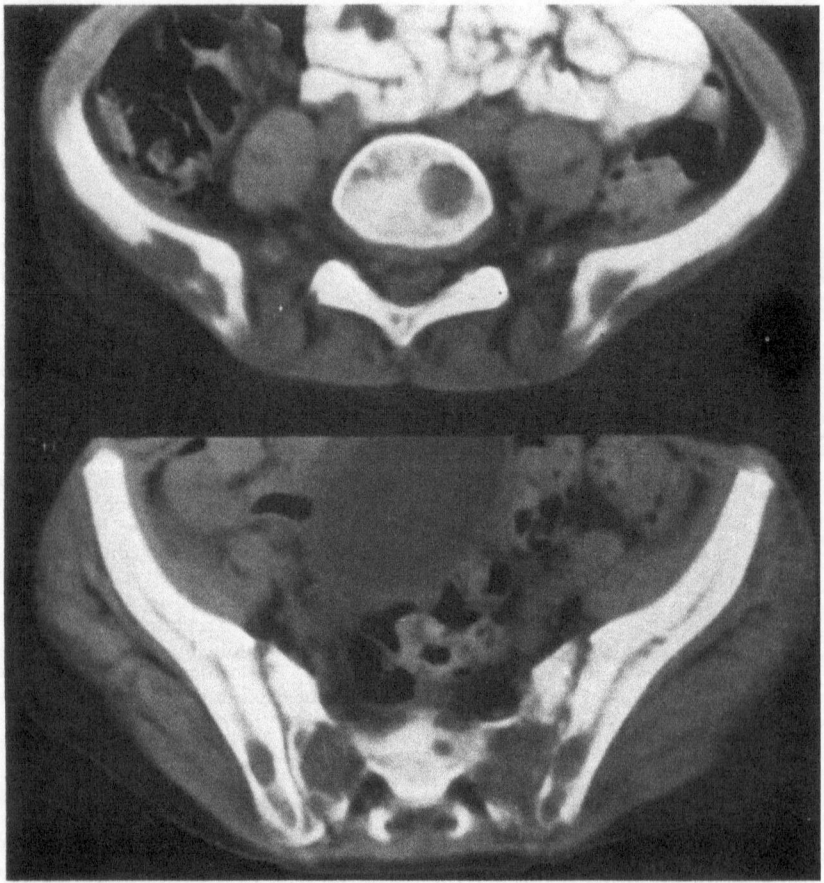

Fig. 22.21. A 10-year-old boy with large pelvic rhabdomyosarcoma. CT performed to reassess the size of the lesion in the left pelvis demonstrates multiple lytic lesions in the body of L-4, sacrum, and both iliac bones. These represent metastatic disease and were asymptomatic at the time of the examination.

Miscellaneous

In scoliosis there are two abnormalities of the vertebral column. These include lateral curvature and vertebral rotation. The lateral curvature is easily assessed on plain radiographs, but CT offers a unique method for the evaluation of the degree of vertebral rotation. With the patient in the supine position a scout radiograph is performed and from this an axial slice is chosen through the apical vertebra. From this slice the rotation of this vertebra to the vertical line through the trunk can be measured. It is hoped that in the follow-up of patients with scoliosis this type of examination, which delivers less radiation than the conventional follow-up radiographs, may be useful.

CT is useful for the guidance of bone biopsy. From the transverse axial scans the most appropriate area to be biopsied can be marked on the patient's skin, and a biopsy can be performed with ease in this manner.

A change of less than 5% in the degree of mineralization of bone can be detected by CT, whereas no change less than 30% can be detected by conventional radiography. Despite this factor, CT has not become widely used in the in vivo measurement of bone mineralization in many pediatric disorders such as renal disease.

References

1. deSantos LA, Bernardino ME, Murray JA (1979) Computed tomography in the evaluation of osteosarcoma: experience with 25 cases. AJR 132:535–540
2. Destouet JM, Gilula LA, Murphy WA (1979) Computed tomography of long-bone osteosarcoma. Radiology 131:439–445
3. Donoghue V, Daneman A, Mancer K, Krajbich I (1985) CT features of reactive periostitis in the humerus: a lesion resembling myositis ossificans. J Comput Assist Tomogr 9(2):401–403
4. Levine E, Lee KR, Neff JR, Maklad NF, Robinson RG, Preston DF (1979) Comparison of computed tomography and other imaging modalities in the evaluation of musculoskeletal tumors. Radiology 131:431–437
5. Lukens JA, McLeod RA, Sim FH (1982) Computed tomographic evaluation of primary osseous malignant neoplasms. AJR 139:45–48
6. Mail JT, Cohen MD, Mirkin LD, Provisor AJ (1985) Response of osteosarcoma to preoperative intravenous high-dose methotrexate chemotherapy: CT evaluation. AJR 144:89–93
7. Mancer K, Daneman A, Soto G, Krajbich I, D'amato C (1985) CT pathological correlation of osteogenic sarcoma in children (unpublished data)
8. Murphy WA, Gilula LA, Destouet JM, Monsees BS, Tailor CC, Totty WG (1983) Musculoskeletal system. In: Lee JKT, Sagel SS, Stanley RJ (eds) Computed body tomography. Raven, New York, pp 453–516
9. Pettersson H, Daneman A, Harwood-Nash DCF (1983) Computed tomography in pediatric orthopedic radiology. In: Boijsen E, Ekelund L (eds) Computed tomography in orthopedic radiology. Thieme, Stuttgart, pp 26–48
10. Riddlesberger MM, Kuhn JP (1983) The role of computed tomography in diseases of the musculoskeletal system. CT 7:85–99
11. Shirkhoda A, Jaffe N, Wallace S, Ayala A, Lindell MM, Zornoza J (1985) Computed tomography of osteosarcoma after intraarterial chemotherapy AJR 144:95–99
12. Somer K, Meurman KOA (1982) Computed tomography of stress fractures. J Comput Assist Tomogr 6:109–115
13. Soto G, Daneman A, Harwood-Nash DCF (1985) An evaluation of the role of CT in primary malignant bone tumors in children. Paper presented at Annual Meeting of the Society for Pediatric Radiology, Boston, April 1985
14. Vanel D, Contesso G, Couanet D, Piekarski JD, Sarrazin D, Masselot J (1982) Computed tomography in the evaluation of 41 cases of Ewing's sarcoma. Skeletal Radiol 9:8–13

Chapter 23

Special Areas

General Introduction

Diseases of various parts of the musculoskeletal system have been described in the two preceding chapters, and certain specific areas have been covered in earlier chapters (chest wall, Chap. 6; miscellaneous, Chap. 17; neck masses, Chap. 20). This chapter deals with certain specific areas that have not been covered previously in this book. These areas have in common extremely complex musculoskeletal anatomy. Because of their complexity the bones and soft tissues of these areas are usually poorly imaged by other modalities either independently or in combination [13, 15]. The bones and soft tissues of these areas often have variations in thickness, unusual angles, and curvatures, and often overlying adjacent structures such as bones, gas, and soft tissues make delineation of these areas difficult. The cross-sectional anatomy provided on CT, with the high-density resolution of the soft tissues, obviates these problems; therefore CT has become the best imaging modality for evaluation of many of these areas.

Although not every complex anatomical area of the body has been included for description in this book, the general principles outlined in this chapter can easily be applied to other areas. Often CT will provide additional information which may not be obtained from a variety of other imaging procedures. These principles may be applied to lesions that are congenital, infectious, neoplastic, or traumatic in origin.

Hips

Introduction

The radiographic evaluation of pediatric hip disease has improved significantly with the development of CT. The literature has centered on the usefulness of CT in congenital dislocation of the hip and, to a lesser extent, on trauma [7, 8, 18]. At the Hospital for Sick Children, Toronto, we have used CT to study children and adolescents with a wide spectrum of hip diseases, including avascular necrosis, congenital dislocation of the hip, trauma, inflammatory arthritis, slipped upper femoral epiphysis, tumors, proximal focal femoral deficiency, and myositis ossificans. In 1984, Donoghue et al. [4] reviewed the clinical and radiographic findings in 49 children and adolescents with suspected hip disease seen at our institution. In some CT was performed only after use had been made of other imaging modalities such as plain radiography, bone scintigraphy, conventional tomography, or arthrography. However, in many of the more recent patients CT has come to replace these other modalities and has been used after plain radiographs only.

In 44 of the 49 patients (i.e., 90%) CT was able to provide the specific answers requested by the clinicians. In the other five CT did not provide the necessary or correct information. This problem related to the limitations of CT in the detection of intra-articular loose bodies (see p. 355). In 41 of the 49 patients (i.e., 84%) CT provided information not available from plain radiographs. The axial display of structures and the high density and spatial resolution afforded by CT allow visualization of small lesions which may otherwise be overlooked or grossly underestimated on plain radiographs. CT added more information in only one of four patients who also had conventional tomography and one of six patients who also had arthrography. In the other patients CT gave the same information as these other modalities.

Our study thus confirmed the usefulness of CT in a wide variety of pathological conditions of the hip in children. However, plain radiography should be performed on all patients as the initial investigation as it contributes essential information concerning the presence of skeletal and soft tissue abnormalities as well as their character and aggressiveness. Radionuclide bone scans show the vascularity of the femoral head and may confirm the presence of skeletal and soft tissue lesions and may establish the local extent, distant spread, or multiplicity of lesions, but they are usually nonspecific. Conventional tomography is now rarely used as a further investigation as it is only slightly more sensitive than plain radiography. More recently, sonography has been used very successfully for evaluation of the pediatric hip. This is particularly true in the infant, when the cartilaginous head and its relationship to the acetabulum can be easily evaluated with this modality.

CT is useful in the following circumstances:

1. In accurately localizing the position of the femoral head and metaphysis and their relationship to one another and to the acetabulum in conditions such as congenital dislocation of the hip, slipped upper femoral epiphysis, and proximal focal femoral deficiency (see Figs. 23.1, 23.2, 23.3, 23.4)

2. In delineating the characteristics of the femoral head, adjacent bones, and soft tissues in Perthes disease, avascular necrosis, inflammatory arthritis, and tumors (see Fig. 23.5)

3. In detecting slight changes in the size of the joint space and the presence of intra-articular obstacles such as (a) loose bodies in trauma and avascular necrosis (see Fig. 23.5) and (b) pulvinar hypertrophy in some cases of inadequate reduction of a congenital dislocation (see Fig. 23.1)

4. In the preoperative planning of surgical procedures by enabling measurement of the angle of declination and the plate/neck angle in the axial plane (see p. 354; see also Figs. 23.3, 23.4).

Congenital Dislocation

Early recognition and treatment of congenital dislocation of the hip (CDH) will ensure normal subsequent development of the hip in the vast majority of affected children [8]. Hernandez has reported his experience with over 200 hip CT examinations in children with CDH [7]. This author does not advocate the routine and indiscriminate use of CT in children with CDH and specifically does not use CT for initial diagnosis, particularly in the neonate and infant with easily reducible CDH. More recently, sonography of the hip has become widely used for this purpose. CT is particularly helpful if the patient is surrounded by a plaster cast making plain radiographs suboptimal and sonography difficult. The cast does not detract from the CT image quality nor does it obscure anatomical detail [7, 18]. The clinically irreducible hip is usually a problem in children over 6 months of age [7]. CT can accurately display the relationship of the proximal femur (head or metaphysis) to the acetabulum. Such anteroposterior relationships are difficult to appreciate on plain radiographs, particularly when the child is in a cast following closed reduction.

When the femoral head is not yet ossified its position may be difficult to appreciate on the transverse axial CT scan. Hernandez [8] has likened the appearance of the upper femur to a foot in a clog (femoral neck and metaphysis) kicking a ball (unossified femoral head) when the patient is in a "frog" leg position (i.e., hips flexed and abducted). The upturn of the tip of the clog indicates the position of the femoral head. With this image in mind it is easier to appreciate the position of the unossified head. CT plays a major role in determining whether the femoral head has been concentrically reduced, particularly when the head is unossified or if the patient is surrounded by a cast. Reasons for failing to obtain satisfactory reduction of the hip include pulvinar hypertrophy, inverted limbus, capsular adhesions, pericephalic insertion of the capsule, redundant ligamentem teres, and a tight iliopsoas tendon, or a combination of several of these [7, 18]. A tight iliopsoas tendon is the commonest of these complications. This tendon can be visualized easily on CT, and therefore this modality is extremely valuable for determining its position. When the hip dislocates, the ilio-psoas, which is intimately associated with the joint capsule, interposes between the head and the acetabulum and causes a crease in the capsule. It thus divides the capsule into acetabular and capital parts divided by an isthmus. The size of the isthmus will determine the success of an attempted closed reduction as the femoral head has to pass through this isthmus. The infolding

of the capsule can sometimes keep the head outside the acetabulum.

Intra-articular obstacles may also contribute to persistent subluxation of the femoral head [7, 18]. The pulvinar (fibrofatty tissue at the apex of the acetabulum) may hypertrophy in CDH and will cause a decrease in the capacity of the acetabulum. The fatty nature of this tissue is easily documented by CT (Fig. 23.1), and the

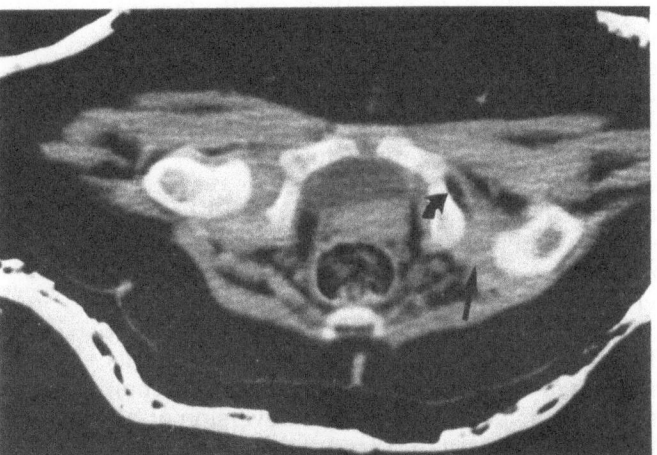

a

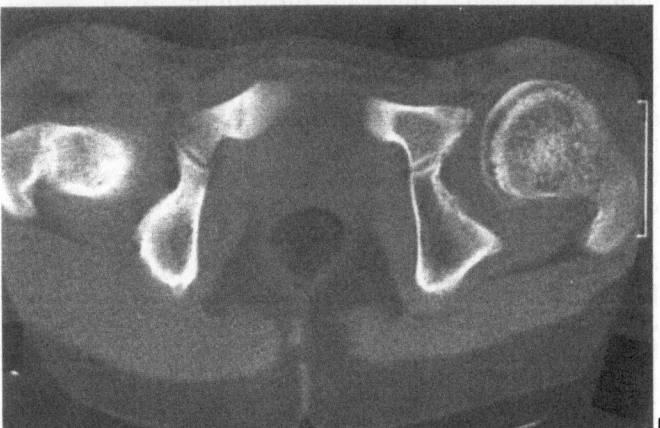

b

Fig. 23.1. a A 6-month-old boy with congenital dislocation of the left hip treated by closed reduction. The left femoral head is dislocated posteriorly (*arrow*). There is left pulvinar hypertrophy (the tissue of fatty negative attenuation lying deep in the acetabulum) (*curved arrow*). The child is in a plaster cast, which can be seen peripherally. The changes on CT were not evident on plain radiographs. b A 2-year-old boy with congenital dislocation of the left hip. CT shows anteversion and subluxation of the femoral head. The femoral head is larger than the size of the acetabulum and there is acetabular irregularity. c A 23-year-old woman with previously treated congenital dislocation of the left hip. The left femoral head is in a normal position, but there are marked degenerative changes with osteophyte formation noted on both sides of the joint. The right hip appears normal. In b and c the muscles on the involved side show disuse atrophy.

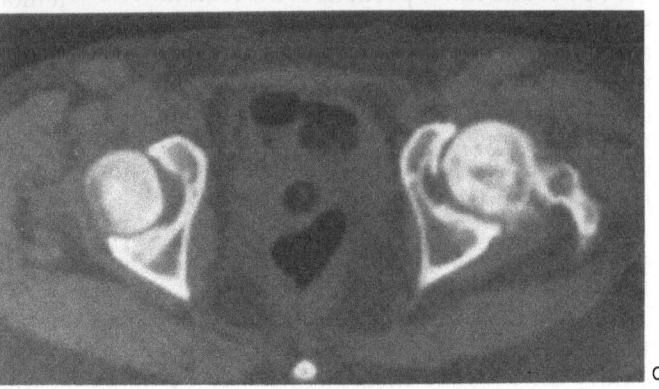

c

cause for the persistent subluxation is easily appreciated. Interposition of other interarticular soft tissue may be better defined by a combination of CT and arthrography [18]. Iatrogenic causes of persistent subluxation include metallic pins, which may project from the innominate bone into the acetabulum, displacing the femoral head outward.

Dislocation of the femoral head may be lateral or posterior. Lateral displacement may be due to obstacles such as a fold of capsule or a tight iliopsoas tendon interposed between the femoral head and acetabulum. On CT, the proximal femur is well orientated toward the acetabulum but is not adequately seated in the socket of the acetabulum [8]. In posterior dislocation the femoral metaphysis approximates to the posterior aspect of the acetabulum, a mass (the unossified femoral head) projects behind the ischium, and the fat plane anterior to the gluteus maximus is deformed, to be displaced posteriorly [8].

Excessive anteversion of the femoral neck (femoral torsion) is important in CDH [7] and its measurement is useful when surgical correction is contemplated. The angle of anteversion of the hip is the angle that the plane of the femoral neck forms in relation to the plane through the distal femoral condyle [7]. The normal range is 30°–50° in the fetus and newborn. This decreases with weight bearing and is approximately 10°–15° at 6–12 years of age. A derotational osteotomy may be required if this angle is abnormal, not only in CDH but also in such conditions as Legg–Perthes disease and some neuromuscular disorders.

Determination of this angle of anteversion by conventional radiographic techniques is difficult [7, 18]. Reproducible landmarks are difficult to establish, complex limb positioning and immobilization is required, and distortion and magnification are encountered. Measurement with CT is very much easier because of the axial display of the upper and lower portions of the femora. Two scans are necessary for measurement of the angle: (1) a scan at the level of the pubic symphysis which includes the femoral head, neck, and trochanteric region; and (2) a scan through the distal femur that includes the broadest diameter of the condyles (obtained at a level just below the upper margin of the patella).

Hernandez [7] has devised a special foot-board with a Velcro surface and several sizes of open-toe shoes with Velcro soles to achieve correct symmetrical positioning and immobilization of the patient for adequate scanning. This is mandatory for accurate measurements to be made

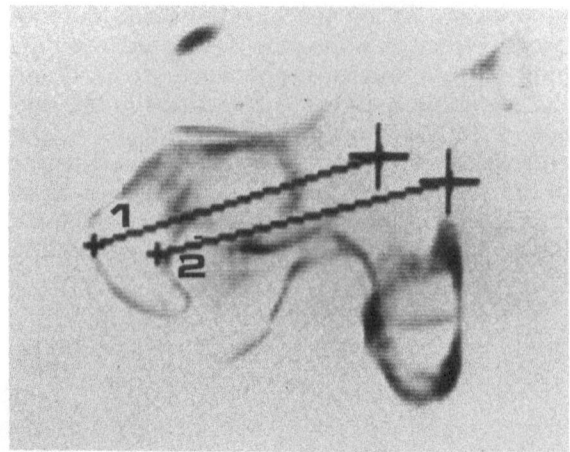

Fig. 23.2. Assessment of femoral anteversion in a 14-year-old boy. The image illustrated shows superimposition of CT images through the femoral head, neck, and trochanteric region superimposed on an image through the femoral condyle on the right. *Line 1* is the axis of the femoral neck. *Line 2* is the transcondylar axis, which bisects the lines tangential to the anterior and posterior margins of the condyles. The angle of femoral anteversion is defined as the angle between *lines 1* and *2* (Pettersson and Harwood-Nash 1982 [15])

from the two scans obtained. The device ensures no rotational motion between the two scans. The method we have used to measure the angle of anteversion or declination is that described by Hernandez et al. [7] (Fig. 23.2). The two images obtained are double exposed on the same film. If the table height is not changed between the two scans, the upper and lower portions of the femur will not be at the same position on the film. If they overlap, it may be easier to magnify each image and relocate them to facilitate measurements [7]. Measurements are most easily made with images viewed with a wide window setting to eliminate soft tissues and provide an outline of the bone.

A line is drawn through the long axis of the femoral neck in the superior scan. This line should not include the greater trochanter, which lies posterior to it. The neck may be difficult to define in infants, in whom it is short, or following surgery. In the inferior scan the transcondylar axis is that line which bisects the angle between lines drawn tangential to the anterior and posterior margins of the condyles. The lines of the femoral neck and transcondylar axes are made to intersect, and the angle between these two is considered the angle of anteversion. If the two lines meet lateral to the symphysis pubis there is anteversion. If they meet medially toward the symphysis there is retroversion [7].

Using this technique, Hernandez [7] found that the intraobserver variation varied from 0° to 8° (mean 2°) and the interobserver error from 0° to 8° (mean 3°). The greatest errors were noted in children with severe femoral neck abnormalities and in postsurgical patients. Another difficult situation is in patients with extensive rotation causing a vertical orientation of the femoral neck, because the axis of the neck may be difficult to find [7].

CT accurately displays the depth and size of the anterior and posterior acetabular lips. This is particularly important in the older child with previous dislocation when pelvic osteotomy is considered to provide better coverage of the femoral head by increasing the capacity of the acetabulum [7]. The angle of acetabular torsion is the angle between a line connecting the anterior and posterior lips of the acetabulum to the sagittal plane. Anteversion is present when the angle inclines forward and is seen in patients with CDH [7]. In conditions that result in deformity of the femoral head such as CDH and Legg–Perthes disease it is important to know the degree of eccentricity of the femoral head and its symmetry in relationship to the acetabulum (see Fig. 23.1). Hip CT provides this information and obviates the need for arthography. However, the cartilaginous rim is better shown with arthrography combined with CT [18].

The value of CT in patients with CDH can thus be summarized as follows:

1. *To evaluate concentricity of reduction of the femoral head after an attempted closed reduction.* This is particularly important if the clinical findings or plain radiographs raise the possibility that the hip is not concentrically reduced. CT will accurately display the relationship of the femoral head to the acetabulum and often reveals the cause for the persistent dislocation or subluxation such as a tight iliopsoas tendon, or intra-articular obstacles such as pulvinar hypertrophy, or intra-articular soft tissue interposition and metallic pins.

2. *To determine the degree of femoral torsion and the configuration of the acetabulum when surgical procedures are required.*

Proximal Focal Femoral Deficiency

Proximal focal femoral deficiency is a rare congenital skeletal anomaly characterized by failure of normal development of a variable portion of the proximal femur. The etiology is obscure and diagnosis may only be evident on radiological study. No previous report has described the use of CT in this condition. We have found that CT may be of value in determining the relationship of the remaining femoral shaft to the acetabulum, particularly when there is still only poor ossification in the femoral head (Fig. 23.3) which may not be detected on plain radiographs. The transverse axial scans of CT may show the anteroposterior relationships at the level of the upper thigh and acetabulum more accurately than plain radiographs.

Slipped Upper Femoral Epiphysis

The CT appearances in slipped upper femoral epiphysis have not previously been described. The studies performed on our four patients con-

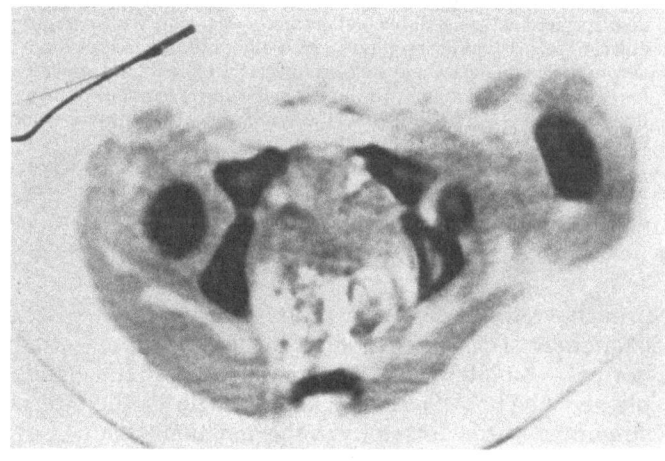

Fig. 23.3. A 1-year-old boy with left proximal focal femoral deficiency. CT shows the position of the small left femoral head in the acetabulum and the relationship to the upper part of the femoral shaft, which is displaced superiorly. The femoral head and its relationship to the adjacent shaft was extremely poorly delineated with plain radiography.

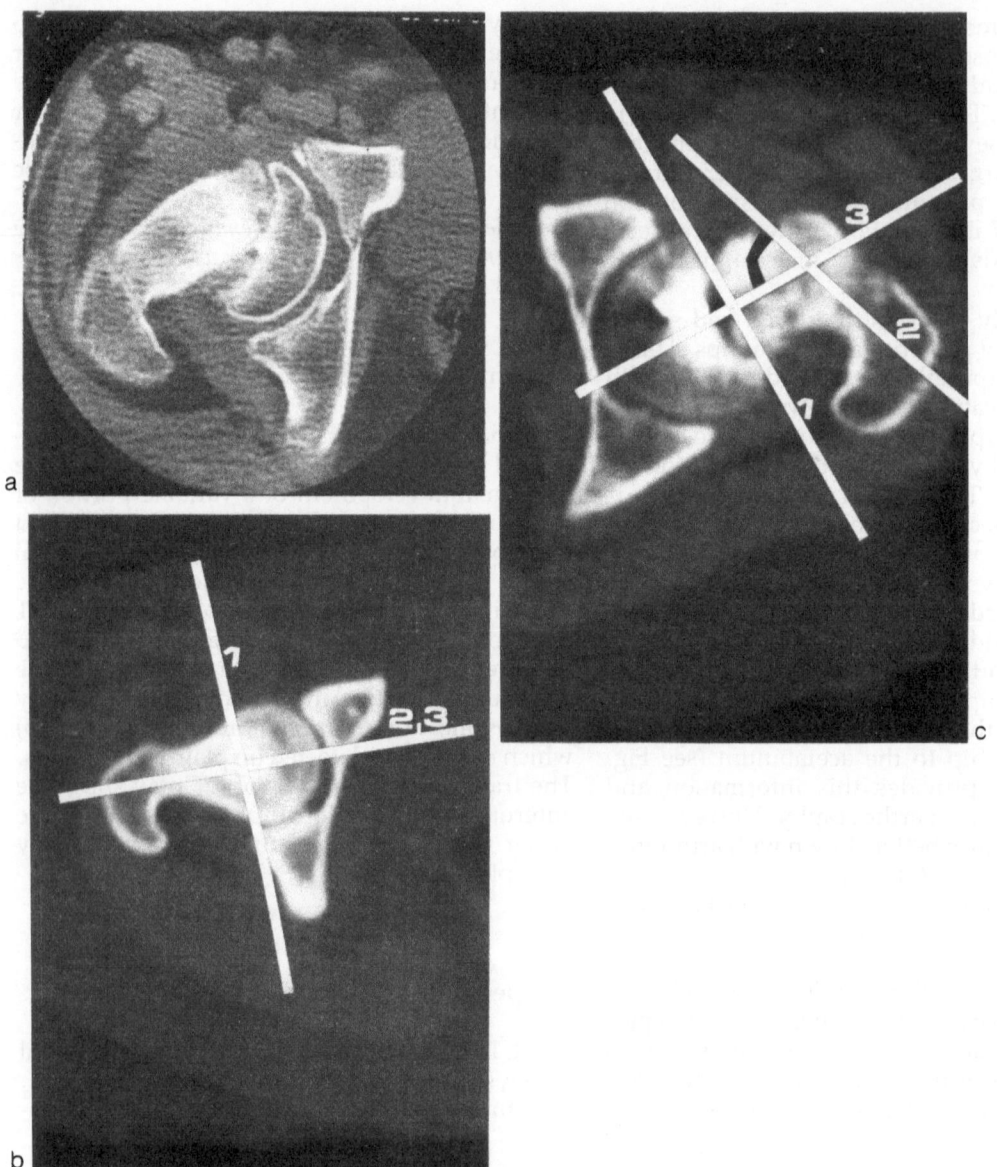

Fig. 23.4. a Slipped upper femoral epiphysis. The femoral epiphysis lies within the acetabular cavity, but there is marked displacement of the metaphysis at the epiphyseal plate with external rotation deformity. Note the irregularity of the bone with adjacent sclerosis at the epiphyseal plate (Pettersson and Harwood-Nash 1982 [15]). **b, c** Measurement of the upper femoral epiphyseal plate/neck angle. *Line 1* connects the edges of the upper femoral epiphysis. *Line 2* is drawn along the long axis of the femoral neck. *Line 3* represents the axis of the upper femoral epiphysis and is a line drawn at right angles to *line 1*, bisecting this line midway between the edges of the femoral epiphysis. A normal hip is shown in **b**. *Lines 2* and *3* are superimposed, making the plate/neck angle 0°. In **c** measurements are shown in a patient with a slipped upper femoral epiphysis. The plate/neck angle between *lines 2* and *3* is shown clearly and this measures the angle of external rotation deformity. Note the relationship of the femoral head to the acetabulum and the rotation of the metaphysis at the epiphyseal plate (Donoghue et al. 1984 [3])

firm that slipped femoral epiphysis is indeed a misnomer. To a large degree the epiphysis is normally situated and it is mainly the metaphysis which slips (Fig. 23.4a). To date, the amount of varus deformity in these patients has been determined from an anteroposterior view of the pelvis showing the hips in a position as nearly neutral as possible. The degree of posterior tilting has been measured on a frog lateral radiograph [3]. These angles determine the wedges of bone to be removed in these planes in patients who require corrective osteotomies. It has been accepted that posterior tilting and external rotation are related. However, the corrective osteotomies that have been performed still leave a significant percentage of these children with persistent out-toeing (external rotation) postoperatively. Orthopedic surgeons have thus been less meticulous about correcting the external rotation deformity except perhaps in a severe deformity. This may be due to the fact that they have not had an adequte method of determining the degree of the deformity. Some of these patients may regain internal rotation of the hip without surgical correction, but this must result in displacement of the femoral head posteriorly in relation to the acetabulum as no remodeling is to be expected in older children.

No previous use has been made of CT images to measure the amount of femoral external rotation in patients with slipped upper femoral epiphysis. With the patient in the supine position we have used the axial CT scans to measure the angle between the upper femoral epiphyseal plate and the femoral neck (plate/neck angle) to assess the amount of femoral rotation. The method requires one scan through the femoral head, neck, and trochanteric region. The angle is measured in the following manner (see Fig. 23.4b,c): Line 1 is drawn to connect the edges of the upper femoral epiphysis. Line 3, which represents the axis of the femoral epiphysis is defined as a line which is at right angles to and bisects line 1 between the edges of the epiphysis. Line 2 represents the axis of the femoral neck and is drawn through the long axis of the neck. The angle measured between lines 2 and 3 is defined as the angle of external or internal rotation deformity of the head on the neck and is close to 0° in the normal pediatric hip.

By using CT to measure the plate/neck angle we can accurately determine the degree of external rotation deformity and thus accurately assess the triple deformity in this condition. This modality is thus of great value when corrective osteotomy is planned.

Loose Bodies

Loose bodies may be present in the hip joint following trauma or in relation to Legg–Perthes disease. Small loose bony fragments in the hip joint may be extremely difficult to document on plain radiographs. Often the only sign of loose fragments within the joint on plain radiography is widening of the joint space compared with the normal side. It has been shown that maximum joint space widening secondary to a single fragment correlates with its position within the joint. The initial radiographs in acutely injured patients may be of suboptimal quality. In addition, rotation of the pelvis may significantly alter the apparent degree of widening [3]. We have found CT to be extremely useful in the acute phase and in those children with persistent hip pain following dislocation and who have had manipulative or spontaneous reduction (Fig. 23.5a). Many of these have disruption of the ligamentum teres with attached bony fragments lying within the joint cavity [3].

We have used CT to document the presence or absence of loose bodies in the hip joints in 15 children with either trauma or Legg–Perthes disease. CT obviated the need for an exploratory hip operation in four of our patients suspected of having a posttraumatic loose body. It proved very useful in detecting the number and position of small ossified loose fragments together with surrounding acetabular injury in six patients (Fig. 23.5a), one of whom had normal plain radiographs.

However, CT does have limitations in the detection of intra-articular loose bodies, particularly in patients with Legg–Perthes disease. One patient had a CT scan which was interpreted as normal following trauma, but at operation was found to have a ruptured ligamentum teres with no attached ossified fragments. In three patients who had Legg–Perthes disease and in whom a loose intra-articular fragment of bone was suspected clinically, CT showed irregular fragments of bone lying in defects in the femoral head (Fig. 23.5b,c). It was impossible to determine whether these were loose or fixed. Some were shown to lie loose in the joint cavity once the femoral head had been dislocated at operation. Perhaps the study should be performed with as much adduction of the hip as possible in children in whom there is a strong clinical suspicion of a loose osteochondral fragment which is still attached to the ligamentum teres. This maneuver elevates the fragment from its bed in the femoral head by traction exerted through the ligamentum teres. Another patient with Legg–Perthes disease had a soft tissue mass containing fragments of bone in the joint space (Fig. 23.5d). At the time of the CT examination this was not appreciated as representing the phase of reossification and was thought to represent loose fragments.

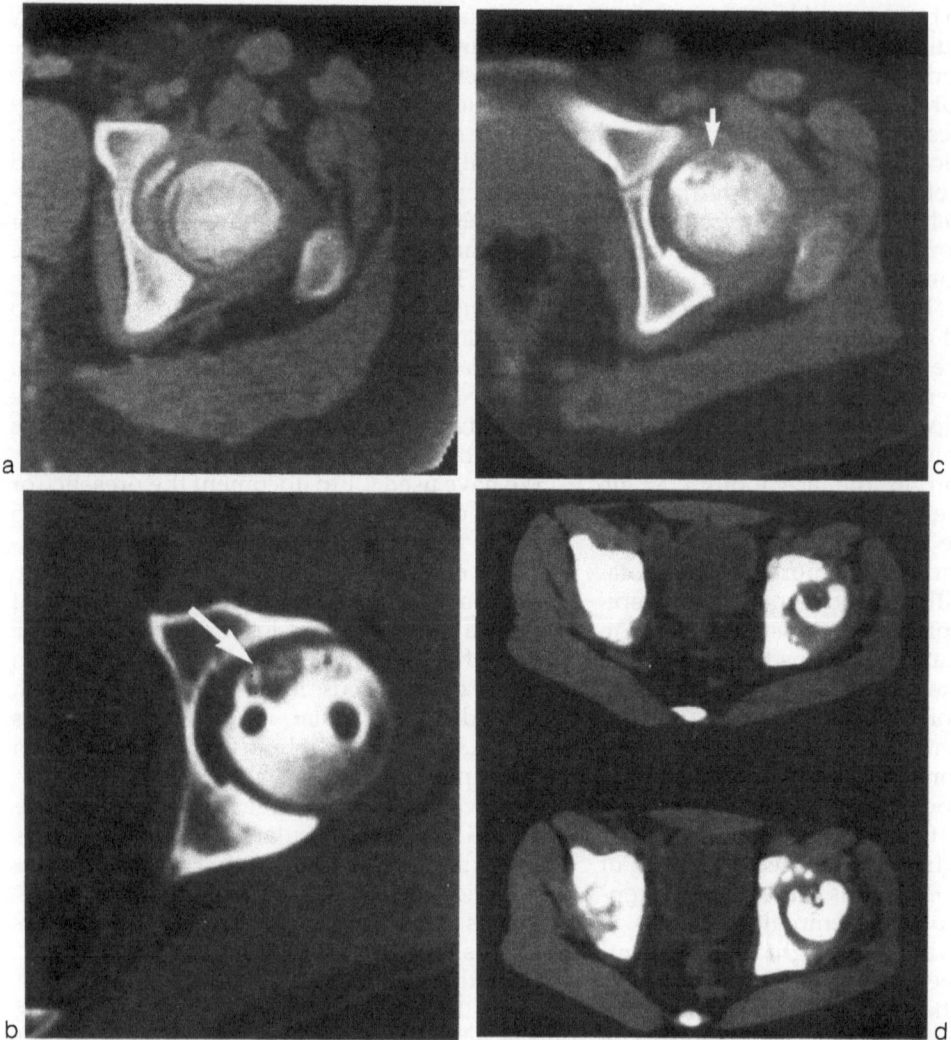

Fig. 23.5a–d. Suspected or proven loose bodies within the hips. **a** A 10-year-old boy with trauma to the left hip 2 months previously. CT shows a loose fragment of bone in the joint space. This fragment was found to be attached to a torn ligamentum teres at operation. **b** Adolescent male with Legg–Perthes disease. Irregular fragments of bone are noted (*arrow*) in a defect in the femoral head. When the femoral head was dislocated at operation, these fragments were found to be lying within the joint but attached to the ligmentum teres. **c** An 11-year-old female with Legg–Perthes disease. Irregular bony fragments are noted lying in a defect in the femoral head (*arrow*). These fragments were not found to be loose at operation. It is not possible to distinguish this appearance from that illustrated in **b**. **d** A 12-year-old boy with Legg–Perthes disease. Fragments of bone are noted within an area of soft tissue attenuation in the joint space. These were thought to represent loose fragments within the joint space but were found to be areas of reossification within the cartilage of the femoral head (Donoghue et al. 1984 [3])

Therefore, although CT is valuable for the detection of intra-articular loose bodies, it does have limitations, which can be summarized as follows: Noncalcified loose bodies may not be visualized, reossification of the femoral head may mimic the presence of loose bodies, and bony fragments lying free in cavities within the femoral head cannot be differentiated from those that are attached to the head.

Miscellaneous

Mention must also be made of various other ways in which CT examination of the hip can be of value. CT accurately provides valuable information required for correct treatment not only in trauma to the femoral head but also in trauma involving the acetabulum and other parts of the bony pelvis [13, 18]. Indeed, CT may provide

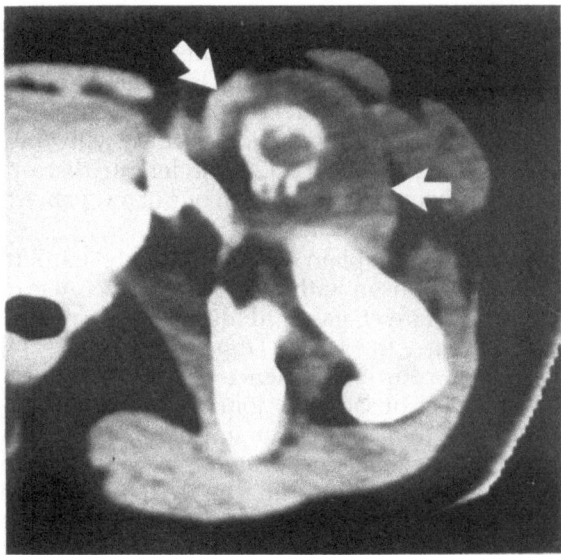

Fig. 23.6. A 17-year-old female with myositis ossificans. CT shows a soft tissue mass (*arrows*) containing a relatively well-defined central area of calcification. The abnormality was not visualized on the plain radiographs (Donoghue et al. 1984 [3])

such as intrapelvic hematomas are also easily documented with CT. In addition, CT is valuable for the delineation of other bone and soft tissue lesions adjacent to the hip. Examples of lesions we have studied are illustrated in Figs. 23.6 and 23.7 (see also Fig. 21.3, p. 316, and Fig. 21.12, p. 324).

Sacroiliac Joints

Introduction

The sacroiliac joints are extremely complex joints with two types of articulation. The anteroinferior third is synovial, and the posterosuperior two-thirds are ligamentous. Both parts of the joint have an undulating surface. Because these joints are angulated to the sagittal plane and because of the large amount of adjacent bone and overlying bowel gas and stool, they are extremely difficult to image with plain radiographs. CT obviates these problems and has been found to be extremely useful in delineating traumatic, neoplastic, infectious, and arthritic changes of the sacroiliac joints. The vast majority of the published literature regarding the value of CT in sacroiliac joint disease concerns adults, and little has been written on the value of CT in pediatric sacroiliac joint disease.

valuable information which cannot be appreciated on conventional studies and which may change the mode of therapy. For example, the treatment of acetabular fractures depends on whether the fracture involves the anterior or posterior column of the acetabulum; this information is easily obtained from the transverse axial images of CT. Adjacent soft tissue injury

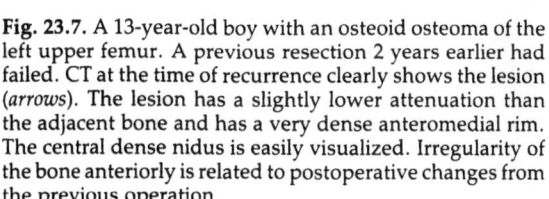

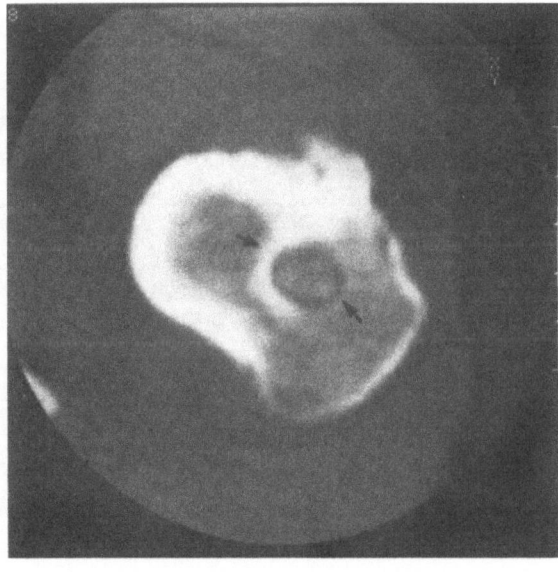

Fig. 23.7. A 13-year-old boy with an osteoid osteoma of the left upper femur. A previous resection 2 years earlier had failed. CT at the time of recurrence clearly shows the lesion (*arrows*). The lesion has a slightly lower attenuation than the adjacent bone and has a very dense anteromedial rim. The central dense nidus is easily visualized. Irregularity of the bone anteriorly is related to postoperative changes from the previous operation.

Lawson et al. [10] have described a useful method for examining the sacroiliac joints with CT. An initial lateral computed radiograph is performed, from which the angle of the sacrum is determined. The gantry is then angulated to correspond as closely as possible to this angle. Scans taken with this gantry angle show the synovial portion of the joint to be orientated vertically on the CT image, while the ligamentus portion is orientated more obliquely (Fig. 23.8). Criteria of normalcy of the sacroiliac joints are that the two sides are symmetrical, that the joint spaces are uniformly thick, and that the cortices are uniformly thin and parallel with no focal erosions. In adults it has been found that CT can detect subtle changes in the joints when plain radiography shows no abnormality [10].

Trauma

Radiographic evidence of disruption of the sacroiliac joint in pelvic trauma in children is uncommon. In a review of 100 cases described by Rang [17] at the Hospital for Sick Children, Toronto, over a 10-year period, 13% were found to have sacroiliac joint disruption. Late development of degenerative changes in the injured adult sacroiliac joint with pain is a common feature, regardless of the initial insult, and may require fusion [9]. Although the long-term results in children have not been systematically studied, the use of a pelvic sling and appropriate traction will generally result in healing of the sacroiliac joint fractures without disability [16].

However, there are unique features associated with traumatic disruption of the sacroiliac joints in the growing pelvis which include undergrowth of the hemipelvis and subsequent sacroiliac joint fusion, and pelvic deformity with limb-length discrepancy [12]. Limb-length discrepancy has been documented in one of our patients 6 months post trauma.

Good-quality plain radiographs are hard to obtain in children with pelvic trauma because of overlying bowel gas and difficulty in patient positioning. In 1985, Donoghue et al. [4] reported our experience with the CT appearances of sacroiliac joint trauma in six children. We found that our impression of radiographic evidence of sacroiliac joint space widening after pelvic injury in five children was confirmed by CT in only one. In three of these children CT showed that the apparent joint space widening was due to a subchondral fracture of the ilium, and the joint space itself was intact (Figs. 23.9, 23.10). In the fifth patient the joint space appeared normal on CT, but both sides of the injured sacroiliac joint were irregular. In the sixth patient plain radiographs showed apparently normal sacroiliac joints, but CT showed a narrow left sacroiliac joint space.

CT scans performed immediately following trauma in children with subchondral fractures may show an appearance suggesting sacroiliac joint widening. However, within several days subchondral new bone begins to form, and scans at this time reveal an intact joint space with new bone at the site of the fracture. Follow-up scans from 3 weeks to 2.5 years post trauma demon-

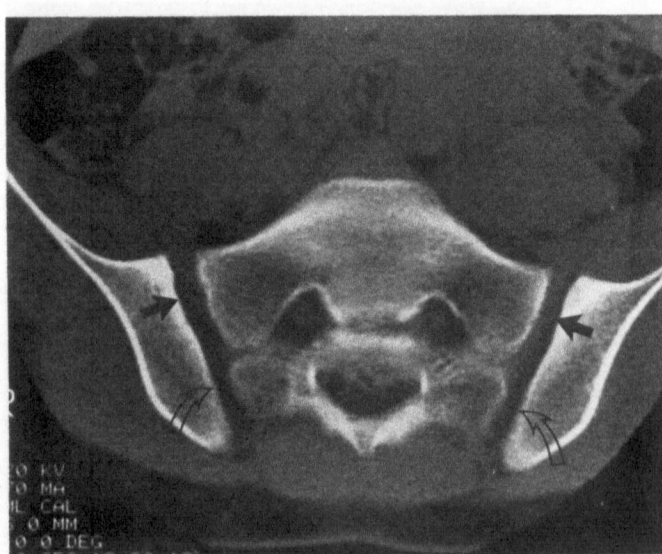

Fig. 23.8a,b. Example of sacroiliac joints. **a** The synovial portions of the joint are indicated by *black arrows* and the ligamentous portions by *curved arrows*.

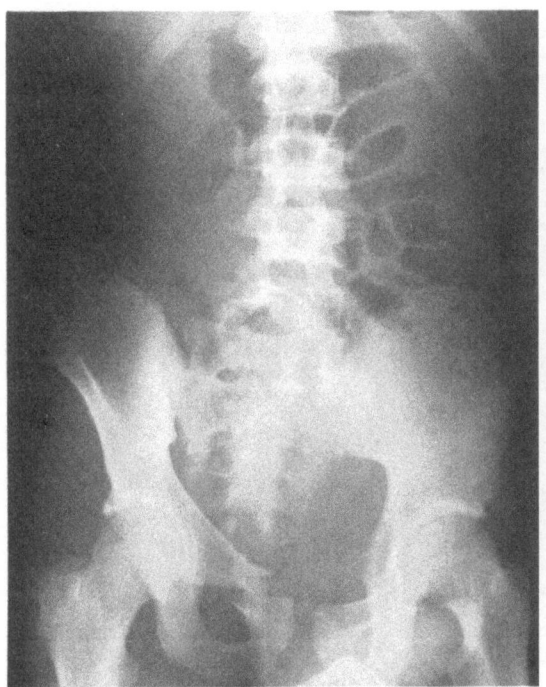
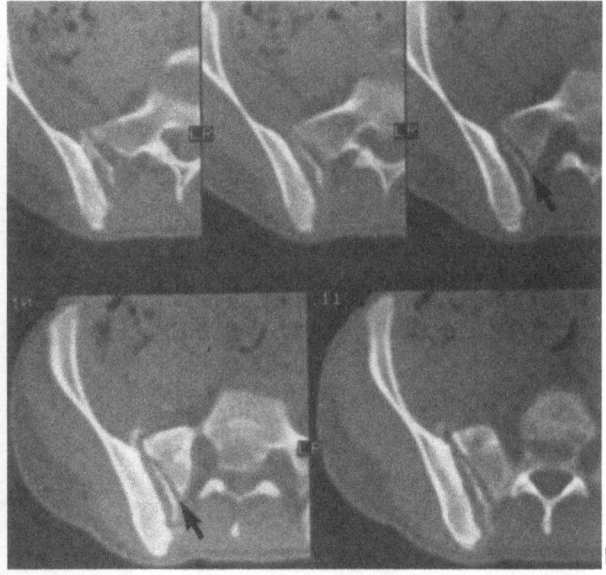

Fig. 23.9a,b. A 15-year-old boy with pelvic trauma from a motor vehicle accident. **a** Plain radiograph shows apparent disruption of the right sacroiliac joint. **b** CT scans 1 month after trauma demonstrate a subchondral fracture of the right ilium and an intact joint space (*arrow*). There is some posterior displacement of the ilium. New bone formation along the anterior surface of the ilium indicates that there has been associated subperiosteal injury at this site.

strated that the injured sacroiliac joint was normal in four patients, slightly narrow in one, and there was partial fusion in the sixth. All except this sixth patient are now symptom free. All three subchondral fractures have shown good healing.

Narrowing of the joint space and subchondral fractures in association with an intact joint space have not previously been reported with sacroiliac joint trauma in children. Sacroiliac joint space narrowing is thought to occur as a result of a compression injury. The subchondral fractures are thought to occur through the structurally weak areas, as defined by our morphological study. This type of injury may explain the good long-term results in children with trauma to this region. Widening of the sacroiliac joint space in association with trauma, as suggested on plain radiographs, may thus not be as common as was previously thought. The narrowed joint space may resemble a Salter type V injury, and the subchondral fracture a Salter type I or II epiphyseal injury. However, the uncommon subsequent narrowing of the joint space and/or fusion may represent a higher grade of epiphyseal type fracture resembling a Salter type III or V injury.

Our observations have correlated with a morphological study in which a normal sacroiliac joint from an autopsy of a human male aged 8 years was studied [4]. The study suggested that the structurally weak areas may represent the zones of cartilage proliferation and provisional calcification in the growing cartilage of the opposing sacroiliac joint surfaces and the zone of cambium layer of the periosteum in the areas of ligamental insertion, as these areas contain relatively fewer collagen fibers.

Neoplasms

Although it is rare for neoplasms to arise within the sacroiliac joint it is not uncommon for them to occur in the adjacent ilium or sacrum. Whenever evaluating such lesions it is always important to assess whether the sacroiliac joint is involved, as this has important therapeutic implications. These lesions include osteogenic sarcoma, Ewing's sarcoma, giant cell tumor, histiocytosis X, and metastases (Fig. 23.11). However, it has been our experience that in the vast majority of these cases the joint space is not violated.

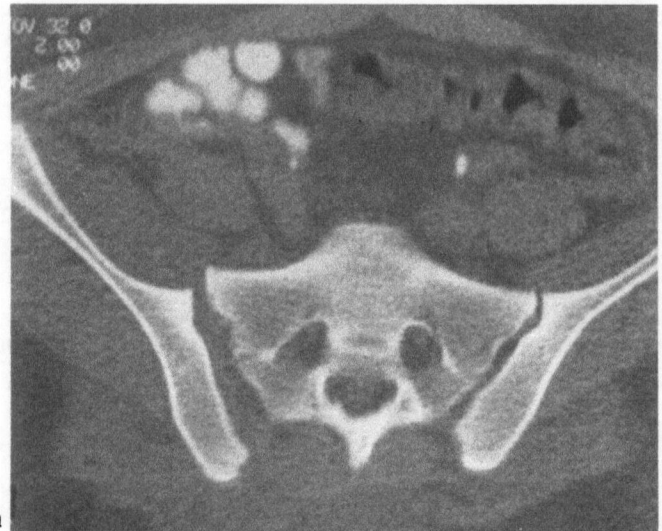

a

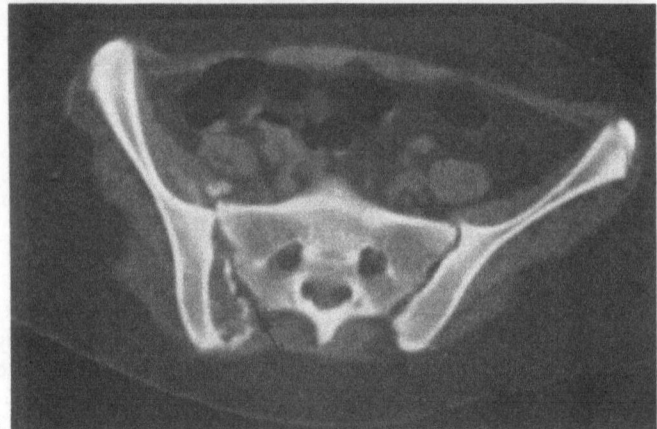

b

Fig. 23.10a,b. A 15-year-old boy with pelvic trauma from a motor vehicle accident. **a** CT immediately after trauma shows apparent disruption of the right sacroiliac joint space. There is some posterior displacement of the right ilium. **b** Follow-up CT 3 weeks later shows a normal-sized sacroiliac joint space (*arrow*) and some healing of the subchondral fracture of the ilium. New bone is noted anterior to the joint space on the right ilium indicating that the fracture extends in a subperiosteal plane along the ilium.

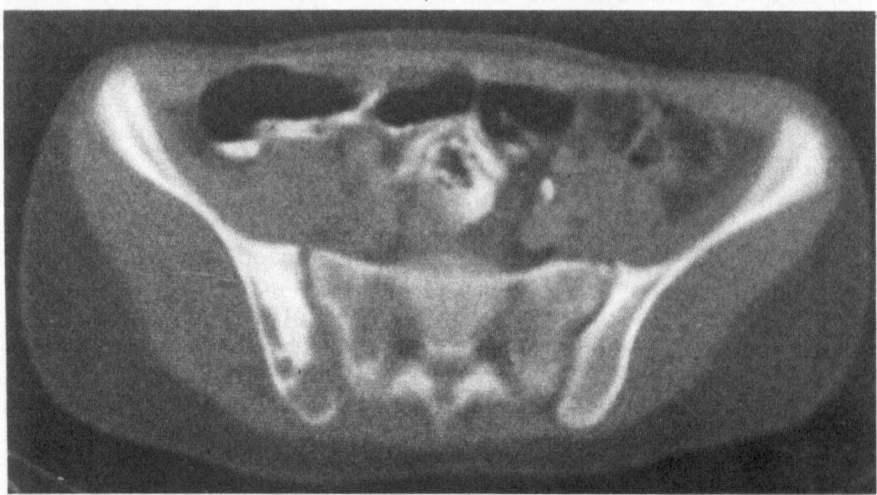

Fig. 23.11. A 6-year-old girl with Hodgkin's disease and metastasis to the posterior aspect of the right ilium. Note the bone destruction in this region and extension through the cortex into the sacroiliac joint posteriorly. CT is a valuable modality in defining accurately the relationship of iliac and sacral neoplasms to the sacroiliac joints.

Infection

The sacroiliac joints are rarely affected by infectious processes, but, when they are, CT provides important information regarding the extent of these infections which may not be easily documented with plain radiography or radionuclide scans. An example is shown by the case illustrated in Fig. 23.12, where infection extended from the sacroiliac joint into the spinal canal. CT also provides useful information for follow-up.

Arthritis

In children, we have rarely used CT to evaluate the sacroiliac joints for arthritic changes. However, CT may be extremely useful when a clinical diagnosis has not been established and con-

ventional radiographs are either normal or equivocal. CT shows more subtle changes than can be appreciated on plain radiographs and is also valuable for follow-up. Manifestations of arthritis include changes in the size of the joint, erosions, sclerosis, fusion, and hypertrophic spur formation [13].

Feet

Introduction

The complex three-dimensional anatomy of the bones and soft tissues of the feet make this region extremely difficult to evaluate. We have found that CT is very useful in the evaluation of disorders of the feet and has provided extra

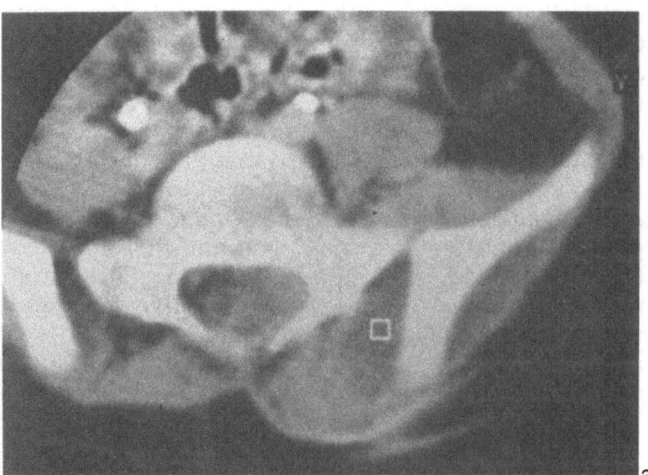

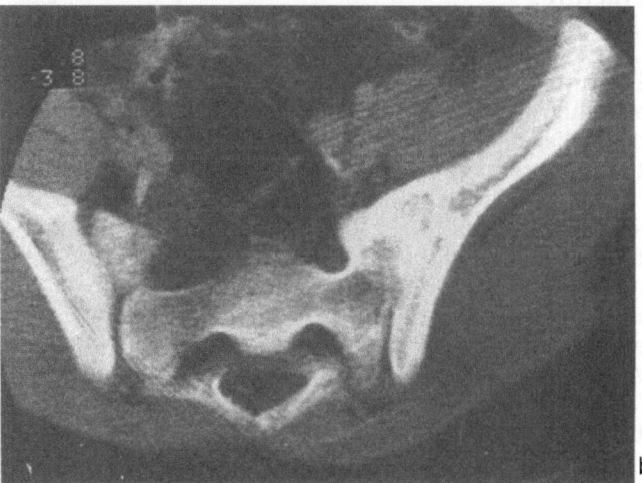

Fig. 23.12a,b. A 10 year old girl with low back pain and fever. **a** CT shows enlargement of the soft tissues anterior and posterior to the left sacroiliac joint. The *square cursor* indicates a large area extending out of the joint that has failed to enhance; this represents an abscess. The remainder of the soft tissue swelling is related to associated muscle inflammation. Note the asymmetry of the tissues in the spinal canal at this level. The increased soft tissue present on the left is due to inflammatory tissue extending into the spinal canal. **b** CT scan at a lower level through the sacroiliac joints shows fusion of the anterior aspect of the left joint with adjacent bony sclerosis.

information which was not obtained from more conventional radiographs. We have used CT to delineate fractures, tumors, tarsal coalition, and foreign bodies in the feet. The examination is very simple but requires meticulous attention to technique. Both feet should be placed in the scanner gantry alongside each other, as symmetrically as possible. The feet can be securely taped together or to the table top. The patient is usually examined in the supine position with the knees flexed and the feet placed with their plantar aspect on the table. It is extremely important to make sure that the patient is comfortable so that there will be no movement during scanning. In order to do this a pillow may be placed under the flexed knees, and the knees can be taped together as well to ensure stability. Patients who have suffered recent trauma to the foot and who are still in pain may not be able to lie in the position described. We have found it useful to examine these patients in the lateral decubitus position with both feet positioned as symmetrically as possible within the gantry. Under these circumstances it may be more difficult to achieve a symmetrical position, and taping of the feet may be more difficult.

Images of the feet should be viewed at both a bone and soft tissue window so that the bones, joints, and adjacent soft tissues can all be evaluated adequately. It is best to have CT sections passing at right angles through the joints that are being examined; other positions than those already described may be more useful when unusual abnormalities of the foot are to be assessed.

Fractures

Fractures of the calcaneus can be very disabling and their treatment is controversial. Knowledge of the basic fracture configuration is essential in the management of these injuries [5,19].

Type I fractures of the calcaneus are isolated or simple fractures in the body, anterior end, or tuberosity, with little displacement and without extension into the articular surfaces. These do not pose a significant clinical problem, except for avulsion fractures of the tuberosity involving the Achilles tendon.

Type II fractures involve the subtalar joints. Essex-Lopresti [5] recognized two patterns of fractures, which he described as (1) tongue-type

and (2) depression-type fractures. In the tongue-type fracture the primary fracture line extends from the posterior aspect of the talocalcaneal joint to the plantar surface of the calcaneus. This is associated with a transverse horizontal fracture extending back to the posterior aspect of the calcaneal tuberosity. The fragment involving the lateral half of the articular surface of the posterior facet and the superior surface of the body of the calcaneus constitutes the tongue. Depending upon the severity of the injury this acts as a seesaw, with the anterior end dipping into the cancellous bone of the body and the posterior end riding superiorly. In the joint depression-type fracture the secondary fracture line extends backward and upward posterior to the articular surface. This fragment is driven down into the cancellous bone depending on the force involved and eventually causes the lateral margin of the calcaneus to burst. This causes displacement of the peroneus longus and brevis tendons.

In the management of fractures of the calcaneus it is generally desirable to restore the normal anatomy. Five recognized causes of persistent pain complicating healed fractures of the calcaneus include (1) scarring and posttraumatic arthritis causing subtalar pain, (2) peroneal tendonitis caused by compression and displacement, (3) plantar calcaneal bone spurs caused by malunion and associated with disruption of the heel fat, (4) arthritis of the calcaneocuboid joint, and (5) nerve entrapment of the medial and lateral plantar branches [2].

Plain lateral radiographs of the calcaneus give good information on the integrity of Bohler's angle [1], and axial views give some idea of the integrity of the medial and lateral surfaces of the calcaneus. However, with impaction, details of the fractures are frequently obscured, and the extent of injury must often be inferred. Because of pain, axial views are sometimes impossible to obtain, and plain films do not give any precise information on the nature of soft tissue involvement.

Examination of the hindfoot with CT has proven useful in cases of healed calcaneal fractures with residual pain and has helped to determine the state of the peroneal tendons and damage to the talocalcaneal articular surfaces [20]. Pablot et al. [14] have recently shown that CT is extremely useful in the assessment of acute comminuted fractures of the calcaneus as it gives graphic visualization of the size and number of fracture fragments, which may not be appreciated on plain films. It also gives information regarding the extent of involvement of the articular surfaces, visualization of the disruption of the medial and lateral walls of the calcaneus, and their relationship to the peroneal tendons laterally (Fig. 23.13). In addition, in one patient the articular surface of the calcaneocuboid joint was shown to be involved, and this could not be appreciated on plain radiographs. CT images should not only be viewed at bony window settings but should also be viewed at soft tissue window settings to assess injuries that may involve the peroneal tendons and the heel fat pad, and possibly the plantar nerves.

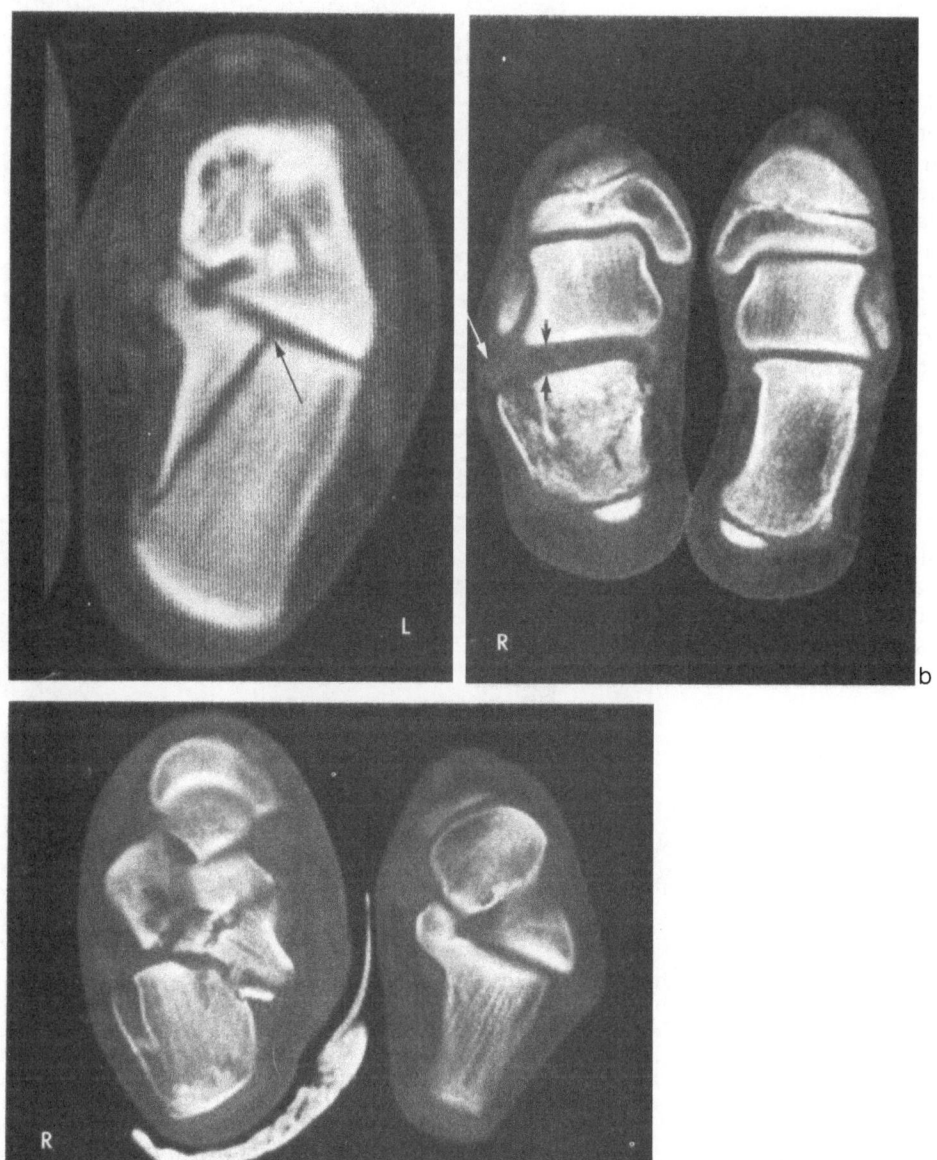

Fig. 23.13a–c. Examples of the value of CT in the assessment of acute fracture of the calcaneus. The three cases illustrated are of young teenage boys who all fell from a height. **a** CT shows a tongue-type fracture line in the left calcaneus passing into the talocalcaneal joint (*arrow*). The fracture fragments are undisplaced and the joint is intact. **b** CT shows a comminuted-type fracture of the right calcaneus with a small eggshell-type fragment laterally. There is marked anteroposterior compression of the right calcaneus with widening of the posterior talocalcaneal joint (*black arrows*). The *white arrow* indicates the proximity of the peroneal tendon to the fracture laterally. **c** CT shows large fracture fragments of the right calcaneus in the subtalar portion of the bone. The medial and lateral margins of the bone are grossly disrupted. Some of the abnormalities delineated by CT, such as the widening or irregularity of joint surfaces and relationship of the peroneal tendons to the fracture site, cannot be delineated on plain radiographs.

The findings on CT have helped to determine whether the treatment of such fractures should be conservative or operative and have also given the surgeon important preoperative information regarding the site of incision and the type of operation necessary. The CT appearances correlate well with the operative findings.

Tumors

We have rarely had the opportunity to study soft tissue or bony tumors arising in the foot. However, CT is useful in certain lesions because of the complex three-dimensional anatomy of the foot. CT scans will display the transverse anatomy of these lesions better than plain radiography and will delineate their soft tissue component very much better (Fig. 23.14). Such studies are not only useful preoperatively but are also useful as a baseline for evaluation of response to therapy.

Tarsal Coalition

We have found CT to be extremely useful in the evaluation of tarsal coalition when plain radiographs are equivocal. When examining the foot for tarsal coalition it is best to have the CT sections at right angles to the joint in question. For evaluation of the subtalar joint the most desir-

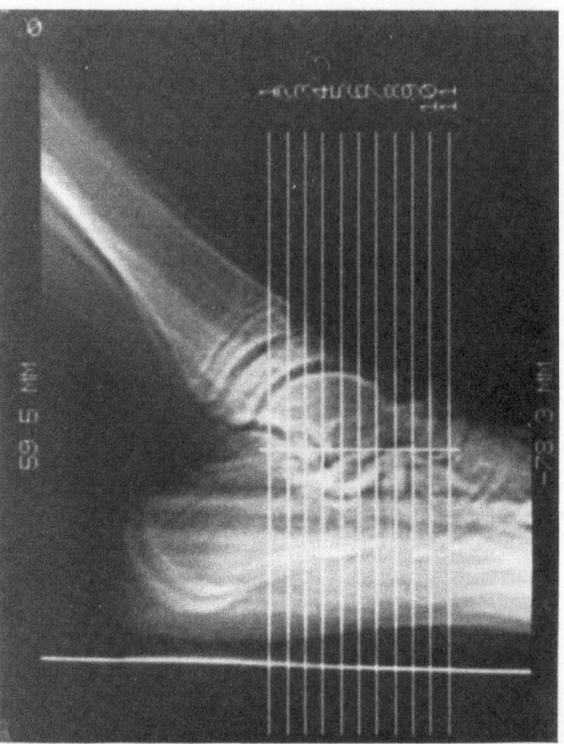

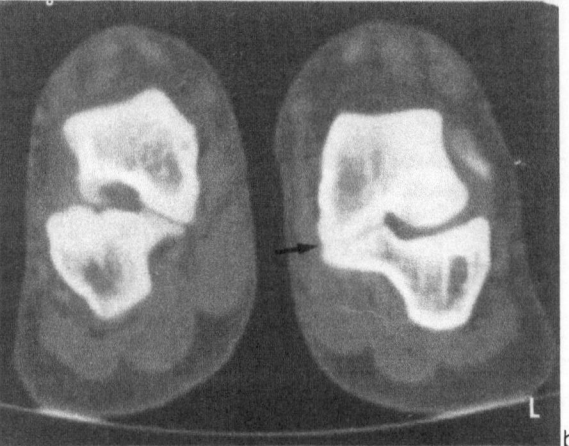

Fig. 23.15. a Lateral scout radiograph shows the position of the foot in the gantry for the detection of talocalcaneal coalition. The *numbered vertical lines* indicate the position of the scans to evaluate the relationship between the talus and the calcaneus. Different positions may be required to evaluate coalition at other intertarsal joints. **b** CT shows talocalcaneal coalition on the left (*arrow*). The right joint shows a normal smooth surface, but the left joint shows irregularity of this joint surface, narrowing of the joint space, and increased sclerosis adjacent to the joint. Coalition at the joint is usually associated with a slightly more oblique angle of the joint than normal.

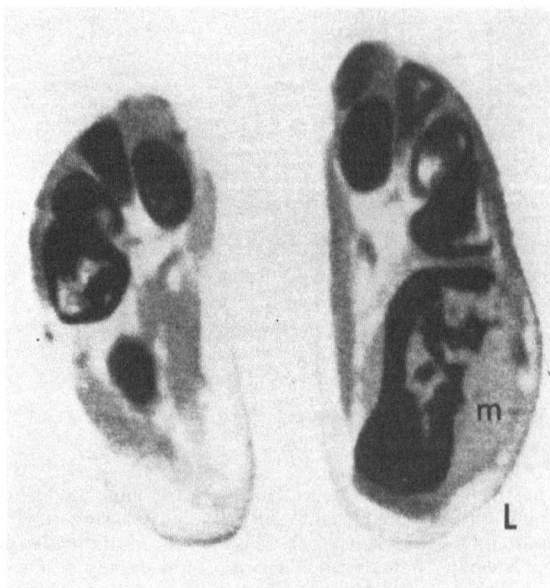

Fig. 23.14. A 6-year-old boy with Ewing's sarcoma of the left calcaneus. The bone shows destruction, and a soft tissue mass (*m*) is noted laterally.

able position is that with the patient lying supine, with knees flexed and the plantar aspect of the foot placed on the table. Sections of 5 mm thickness can be easily obtained through the joint, and any coalition can be easily visualized (Fig. 23.15). Comparison should always be made with the opposite side. Tarsal coalition may often be bilateral.

Miscellaneous

The use of CT has proved of immense value in the assessment of the soft tissues when foreign bodies are suspected and are not visible on plain radiographs. The higher density resolution of CT will often delineate these foreign bodies extremely easily.

Spine

In the Radiology Department at the Hospital for Sick Children, Toronto, CT studies of the spinal cord are primarily supervised by our pediatric neuroradiologists. The reason for this is that many of the studies are performed after the injection of dilute metrizamide into the subarachnoid space [6, 15]. The description of this type of examination has thus been excluded from this book and for a detailed account of these studies the reader is referred to *CT and Myelogra-phy of the Spine and Cord*, authored by Drs. Holger Pettersson and Derek Harwood-Nash [15]. This book reflects our departmental approach to CT of the spine in children. The relationship of CT metrizamide myelography to general body CT studies, particularly as it applies to posterior mediastinal (see Chap. 4, p. 44) and adrenal and retroperitoneal masses (see Chap. 10, p. 127), has been referred to previously.

In many children, however, CT of the vertebrae is required and can be accomplished successfully without metrizamide myelography [11]. In these instances radiologists not involved with neuroradiology occasionally supervise the studies. This distinction is somewhat artificial but we have found that it works well in our department. Examples of some of these cases are shown in Figs. 23.16–23.23. Two examples have also had metrizamide myelography. CT of the spine is invaluable in the delineation of congenital, traumatic, inflammatory, and neoplastic diseases of the vertebrae just as it is elsewhere in the musculoskeletal system. The axial images of CT are an ideal way to view the complex bony anatomy of the spine and adjacent tissue. In smaller patients direct sagittal scans can be obtained by directly positioning the patient in the gantry (see Fig. 4.29, p. 42). Plain radiographs of the spine are mandatory prior to CT of this region and in many instances bone scintigraphy is also required. Conventional tomography is rarely, if ever, necessary. Magnetic resonance imaging in different planes offers an even more sophisticated manner of imaging the complex anatomy of the spine and cord.

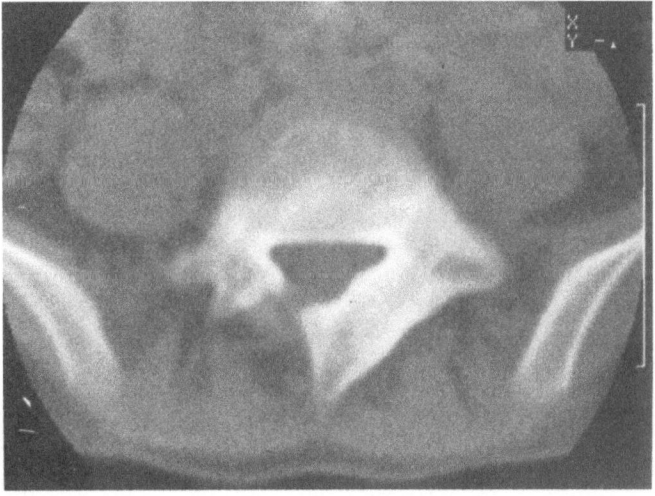

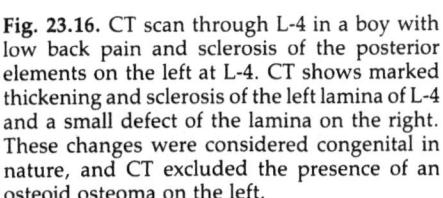

Fig. 23.16. CT scan through L-4 in a boy with low back pain and sclerosis of the posterior elements on the left at L-4. CT shows marked thickening and sclerosis of the left lamina of L-4 and a small defect of the lamina on the right. These changes were considered congenital in nature, and CT excluded the presence of an osteoid osteoma on the left.

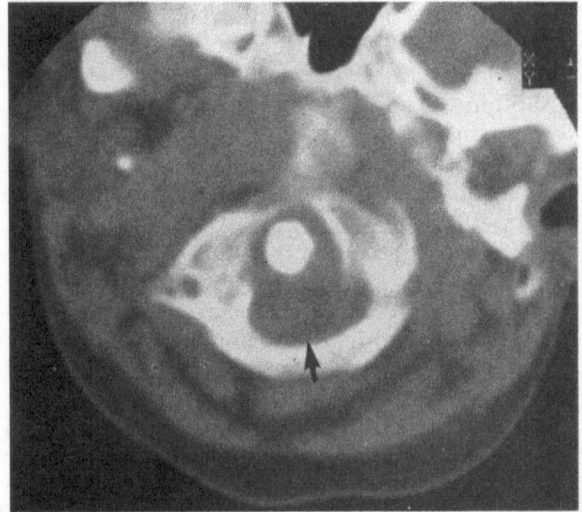

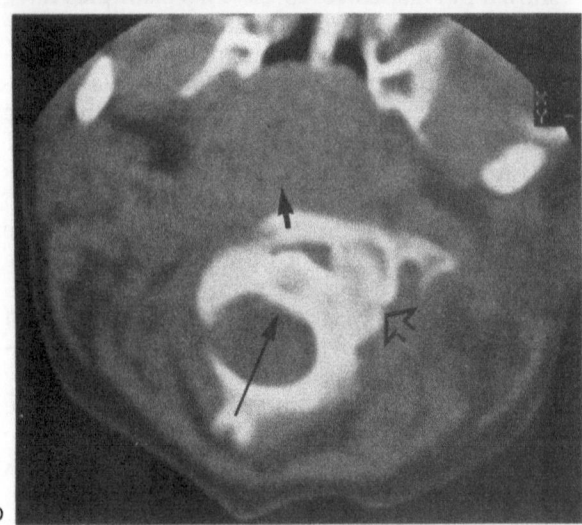

a

b

Fig. 23.17a,b. A 5-year-old girl with rotatory subluxation at the C-1/C-2 level. In **a** and **b** the *short arrow* indicates the anteroposterior axis of the C-1 vertebral ring. The *long arrow* in **b** indicates the anteroposterior axis of C-2. The *open arrow* indicates the subluxation of the articular facets on the left of C-1 and C-2, as both have been included in scan **b**. CT offers an easy method of examination of the craniocervical junction.

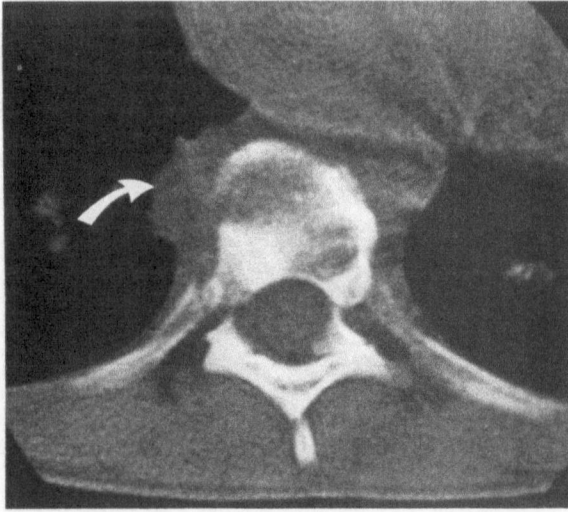

Fig. 23.18. Osteomyelitis of one of the mid-thoracic vertebral bodies. Note the destruction of the vertebral body, particularly anteriorly, on the right and a soft tissue mass extending into the posterior mediastinum (*curved arrow*).

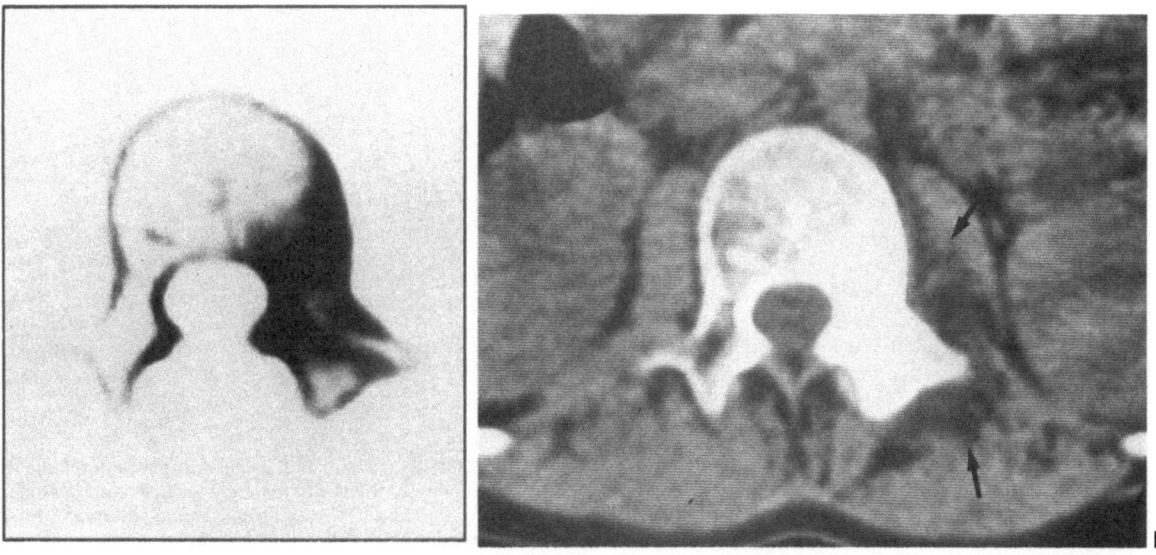

a   b

Fig. 23.19a,b. A 14-year-old boy who was found to have a scoliosis during a routine pre-camp medical examination. Plain radiograph of the lumbar spine showed sclerosis of the pedicle of L-2. **a** CT through L-2 shows marked sclerosis of the left pedicle and adjacent vertebral body. Centrally a nidus of low attenuation is evident, and this appearance is typical of that of an osteoid osteoma. **b** Same scan as **a** but viewed at a soft tissue window shows low-attenuation areas in the adjacent psoas and erector spinae muscles on the left (*arrows*). These areas have the attenuation values of fat and were thought to represent adjacent muscle atrophy. (McConnell and Daneman 1984 [11])

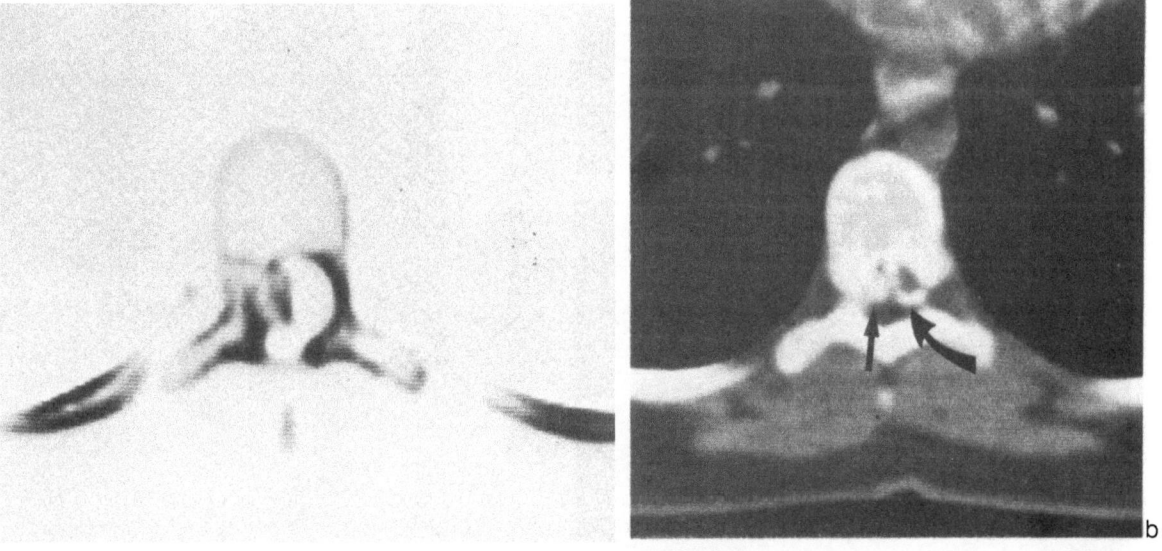

a   b

Fig. 23.20a,b. A 12-year-old girl who had been diagnosed as having acute lymphocytic leukemia at 6 years of age and had been treated with craniospinal irradiation. At the time of presentation she had developed an unsteady gait, and plain radiographs revealed a small sclerotic lesion just to the right of the midline at the level of the T-9 vertebral body. A scoliosis was present convex to the right. **a** CT shows a bony protuberance extending into the spinal canal from the right pedicle of T-9. **b** The scan has been performed after intrathecal injection of metrizamide, which has outlined the dural sac (*curved arrow*). The sac is displaced markedly to the left and is compressed by the bony lesion on the right (*straight arrow*). The lesion was removed and found to be a benign osteochondroma, which is believed to have been radiation induced.

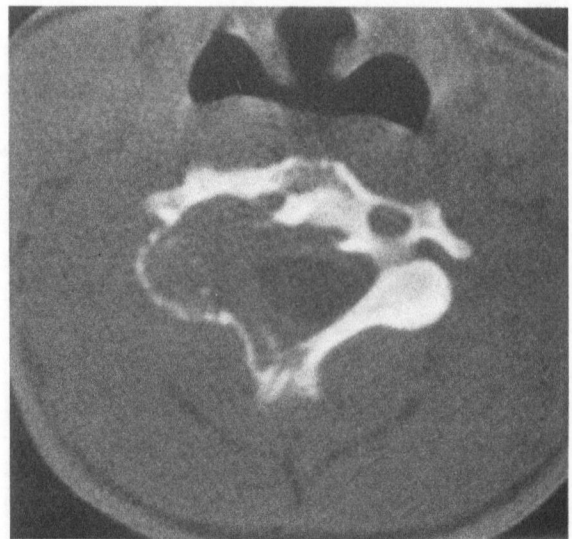

Fig. 23.21. Histiocytosis X of a cervical vertebra. Note the destruction of the vertebral body, pedicle, and lamina on the right. The dural sac can be seen as an area of lower attenuation within the spinal canal.

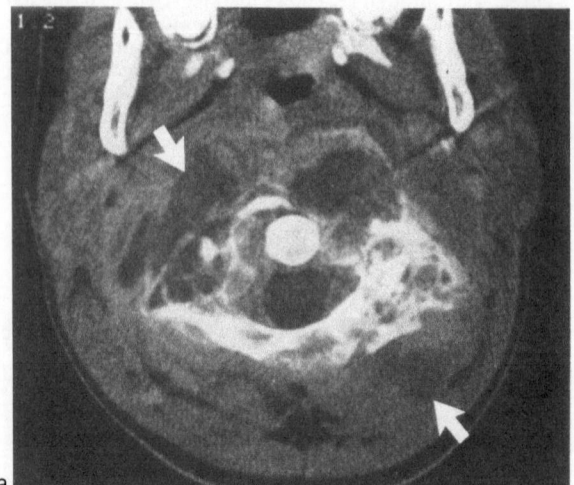

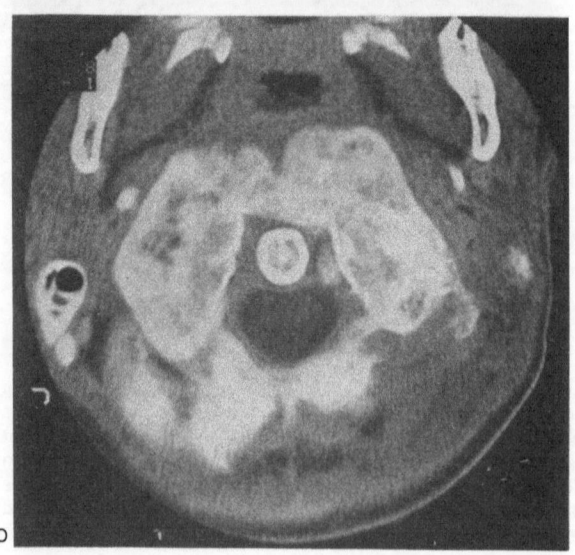

Fig. 23.22a,b. A 12-year-old boy with small cell sarcoma of the C-1 vertebra. **a** The scan shows marked destruction of the C-1 ring and marked soft tissue extension of the tumor (*arrows*). **b** Following intensive chemotherapy and radiotherapy there has been healing of C-1, which now appears to be sclerotic and expanded because of the new bone formation in the previous tumor.

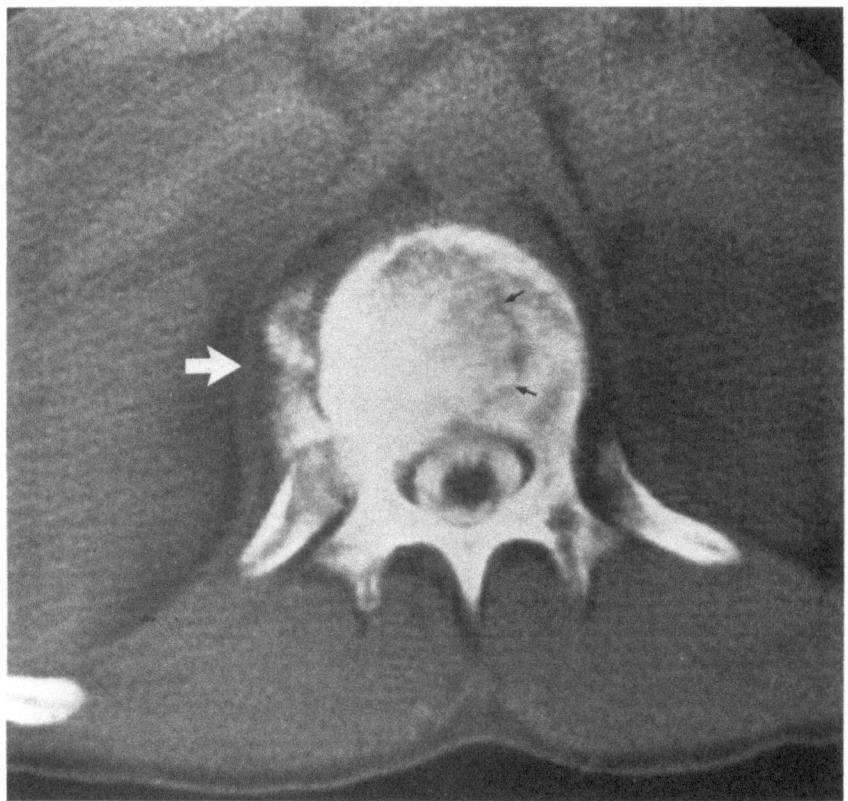

Fig. 23.23. A 16-year-old boy with previous osteogenic sarcoma of the proximal humerus. Follow-up chest radiograph revealed a paravertebral mass to the right of the T-12 vertebra. CT after intrathecal injection of metrizamide shows a sclerotic metastatic lesion replacing most of the body of T-12 (*small arrows*) and extending beyond the limits of the vertebra to the right into the retrocrural region. *White arrow*, right crus of the diaphragm. Note the slight extension into the spinal canal with slight asymmetry of the dural sac.

References

1. Bohler L (1931) Diagnosis: pathology and treatment of the os calcis. J Bone Joint Surg 13:75–89
2. Deyerle WM (1973) Long term follow-up of fractures of the os calcis. Diagnostic peroneal synoviogram. Orthop Clin North Am 4:213–227
3. Donoghue VB, Daneman A, Stringer DA, O'Brien T (1984) The value of CT in pediatric hip disease: special reference to slipped proximal femoral epiphysis and intra-articular loose bodies. Paper presented at the 70th Annual Meeting of the Radiological Society of North America, Chicago, November 1984
4. Donoghue VB, Daneman A, Krajbich I, Smith CR (1985) CT appearance of sacroiliac joint trauma in children. J Comput Assist Tomogr 9(2):352–356
5. Essex-Lopresti P (1952) The mechanism, reduction technique and results in fractures of the os calcis. Br J Surg 39:395–419
6. Harwood-Nash DCF (1981) Computed tomography of the pediatric spine: a protocol for the 1980s. Radiol Clin North Am 19:479–494
7. Hernandez RJ (1983) Evaluation of congenital hip dysplasia and tibial torsion by computed tomography. J Comput Tomogr 7:101–108
8. Hernandez RJ (1984) Concentric reduction of the dislocated hip. Radiology 150:266–268
9. Langloh ND, Johnson EW, Jackson CB (1972) Traumatic sacroiliac disruptions. J Trauma 12:931–935
10. Lawson TL, Foley WD, Carrera GF, Berland LL (1982) The sacroiliac joints: anatomic, plain roentgenographic, and computed tomographic analysis. J Comput Assist Tomogr 6:307–314
11. McConnell JR, Daneman A (1984) Fatty replacement of muscles adjacent to spinal osteoid osteoma. J Comput Assist Tomogr 8(1):147–148
12. McDonald GA (1980) Pelvic disruptions in children. Clin Orthop 151:130 134
13. Murphy WA, Gilula LA, Destouet JM, Monsees BS, Tailor CC, Totty WG (1983) Musculoskeletal system. In: Lee JKT, Sagel SS, Stanley RJ (eds) Computed body tomography. Raven Press, New York, pp 486–487
14. Pablot SM, Daneman A, Stringer DA, Carroll N (1985) The value of computed tomography in the early assessment of comminuted fractures of the calcaneus: a review of three patients. J Pediatr Orthop 5:435–438
15. Pettersson H, Harwood-Nash DCF (1982) CT and

myelography of the spine and cord. Techniques, anatomy and pathology in children. Springer, Berlin Heidelberg New York

16. Quinby WC (1966) Fractures of the pelvis and associated injuries in children. J Pediatr Surg x:353–364

17. Rang M (1975) Children's fractures. Lippincott, Toronto, pp 233–241

18. Riddlesberger M, Kuhn JP (1983) The role of computed tomography in diseases of the musculoskeletal system. J Comput Tomogr 7:85–99

19. Rockwood CA, Green DP (1984) Fractures, Vol 2, 2nd edn. Lippincott, Philadelphia

20. Smith RW, Staple TW (1982) Cat-scan evaluation of the hindfood anatomical and clinical study. Foot Ankle 2(6):346

Subject Index